LUNG CANCER DIFFERENTIATION

LUNG BIOLOGY IN HEALTH AND DISEASE

Executive Editor

Claude Lenfant
Director, National Heart, Lung, and Blood Institute
National Institutes of Health
Bethesda, Maryland

1. Immunologic and Infectious Reactions in the Lung, *edited by Charles H. Kirkpatrick and Herbert Y. Reynolds*
2. The Biochemical Basis of Pulmonary Function, *edited by Ronald G. Crystal*
3. Bioengineering Aspects of the Lung, *edited by John B. West*
4. Metabolic Functions of the Lung, *edited by Y. S. Bakhle and John R. Vane*
5. Respiratory Defense Mechanisms (in two parts), *edited by Joseph D. Brain, Donald F. Proctor, and Lynne M. Reid*
6. Development of the Lung, *edited by W. Alan Hodson*
7. Lung Water and Solute Exchange, *edited by Norman C. Staub*
8. Extrapulmonary Manifestations of Respiratory Disease, *edited by Eugene Debs Robin*
9. Chronic Obstructive Pulmonary Disease, *edited by Thomas L. Petty*
10. Pathogenesis and Therapy of Lung Cancer, *edited by Curtis C. Harris*
11. Genetic Determinants of Pulmonary Disease, *edited by Stephen D. Litwin*
12. The Lung in the Transition Between Health and Disease, *edited by Peter T. Macklem and Solbert Permutt*
13. Evolution of Respiratory Processes: A Comparative Approach, *edited by Stephen C. Wood and Claude Lenfant*
14. Pulmonary Vascular Diseases, *edited by Kenneth M. Moser*
15. Physiology and Pharmacology of the Airways, *edited by Jay A. Nadel*
16. Diagnostic Techniques in Pulmonary Disease (in two parts), *edited by Marvin A. Sackner*
17. Regulation of Breathing (in two parts), *edited by Thomas F. Hornbein*
18. Occupational Lung Diseases: Research Approaches and Methods, *edited by Hans Weill and Margaret Turner-Warwick*
19. Immunopharmacology of the Lung, *edited by Harold H. Newball*
20. Sarcoidosis and Other Granulomatous Diseases of the Lung, *edited by Barry L. Fanburg*
21. Sleep and Breathing, *edited by Nicholas A. Saunders and Colin E. Sullivan*

22. *Pneumocystis carinii* Pneumonia: Pathogenesis, Diagnosis, and Treatment, *edited by Lowell S. Young*
23. Pulmonary Nuclear Medicine: Techniques in Diagnosis of Lung Disease, *edited by Harold L. Atkins*
24. Acute Respiratory Failure, *edited by Warren M. Zapol and Konrad J. Falke*
25. Gas Mixing and Distribution in the Lung, *edited by Ludwig A. Engel and Manuel Paiva*
26. High-Frequency Ventilation in Intensive Care and During Surgery, *edited by Graziano Carlon and William S. Howland*
27. Pulmonary Development: Transition from Intrauterine to Extrauterine Life, *edited by George H. Nelson*
28. Chronic Obstructive Pulmonary Disease: Second Edition, Revised and Expanded, *edited by Thomas L. Petty*
29. The Thorax (in two parts), *edited by Charis Roussos and Peter T. Macklem*
30. The Pleura in Health and Disease, *edited by Jacques Chrétien, Jean Bignon, and Albert Hirsch*
31. Drug Therapy for Asthma: Research and Clinical Practice, *edited by John W. Jenne and Shirley Murphy*
32. Pulmonary Endothelium in Health and Disease, *edited by Una S. Ryan*
33. The Airways: Neural Control in Health and Disease, *edited by Michael A. Kaliner and Peter J. Barnes*
34. Pathophysiology and Treatment of Inhalation Injuries, *edited by Jacob Loke*
35. Respiratory Function of the Upper Airway, *edited by Oommen P. Mathew and Giuseppe Sant'Ambrogio*
36. Chronic Obstructive Pulmonary Disease: A Behavioral Perspective, *edited by A. John McSweeny and Igor Grant*
37. Biology of Lung Cancer: Diagnosis and Treatment, *edited by Steven T. Rosen, James L. Mulshine, Frank Cuttitta, and Paul G. Abrams*
38. Pulmonary Vascular Physiology and Pathophysiology, *edited by E. Kenneth Weir and John T. Reeves*
39. Comparative Pulmonary Physiology: Current Concepts, *edited by Stephen C. Wood*
40. Respiratory Physiology: An Analytical Approach, *edited by H. K. Chang and Manuel Paiva*
41. Lung Cell Biology, *edited by Donald Massaro*
42. Heart–Lung Interactions in Health and Disease, *edited by Steven M. Scharf and Sharon S. Cassidy*
43. Clinical Epidemiology of Chronic Obstructive Pulmonary Disease, *edited by Michael J. Hensley and Nicholas A. Saunders*
44. Surgical Pathology of Lung Neoplasms, *edited by Alberto M. Marchevsky*
45. The Lung in Rheumatic Diseases, *edited by Grant W. Cannon and Guy A. Zimmerman*

46. Diagnostic Imaging of the Lung, *edited by Charles E. Putman*
47. Models of Lung Disease: Microscopy and Structural Methods, *edited by Joan Gil*
48. Electron Microscopy of the Lung, *edited by Dean E. Schraufnagel*
49. Asthma: Its Pathology and Treatment, *edited by Michael A. Kaliner, Peter J. Barnes, and Carl G. A. Persson*
50. Acute Respiratory Failure: Second Edition, *edited by Warren M. Zapol and Francois Lemaire*
51. Lung Disease in the Tropics, *edited by Om P. Sharma*
52. Exercise: Pulmonary Physiology and Pathophysiology, *edited by Brian J. Whipp and Karlman Wasserman*
53. Developmental Neurobiology of Breathing, *edited by Gabriel G. Haddad and Jay P. Farber*
54. Mediators of Pulmonary Inflammation, *edited by Michael A. Bray and Wayne H. Anderson*
55. The Airway Epithelium, *edited by Stephen G. Farmer and Douglas Hay*
56. Physiological Adaptations in Vertebrates: Respiration, Circulation, and Metabolism, *edited by Stephen C. Wood, Roy E. Weber, Alan R. Hargens, and Ronald W. Millard*
57. The Bronchial Circulation, *edited by John Butler*
58. Lung Cancer Differentiation: Implications for Diagnosis and Treatment, *edited by Samuel D. Bernal and Paul J. Hesketh*

ADDITIONAL VOLUMES IN PREPARATION

Pulmonary Complications of Systemic Disease, *edited by John F. Murray*

Lung Vascular Injury: Molecular and Cellular Response, *edited by Arnold Johnson and Thomas J. Ferro*

Cytokines of the Lung, *edited by Jason Kelley*

The Mast Cell in Health and Disease, *edited by Michael A. Kaliner and Dean Metcalfe*

Pulmonary Disease in the Elderly Patient, *edited by Donald A. Mahler*

LUNG CANCER DIFFERENTIATION

IMPLICATIONS FOR DIAGNOSIS AND TREATMENT

Edited by

Samuel D. Bernal
Paul J. Hesketh

Boston University Medical Center
Boston, Massachusetts

MARCEL DEKKER, INC.   New York • Basel • Hong Kong

Library of Congress Cataloging-in-Publication Data

Lung Cancer differentiation : implications for diagnosis and treatment / edited by Samuel D. Bernal, Paul J. Hesketh.
p. cm. -- (Lung biology in health and disease ; v. 58)
Includes bibliographical references and index.
ISBN 0-8247-8638-6 (alk. paper)
1. Lungs--Cancer. 2. Cancer cells--Growth. 3. Lungs--Cancer--Treatment. 4. Tumor markers. I. Bernal, Samuel D. II. Hesketh, Paul J. III. Series.
[DNLM: 1. Cell Differentiation--congresses. 2. Cell Transformation, Neoplastic--congresses. 3. Lung--cytology--congresses. 4. Lung Neoplasms--diagnosis--congresses. 5. Lung Neoplasms--therapy--congresses. 6. Tumor Markers, Biological--congresses. W1 LU62 v.58]
RC280.L8L776 1992
616.99'424--dc20
DNLM/DLC
for Library of Congress 92-9996
CIP

This book is printed on acid-free paper.

MARCEL DEKKER, INC.
270 Madison Avenue, New York, New York 10016

Current printing (last digit):
10 9 8 7 6 5 4 3 2 1

PRINTED IN THE UNITED STATES OF AMERICA

This book is dedicated to my parents, Teofilo and Loreto Bernal,
and to my children, Ariel, Elise, and Laure

SDB

To my wife, Ann Marie, and my son, Matthew,
for their sustaining love and support

PJH

INTRODUCTION

> But it is clearer than ever that cancer is a solvable problem, solvable by a human thought-and-action process that we call scientific research, and within the capability of human intelligence with which man was endowed by his creator.
>
> *M. B. Shimkin, 1973*

This volume, *Lung Cancer Differentiation: Implications for Diagnosis and Treatment*, is the fourth monograph of the Lung Biology in Health and Disease series that is entirely devoted to lung cancer. In addition, several other volumes of the series include chapters or sections with a focus on lung cancer.

Why, one might ask, is such emphasis placed on this disease? I believe the answer is simple. First, cancer of the lung remains an ever-increasing major public health problem. The annual statistics published by the United States Public Health Service, by other countries, and by the World Health Organization continually remind us of the magnitude of the problem.

The very sad thing is that, by and large, lung cancer is a self-inflicted problem caused by cigarette smoking. It is no wonder that public health officials and planners are sponsoring a major research program to find ways to treat lung cancer, as so many people seem unable to help themselves by avoiding the known cause of this disease. This continuing research effort constitutes the second reason for making lung cancer a topic of such importance in this series of monographs.

Indeed, the research effort on lung cancer is remarkable for its magnitude and productivity. Not only have many forms of cancer greatly benefited from this research, but many other research areas have benefited as well. Few research pursuits have brought together the best basic scientists and the best clinical investigators as has lung cancer.

This volume, edited by Drs. Samuel Bernal and Paul Hesketh, illustrates and exemplifies the superb outcomes of pioneering cancer research. Certainly, its content reassures us that Shimkin's prediction is closer than ever to becoming a reality. While much more remains to be done, we can be confident that "the thought-and-action process," as well as "human intelligence," will someday lead us to success.

Researchers from many laboratories and from several countries have contributed to this volume. The result testifies to the great value of international cooperation and exchange. This research is at the cutting edge of science: doubtless it will inspire other investigators. One of the most valuable features of this volume is that it brings the outcome of basic research to the "bedside"; that is, it offers a scientific rationale for novel therapeutic regimens.

The readership of this series will undoubtedly welcome this new addition. Personally, I am indebted to Drs. Bernal and Hesketh for their efforts and for bringing together such a distinguished roster of contributors. All together, they have produced this volume, which I view as a great asset to the series and, more important, a contribution to the welfare of many patients who suffer from lung cancer.

Claude Lenfant, M.D.
Bethesda, Maryland

PREFACE

This volume on lung cancer differentiation in the Lung Biology in Health and Disease Series emphasizes the implications of cell differentiation for the diagnosis and therapy of lung cancer. We have brought together the work of basic scientists who study the differentiation of normal and neoplastic lung epithelial cells and of clinicians who base their diagnostic and therapeutic modalities on the differentiation characteristics of lung cancer cells. Most of the authors in this book presented their data at the International Conference on Lung Cancer on November 9–11, 1990, which was organized by the Evans Memorial Department of Clinical Research at Boston University with the cooperation of the International Association for the Study of Lung Cancer.

In Part I, five chapters cover basic studies on differentiation of normal and neoplastic lung epithelial cells and on links between differentiation and drug resistance. In Part II, oncogenes and growth factors important in the expression of differentiation phenotypes are described in four chapters. Part III consists of four chapters on biochemical markers of lung cancer differentiation, including small-cell lung cancer antigens recently clustered at an international workshop. Part IV covers in three chapters the applications of differentiation markers in the diagnosis of lung cancer, including strategies for reversal of preneoplastic changes in upper-respiratory epithelium. Part V and Part VI include a total of nine chapters describing therapeutic protocols directed at non-small-cell lung cancers (squamous, glandular, or large-cell undifferentiated cancers). In Part VII, two chapters describe strategies and problems in the treatment of small-cell lung cancers. By separating small-cell from non-small-cell lung cancers, clinicians have long recognized that the differentiation characteristics of lung cancers are important in the natural history, prognosis, and responsiveness of lung cancers to chemotherapy and radiation. Future studies will be directed at the identification of the specific molecular links between differentiation and clinical behavior of lung cancers.

We hope that this book is of interest to basic researchers who are concerned not only with molecular approaches to lung cell differentiation, but also with the clinical implications of lung cancer differentiation. Furthermore, we hope that clinicians will gain from this book not only a perspective on the importance of cell differentiation in the current state of diagnosis and therapy of lung cancer, but also an overview of the regulation and molecular events during differentiation of lung epithelial cells.

Many of the contributors to this volume initially presented their work at the International Lung Cancer Conference held in Boston, Massachusetts from November 9–11, 1990. We gratefully acknowledge the help of Ms. Mary Hill in the Department of Continuing Medical Education at Boston University and Dr. Heine Hansen, President of the International Association for the Study of Lung Cancer, in the organization and execution of this conference. We also are very appreciative of the support provided through educational grants from Bristol-Myers Company and Glaxo Pharmaceuticals and grants-in-aid from Affinity BioReagents, Inc., The Purdue Frederick Company, and Schering Corporation.

Finally we would like to acknowledge the unceasing encouragement and support we have received from Dr. Ronald McCaffrey, Chief of the Section of Medical Oncology, Boston University Medical Center, in bringing this project to fruition.

Samuel D. Bernal
Paul J. Hesketh

CONTRIBUTORS

Ross Abrams, M.D. Radiation Oncologist, Department of Radiation Oncology, Johns Hopkins University Oncology Center, Johns Hopkins Oncology Center, Baltimore, Maryland

David K. Ahn, Ph.D. Northern California Oncology Group, Belmont, California

Phyllis G. Andrews Environmental Health Research and Testing, Inc., Research Triangle Park, North Carolina

Edward D. Ball, M.D. Department of Microbiology and Department of Medicine, Dartmouth Medical School, Hanover, New Hampshire

Mark S. Bankoff, M.D. Chief of CT and Body MRI, Department of Radiology, Tufts University/New England Medical Center, Boston, Massachusetts

Ma-Teresa Barzaga, M.D.* Section of Medical Oncology, Boston University Medical Center, Boston, Massachusetts

Samuel D. Bernal, M.D., Ph.D. Associate Professor of Medicine, Section of Medical Oncology, Boston University Medical Center, Boston, Massachusetts

H. Bischoff, M.D. Department of Internal Medicine/Oncology, Chest Hospital, Heidelberg, Germany

Jacob D. Bitran, M.D. Clinical Professor of Medicine, Section of Hematology/Oncology, University of Chicago, Chicago, Illinois

---

**Present affiliation*: Staff Pathologist, Lung Center of the Philippines, Quezon City, Philippines

M. J. Buffo, B.S. Flow Cytometry Supervisor, Department of Medicine, Allegheny Singer Research Institute, Pittsburgh, Pennsylvania

R. Carey, M.D. Associate Clinical Professor, Department of Medical Oncology, Massachusetts General Hospital, Boston, Massachusetts

N. Choi, M.D. Associate Professor of Medicine, Department of Radiation Oncology, Massachusetts General Hospital, Boston, Massachusetts

Stephen G. Combs, M.D.† Department of Pathology, MacNeal Hospital, Berwyn, Illinois

Frank Cuttitta The NCI-Navy Medical Oncology Branch, National Navy Medical Center, Bethesda, Maryland

M. Dalbow, M.S. Consultant, Department of Ophthalmology, Allegheny Singer Research Institute, Pittsburgh, Pennsylvania

Benedict D.T. Daly, M.D. Professor of Cardiothoracic Surgery, Tufts University/New England Medical Center, Boston, Massachusetts

Albert B. Deisseroth, M.D., Ph.D. Professor and Chairman, Department of Hematology, The University of Texas M. D. Anderson Cancer Center, Houston, Texas

James T. Diehl, M.D. Associate Professor of Surgery, Department of Cardiothoracic Surgery, Tufts University/New England Medical Center, Boston, Massachusetts

Nancy A. DiMartino, M.D. Chief, Department of Hematology/Oncology, Boston VA Medical Center, Boston, Massachusetts

L. Austin Doyle, M.D. Associate Professor of Medicine, University of Maryland Cancer Center, Baltimore, Maryland

P. Drings, M.D., Ph.D. Professor, Department of Internal Medicine/Oncology, Chest Hospital, Heidelberg, Germany

Chris English, B.S.N. Clinical Specialist—Chest Oncology, Department of Medicine, Section of Hematology/Oncology, University of Chicago, Chicago, Illinois

---

†Deceased.

L. Jack Faling, M.D. Associate Chief of Medicine, Department of Medicine, Boston VA Medical Center, and Associate Professor of Medicine, Tufts University School of Medicine, Boston, Massachusetts

Barry Fanburg, M.D. Chief, Pulmonary Division, Tufts University/New England Medical Center, Boston, Massachusetts

J. R. Fischer, M.D. Department of Internal Medicine/Oncology, Chest Hospital, Heidelberg, Germany

A. Fisseler-Eckhoff, M.D. Institute of Pathology, Berufsgenossenschaftliche Krankenanstalten "Bergmannsheil," University Clinic Bochum, Bochum, Germany

David R. Gandara, M.D. Associate Professor of Medicine, Department of Hematology/Oncology, University of California, Davis, VA Medical Center, Martinez, California and Northern California Oncology Group, Belmont, California

Ghanashyam Ghadge, Ph.D. Postdoctoral Research Associate, Department of Microbiology/Immunology, Northwestern University, VA Lakeside Medical Center, Chicago, Illinois

Harvey M. Golomb, M.D. Professor, Department of Medicine, and Director, Section of Hematology/Oncology, University of Chicago, Chicago, Illinois

M. Goutsou Department of Biostatistics, Harvard School of Public Health, Boston, Massachusetts

William Gradishar, M.D. Assistant Professor of Medicine, Department of Medicine, Section of Hematology/Oncology, University of Chicago, Chicago, Illinois

Stefan C. Grant, M.D., B.Ch. Research Fellow, Thoracic Oncology Service, Department of Medicine, Memorial–Sloan Kettering Cancer Center, New York, New York

F. Anthony Greco, M.D. Professor of Medicine, and Director, Department of Medical Oncology, Vanderbilt University, Nashville, Tennessee

M. Green, M.D. Professor of Medicine, University of California Medical Center, San Diego, California

G. Kenneth Haines, M.D. Chief Resident, Department of Pathology, Northwestern University, VA Lakeside Medical Center, Chicago, Illinois

John D. Hainsworth, M.D. Associate Professor, Department of Medicine, Vanderbilt University, Nashville, Tennessee

Heine H. Hansen, M.D. Physician-in-Chief, Department of Oncology, Finsen Institute, Rigshospitalet, Copenhagen, Denmark

Suzanne K. Hansen, B.S., M.S.* Environmental Health Research and Testing, Inc., Research Triangle Park, North Carolina

Richard Heidbreder, M.D. Instructor of Radiation Oncology and Radiotherapist, Department of Radiation Oncology, Tufts University/New England Medical Center, Boston, Massachusetts

Paul J. Hesketh, M.D. Associate Professor of Medicine and Clinical Director, Section of Medical Oncology, Boston University Medical Center, Boston, Massachusetts

Setsuo Hirohashi, M.D. Chief, Pathology Division, National Cancer Center Research Institute, Tokyo, Japan

Philip C. Hoffman, M.D. Associate Professor, Department of Medicine, Section of Hematology/Oncology, University of Chicago, Chicago, Illinois

Waun K. Hong, M.D. Professor of Medicine, and Chief, Section of Head/Neck and Thoracic Medical Oncology, The University of Texas M. D. Anderson Cancer Center, Houston, Texas

Anton M. Jetten, M.D. Head, Cell Biology Group, Laboratory of Pulmonary Pathobiology, National Institute of Environmental Health Sciences, Research Triangle Park, North Carolina

David H. Johnson, M.D. Associate Professor of Medicine, Department of Medicine, Division of Oncology, Vanderbilt University, Nashville, Tennessee

**Present affiliation*: Sphinx Biotechnologies Corporation, Durham, North Carolina

Mika Kakefuda, M.D.* Section of Medical Oncology, Boston University Medical Center, Boston, Massachusetts

Daniel D. Karp, M.D. Director of Head/Neck and Thoracic Services Medical Oncology, Department of Hematology/Oncology, Tufts University/New England Medical Center, Boston, Massachusetts

E. C. Klein, V.M.D. Assistant Professor, Division of Laboratory Animal Resources, University of Pittsburgh, Pittsburgh, Pennsylvania

A. M. C. Koros, Ph.D. Assistant Research Professor, Department of Infectious Diseases and Microbiology, Graduate School of Public Health, University of Pittsburgh, Pittsburgh, Pennsylvania

Mark G. Kris, M.D. Chief, Thoracic Oncology Service, Division of Solid Tumor Oncology, Memorial–Sloan Kettering Cancer Center, New York, New York

Paul E. G. Kristjansen, M.D. Department of Oncology, Finsen Institute, Rigshospitalet, Copenhagen, Denmark

Scott M. Lippman, M.D. Assistant Professor of Medicine, Department of Medical Oncology, The University of Texas M. D. Anderson Cancer Center, Houston, Texas

Mack Mabry, M.D. Assistant Professor, Department of Medical Oncology, Johns Hopkins Oncology Center, Baltimore, Maryland

C. Manegold, M.D., Ph.D. Consultant of Medical Oncology, Department of Internal Medicine/Oncology, Chest Hospital, Heidelberg, Germany

D. Mathisen, M.D. Associate Chief of Thoracic Surgery, Department of Thoracic Surgery, Massachusetts General Hospital, Boston, Massachusetts

Yoshihiro Matsuno, M.D. Research Member, Pathology Division, National Cancer Center Research Institute, Tokyo, Japan

Caron Modeas Chief Database Manager, Frontier Science and Technology Research Foundation, Inc., Amherst, New York

---

**Present affiliation*: Staff Physician, Department of Medicine, Johns Hopkins Hospital, Baltimore, Maryland

K.-M. Müller, M.D. Ph.D. Professor, Institute of Pathology, Berufsgenossenschaftliche Krankenanstalten "Bergmannsheil," University Clinic Bochum, Bochum, Germany

James L. Mulshine, M.D. Chief, Biomarkers and Prevention Research Branch, Education and Community Oncology Program, Division of Cancer Prevention and Control, National Cancer Institute, Bethesda, Maryland

Masayuki Noguchi, M.D. Research Member, Pathology Division, National Cancer Center Research Institute, Tokyo, Japan

Timothy O'Connor, M.D. Newton-Wellesley Hospital, Newton, Massachusetts

Sara E. Owens Environmental Health Research and Testing, Inc., Research Triangle Park, North Carolina

Edith A. Perez, M.D. Assistant Professor of Clinical Medicine, Department of Hematology/Oncology, University of California, Davis, VA Medical Center, Martinez, California and Northern California Oncology Group, Belmont, California

M. Peukert, M.D. Department of Clincal Cancer Research, Asta Medical AG, Frankfurt, Germany

Theodore Phillips, M.D. Professor and Chairman, Department of Radiation/Oncology, University of California, San Francisco, California, and Northern California Oncology Group, Belmont, California

K. Propert Assistant Professor of Medicine, Department of Biostatistics, Harvard School of Public Health, Boston, Massachusetts

James A. Radosevich, Ph.D. Associate Professor, Department of Medicine, Division of Allergy and Immunology, Northwestern University, VA Lakeside Medical Center, Chicago, Illinois

R. Raikow, Ph.D. Scientist, Department of Ophthalmology, Allegheny Singer Research Institute, Pittsburgh, Pennsylvania

V. Rege, M.D. Associate Director, Department of Medical Oncology, Rhode Island Hospital, Providence, Rhode Island

Mack Roach, III, Ph.D. Assistant Professor of Medicine, Department of Radiation/Oncology, University of California, San Francisco, California

Nicholas J. Robert, M.D. Hematologist, Oncologist, and Pathologist, Division of Hematology/Oncology, Fairfax Hospital, Falls Church, Virginia

Steven T. Rosen, M.D. Director, Department of Medicine, and Genevieve Teuton Professor, Northwestern University Cancer Center, Chicago, Illinois

A. Schmähl, M.D. Department of Internal Medicine/Oncology, Chest Hospital, Heidelberg, Germany

D. Sherman, M.D. Director, Department of Radiation Oncology, St. Joseph's Hospital, Milwaukee, Wisconsin

Nobuyoshi Shimizu, Ph.D. Department of Molecular Biology, Keio University School of Medicine, Tokyo, Japan

Yukio Shimosato, M.D. Chief, Clinical Laboratory Division, National Cancer Center Research Institute, Tokyo, Japan

Jill M. Siegfried, Ph.D. Assistant Professor, Department of Pharmacology, University of Pittsburgh, Pittsburgh, Pennsylvania

Robert L. Souhami, M.D., F.R.C.P. Professor of Clinical Oncology, Department of Oncology, University College and Middlesex School of Medicine, London, England

G. Strauss, M.D. Instructor of Medicine, Brigham and Women's Hospital/Harvard Medical School, and Medical Oncologist, Harvard Community Health Plan, Boston, Massachusetts

Bayar Thimmapaya, Ph.D. Associate Professor, Department of Microbiology/Immunology, Northwestern University, VA Lakeside Medical Center, Chicago, Illinois

Melvyn S. Tockman Environmental Health Sciences, The Johns Hopkins School of Hygiene and Public Health, Baltimore, Maryland

Yoshiya Tome, B.S., C.T. Technologist, Clinical Laboratory Division, National Cancer Center Research Institute, Tokyo, Japan

Andrew T. Turrisi, III, M.D. Associate Professor, Department of Radiation Oncology, University of Michigan Medical Center, Ann Arbor, Michigan

Godofredo Urbano Section of Medical Oncology, Boston University Medical Center, Boston, Massachusetts

Frank H. Valone, M.D. Department of Hematology/Oncology, University of California, San Francisco, California, and Northern California Oncology Group, Belmont, California

Everett E. Vokes, M.D. Associate Professor of Medicine, Section of Hematology/Oncology, University of Chicago, Chicago, Illinois

James J. Vredenburgh Department of Medicine, Dartmouth Medical School, Hanover, New Hampshire

Frank S. Walsh, Ph.D. Professor, Department of Experimental Biology, UMDS Guy's Hospital, London, England

David Wazer, M.D. Assistant Professor, and Clinical Director, Department of Radiation Oncology, Tufts University/New England Medical Center, Boston, Massachusetts

Bernard Willett, M.D., F.A.C.S. Chief, Department of Radiation Oncology, Boston VA Medical Center, and Assistant Professor of Radiation/Oncology, Tufts University School of Medicine, Boston, Massachusetts

Yuk-Chor Wong, Ph.D. Assistant Research Professor of Medicine, Evans Memorial Department of Clinical Research, Boston University Medical Center, Boston, Massachusetts

CONTENTS

Part II ONCOGENES AND GROWTH FACTORS IN LUNG CANCER

Part VI NON-SMALL-CELL LUNG CANCER: NEW THERAPEUTIC AGENTS

PART I

DIFFERENTIATION OF NORMAL AND NEOPLASTIC LUNG EPITHELIAL CELLS

1

Proliferation and Differentiation in Normal and Neoplastic Tracheobronchial Epithelial Cells

ANTON M. JETTEN

National Institute of Environmental Health Sciences
Research Triangle Park, North Carolina

I. Introduction

Lung cancer is one of the most frequently diagnosed malignant neoplasms throughout the world and is the most frequent cause of death due to cancer in industrialized countries (Hammar, 1988; Jett et al., 1983; Silverberg and Lubera, 1987, Rosen et al., 1987). Environmental factors, cigarette smoke in particular, in conjunction with genetic factors are important determinants of this disease (Hammar, 1988; Hammond and Horn, 1958; Fielding, 1985). The bronchial epithelium is the most common site for tumor formation in the lung. The four main histopathologic types of lung neoplasms (adenocarcinoma, squamous cell carcinoma, small cell carcinoma, and large cell carcinoma) account for, respectively, 26%, 35%, 20%, and 15% of all lung tumors (McDowell et al., 1982; Melamed and Zaman, 1982; World Health Organization, 1982). Cells in these tumors often retain many characteristics of normal cells: adenocarcinoma cells exhibit features of mucous secretory cells, squamous carcinoma cells resemble basal cells, and small cell carcinomas contain cells with neuroendocrine characteristics. Most lung tumors exhibit histologic heterogeneity, which complicates the diagnosis of lung neoplasms by histologic criteria (Roggli et al., 1985). The histogenesis of common lung neoplasms is poorly understood. The observed divergence of histologic appearance in the same neoplasm has led to the interpretation that all cell types and tumor types may be derived from a common stem cell (McDowell et al., 1982; Yesner, 1978). Aberrations in the tracheobronchial stem cell could account for the great heterogeneity and diversity in lung tumors. Identification and characterization of the stem cell(s) in the tracheobronchial epithelium and elucidation of the regulation of the pathways of differentiation in these cells will be necessary to allow us to fully understand the process of carcinogenesis in the lung.

Aberrant cell proliferation and differentiation are consistent and important characteristics of malignant cells (McDowell et al., 1982; Rosen et al., 1987; Pierce and Speers, 1988). Defects in the control of proliferation and differentiation are thought to be important steps in the process of carcinogenesis. Constitutive production of positive growth regulators, loss of the response to negative growth regulators, altered response to factors that regulate differentiation, activation of specific oncogenes, or loss of suppressor genes are all defects that could lead to uncontrolled cell growth and a reduced probability of cellular differentiation. Therefore, it is critical to obtain a clear insight into the basic mechanisms that regulate proliferation and differentiation of normal epithelial cells in order to identify the various types of defects in malignant cells at the molecular level. A better understanding of the aberrations in the control of these processes offers hope that effective strategies to fight neoplastic diseases of the lung will be discovered.

II. Pathways of Differentiation

A. Stem Cells

Many epithelia, the tracheobronchial epithelium included, are continually renewing themselves. Terminally differentiated cells are replaced throughout the proliferation and differentiation of a distinct population of cells, defined as stem cells. Stem cells are considered to have an unlimited, at least with respect to the life span of the species, capacity for self-renewal and to have the potential to produce progeny that is committed to differentiate into one or more lineages (Fig. 1). For example, epidermal basal cells appear to undergo only a single pathway of squamous cell differentiation (Watt, 1988; Jetten, 1989) and are considered unipotent. Hematopoietic stem cells (Dexter and Spooncer, 1987; Ogawa, 1989), mesenchymal stem cells (Taylor and Jones, 1979; Pinney and Emerson, 1989), and intestinal stem cells (Potten, 1983) are pluripotent, giving rise to many differentiated cell types. In several tissues the differentiation of stem cells into terminally differentiated cells appears to occur via transit-amplifying progenitor populations that have a limited capacity for self-renewal and are committed to terminal differentiation. Under normal, steady-state conditions, most stem cells are not engaged in active proliferation and appear to remain in the G_0 phase of the cell cycle; much of the turnover may occur via the transit-amplifying population. A

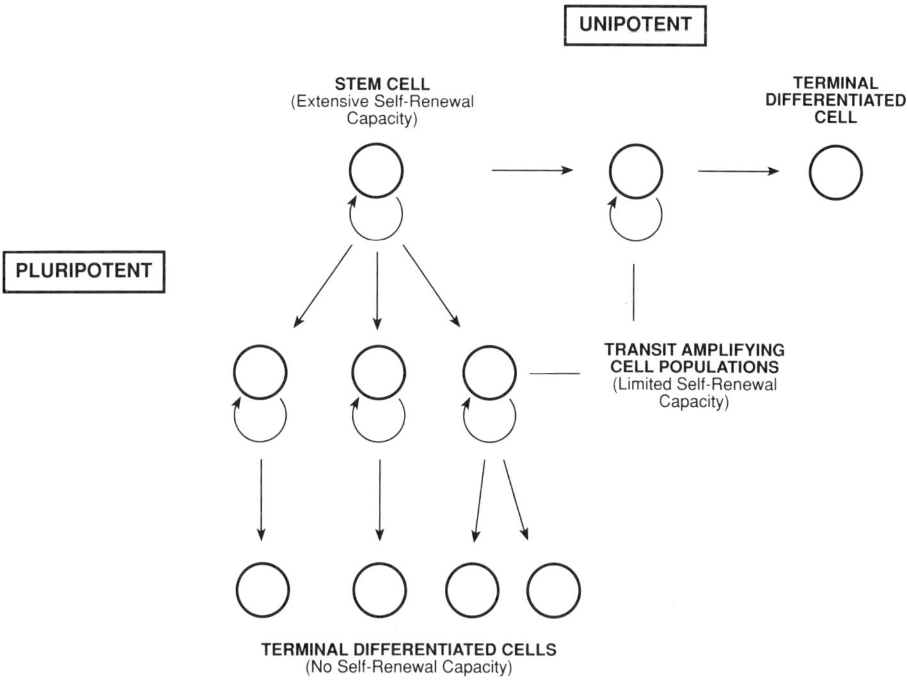

Figure 1 Differentiation of unipotent and pluripotent stem cells. Stem cells have an extensive self-renewal capacity and can differentiate via one or more pathways into cells with a much more limited proliferative capacity (transit-amplifying population) and that are committed to undergo terminal differentiation.

balance exists between stem cell renewal and differentiation, which suggests that the control of these processes is tightly coordinated. The commitment of stem cells to produce stem cells or differentiated cells could be controlled in a predetermined manner (stem cells yield one daughter stem cell and one differentiated daughter cell with each asymmetrical division) or can be stochastic (a stem cell can produce either two daughter stem cells, or one daughter stem cell and one differentiated daughter cell, or two differentiated daughter cells; Holtzer, 1978; Hall and Watt, 1989). The latter process may be controlled by specific factors that regulate proliferation and differentiation and/or by fluctuations in the heterogeneity of the stem cell population.

B. Bronchiolar and Tracheobronchial Stem Cells

The tracheobronchial lining consists of a pseudostratified epithelium containing different cell types (Breeze and Wheeldon, 1977). The main cell types of this epithelium are the ciliated cell, basal cell, and a variety of secretory cells (mucous secretory, Clara, serous, and neuroendocrine cells). The relationship between these different cell types and the exact pathways of differentiation is not precisely known. The neuroendocrine cell is a cell type with proliferative capacity; however, little is known about its differentiation (Sorokin and Hoyt, 1989). The ciliated cell appears unable to undergo mitosis and is likely to constitute a terminally differentiated cell.

Clara cells, which, together with ciliated cells form the lining of the bronchioles (Massaro, 1989), are also found in the tracheobronchial epithelium of many species. To what degree the bronchiolar Clara cells and the tracheobronchial Clara cells are identical needs further study. The Clara cells contain high levels of the P-450-dependent mono-oxygenase system and metabolize xenobiotics. Clara cells are secretory cells that contain dense cytoplasmic granules (Hook et al., 1990). The major secretory protein has been identified as uteroglobin (Aumuller et al., 1985). Although the role of uteroglobin is not yet fully established, evidence has been presented suggesting that it might function as a phospholipase A_2 inhibitor (Miele et al., 1988). Studies of Clara cells in vivo have demonstrated that these cells are unable to undergo cell division and have the potential to differentiate into ciliated cells (Evans, 1983; Evans et al., 1986). Recent studies by Hook et al. (1987) and Brody et al. (1987) have confirmed these observations, and have shown that cells from 90–95% pure Clara cell preparations isolated from rabbit lungs are able to repopulate denuded tracheas transplanted onto the backs of nude mice, and to establish an epithelium with Clara and ciliated cells resembling the bronchiolar epithelium. The proliferative capacity of Clara cells was further shown by the cultivation and growth of Clara cells in vitro (Jetten and Hook, unpublished observations). These studies indicate that Clara cells are the stem cells of the bronchiolar epithelium that exhibit self-renewal capacity and the ability to undergo terminal differentiation into ciliated cells (Fig. 2A). Whether Clara cells are unipotent stem cells or have the ability to differentiate into other cell types needs further study. In vitro studies have indicated that Clara cells do not have the ability to undergo squamous cell differentiation (Jetten and Hook, unpublished observations).

One of the functions of the mucosecretory cell is the synthesis and secretion of mucuslike glycoproteins (Basbaum and Finkbeiner, 1989). It has been shown that these cells have an extensive proliferative capacity (Keenan et al., 1982). These cells are able to differentiate into mature mucous–secretory cells or goblet cells and into ciliated cells (McDowell et al., 1984). The differentiation into goblet cells may be a nonterminal, reversible process, whereas the differentiation into ciliated cells appears to constitute a terminal pathway of differentiation (Fig. 2B).

Several morphological features distinguish the basal cell from the columnar cells: the basal cell forms hemidesmosomes with the basement membrane, has a large nucleus/cytoplasm ratio, contains extensive tonofilaments, and does not

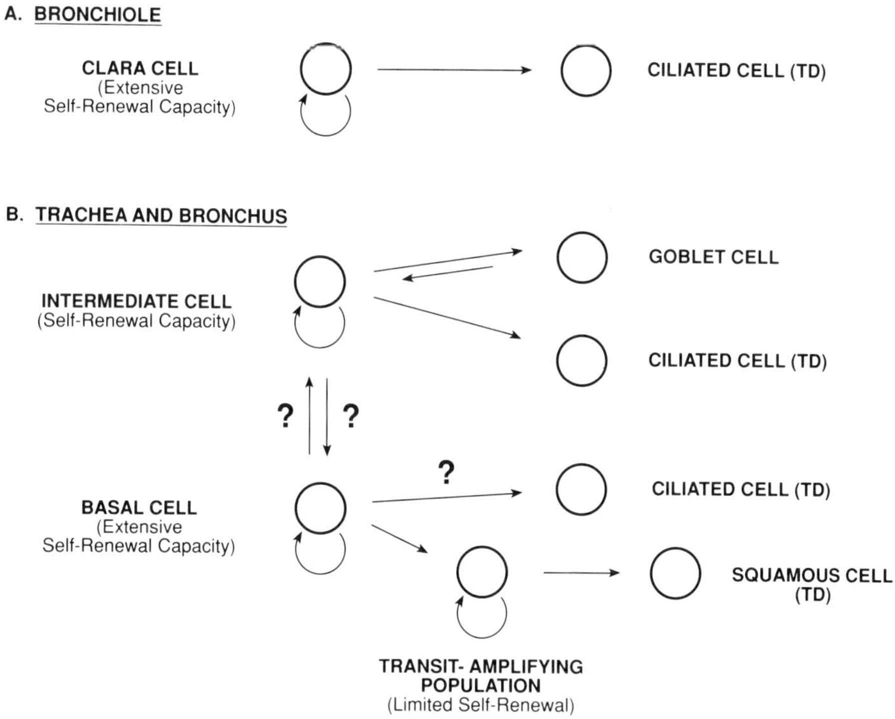

Figure 2 Putative pathways of differentiation of (A) bronchiolar and (B) tracheobronchial epithelial cells. TD, terminal differentiation.

extend all the way to the tracheobronchial lumen. In addition, it expresses a specific pattern of keratin intermediate filaments and specific cell surface antigens. The lectin *Griffonia simplicifolia* I-B4 has been reported to bind specifically to basal cells (Flint et al., 1986). Like some of the columnar cells, basal cells have been shown to be able to undergo cell division. Basal cells isolated from the rabbit trachea can be cultured efficiently in vitro in Ham's F12 medium supplemented with growth factors (Jetten et al., submitted). Observations in vivo and in vitro have shown that these cells can undergo squamous cell differentiation and appear to be the major cell type involved in epidermoid metaplasia (Wong and Buck, 1971; Chopra, 1982; Jetten, 1989). Basal cells have long been considered as the stem cell in the tracheobronchial epithelium (Jeffery et al., 1982; Chopra, 1982). This view appears to be supported by recent studies by Inayama et al. (1988a,b), which examined the ability of rabbit tracheal basal cells to repopulate tracheal grafts denuded of their own epithelium and transplanted onto the backs of nude mice. Highly purified suspensions of basal cells were able to establish a new columnar, pseudostratified epithelium, which suggests that the basal cells are the main stem cells in the large airways of rabbits. However, this hypothesis has been challenged by several other investigations. Studies examining the formation of the tracheobronchial epithelium during fetal development have indicated that during development the columnar preciliated and presecretory cells appear before or at the same time as the prebasal cells (McDowell et al., 1985a,b; Cutz, 1986; Plopper et al., 1986). These findings have been interpreted to indicate that a presecretory, columnar cell (intermediate cell) and not the basal cell is the stem cell in the tracheobronchial epithelium (Evans and Shami, 1989). Recent studies by Johnson et al. (1990) appear to be in agreement with this concept. Their experiments have shown that secretory cells isolated from the rat trachea establish an epithelium containing basal, secretory, and ciliated cells when inoculated into denuded tracheal grafts transplanted onto the backs of nude mice. In contrast, isolated basal cells form an epithelium consisting of only basal and ciliated cells. Recently, an additional role for the basal cell in the adhesion of columnar cells has been proposed (Evans and Plopper, 1988). The basal cells, which are attached to the basement membrane through hemidesmosomes and to the columnar cells via desmosomal junctions, may increase via these junctions the adherence of the columnar cells to the basement membrane.

A scheme of the putative pathways of differentiation of tracheobronchial epithelial cells is presented in Figure 2B and shows that both the basal and the intermediate cells are pluripotent. The intermediate cells have self-renewal capacity and can differentiate further into ciliated cells and mucous or goblet cells, and possibly basal cells. Basal cells also exhibit an extensive self-renewal capacity and can undergo differentiation into either squamous cells or ciliated cells, and possibly intermediate cells. Conflicting findings on the differentiation capacity of basal cells have made it impossible to give a definite answer on the question of which of the two cell types, the intermediate or the basal cell, is the true stem cell in the tracheobronchial epithelium (McDowell et al., 1985a; Inayama et al., 1988a,b; Johnson, 1990).

III. Expression of Intermediate Filaments

The expression of each of the five classes of intermediate filaments in eukaryotic cells is limited to very specific cell types. For example, vimentin is mostly found in mesenchymal cells, and neurofilaments are mostly found in neuronal cells including the neuroendocrine cells in the lung (Lehto et al., 1983). Keratins are the structural elements of intermediate filaments in most epithelial cells. These proteins have been classified into two families, acidic or type I and basic or type II keratins, on the basis of their biochemical, immunologic, and molecular properties (Moll et al., 1982; Sun et al., 1983). The expression of keratins has been shown to depend on the cell type and the differentiated state of the cells. Also in the tracheobronchial epithelium, different cell types express different sets of keratins. Figure 3 shows a comparison between the keratin profiles of freshly isolated and cultured basal and Clara cells (Jetten and Hook, unpublished observations). Freshly isolated basal cells express three major keratins that have been identified as keratins K5, K14, and K19, on the basis of their immunoreactivity with two antikeratin monoclonal antibodies, AE1 and AE3 (Fig. 3A). During culture these cells also express keratins K6 and K16. Analysis of keratins via immunohistochemical staining has confirmed that K5 and K14 are the major keratins in basal cells. These keratins are also found in squamous metaplastic foci but not normally in secretory or ciliated cells. Analysis of the expression of keratins in freshly isolated Clara cells via two-dimensional electrophoresis and via immunoblot analysis showed that these cells contain keratins K7, K8, K17, K18, and K19 (Fig. 3B). Clara cells in culture express the same keratin profile as freshly isolated cells. Immunohistochemical studies have shown that, like the Clara cells, the mucosecretory and ciliated cells express a keratin profile that is typically found in simple epithelia and include the expression of keratins K7, K8, K18, and K19 (Blobel et al., 1984; Rutten et al., 1988; Broers et al., 1989). The expression of keratins in the human tracheobronchial epithelium has been reported to be dependent on the stage of fetal development (Broers et al., 1989). At early stages (9–10 weeks of gestation), cells of the tracheobronchial epithelium express only keratins of so-called simple epithelia (K7, K8, K18) and coexpression is observed with vimentin. At later stages keratin expression becomes more complex, vimentin expression is reduced, and basal cells start to express K14. These studies on keratin expression are in agreement with the observations that the basal cells appear during development after the columnar cells (McDowell et al., 1985; Cutz, 1986; Plopper et al., 1986), which suggests that they are derived form the presecretory (intermediate) cell and may not be the true stem cell in the tracheobronchial epithelium. Table 1 shows a summary of the keratin expression by adult tracheobronchial epithelial cells.

Expression of intermediate filaments in neoplastic cells has been extensively studied (Blobel et al., 1982; Banks-Schlegel et al., 1984; Banks-Schlegel et al., 1985; Gould et al., 1986; De Ley et al., 1987; Broers et al., 1988) and has been shown to depend on the extent and type of differentiation. Correlation of keratin expression with a specific type of neoplasm has been often complicated by the lack of suitable markers other than histologic findings to identify the neoplasm. The expression of intermediate filaments in small cell carcinomas falls into two classes: the classic small cell carcinomas contain only keratins, whereas the variant small cell carcinomas do not express keratins but occasionally neurofilaments. In general, adenocarcinomas contain a keratin profile similar to that of simple epithelia. Squamous cell carcinomas are characterized by a very complex pattern, including simple epithelium-type keratins and keratins expressed by stratified epithelia. Large cell carcinomas contain either a keratin pattern similar

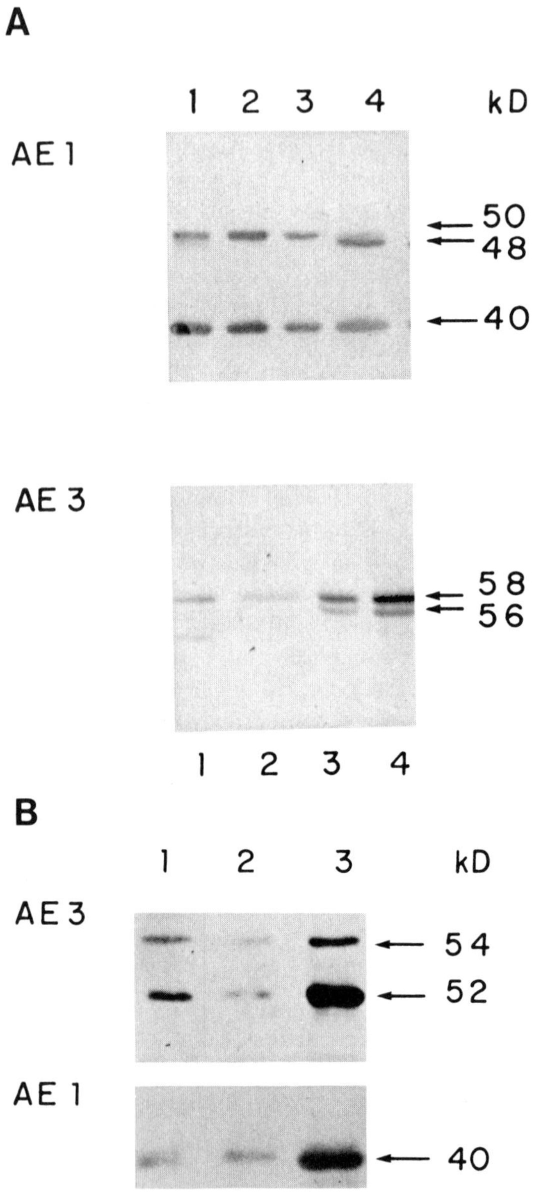

Figure 3 Comparison of keratin expression in freshly isolated and cultured (A) Clara and (B) basal cells from the rabbit tracheobronchial epithelium. Keratin expression was analyzed by immunoblot analysis using monoclonal antibodies AE1 and AE3. Lanes 1, Freshly isolated 95% pure basal or Clara cell preparation; 2, 24 hr after plating; 3, 6 days after plating; 4, 8 days after plating.

Table 1 Comparison of Keratin Expression in Tracheobronchial Epithelial Cells

Keratin	MW	Immunoreactivity	Basal cell A	Basal cell B	Mucous/ciliated/ Clara cell
K5	58	AE3	+	+	−
K6	56	AE3	−	+	−
K7	54	AE3	−	−	+
K8	50	AE3	−	−	+
K14	50	AE1	+	+	−
K16	48	AE1	−	+	−
K17	46		−	−	+
K18	45		−	−	+
K19	40	AE1	+	+	+

A, cells in vivo; B, cells cultured in vitro.

to that found in adenocarcinomas or squamous cell carcinomas. Many neoplastic cells have been shown to coexpress keratins and vimentin (Banks-Schlegel et al., 1985).

IV. Hyperplasia

A. In Vivo

Cells in the normal tracheobronchial epithelium slough off into the lumen and are continually replaced through the proliferation and differentiation of the stem or progenitor cells. Under normal conditions the rates of proliferation, differentiation, and cell loss must be equal to create a balance. The maintenance of such a delicate balance requires that the controls of proliferation and differentiation be regulated in a coordinated fashion, and very likely involves an equilibrium between positive and negative growth and differentiation factors including TGF-α, TGF-β, and retinoids. The turnover in the normal tracheobronchial epithelium occurs at a rather slow rate as indicated by the low incorporation of [^{3}H]thymidine into nuclei (labeling index; Lane and Gordon, 1974; Boren and Paradise, 1978; Donnelly et al., 1982; Keenan et al., 1982; Evans and Shami, 1989) and could be related to the presence of very low levels of (activated) positive growth factors.

Mechanical or toxic injury and vitamin A deficiency have been shown to induce hyperplasia and squamous metaplasia (Wolbach and Howe, 1926; Wong and Buck, 1971; Sporn et al., 1975; Harris et al., 1973; Chopra, 1982; Klein-Szanto et al., 1980; Woodworth et al., 1983; Keenan, Wilson and McDowell, 1983). These conditions increase dramatically the mitotic rate of tracheal cells (Lane and Gordon, 1974; Keenan et al., 1982). We have proposed (Floyd and

Jetten, 1988; Jetten, 1989; Vollberg et al., 1990) that in the normal tracheobronchial epithelium many cells are not continuously participating in the turnover of the epithelium and remain in the quiescent (G_0) phase of the cell cycle (Fig. 4). During the hyperproliferative response these resting cells may be recruited and re-enter the cell cycle. This induction of proliferation may be caused by a disturbance of the balance between positive and negative growth regulatory factors. For example, an increase in the production of TGF-α by tracheobronchial epithelial cells could stimulate cellular proliferation via an autocrine manner. The suggested role of EGF/TGF-α in hyperplasia finds support in the studies showing that intravenous administration of epidermal growth factor to fetal lambs can result in hyperplasia of the tracheobronchial epithelium (Stahlman et al., 1988). An alternative way to induce hyperplasia could be a reduction in the levels of negative growth factors. Hyperplasia induced during vitamin A deficiency could be related to reduced TGF-β levels, whereas retinoids may increase TGF-β levels and antagonize hyperplasia (Glick et al., 1989). In many tissues, including the lung, epithelial cells communicate with other cell types such as mesenchymal cells and inflammatory cells. Factors secreted by mesenchymal cells or lung macrophages can influence the proliferation and differentiation of epithelial cells in a paracrine manner. For example, mesenchymal cells have been demonstrated to secrete keratinocyte growth factor KGF, a FGF-like growth factor (Finch et al., 1989), that can stimulate the growth of certain epithelial cells including tracheobronchial epithelial cells. Embryonic lung fibroblasts have been shown to synthesize insulin growth factor I, IGF-I, which could stimulate the growth of lung epithelial cells

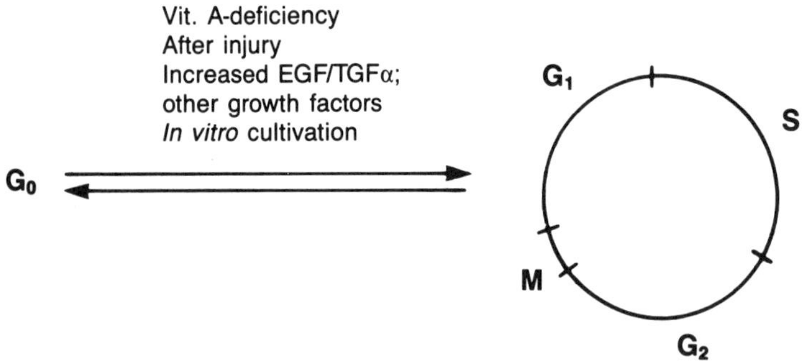

Figure 4 Schematic view of the induction of hyperplasia. In the normal tracheobronchial epithelium many cells remain quiescent (in the G_0 phase of cell cycle). Under certain conditions, such as vitamin A deficiency or mechanical or toxic injury, these cells are recruited and re-enter the cell cycle resulting in hyperplasia. This probably involves increased syntheses or activation of positive growth factors (EGF/TGFα, IGF-I, etc.). Cells mimic the hyperproliferative response when cultured in vitro in the presence of excess growth factors.

during development (Stiles and Moats-Staats, 1989). Proliferation of epithelial cells may also be influenced by growth regulatory factors secreted by macrophages. Macrophages have been shown to produce and secrete a host of growth factors including TGF-α and TGF-β (Nathan, 1987). During injury or conditions that induce hyperplasia, the production or activation of positive growth factors by mesenchymal cells and/or macrophages may increase and stimulate proliferation of epithelial cells in a paracrine manner. Higher levels of autocrine and paracrine growth factors may also be required during embryonic and fetal development when tissues are rapidly expanding.

B. In Vitro

Several in vitro culture systems have been established to study the proliferation and differentiation of tracheobronchial epithelial cells at the biochemical and molecular level (Lechner et al., 1981; Wu et al., 1982; Lechner and LaVeck, 1985; Jetten and Smits, 1985; Kim et al., 1985; Thomassen et al., 1986; Wu, 1987; Chopra et al., 1987). Our laboratory has been concentrating on epithelial cells from the rabbit trachea and the human bronchus. Rabbit tracheal epithelial cells (RbTE), obtained after pronase digestion of the tracheal epithelium, and human bronchial epithelial (HBE) cells, obtained from outgrowths of explants of human bronchus, when plated and grown in serum-free media proliferate with doubling times of approximately 19 and 24 hr, respectively (Lechner et al., 1981, 1984; Jetten and Shirley, 1985; Jetten and Smits, 1985). Epidermal growth factor (EGF) and insulin are two major growth-stimulatory factors for tracheobronchial epithelial cells. TGFα, which, like EGF, acts through the EGF receptor, can be substituted for EGF. IGF-I can be substituted for insulin. IGF-I stimulates proliferation at almost 100-fold lower concentrations than insulin (Jetten, unpublished observations). It is likely that both the insulin and IGF-I-stimulated growth response are mediated through the IGF-I receptor. The recently discovered keratinocyte growth factor (KGF), which appears to be a member of the FGF growth factor family, can also stimulate the growth of tracheobronchial epithelial cells (Finch et al., 1989).

The hyperproliferative response of tracheobronchial epithelial cells in culture is probably comparable to the hyperproliferative response of cells in vivo. Many of the freshly isolated tracheobronchial epithelial cells are quiescent and reenter the cell cycle and undergo hyperproliferation when placed in culture in medium containing an excess of positive growth factors such as insulin/IGF-I and EGF/TGFα (Fig. 4).

C. Neoplastic Cells

Neoplastic cells have been shown to exhibit alterations in the mechanisms that control their growth. The aberrations in the growth control have been related to genetic changes in genes (e.g., proto-oncogenes and tumor suppressor genes) that regulate proliferation and differentiation of tracheobronchial epithelial cells. Expression of oncogenes have been categorized as growth factors (e.g., *sis*); growth factor receptors (e.g., *erb*B); *tyr*- or thr/ser kinases (e.g., *abl*, *src*, *raf*, *erb*B); GTP-binding proteins (e.g., *ras*-family); nuclear proteins (e.g., *erb*A, *myc*-family, *fos*). Activation or amplification of many of these oncogenes has been found in lung carcinomas (Nau et al., 1986; Rodenhuis et al., 1987; Johnson et al., 1987; Kaul, 1987; Rapp et al., 1988; Havemann et al., 1988) and related to altered growth properties as well as to the expression of other characteristics of tumor cells including invasiveness (Bonfil et al., 1989). In contrast to the growth of normal cells, which is dependent on exogenous signals, neoplastic cells can grow independently of exogenous signals (Fig. 5). For example, the growth of normal cells is strongly dependent on the presence of EGF or TGFα, whereas many neoplastic cells have become independent of exogenous EGF/TGFα. This independence of exogenous growth factors found in many neoplastic cells could be related to a mutation in the EGF receptor (c-*erb*B) resulting in constitutive activation of the receptor and stimulation of cell growth (Fig. 5B; Havemann et al., 1988). As an alternative, constitutive synthesis and secretion of high levels of active TGF-α could induce proliferation of these cells in an autocrine manner (Siegfried, 1987; Jetten, unpublished observations). The growth of tracheobronchial epithelial cells expressing the v-Ha-*ras* oncogene is independent of the presence of EGF and is related to the synthesis and secretion of high levels of TGF-α (Fig. 5B; Jetten, unpublished observations). Other examples of constitutive TGF-α synthesis are the adenocarcinoma cell lines A549 and PC-9; addition of anti-TGF-α antibodies has been shown to inhibit the growth of these cells (Siegfried and Owens, 1988; Imanishi et al., 1989).

Many neoplastic cells are resistant to negative growth regulatory factors such as TGF-β or lose the responsiveness to differentiation inducers such as protein kinase C activators (see below). Such changes make cells escape the normal negative growth regulatory mechanisms and result in uncontrolled proliferation. One category of tumor suppressor genes may constitute genes involved in controlling growth suppression. The retinoblastoma (RB) gene and the p53 gene are tumor suppressor genes that encode nuclear proteins that appear to be involved in negative growth regulation (Huang et al., 1988; Eliyahu et al., 1989). The loss of expression of these proteins has been observed in many lung carcinomas (Yokota et al., 1988; Takahashi et al., 1989) and may be related to the uncontrolled growth of these cells.

V. Squamous Differentiation

A. Irreversible Growth Arrest

The morphologic and biochemical changes that accompany squamous differentiation in cultured tracheobronchial epithelial cells are very similar to those observed

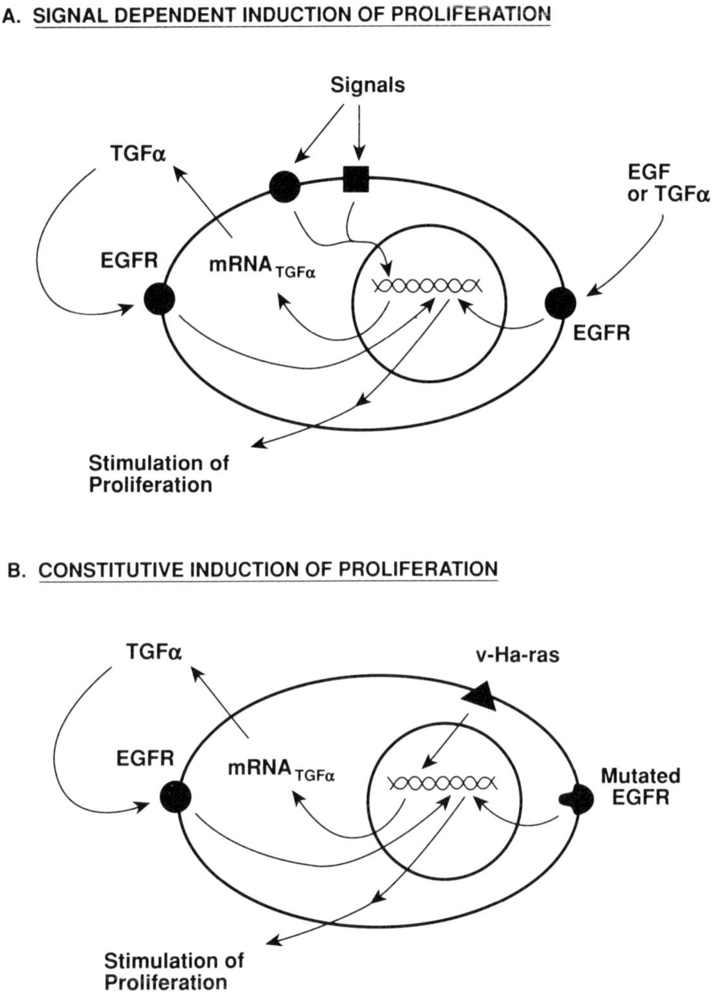

Figure 5 Control of proliferation in normal and tumorigenic tracheobronchial epithelial cells. (A) The proliferation of normal cells is dependent on external signals (growth factors, hormones etc.). (B) In malignant cells growth regulation is uncoupled from the normal growth regulatory signals, for example, through the expression of a mutated EGF receptor (EGFR/c-*erb*B) or the expression of v-Ha-*ras* or mutated Ha-*ras*.

during squamous metaplasia in vivo. Cultured tracheobronchial epithelial cells undergo squamous differentiation when reaching confluence (Jetten and Smits, 1985; Jetten and Shirley, 1985; Rearick et al., 1987c): cells become larger and flatten, the nucleus to cytoplasm ratio is reduced, and desmosomal junctions are established. The proliferative capacity of the cells is also altered at confluence. During the exponential phase, more than 95% of the cells incorporate [^{3}H]thymidine into their nucleus and have a relatively high colony forming efficiency, whereas cells at confluence are unable to incorporate [^{3}H]thymidine into the nucleus or to form colonies after subculture. These results indicate that at confluence tracheobronchial epithelial cells lose the ability to undergo mitosis or, in other words, undergo irreversible growth arrest (terminal cell division). Irreversible growth arrest is accompanied by decreased levels of inositol phosphates, and the commitment to terminal cell division appears to be a requirement for the expression of the squamous differentiated phenotype. Little is known about the molecular mechanisms that control irreversible growth arrest. However, reduced probability that cells will undergo irreversible growth arrest either during differentiation or senescence (immortalization) is an important step in the carcinogenesis process (Barrett and Wiseman, 1987). Expression of so-called immortalizing genes, like those encoding the viral proteins Ela and SV40 large T antigen, may interfere with mechanisms that control growth suppression. It is of interest that these genes interact with the retinoblastoma (RB) gene (Ludlow et al., 1989; Egan et al., 1989), which appears to be involved in the regulation of proliferation.

B. Expression of the Squamous Phenotype

1. Biochemical Markers

Squamous cell differentiation constitutes an abnormal pathway of differentiation in the tracheobronchial epithelium and follows hyperplasia induced after toxic or mechanical injury, or during vitamin A deficiency (Jetten, 1989). It can also be observed in squamous cell carcinomas. Squamous differentiation in tracheobronchial epithelial cells has many morphologic similarities to squamous differentiation in epidermal keratinocytes (Jetten, 1989) and is therefore associated with many of the same squamous cell markers. As do epidermal keratinocytes, tracheobronchial epithelial cells form cross-linked envelopes, layers of covalently linked protein deposited just beneath the plasma membrane (Rice and Green, 1977; Simon and Green, 1985; Jetten and Shirley, 1985; Jetten et al., 1987b). The enzyme transglutaminase type I catalyzes the cross-linking of the protein precursors via the formation of a covalent linkage between the ϵ-NH2 of lysine and the γ-NH2 of glutamine (Thacher and Rice, 1985). Cultured RbTE and HBE cells express very low levels of transglutaminase type I activity during the exponential growth phase (Jetten and Shirley, 1985; Jetten and George, submitted). At this stage, HBE cells contain relatively high levels of transglutaminase type II activity, whereas very little type II activity could be detected in RbTE cells. The two transglutaminases can be differentiated from each other immunologically and by the difference in their cellular distribution: type I is membrane-associated, whereas type II is a cytosolic enzyme. At confluence, the level of transglutaminase type I rapidly increases in HBE and RbTE cells; in HBE cells this is accompanied by a simultaneous decrease in type II transglutaminase (Fig. 6; Jetten et al., 1990). High levels of transglutaminase type I can also be observed in the upper layers of squamous metaplastic foci in tracheas from vitamin-A-deficient hamsters (Jetten et al., 1987b). Thus the induction of transglutaminase type I activity functions as a biochemical marker for squamous differentiation of tracheobronchial epithelial cells in vivo as well as in vitro. Recently, we have isolated a cDNA clone, pTG-7, encoding rabbit type I transglutaminase (Floyd and Jetten, 1989). Northern blot analysis using pTG-7 as a probe has shown that the increase in transglutaminase type I activity is related to an increase in corresponding mRNA levels. The stimulation of type I transglutaminase activity is accompanied by an increase in the formation of cross-linked envelopes (Fig. 5). Several cross-linked envelope precursors have been identified. HBE cells synthesize involucrin when undergoing squamous differentiation (Said et al., 1983). In RbTE cells a 35 kD cytosolic protein has been identified that is a substrate for transglutaminase type I and is a constituent of the cross-linked envelope (Jetten and Smits, unpublished observations).

Recently, we have discovered that the accumulation of cholesterol sulfate functions as a marker of squamous differentiation in cells from several tissues (Rearick and Jetten, 1986; Rearick et al., 1987c; Rearick et al., 1988; Jetten et al., 1989a). RbTE and HBE cells contain low levels of cholesterol sulfate during the exponential growth phase. When cultures reach the confluent phase of the growth curve the levels of cholesterol sulfate rapidly increase in parallel with the increase in transglutaminase type I activity. We have demonstrated that this stimulation of the accumulation of cholesterol sulfate is related to an increase in the cholesterol sulfotransferase activity (Rearick et al., 1987a). The function of cholesterol sulfate in the differentiation process is not yet known. Possibly this lipid alters the membrane fluidity thereby modulating the activity of enzymes or receptors. As an alternative, cholesterol sulfate may function as a receptor for cross-linked envelope precursors and thereby assist in the formation of the cross-linked envelopes.

RbTE and HBE cells in culture exhibit a keratin profile that is characteristic for stratified epithelia. During the exponential growth phase, RbTE cells are undifferentiated and express three major keratins, K5, K14, and K19, and two minor keratins, K6 and K16 (Jetten et al., 1989). At confluence, cells undergo squamous differentiation and show an increased expression of keratins K6, K13, K16, and K19 (Fig. 7). These keratins were identified on basis of their molecular weight, isoelectric point, and their reactivity with several monoclonal antibodies against specific keratins. Keratins K5 and K6 reacted with monoclonal antibody

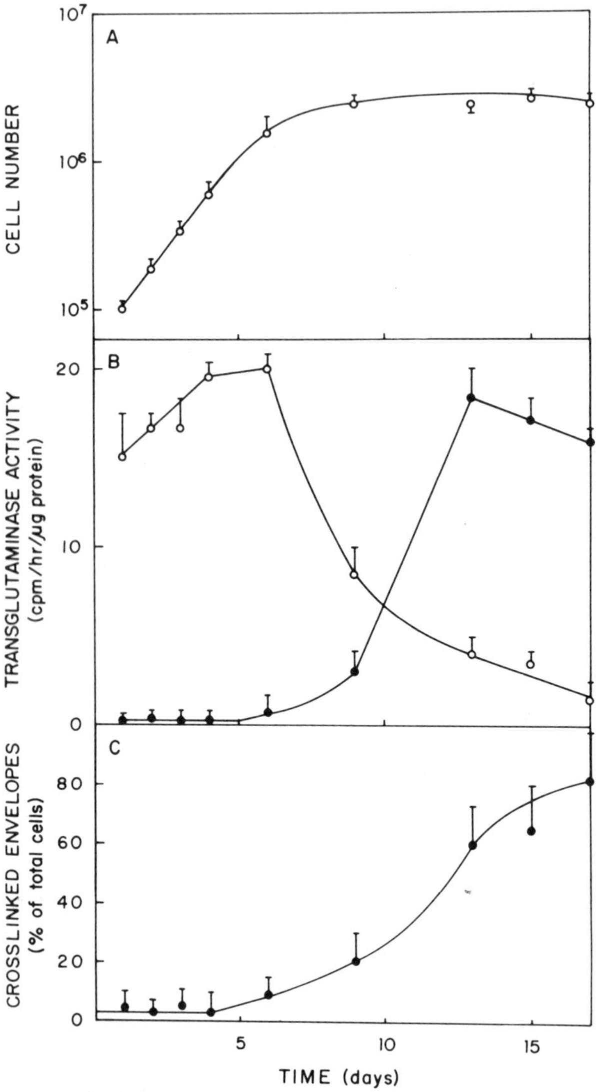

Figure 6 Alterations in transglutaminase type I and type II activity during squamous differentiation of HBE cells. HBE cells were grown in HBE-medium in 60 mm dishes and at different stages of the growth curve the cell number (A) and transglutaminase activity (B)—type I (B, ●) and type II (B, ○) transglutaminase activity, and the number of cross-linked envelopes (C) were determined. At confluence, HBE cells undergo squamous differentiation, which is accompanied by a decrease in transglutaminase type II activity and an increase in type I activity and cross-linked envelope formation. (From Jetten et al., 1991).

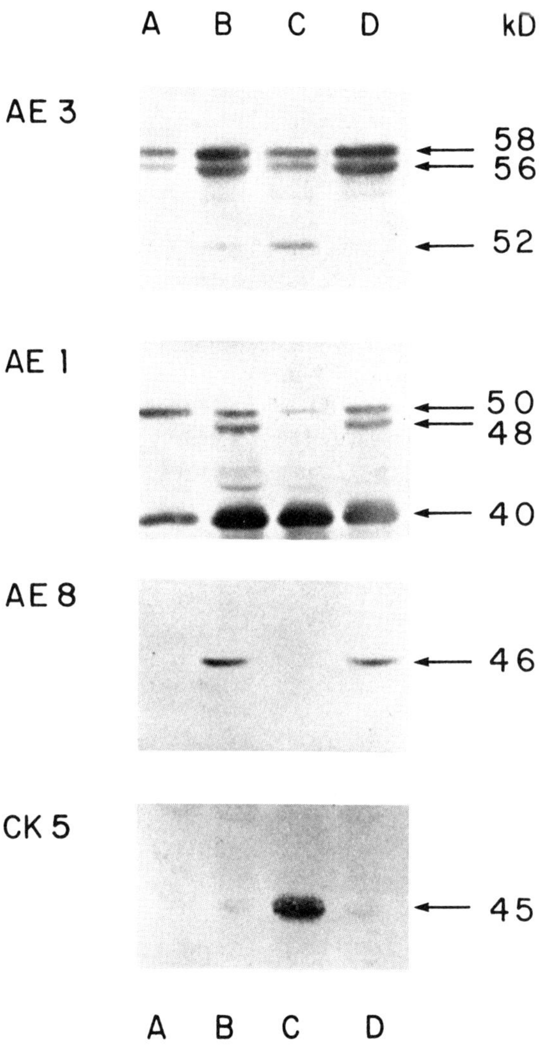

Figure 7 Keratin expression in rabbit tracheal epithelial (RbTE) cells in relation to squamous differentiation. RbTE cells were grown in culture under various conditions and then analyzed for keratin expression by immunoblot analysis using the antikeratin monoclonal antibodies AE1, AE3, AE8, CK5. (A) Proliferative RbTE cells; (B) Confluent squamous differentiated cells; (C) Confluent retinoic acid treated cells; (D) confluent Ca^{2+} (1.8 mM)-treated cells. The AE3 reactive keratins are K5(58 kD), K6(56 kD); the AE1-reactive keratins are K14(50 kD), K16(48 kD), and K19(40 kD); the AE8-reactive keratin is K13(46 kD), and the CK5-reactive keratin K18(45 kD). (From Jetten et al., 1989b).

AE3, keratins K14, K16, and K19 with antibody AE1, keratins K16 and K13 with antibody 8.12 (not shown), whereas the antibody AE8 was specific for keratin K13. High calcium concentration in the medium did not affect the keratin expression. In particular, the induction of the keratin K13 functions as a strong biochemical marker for the expression of the squamous differentiated phenotype in tracheobronchial epithelial cells. This is confirmed by immunohistochemical studies showing staining for this keratin in the suprabasal layers of squamous metaplastic foci in the trachea of vitamin-A-deficient hamsters (Roop, personal communication). The induction of keratin K13 appears to be specific for squamous differentiation of the tracheobronchial epithelium since it is not induced during epidermal differentiation. HBE cells in culture synthesize keratins K5, K6, K14, K16, and K19 (Gilfix and Eckert, 1985; Wu and Wu, 1986; Jetten, unpublished results); however, if any of these keratins is differentially expressed during differentiation of HBE cells has to be established. The pattern of keratin expression of cultured RbTE and HBE cells is very similar to that of basal cells, in agreement with the concept that the clonogenic cells in culture either are basal cells or are closely related to basal cells. Moreover, more than 95% of RbTE cells in culture bind the lectin *Griffonia simplicifolia* (GSA I-B4) that specifically reacts with basal cells. These studies suggest that it is the basal cell that undergoes squamous cell differentiation in vitro and probably is also the cell type that is involved in squamous metaplasia in vivo.

2. Molecular Markers

To study the regulation of gene expression during squamous differentiation, a cDNA library was constructed from mRNA isolated from squamous differentiated RbTE cells. Screening of the cDNA library was aimed at identifying RNAs that are abundant in squamous differentiated cells and are expressed at low frequency in undifferentiated cells (Smits et al., 1987). Three different cDNA clones, SQ10, SQ37, and C12, were obtained encoding RNAs that are present at approximately 50-fold higher levels in squamous differentiated cells than in undifferentiated cells (Fig. 8). The cDNA clone SQ37 has been sequenced and contains a tandem repeat of the amino acid sequence PKVPEPCQ. The function of this gene product is not known. The two other clones, SQ10 and C12, have been partially sequenced and also represent unknown squamous cell-specific gene products. A different strategy has been followed to isolate a cDNA for the transglutaminase type I. This transglutaminase is a member of a larger family of transglutaminases that include Type II (tissue) transglutaminase, and factor XIII, which plays a role in blood clotting. Comparison of the full-length coding sequences of both of these transglutaminases showed that the active site, consisting of eight amino acids, is 100% homologous (Floyd and Jetten, 1989). A mixture of oligonucleotides encoding this active site was used to screen a cDNA library prepared from poly(A)$^+$ RNA

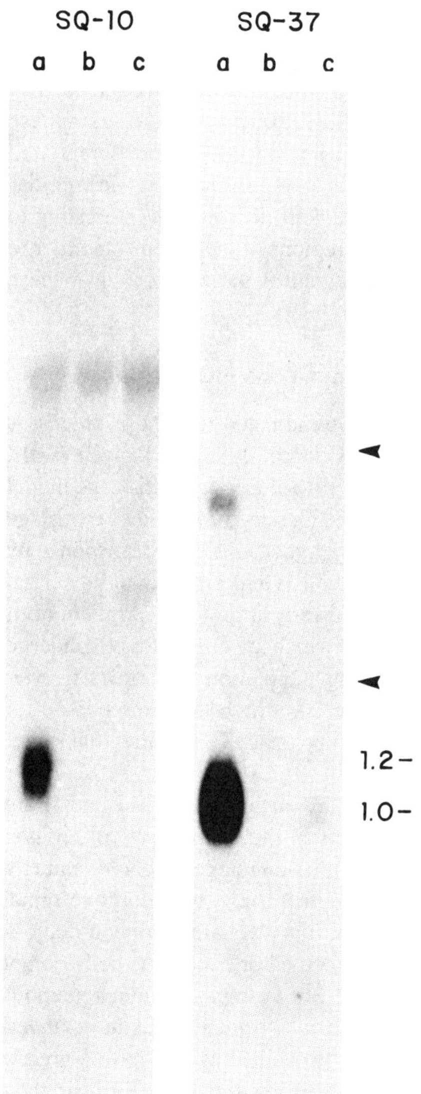

Figure 8 Expression of two squamous cell-specific mRNAs, SQ10 and SQ37, in RbTE cells. Northern blot analysis. (A) Poly(A)$^+$ RNA isolated from confluent squamous differentiated cells; (B) Poly(A)$^+$ RNA isolated from proliferative cells; (C) Poly(A)$^+$ RNA from confluent retinoic acid-treated cells. RNAs hybridizing to SQ10 and SQ37 are only abundant in squamous cells. (From Smits et al., 1987).

isolated from squamous differentiated RbTE cells. From the five clones that were obtained and sequenced, four appeared to be encoding the transglutaminase type I. The fifth clone, pTG-15, appeared to be another squamous cell-specific mRNA encoding an unknown gene product. The SQ10, SQ37, C12, the transglutaminase type I, and pTG-15 genes all are expressed at low levels in undifferentiated tracheobronchial cells and at high levels when cells undergo squamous differentiation, and could be regulated via a common mechanism. It would be interesting to compare the regulatory elements in the promoter regions of these genes in order to determine whether common enhancer elements control the expression of these genes.

C. Multi-Stage Model of Hyperplasia/Squamous Metaplasia

Studies of hyperplasia/squamous metaplasia have indicated that these processes occur in several steps (Wong and Buck, 1971; Chopra, 1982; McDowell et al., 1984). Based on these observations and on our in vitro studies a multi-stage model of hyperplasia/squamous metaplasia was proposed (Jetten, 1989; Fig. 9). In stage I, quiescent cells (probably basal cells) undergo a hyperproliferative response by reentering the cell cycle. Cell division of basal cells yield either daughter basal cells with extensive proliferative capacity or a transit amplifying population of cells that have a limited proliferative capacity and which are committed to undergo squamous differentiation. The transit amplifying population undergoes irreversible growth arrest (terminal cell division; stage II), which is a prerequisite for expression of the squamous differentiated phenotype (stage III). In the final stage, cells cornify.

From this model it can be predicted that, in particular, stage I and II are relevant to the development of neoplasm. Defects in the control of proliferation (stage I) and the commitment to terminal differentiation (stage II) could lead to a constitutive induction of proliferation and reduced probability to undergo terminal differentiation and result in uncontrolled growth. This has already been demonstrated in many tumor cell lines. However, transformed or neoplastic cells do not always lose the ability to undergo differentiation. For example, certain squamous cell carcinomas are well-differentiated tumors in which many cells have undergone terminal differentiation. However, these tumor cells may still have a greatly reduced ability to undergo differentiation in combination with aberrations in their growth control.

VI. Modulators of Cell Proliferation and Differentiation

A. Retinoids

Retinoids, analogues of vitamin A, are regulators of proliferation and differentiation in many cell systems including tracheobronchial epithelial cells (Sporn et al.,

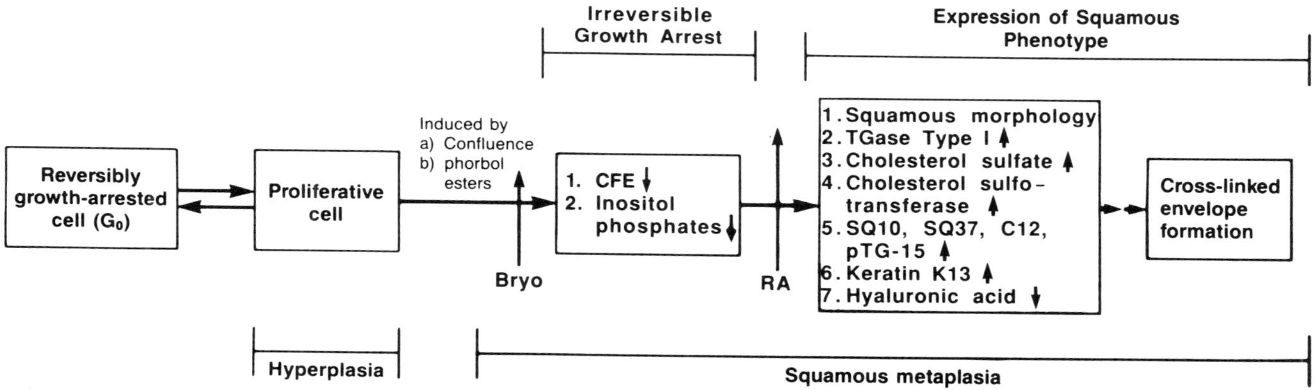

Figure 9 Schematic view of the multistage program of squamous cell differentiation in tracheobronchial epithelial cells in vivo and in vitro. In stage I, quiescent cells re-enter the cell cycle and become hyperproliferative. In vivo, this stage is equivalent to hyperplasia. In stage II, cells become committed to irreversible growth arrest (terminal cell division). In stage III, cells start to express the squamous differentiated phenotype and several biochemical and molecular squamous cell markers are induced. In the final stage, cells form cross-linked envelopes. The tumor promoter phorbol 12-myristate-13-acetate (PMA) induces a commitment to squamous cell differentiation. This induction is inhibited by bryostatins (Bryo) at stage II. Retinoids (RA) block the differentiation process at stage III. TGase, transglutaminase type I.

1984; Sherman, 1986). In vivo, retinoids are important in maintaining the normal pathway of differentiation in the tracheobronchial epithelium: vitamin A-deficiency induces hyperplasia and squamous metaplasia in animals (Wolbach and Howe, 1926; Wilhelm, 1954; Wong and Buck, 1971; Sporn et al., 1975; McDowell et al., 1984), which can be reversed after treatment with vitamin A. Studies with tracheobronchial cells in culture have shown that retinoids can inhibit squamous differentiation and stimulate the expression of a secretory phenotype (Jetten et al., 1987; Rearick et al., 1987b). RbTE cells, when grown on a collagen gel matrix in the absence of retinoids, undergo squamous differentiation; however, in the presence of retinoids, cells form tight junctions and have secretory granules containing mucous-like glycoconjugates. Retinoids appear to affect differentiation of tracheobronchial cells at different stages. These agents antagonize the induction of a hyperproliferative response (hyperplasia), promote expression of the mucociliary phenotype, and inhibit squamous differentiation. Controls of these three processes are likely to be interrelated.

Retinoids are very potent inhibitors of squamous differentiation in cultured HBE and RbTE cells (Jetten and Shirley, 1985; Rearick and Jetten, 1986; Rearick et al., 1987c). These compounds influence the multistage program of squamous differentiation at very specific stages. Retinoids appear to influence the first stage since the absence of retinoids induces hyperplasia in vivo, which is reversed after retinoid treatment. Little is known about the mechanisms by which retinoids control the switch that determines whether the cells undergo normal differentiation or hyperplasia. The commitment to irreversible growth arrest (stage II; Fig. 9) that precedes the expression of the squamous differentiated phenotype is not affected by retinoids. However, retinoids block the induction of the squamous differentiated markers (stage III; Fig. 9). Treatment of tracheobronchial epithelial cells with retinoids inhibits the increase in transglutaminase type I (Jetten and Shirley, 1985) and cholesterol sulfotransferase activity and the accumulation of cholesterol sulfate (Rearick and Jetten, 1986; Rearick et al., 1987a). Retinoids also inhibit the expression of keratins K5, K6, and K16 in both RbTE and HBE cells and block the expression of keratin K13 in RbTE cells (Fig. 7; Gilfix and Eckert, 1985; Wu and Wu, 1986; Huang et al., 1988; Jetten et al., 1989b). Retinoids induce keratin K18, which is usually expressed in mucociliary cells. This observation is in agreement with the concept that retinoids promote mucociliary differentiation. The suppression of the induction of transglutaminase type I and several keratin proteins by retinoids reflects the levels of corresponding mRNA (Gilfix and Eckert, 1985; Jetten et al., 1989b; Floyd and Jetten, 1989). Retinoids also suppress the expression of the squamous cell-specific mRNAs, SQ10, SQ37, C12, and pTG-15 in RbTE cells (Fig. 7; Smits et al., 1987; Jetten, unpublished observations).

The mechanism by which retinoids exert their action has not yet been fully elucidated. The inhibition of squamous differentiation in HBE and RbTE cells and the induction of the secretory phenotype in RbTE cells by retinoids occur at nanomolar concentrations. Moreover, specific structural requirements are critical for the biological activity of retinoids (Jetten et al., 1987a). These observations suggest that the action of retinoids is mediated via high affinity retinoid receptors. Several specific cytosolic retinoid binding proteins and nuclear retinoic acid receptors have been found to be expressed in eukaryotic cells (Chytil and Ong, 1979, 1983; Petkovich et al., 1987; Giguere et al., 1987). Thus far three nuclear retinoic acid receptors, RARα, RARβ, and RARγ have been identified (Petkovich et al., 1987; Giguere et al., 1987; Benbrook et al., 1988; Brand et al., 1988; Krust et al., 1989; Zelent et al., 1989). These receptors are members of a superfamily of nuclear receptors, which includes the receptors for steroid and thyroid hormones and for vitamin D3 (Evans, 1988). The RAR receptors have a molecular weight of 50,000 daltons and are localized almost solely in the nucleus (Nervi et al., 1989; Gaub et al., 1989). Like the other members of this family, the nuclear retinoic acid receptors act as ligand-dependent transacting enhancing factors. After binding of the retinoid to the RAR receptor, a dimer is formed that interacts with regulatory sequences (retinoic acid response elements) of specific genes and, through the interaction with other nuclear proteins induces changes in the rate of their transcription (Fig. 10; Jetten, 1990). The retinoic acid-RAR complex is able to form not only a homodimeric complex but also a heterodimeric complex with the closely related thyroid hormone receptor (T3R) (Glass et al., 1989), and possibly with different RARs as well (Fig. 10). Tracheobronchial epithelial cells in culture express both RARα and RARγ but not RARβ (Jetten, unpublished results). Based on the structure-activity relationship, it appears likely that the suppression of squamous differentiation and the induction of the mucosecretory phenotype by retinoids is mediated via the RAR receptors. However, if the suppression of the SQ10, SQ37, C12, transglutaminase type I, pTG-15, and keratin 13 genes, and the induction of mucous glycoproteins occur directly via the retinoic acid response elements in the promoter regions of these genes or indirectly via the suppression or activation of another regulatory protein has to be established.

Tracheobronchial epithelial cells contain very low levels of the cytosolic retinoic acid-binding protein (CRABP) and retinol-binding protein (CRBP). Several functions for CRBP and CRABP have been proposed. Bhat and Jetten (1987) have shown that RbTE cells have the ability to metabolize retinol into retinyl esters and retinoic acid. The CRBP may mediate the transport of retinol to the endoplasmic reticulum, where it is metabolized to retinyl esters and to retinoic acid, as has been demonstrated in rat liver (Yost et al., 1988). CRABP could have a similar function. Through binding retinoic acid and possibly facilitating its metabolism into less active retinoids, CRABP may control the effective retinoic acid concentration (Maden et al., 1988). In this way, CRABP could reduce the binding of retinoic acid to the RAR receptors and thereby antagonize the RAR-mediated action of retinoic acid on gene expression.

Since retinoic acid affects the proliferation and differentiation of tracheo-

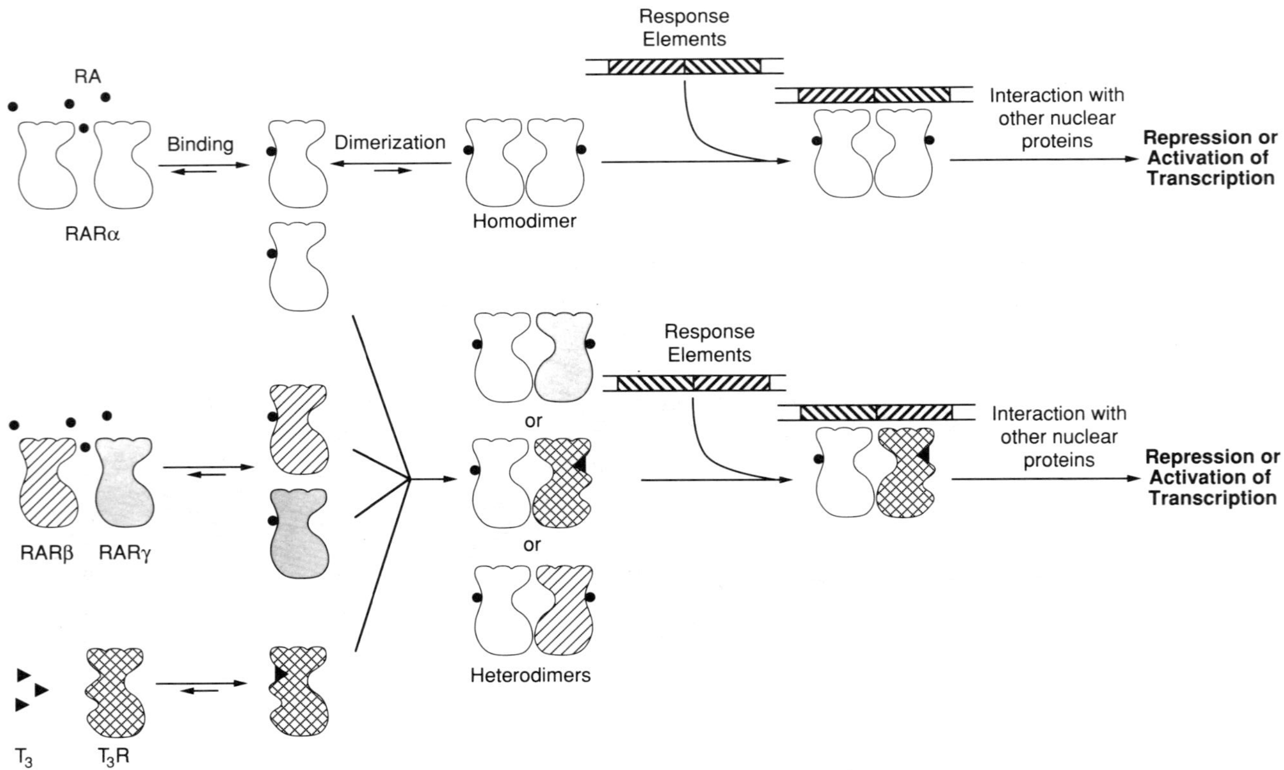

Figure 10 Schematic presentation of the mechanism of action of retinoic acid. Retinoic acid binds, for example, to the RARα receptor and forms a homodimer, or heterodimer with either T3R, or RARβ or RARγ. These dimers, after binding to specific response elements and interacting with other nuclear proteins, influence gene transcription in a positive or negative manner. RA, retinoic acid; RAR, nuclear retinoic acid receptor; T3R, thyroid hormone receptor; T3, thyroid hormone.

bronchial epithelial cells, alterations in the activity or synthesis of the RAR receptors could play a role in the induction of neoplasia. Such an involvement has already been established for the thyroid hormone receptors (c-*erb*A), which are closely related to the RAR receptors (Jetten, 1990). For example, the viral oncogene v-*erb*A, which inhibits the differentiation of erythroblasts into erythrocytes, has been demonstrated to be able to enhance the transformed phenotype of certain eukaryotic cells in conjunction with other oncogenes (Venstrom et al., 1980). This oncogene is unable to bind thyroid hormone but can bind to the thyroid hormone response element, thereby inhibiting the binding of the thyroid hormone-thyroid hormone receptor complex (Damm et al., 1989). The RARs could function as proto-oncogenes, in a manner similar to that described for v-*erb*A. Alternatively, since retinoids inhibit hyperplasia, RARs could act as tumor suppressor genes; loss of an RAR receptor results in the loss of a growth suppressor gene and results in uncontrolled proliferation.

Little is known about the expression of RAR and CRABP receptors in neoplastic cells. Expression of RARα, β, and γ has been observed in adeno and squamous cell carcinomas. Small cell carcinoma H-69 cells expressed only the RARβ (Jetten, unpublished observations).

B. Activators of Protein Kinase C

The Ca^{2+}- and phospholipid-dependent protein kinase, protein kinase C, consists of a family of isoenzymes that exhibit a high degree of homology and are encoded by different genes (Nishizuka, 1984; Blumberg, 1988; Nishizuka, 1988; Kikkawa et al., 1989). Diacylglycerols are the endogenous ligands of protein kinase C. These enzymes function in signal transduction for a variety of external stimuli that interact with specific cell surface receptors, resulting in the activation of phospholipase C and the generation of diacylglycerol from phosphatidylinositol. Protein kinase C can be activated directly by a variety of exogenous agents. Addition of certain diacylglycerol analogs to the culture medium can activate protein kinase C in several cell types. The major responses of cells to the tumor promotors, phorbol esters, and the macrocyclic lactones, bryostatins (Pettit et al., 1982; Blumberg, 1988) are mediated through protein kinase C.

Phorbol esters induce a variety of biological and biochemical changes in cells from many tissues. They function as tumor promoters in the mouse skin carcinogenesis model (Slaga, 1984) and enhance tracheal carcinogenesis in rats (Topping and Nettesheim, 1980; Steele et al., 1984). In a transformed rat tracheal epithelial cell line, 2C5, the phorbol ester phorbol 12-myristate 13-acetate (PMA) reduces the binding of EGF and induces ornithine decarboxylase activity (Jetten and Shirley, 1985; Jetten et al., 1985). In normal tracheobronchial epithelial cells, phorbol esters induce squamous cell differentiation (Willey et al., 1984; Hesterberg et al., 1987; Jetten et al., 1989). Cells treated with PMA spread out, exhibit extended processes, and become irreversibly growth-arrested (undergo terminal cell division). PMA-treated HBE cells start to express transglutaminase type I activity and increased cholesterol sulfate accumulation, which are biochemical markers of squamous cell differentiation (Rearick et al., 1987c; Jetten et al., 1989c). In addition, PMA increases the formation of cross-linked envelopes (Willey et al., 1984; Hesterberg et al., 1987). The response of human tracheobronchial epithelial cells to phorbol esters is heterogeneous; at low concentrations of PMA a small subpopulation of cells does not undergo terminal differentiation (Hesterberg et al., 1987; Jetten, unpublished observations). This subpopulation, consisting of cells with the lowest probability of undergoing differentiation, appears to represent the smallest tracheobronchial epithelial cells and may represent stem cells.

Diacylglycerols, the endogenous ligands of protein kinase C, induce many of the same responses in eukaryotic cells as phorbol esters do. In the rat tracheal cell line 2C5 diacylglycerol, added either exogenously or derived after treatment of the cells with phospholipase C, reduces EGF-binding and induces ornithine decarboxylase activity, as does treatment with PMA (Jetten et al., 1985). However, diacylglycerol does not mimic all the actions of PMA. In promyelocytic leukemia HL60 cells, diacylglycerols are unable to induce monocytic differentiation (Yamamoto et al., 1985). In HBE cells, the diacylglycerol analogs, dioctanoylglycerol and didecanoylglycerol, at high concentrations can induce irreversible growth arrest and expression of the squamous differentiated phenotype (Jetten et al., 1989c).

Recently, it has been shown that bryostatins, macrocyclic lactones isolated from the marine bryozoan *Bugula neritina*, bind to and activate protein kinase C (Pettit et al., 1982). However, the bryostatins mimic several but not all of the effects of phorbol esters (Kraft et al., 1986; Sako et al., 1987; Kraft and May, 1987). In contrast to phorbol esters, bryostatins do not induce irreversible growth arrest and do not increase type I transglutaminase activity or cholesterol sulfate levels (Jetten et al., 1989c), which indicates that these agents do not induce squamous cell differentiation. The bryostatin not only failed to induce squamous cell differentiation, but in HBE cells it also antagonized the PMA-induced commitment to terminal differentiation. Bryostatin 1 blocked both phorbol ester-induced irreversible growth arrest (terminal cell division) and the expression of the differentiated phenotype (Fig. 11), and appeared to block the multistage program of squamous differentiation at stage II. Retinoids are also able to antagonize PMA action. However, in contrast to bryostatins, retinoids do not inhibit PMA-induced irreversible growth arrest but can inhibit expression of the squamous cell markers, which is in agreement with the concept that retinoids block stage III of the squamous differentiation pathway.

Bryostatin is able to inhibit the commitment to differentiation in PMA-treated cells long after the addition of PMA: 9 hr after the addition of PMA, bryostatin 1 still inhibits differentiation in about 50% of the cells (Jetten et al., 1989c). These findings suggest that the commitment to terminal differentiation

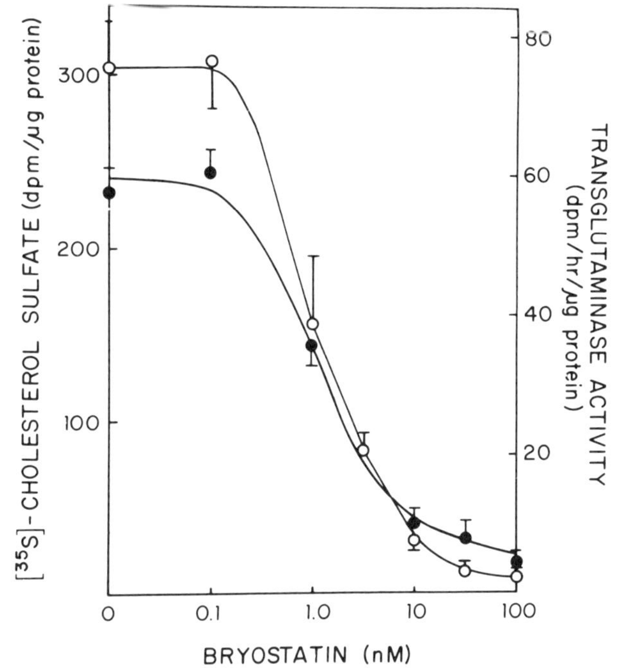

Figure 11 Antagonistic effects of the phorbol ester PMA and bryostatin 1 on squamous differentiation of HBE cells. HBE cells were treated simultaneously with PMA (10 nM) and with bryostatin 1 at the concentrations indicated. After 48 hr incubation, cells were harvested and the accumulation of cholesterol sulfate (○), and the level of transglutaminase type I activity (●) determined.

induced by PMA is a relatively late event in many cultured HBE cells. The delayed response to phorbol esters may be related to the possibility that PMA acts in a specific phase of the cell cycle and therefore brings about a gradual induction of the commitment to terminal differentiation in asynchronous cell cultures. The mechanism of the antagonism between phorbol esters and bryostatins is still poorly understood. Bryostatin may selectively activate one protein kinase C isozyme, thereby generating a response that antagonizes the signal transduction of another protein kinase C isozyme (Blumberg, 1988; Fields et al., 1988).

Several studies have shown that neoplastic tracheobronchial epithelial cells exhibit an altered response to phorbol esters. In general, neoplastic or transformed tracheobronchial epithelial cells are resistant to PMA-induced terminal differentiation (Willey et al., 1984; Sanchez et al., 1987; Jetten et al., 1989c). PMA does not induce irreversible growth arrest or expression of squamous cell markers indicating that these cells acquired defects in their differentiation control mechanism.

C. TGF-β

Transforming growth factor β1 (TGF-β1) is a hormonally active polypeptide that belongs to a family of closely related, but functionally distinct proteins (Roberts and Sporn, 1989). TGF-β1 is synthesized as a 390 amino acid precursor protein, which, after proteolytic cleavage at the carboxy terminus, yields the mature 112 amino acid TGF-β1 monomer. Active TGF-β1 consists of two identical monomers linked by disulfide bridges. TGF-β1 is secreted as a latent high-molecular weight complex and can be activated by specific proteases. TGF-β1 has been shown to regulate proliferation and differentiation of many cell types, including tracheobronchial epithelial cells (Masui et al., 1986; Jetten et al., 1986). The cellular responses to TGF-β1 are mediated via specific cell surface receptors (Wakefield et al., 1987; Cheifetz et al., 1987, 1988).

Normal human bronchial epithelial cells and many lung carcinoma cell lines have been shown to produce and secrete the latent form of TGF-β (Wakefield et al., 1987). This form does not bind to the TGF-β receptor and therefore does not induce a response in these cells. The addition of active TGF-β1 induces diverse effects in tracheobronchial epithelial cells. When RbTE and HBE cells are treated with TGF-β1 at low cell density, terminal cell division and squamous differentiation are induced (Masui et al., 1986; Jetten et al., 1986). At high cell density (more than 105 cells/60 mm dish), TGF-β1 inhibits cell growth but does not induce squamous cell differentiation. In contrast, TGF-β1 appears to inhibit squamous differentiation when HBE cells reach confluence. At high densities TGFβ does not induce transglutaminase type I activity or cholesterol sulfate, which are biochemical markers for squamous differentiation. However, TGF-β1 increases the synthesis of several other gene products, including transglutaminase type II and fibronectin. The stimulation in transglutaminase type II activity by TGF-β1 is related to an increase in type II transglutaminase protein and mRNA (George et al., 1990; Jetten et al., 1991; Fig. 12). The significance of this enhancement in transglutaminase type II activity is not fully understood. An increase in the levels of this enzyme has been found to be associated with apoptosis, a process of programmed cell death involved in the regression of tissue following hyperplasia, and may be an important mechanism to control tissue size. This raises the question of whether TGF-β functions as a regulator of hyperplasia by inducing apoptosis. TGF-β1 can affect gene expression at the level of transcription as well as at the level of the stability of the RNA. The stimulation of fibronectin and collagen α2(1) mRNA in fibroblasts and the increase of fibronectin in lung carcinoma A549 cells (Keski-Oja et al., 1988) have been shown to be dependent on protein synthesis. The transcriptional factor, nuclear factor 1 (NF1), has been implicated in the regulation of these genes by TGF-β1 (Rossi et al., 1988; Dean, 1989). The increase in type II transglutaminase mRNA by TGF-β1 is abrogated by cycloheximide, which suggests that this increase is also dependent on protein synthesis. Studies

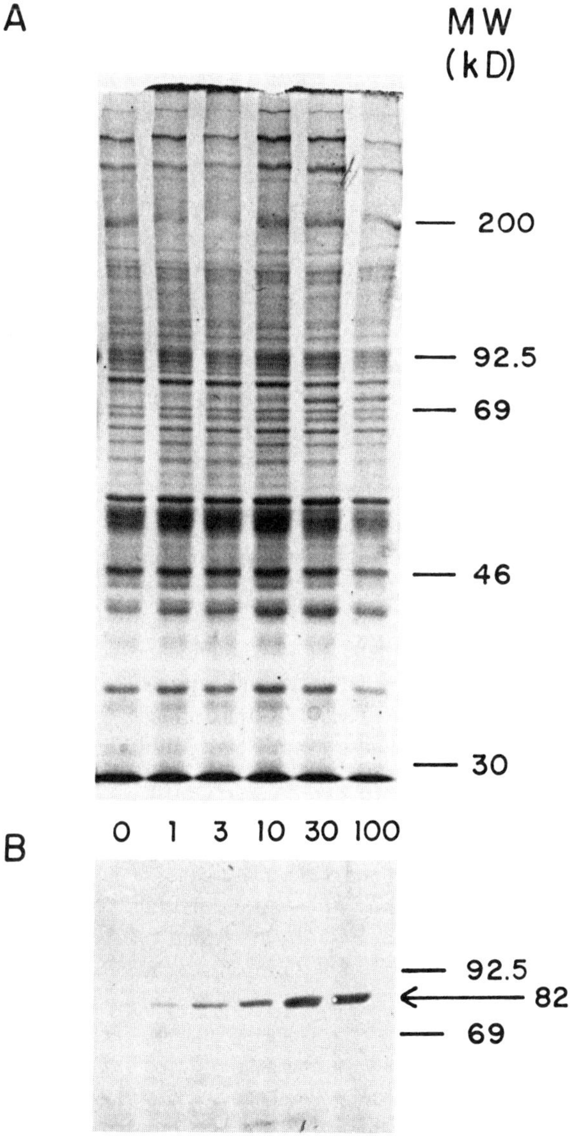

Figure 12 Action of TGF-β1 on transglutaminase type II. Human bronchial epithelial cells were treated for 3 days with varying concentrations of TGF-β1 and then assayed for transglutaminase type II protein via immunoblot analysis. (A) Coomassie brilliant blue staining; (B) immunoblot using a specific antitransglutaminase type II monoclonal antibody. (From Jetten et al., 1991).

are in progress to determine whether nuclear factor 1 is involved in the regulation of the transglutaminase type II gene.

Many of the responses in tracheobronchial epithelial cells induced by TGF-b1 are mimicked by TGF-β2 treatment and are probably mediated via a common receptor (Roberts and Sporn, 1989). Wakefield et al. (1987) have reported that normal human tracheobronchial epithelial cells contain approximately 10^4 high-affinity TGF-β receptors per cell. The apparent differentiation constant (Kd) for the binding of TGF-β was 10 pM.

Many transformed cell lines remain responsive to TGF-β1. For example, lung carcinoma A549 cells are growth inhibited and show increased type II transglutaminase, fibronectin, plasminogen activator (PA) and plasminogen activator inhibitor (PAI) production after the addition of TGF-b (Keski-Oja et al., 1988; Jetten, unpublished observations). PA plays an important role in the degradation of extracellular matrix components either by degrading extracellular proteins directly, or through the activation of other proteases such as collagenase. In contrast, PAI may serve to protect the matrix from proteolytic degradation. It has been suggested (Keski-Oja et al., 1988) that in normal cells the production of PAI may prevail, whereas in carcinoma cells the production of PA is dominant resulting in a more malignant (greater invasiveness) phenotype. Certain transformed cells have been shown to be much more resistant to TGF-β1 than normal cells (Masui et al., 1986; Jetten et al., 1986). These tumor cells do not show increased levels of transglutaminase type II activity after TGF-β1 treatment and are not growth inhibited. TGF-β1 inhibits the growth of SV40-large T transformed cells during early passages, and stimulates transglutaminase type II activity like in normal HBE cells. The resistance to TGF-β1 is not simply due to a lack of receptors, since many neoplastic cells contain TGF-b1 receptors (Masui et al., 1986; Wakefield et al., 1987). This resistance may be related to aberrations in the signal transduction mechanism of TGF-β1 or to the expression of one of the target genes of TGF-β1. In a xenograft of human lung adenocarcinoma A549 cells, TGF-β1 inhibits growth and stimulates differentiation into goblet-like cells (Twardzik et al., 1989). These results suggest a role for TGF-β1 in the induction of normal differentiation. In this regard, the action of TGF-β1 resembles that of retinoic acid. It is interesting that retinoic acid has been shown to induce TGF-β2 synthesis in mouse epidermal keratinocytes (Glick et al., 1989). Some of the retinoic acid induced-responses in tracheobronchial epithelial cells may be mediated via an increase in TGF-β2 synthesis. The latter may constitute a mechanism by which retinoids control hyperplasia and normal differentiation.

VII. Summary

Much has been learned about the various factors that regulate proliferation and differentiation of tracheobronchial epithelial cells, as well as about the biochemical and molecular changes that accompany squamous differentiation. Some regulators, such as the various growth factors, act via specific receptors that, after activation, set in motion a signal transduction mechanism that ultimately affect gene expression. Others, such as the retinoids, affect gene expression more directly via binding to specific nuclear receptors. A multistage model for hyperplasia/squamous metaplasia has been proposed. In this model, modulators of squamous differentiation affect the process at very specific stages. From this model it can be predicted that two stages (stage I and II) are particularly important to the carcinogenesis process. Constitutive activation of the proliferative response and the loss of irreversible growth arrest (immortalization) will lead to uncontrolled growth. Determining the biochemical and molecular mechanisms that underlie these two processes will help to understand the regulation of growth in normal and neoplastic cells.

Acknowledgments

The author gratefully acknowledges the many scientific contributions and valuable discussions by M. D. George and by Drs. H. L. Smits, E. E. Floyd, C. Nervi, J. I. Rearick, T. M. Vollberg, P. Nettesheim, and G. E. R. Hook.

References

Aumuller, G., Seitz, J., Heyns, W., and Kirchner, C. (1985). Ultrastructural localization of uteroglobin immunoreactivity in rabbit lung and endometrium, and rat ventral prostate. *Histochem.* **83:**413–417.

Banks-Schlegel, S., Gazdar, A. F., and Harris, C. C. (1985). Intermediate filament and cross-linked envelope expression in human lung tumor cell lines. *Cancer Res.* **45:** 1187–1197.

Banks-Schlegel, S. P., McDowell, E. M., Wilson, T. S., Trump, B. F., and Harris, C. C. (1984). Keratin proteins in human lung carcinomas. Combined use of morphology, keratin immunochemistry, and keratin immunoprecipitation. *Am. J. Pathol.* **114:** 273–286.

Barrett, J. C., and Wiseman, R. W. (1987). Cellular and molecular mechanisms of multistep carcinogenesis: relevance to carcinogen risk assessment. *Environ. Health Perspec.* **76:**65–70.

Basbaum, C. B., and Finkbeiner, W. E. (1989). Mucus-producing cells of the airways. In *Lung Cell Biology*. Edited by D. Massaro. New York, Marcel Dekker, Vol 41, pp. 37–79.

Benbrook, D., Lernhardt, E., and Pfahl, M. (1988). A new retinoic acid receptor identified from a hepatocellular carcinoma. *Nature* **333:**669–672.

Bhat, P. V., and Jetten, A. M. (1987). Metabolism of all-trans-retinol and all-trans-retinoic acid in rabbit tracheal epithelial cells in culture. *Biochim. Biophys. Acta.* **922:**18–27.

Blobel, G. A., Moll, R., Franke, W. W., Vogt-Moykopf, I. (1984). Cytokeratins in normal lung and lung carcinomas. I. Adenocarcinomas, squamous carcinomas and cultured cell lines. *Virchows Arch. B* **45:**407–429.

Blumberg, P. M. (1988). Protein kinase C as the receptor for the phorbol ester tumor promotors: Sixth Rhoads Memorial Award Lecture. *Cancer Res.* **48:**1–8.

Bonfil, R. D., Reddel, R. R., Ura, H., Reich, R., Firdman, R., Harris, C. C., Klein-Szanto, A. J. P. (1989). Invasive and metastatic potential of a v-Ha-ras-transformed human bronchial epithelial cell line. *J. Natl. Cancer Inst.* **81:**587–594.

Boren, H. G., and Paradise, L. J. (1978). Cytokinetics of lung. In *Pathogenesis and Therapy of Lung Cancer*. Edited by C. C. Harris. New York, Marcel Dekker, pp. 369–418.

Brand, N., Petkovich, M., Krust, A., Chambon, P., de The, H. D., Marchio, A., Tiollais, P., and Dejean, A. (1988). Identification of a second human retinoic acid receptor. *Nature* **332:**850–853.

Breeze, R. G., and Wheeldon, E. B. (1977). The cells of the pulmonary airways. *Am. Rev. Respir. Dis.* **116:**705–777.

Brody, A. R., Hook, G. E. R., Cameron, G., Jetten, A. M., Butterick, C., and Nettesheim, P. (1987). The differentiation capacity of Clara cells isolated from the lungs of rabbits. *Lab. Invest.* **57:**219–229.

Broers, J. L. V., de Leij, L., Klein Rot, M., ter Haar, A., Lane, E. B., Leigh, I. M., Wagenaar, S., Vooijs, G. P., and Ramaekers, F. C. S. (1989). Expression of intermediate filament proteins in fetal and adult human tissues. *Differentiation* **40:** 119–128.

Broers, J. L. V., Ramaekers, F. C. S., Klein Rot, M., Oostendorp, T., Huysmans, A., van Muyen, G. N. P., Wagenaar, S., and Vooijs, G. P. (1988). Cytokeratins in different types of lung cancer as monitored by chain-specific monoclonal antibodies. *Cancer Res.* **48:**3221–3229.

Cheifetz, S. J., Bassols, A., Stanley, K., Ohta, M., Greenberger, J., and Massague, J. (1988). Heterodimeric transforming growth factor β. *J. Biol. Chem.* **263:**10783-10789.

Cheifetz, S. J., Weatherbee, M. L., Tsang, J. K., Anderson, J. E., Mole, R., Lucas, R., and Massague, J. (1987). The transforming growth factor-beta system, a complex pattern of cross-reactive ligands and receptors. *Cell* **48:**409–415.

Chopra, D. P. (1982). Squamous metaplasia in organ culture of vitamin A-deficient hamster trachea: cytokinetic and ultrastructural alterations. *J. Natl. Cancer Inst.* **69:**895–905.

Chopra, D. P., Sullivan, J., Wille, J. J., and Siddiqui, K. M. (1987). Propagation of differentiating normal human tracheobronchial epithelial cells in serum free medium. *J. Cell. Physiol.* **130:**173–181.

Chytil, F., and Ong, D. E. (1983). Cellular retinol and retinoic acid binding proteins. *Adv. Nutr. Res.* **5:**13–29.

Chytil, F., and Ong, D. E. (1979). Cellular retinol and retinoic acid binding proteins in vitamin A action. *Fed. Proc.* **38:**2510–2514.

Cutz, E. (1986). Cytomorphology and differentiation of airway epithelium in developing human lung. In *Lung Carcinomas*. Edited by E. M. McDowell. Edinburgh, Churchill Livingstone.

Damm, K., Thompson, C. C., and Evans, R. M. (1989). Protein encoded by v-erbA functions as a thyroid-hormone receptor antagonist. *Nature* **339:**593-597.

Dean, D. C. (1989). Expression of the fibronectin gene. *Am. J. Respir. Cell. Mol. Biol.* **1:**5–10.

De Ley, L., Broers, J., Ramaekers, F., Berendsen, H., and Wagenaar, S. (1987). Monoclonal antibodies in clinical and experimental pathology of lung cancer. In *Application of Monoclonal Antibodies in Tumor Pathology*. Edited by D. J. Ruiter, G. J. Fleuren, and S. O. Warnaar. Dordrecht, Martinus Nijhoff, pp. 191–210.

Dexter, T. M., and Spooncer, E. (1987). Growth and differentiation in the hemopoietic system. *Annu. Rev. Cell. Biol.* **3:**423–441.

Donnelly, G. M., Haack, D. G., and Heird, C. S. (1982). Tracheal epithelium: Cell kinetics and differentiation in normal rat tissue. *Cell Tissue Kinet.* **15:**119–130.

Egan, C., Bayley, S. T., and Branton, P. E. (1989). Binding of the Rbl protein to E1A products is required for adenovirus transformation. *Oncogene* **4:**383–388.

Eliyahu, D., Michalovitz, D., Eliyahu, S., Pinhasi-Kimhi, O., and Oren, M. (1989). Wild-type p53 can inhibit oncogene-mediated focus formation. *Proc. Natl. Acad. Sci. USA* **86:**8763–8767.

Evans, M. J. (1983). Cell death and cell renewal in small airways and aveoli. In *Mechanisms in Respiratory Toxicology*, Volume I. Edited by H. Witschi and P. Nettesheim. Boca Raton, FL, CRC Press, pp. 189–218.

Evans, M. J., and Plopper, C. G. (1988). The role of basal cells in adhesion of columnar epithelium to airway basement membrane. *Am. Rev. Respir. Dis.* **138:**481–483.

Evans, M. J., Shami, S. G., Cabral-Anderson, L. J., and Dekker, N. P. (1986). Role of nonciliated cells in renewal of the bronchial epithelium of rats exposed to NO2. *Am. J. Pathol.* **123:**126–133.

Evans, M. J., and Shami, S. G. (1989). Lung cell kinetics. In *Lung Cell Biology*. Edited by D. Massaro. New York, Marcel Dekker, Vol 41, pp. 1–31.

Evans, R. M. (1988). The steroid and thyroid hormone receptor superfamily. *Science* **240:** 889–895.

Fields, A. P., Pettit, G. R., and Stratford-May, W. (1988). Phosphorylation of lamin B at the nuclear membrane by activated protein kinase. *C. J. Biol. Chem.* **263:**8253–8260.

Fielding, J. E. (1985). Smoking: health effects and control. *N. Engl. J. Med.* **313:**491–498.

Finch, P. W., Rubin, J. S., Miki, T., Ron, D., and Aaronson, S. A. (1989). Human KGF is FGF-related with properties of a paracrine effector of epithelial cell growth. *Science* **245:**752–755.

Flint, F., Schulte, B. A., and Spicer, S. S. (1986). Glycoconjugate with a galactose. A property common to basal cells and a subpopulation of columnar cells of numerous epithelia in mouse and rat. *Histochemistry* **84:**387–395.

Floyd, E. E., and Jetten, A. M. (1988). Retinoids, growth factors, and the tracheobronchial epithelium. *Lab. Invest.* **59:**1–4.

Floyd, E. E., and Jetten, A. M. (1989). Regulation of type I (epidermal) transglutaminase mRNA levels during squamous differentiation: down regulation by retinoids. *Mol. Cell. Biol.* **9:**4846–4851.

Gaub, M. P., Lutz, Y., Ruberte, E., Petkovich, M., Brand, N., and Chambon, P. (1989). Antibodies specific to the retinoic acid human nuclear receptors α and β. *Proc. Natl. Acad. Sci. USA* **86:**3089–3093.

George, M. D., Vollberg, T. M., Floyd, E. E., Stein, J. P., and Jetten, A. M. (1990). Regulation of transglutaminase type II by TGF-β in normal and transformed human epidermal keratinocytes. *J. Biol. Chem.* **265:**11098–11104.

Giguere, V., Ong, E. S., Segui, P., and Evans, R. M. (1987). Identification of a receptor for the morphogen retinoic acid. *Nature* **330:**620–629.

Gilfix, B. M., and Eckert, R. L. (1985). Coordinate control by vitamin A of keratin gene expression in human keratinocytes. *J. Biol. Chem.* **260:**14026–14029.

Glass, C. K., Lipkin, S. M., Devary, O. V., and Rosenfeld, M. G. (1989). Positive and negative regulation of gene transcription by a retinoic acid-thyroid hormone receptor heterodimer. *Cell* **59:**697–708.

Glick, A. B., Flanders, K. C., Danielpour, D., Yuspa, S. H., and Sporn, M. B. (1989). Retinoic acid induces transforming growth factor-β2 in cultured keratinocytes and mouse epidermis. *Cell Regulation* **1:**87–97.

Gould, V. E., Moll, R., Chejfec, G., Franke, W. W. (1986). Cytoskeletal characteristics of epithelial neoplasms of the lung. In *Biology of Lung Cancer*, volume 37. Edited by S. T. Rosen, J. L. Mulshine, F. Cuttitta, and P. G. Abrams. New York, Marcel Dekker, pp. 121–153.

Hall, P. A., and Watt, F. M. (1989). Stem cells: the generation and maintenance of cellular diversity. *Development* **106:**619–633.

Hammar, S. P. (1988). Common Neoplasms. In *Pulmonary Pathology*. Edited by S. P. Hammar. New York, Springer Verlag, pp. 727–845.

Hammond, E. C., and Horn, D. (1958). Smoking and death rates: report on forty-four months of follow-up of 187,783 men. *JAMA* **166:**1294–1308.

Harris, C. C., Silverman, T., Jackson, F., and Boren, H. G. (1973). Proliferation of tracheal epithelial cells in normal and vitamin A-deficient Syrian golden hamsters. *J. Natl. Cancer Inst.* **51:**1059–1062.

Havemann, K., Kiefer, P., Haeder, M., Hartogh, G., Heimann, Moelling, K., and Bepler, G. (1988). Oncogene expression in the spectrum of pulmonary carcinoma. *Lung Cancer* **4:**155–161.

Hesterberg, T. W., Maness, S. C., Iglehart, J. D., Sanchez, J. H., and Boreiko, C. J. (1987). Subpopulations of human bronchial epithelial cells in culture respond heterogeneously to 12-0-tetradecanoylphorbol-13-acetate (TPA) and other modulators of differentiation. *Carcinogenesis* **8:**1511–1515.

Holtzer, H. (1978). Cell lineages, stem cells and the 'quantal' cell cycle concept. In *Stem Cells and Tissue Homeostasis*. Edited by B. I. Lord, C. S. Potten, and R. J. Cole. Cambridge, Cambridge University Press, pp. 1–27.

Hook, G. E. R., Brody, A. R., Cameron, G. S., Jetten, A. M., Gilmore, L. B., and Nettesheim, P. (1987). Repopulation of denuded tracheas by Clara cells isolated from the lungs of rabbits. *Exp. Lung Res.* **12:**311–330.

Hook, G. E. R., Gilmore, L. B., Gupta, R. P., Patton, S. E., Jetten, A. M., and Nettesheim, P. (1990). The functions of pulmonary Clara cells. In *Biology, Toxicology and Carcinogenesis of Respiratory Epithelium*. Edited by D. S. Thomassen, and P. Nettesheim. New York, Hemisphere Publishing, pp. 38–59.

Huang, F. L., Roop, D. R., and DeLuca, L. M. (1986). Vitamin A deficiency and keratin biosynthesis in cultured hamster trachea. *In Vitro Cell. Dev. Biol.* **22:**223–230.

Huang, H., Yee, J., Shew, J., Chen, P., Bookstein, R., Friedmann, T., Lee, E. Y., and Lee, W. (1988). Suppression of the neoplastic phenotype by replacement of the RB gene in human cancer cells. *Science* **242:**1563–1566.

Imanishi, K., Yamaguchi, K., Kuranami, M., Kyo, E., Hozumi, T., and Abe, K. (1989). Inhibition of growth of human lung adenocarcinoma cell lines by anti-transforming growth factor-α monoclonal antibody. *J. Natl. Cancer Inst.* **81:**220–223.

Inayama, Y., Hook, G. E. R., Brody, A. R., Cameron, G., Jetten, A. M., Gilmore, L. B., Gray, T., and Nettesheim P. (1988). The differentiation potential of tracheal basal cells. *Lab. Invest.* **58:**706–717.

Inayama, Y., Hook, G. E. R., Brody, A. R., Jetten, A. M., Gray, T., and Nettesheim, P. (1989). In vitro and in vivo growth and differentiation of clones of tracheal basal cells. *Amer. J. Pathol.* **134:**539–550

Jeffery, P. K., Ayers, M., and Rogers, D. (1982). The mechanisms and control of bronchial mucous cell hyperplasia. In *Mucus in Health and Disease II*. Edited by E. N. Chantler, J. B. Elder, and M. Elstein. New York, Plenum Press, pp. 399–409.

Jett, J. R., Cortese, D. A., and Fonatana, R. S. (1983). Lung cancer: current concepts. *CA* **33:**74–76.

Jetten, A. M. (1989). Multistep process of squamous differentiation of tracheobronchial epithelial cells in vitro. Analogy with epidermal differentiation. *Environ. Health Perspect.* **80:**149–160.

Jetten, A. M. (1990). Regulation of gene expression by retinoic acid embryonal carcinoma cell differentiation. In *Mechanisms of Differentiation*. Edited by P. B. Fisher. Boca Raton, FL, CRC Press. **I:**49–74.

Jetten, A. M., and Shirley, J. E. (1985). Retinoids antagonize the induction of ornithine decarboxylase activity by phorbol esters and phospholipase C in rat tracheal epithelial cells. *J. Cell. Physiol.* **123:**386–394.

Jetten, A. M., and Shirley, J. E. (1986). Characterization of transglutaminase activity in rabbit tracheal epithelial cells. Regulation by retinoids. *J. Biol. Chem.* **261:**15097–15101.

Jetten, A. M., and Smits, H. (1985). Regulation of differentiation of tracheal epithelial cells by retinoids. In *Retinoids, Differentiation and Disease*. Edited by J. Nugent and S. Clark. CIBA Symposium, London, Pitman, pp. 61–76.

Jetten, A. M., Ganong, B. R., Vandenbark, G. R., Shirley, J. E., and Bell, R. M. (1985). Role of protein kinase C in diacylglycerol-mediated induction of ornithine decarboxylase and reduction of epidermal growth factor binding. *Proc. Natl. Acad. Sci. USA* **82:**1941–1945.

Jetten, A. M., Shirley, J. E., and Stoner, G. (1986). Regulation of proliferation and differentiation of respiratory tract epithelial cells by TGFβ. *Exp. Cell Res.* **147:**539–549.

Jetten, A. M., Anderson, K., Deas, M. A., Kagechika, H., Lotan, R., Rearick, J. I., and Shudo, K. (1987a). New benzoic acid derivatives with retinoid activity: lack of direct correlation between biological activity and binding to cellular retinoic acid protein. *Cancer Res.* **47:**3523–3527.

Jetten, A. M., Brody, A. R., Deas, M. A., Hook, G. E. R., Rearick, J. I., and Thacher, S. M. (1987b). Retinoic acid and substratum regulate the differentiation of rabbit tracheal epithelial cells into squamous and secretory phenotype. *Lab. Invest.* **56:** 654–664.

Jetten, A. M., George, M. A., Nervi, C., Boone, L. R., and Rearick, J. I. (1989a). Increased cholesterol sulfate and cholesterol sulfotransferase activity in relation to the multi-step process of differentiation in human epidermal keratinocytes. *J. Invest. Dermatol.* **92:**203–209.

Jetten, A. M., George, M. A., Smits, H. L., Vollberg, T. M. (1989b). Keratin expression in relation to squamous cell differentiation in rabbit tracheal epithelial cells: regulation by retinoic acid. *Exp. Cell Res.* **182:**622-634.

Jetten, A. M., George, M. A., Pettit, G. R., and Rearick, J. I. (1989c). Effects of bryostatins and retinoic acid on phorbol ester and diacylglycerol-induced squamous differentiation in human tracheobronchial epithelial cells. *Cancer Res.* **49:**3990–3995.

Jetten, A. M., George, M. A., and Vollberg, T. M. (1991). Regulation of transglutaminase activity in human bronchial epithelial cells. *Am. J. Respir. Cell Mol. Biol.* Submitted.

Jetten, A. M., Nettesheim, P., George, M. A., Gilmore, L. B., and Hook, G. E. R. (1991). Isolation, cultivation and biochemical characterization of tracheal basal cells. *Am. J. Physiol.* Submitted.

Johnson, B. E., Ihde, D. C., Makuch, R. W., Gazdar, A. F., Carney, D. N., Oie, H., Russell, E., Nau, M. M., and Minna, J. D. (1987). myc Family oncogene amplification in tumor cell lines established from small cell carcinoma cancer patients and its relationship to clinical status and course. *J. Clin. Invest.* **79:**1629–1634.

Kaul, K. (1987). Oncogenes in human lung cancer. In *Biology of Lung Cancer*. Edited by S. T. Rosen, J. L. Mulshine, F. Cuttitta, and P. G. Abrams. New York, Marcel Dekker, Vol. 37, pp. 155–181.

Keenan, K. P., Combs, J. W., and McDowell, E. M. (1982). Regeneration of hamster tracheal epithelium after mechanical injury. *Virchows Arch. Cell. Pathol.* **41:**215–229.

Keenan, K. P., Wilson, T. S., and McDowell, E. M. (1983). Regeneration of hamster tracheal epithelium after mechanical injury. IV Histochemical, immunocytochemical and ultrastructural studies. *Virchows Arch. Cell Pathol.* **43:**213–240.

Keski-Oja, J., Raghow, R., Sawdey, M., Loskutoff, D. J., Postletwaite, A. E., Kang, A. H., and Moses, H. L. (1988). Regulation of mRNAs for type-1 plasminogen activator inhibitor, fibronectin, and type I procollagen by transforming growth factor-β. *J. Biol. Chem.* **263:**3111–3115.

Kikkawa, U., Kishimoto, A., and Nishizuka, Y. (1989). The protein kinase C family: heterogeneity and its implications. *Annu. Rev. Biochem.* **58:**31–44.

Kim, K. C., Rearick, J. I., Nettesheim, P., and Jetten, A. M. (1985). Biochemical characterization of mucous glycoproteins synthesized and secreted by hamster tracheal epithelial cells in primary culture. *J. Biol. Chem.* **260:**4021–4027.

Klein-Szanto, A. J. P., Topping, D. C., Heckman, C. A., and Nettesheim, P. (1980). Ultrastructural characteristics of carcinogen-induced dysplastic changes in tracheal epithelium. *Am. J. Pathol.* **98:**83–100.

Kraft, A. S., and May, W. S. (1987). Bryostatin induces changes in protein kinase C location and activity without altering c-myc gene expression in human promyelocytic leukemia cells (HL-60). *Oncogene* **1:**111–118.

Kraft, A. S., Smith, J. B., and Berkow, R. L. (1986). Bryostatin, an activator of the calcium phospholipid-dependent protein kinase, blocks phorbol ester-induced differentiation of human promyelocytic leukemia cells HL-60. *Proc. Natl. Acad. Sci. USA* **83:**1334–1338.

Krust, A., Kastner, P. H., Petkovich, M., Zelent, A., and Chambon, P. (1989). A third human retinoic acid receptor, RARγ. *Proc. Natl. Acad. Sci. USA* **86:**5310–5314.
Lane, B. P., and Gordon, R. E. (1974). Regeneration of rat tracheal epithelium after mechanical injury. I. The relationship between mitotic activity and cellular differentiation. *Proc. Soc. Exp. Biol. Med.* **145:**1139–1144.
Lechner, J. F., Haugen, A., Autrup, H., McClendon, I. A., Trump, B. F., and Harris, C. C. (1981). Clonal growth of epithelial from normal human bronchus. *Cancer Res.* **41:** 2294–2304.
Lechner, J. F., Haugen, A., McClendon, L. A., and Shamsuddin, A. M. (1984). Induction of squamous differentiation of normal human bronchial epithelial cells by small amounts of serum. *Differentiation* **25:**229–237.
Lechner, J. F., and LaVeck, M. A. (1985). A serum-free method for culturing normal bronchial epithelial cells. *J. Tissue Cult. Meth.* **9:**43–48.
Lehto, V-P., Stenman, S., Miettinen, M., Dahl, D., and Virtanen, I. (1983). Expression of a neural type of intermediate filament as a distinguishing feature between oat cell carcinoma and other lung cancers. *Am. J. Pathol.* **110:**113–118.
Ludlow, J. W., DeCaprio, J. A., Huang, C., Lee, W-H., Paucha, E., and Livingston, D. M. (1989). SV40 large T antigen binds preferentially to an under phosphorylated member of the retinoblastoma susceptibility gene product family. *Cell* **56:**57–65.
Maden, M., Ong, D. E., Summerbell, D., and Chytil, F. (1988). Spatial distribution of cellular protein to retinoic acid in the chick limb bud. *Nature* **335:**733–735.
Massaro, G. D. (1989). Nonciliated bronchiolar epithelial (Clara) cells. In *Lung Cell Biology*. Edited by D. Massaro. New York, Marcel Dekker, Vol. 41, pp. 81–114.
Miele, L., Cordella-Miele, E., and Mukherjee, A. B. (1987). Uteroglobin: structure, molecular biology, and new perspectives on its function as a phospholipase A2 inhibitor. *Endocrine Rev.* **8:**474–490.
Masui, T., Wakefield, L. M., Lechner, J. F., LaVeck, M. A., Sporn, M. B., and Harris, C. C. (1986). Type b transforming growth factor is the primary differentiation inducing serum factor for normal human bronchial epithelial cells. *Proc. Natl. Acad. Sci. USA* **83:**2438–2442.
McDowell, E. M., Keenan, K. P., and Huang, M. (1984). Restoration of mucociliary tracheal epithelium following deprivation of vitamin A. A quantitative morphologic study. *Virchow Arch.* **45:**221–240.
McDowell, E. M., Harris, C. C., and Trump, B. F. (1982). Histogenesis and morphogenesis of bronchial neoplasms. In *Morphogenesis of Lung Cancer*. Edited by Y. Shimosato, M. R. Melamed, and P. Nettesheim. Boca Raton, FL, CRC Press, Vol. II, pp. 1–37.
McDowell, E. M., Newkerk, C., and Coleman, B. (1985a). Development of hamster tracheal epithelium: a quantitative morphologic study in the fetus. *Anat. Rec.* **213:** 429–447.
McDowell, E. M., Newkerk, C., and Coleman, B. (1985b). Development of hamster tracheal epithelium: II cell proliferation in the fetus. *Anat. Rec.* **213:**448–456.
Melamed, M. R., and Zaman, M. B. (1982). Pathogenesis of epidermoid carcinoma of lung. In *Morphogenesis of Lung Cancer* Edited by Y. Shimosato, M. R., Melamed, and P. Nettesheim. Boca Raton, FL, CRC Press. Vol. II, pp. 37–65.
Moll, R., Franke, W. W., Schiller, D. L., Geiger, B., and Krepler, R. (1982). The catalog of

human cytokeratins: patterns of expression in normal epithelia, tumors and cultured cells. *Cell* **31:**11–24.

Nathan, C. F. (1987). Secretory products of macrophages. *J. Clin. Invest.* **79:**319–326.

Nau, M. M., Brooks, B. J., Carney, D. N., Gazdar, A. F., Battey, J. F., Sausville, E. A., and Minna, J. D. (1986). Human small-cell lung cancers show amplification and expression of the N-myc gene. *Proc. Natl. Acad. Sci. USA* **83:**1092–1096.

Nervi, C., Grippo, J. F., Sheman, M. I., George, M. D., and Jetten, A. M. (1989). Identification and characterization of nuclear retinoic acid-binding activity in human myeloblastic leukemia HL-60 cells. *Proc. Natl. Acad. Sci. USA* **86:**5854–5858.

Nishizuka, Y. (1988). The molecular heterogeneity of protein kinase C and its implications for cellular regulation. *Nature* **334:**661–665.

Ogawa, M. (1989). Hemopoietic stem cells: stochastic differentiation and humoral control of proliferation. *Environ. Hlth. Perspec.* **80:**199–208.

Petkovich, M., Brand, N., Krust, A., and Chambon, P. (1987). A human retinoic acid receptor which belongs to the family of nuclear receptors. *Nature* **330:**444–450.

Pettit, G. R., Herald, C. L., Doubek, D. L., and Herald, D. L. (1982). Isolation and structure of bryostatin. *J. Am. Chem. Soc.* **1204:**6846–6848.

Pierce, G. B., and Speers, W. C. (1988). Tumors as caricatures of the process of tissue renewal: prospects for therapy by directing proliferation. *Cancer Res.* **48:**1996–2004.

Pinney, D. F., and Emerson, C. P. (1989). 10T1/2 cells: an in vitro model for molecular genetic analysis of mesodermal determination and differentiation. *Environ. Hlth. Perspec.* **80:**221–228.

Plopper, C. G., Alley, J. L., and Weir, A. J. (1986). Differentiation of tracheal epithelium during fetal lung maturation in the Rhesus monkey Macaca mulatta. *Am. J. Anat.* **175:**59–71.

Potten, C. S. (1983). *Stem Cells: Their Identification and Characterization.* New York, Churchill Livingstone.

Rapp, U. R., Huleihel, M., Pawson, T., Linnoila, I., Minna, J. D., Heidecker, G., Cleveland, J. L., Beck, T., Forchhammer, J., and Storm, S. M. (1988). Role of raf oncogenes in lung carcinogenesis. *Lung Cancer* **4:**162–167.

Rearick, J. I., and Jetten, A. M. (1986) Accumulation of cholesterol 3-sulfate during in vitro squamous differentiation of rabbit tracheal epithelial cells and its regulation by retinoids. *J. Biol. Chem.* **261:**13898–13904.

Rearick, J. I., Albro, P. W., and Jetten, A. M. (1987a). Cholesterol sulfotransferase activity is induced upon squamous differentiation of RTE cells in vitro. *J. Biol. Chem.* **262:** 13069–13074.

Rearick, J. I., Deas, M. A., and Jetten, A. M. (1987b). Synthesis of mucous glycoproteins by rabbit tracheal cells in vitro. *Biochem. J.* **242:**19–25.

Rearick, J. I., Hesterberg, T. W., and Jetten, A. M. (1987c). Human bronchial epithelial cells synthesize cholesterol sulfate during squamous differentiation in vitro. *J. Cell Physiol.* **133:**573–578.

Rearick, J. I., Stoner, G. D., George, M. A., and Jetten, A. M. (1988). Cholesterol sulfate accumulation in tumorigenic and nontumorigenic rat esophageal epithelial cells: evidence for defective differentiation control in tumorigenic cells. *Cancer Res.* **48:** 5289–5295.

Rice, R. H., and Green, H. (1977). The cornified envelope of terminally differentiated human epidermal keratinocytes consists of cross-linked protein. *Cell* **11:**417–422.
Roberts, A. B., and Sporn, M. B. (1990). The transforming growth factor betas. In *Handbook of Experimental Pharmacology. Peptide Growth Factors and Their Receptors.* Edited by M. B. Sporn and A. B. Roberts. Heidelberg, Springer-Verlag. Vol. 95, pp. 419–472.
Rodenhuis, S., van de Wetering, M. L., Mooi, W. J., Evers, S., van Zandwijk, N., and Bos, J. L. (1987). Mutational activation of the K-ras oncogene. *N. Engl. J. Med.* **317:** 929–935.
Roggli, V. L., Volmer, R. T., Greenberg, S. D., McGavran, J. M. H., Spjut, H. J., and Yesner, R. (1985). Lung cancer heterogeneity: a blinded and randomized study of 100 consecutive cases. *Hum. Pathol.* **16:**569–579.
Rosen, S. T., Mulshine, J. L., Cuttitta, F., and Abrams, P. G. Lung biology in health and disease. In *Biology of Lung Cancer.* Edited by C. Lenfant. New York, Marcel Dekker, Vol. 37, 1987.
Rossi, P., Karsenty, G., Roberts, A. B., Sporn, M. B., and de Crombrugghe, B. (1988). A nuclear factor 1 binding site dedicates the transcriptional activation of a type I collagen promoter by transforming growth factor-β. *Cell* **52:**405–414.
Rutten, A. A. J. J. L., Bruyntjes, J. P., and Ramaekers, F. C. S. (1988). Effect of cigarette smoke condensate and vitamin A depletion on keratin expression patterns in cultured hamster tracheal epithelium. *Virchows Archiv. Cell. Pathol.* **56:**111–117.
Said, J. W., Nash, G., Sassoon, A. F., Shintaku, I, P., and Banks-Schlegel, S. (1983). Involucrin in lung tumors: a specific marker for squamous differentiation. *Lab. Invest.* **49:**563–571.
Sako, T., Yuspa, S. H., Herald, C. L., Pettit, G. R., and Blumberg, P. I. (1987). Partial parallelism and partial blockade by bryostatin 1 of effects of phorbol ester tumor promoters on primary mouse epidermal cells. *Cancer Res.* **47:**5445–5450.
Sanchez, J. H., Boreiko, C. J., Furlong, J., and Hesterberg, T. W. (1987). Differential effects of tumour promoters upon the growth of normal human bronchial epithelial cells and human lung tumor cell lines. *Toxicol. In Vitro* **4:**183–188.
Sherman, M. I. (1986). *Retinoids and Cell Differentiation.* Boca Raton, FL, CRC Press.
Siegfried, J. M. (1987). Detection of human lung epithelial cell growth factors produced by a lung carcinoma cell line: use in culture of primary solid lung tumors. *Cancer Res.* **47:**2903–2910.
Siegfried, J. M., and Owens, S. E. (1988). Response of primary human lung carcinomas to autocrine growth factors produced by a lung carcinoma cell line. *Cancer Res.* **48:** 4976–4981.
Silverberg, E., and Lubera, J. (1987). Cancer statistics, 1987. *CA* **37:**2–19.
Simon, M., and Green, H. (1985). Enzymatic cross-linking of involucrin and other proteins by keratinocyte particulates in vitro. *Cell* **40:**685–695.
Slaga, T. J. (ed.) (1984). *Mechanisms of Tumor Promotion.* Boca Raton, FL, CRC Press.
Smits, H. L., Floyd, E. E., and Jetten, A. M. (1987). Molecular cloning of gene sequences regulated during squamous differentiation of tracheal epithelial cells and controlled by retinoic acid. *Mol. Cell Biol.* **7:**4017–4023.
Sorokin, S. P., and Hoyt, R. F. (1989). Neuroepithelial bodies and solitary small-granule

cells. In *Lung Cell Biology*. Edited by D. Massaro. New York, Marcel Dekker, Vol. 41, pp. 191–344.

Sporn, M. R., Clamon, G. H., Dunlop, N. J., Newton, D. L., Smith, J. M., and Saffiotti, U. (1975). Activity of vitamin A analogues in cell cultures of mouse epidermis and organ cultures of hamster trachea. *Nature* **253:**47–49.

Sporn, M. I., Roberts, A. B., and Goodman, D. S. (1984). *The Retinoids*, Vols. 1 and 2. New York, Academic Press, Inc.

Stahlman, M. T., Gray, M. E., Chytil, F., and Sundell, H. (1988). The effect of retinol on fetal lamb tracheal epithelium with and without epidermal growth factor: a model for the effect of retinol on the healing lung of human premature infants. *Lab. Invest.* **59:** 25–35.

Steele, V. E., Marchok, A. C., and Nettesheim, P. (1980). Enhancement of carcinogenesis in cultured respiratory tract epithelium by 12-0-tetradecanoylphorbol-13-acetate. *Int. J. Cancer* **26:**343–348.

Stiles, A. D., and Moats-Staats, B. M. (1989). Production and action of insulin-like growth factor somatomedin C in primary cultures of fetal lung fibroblasts. *Am. J. Respir. Cell Mol. Biol.* **1:**21–26.

Sun, T-T., Eichner, R., Nelson, W. G., Tseng, S. C. G., Weiss, R. A., Jarvinen, M., and Woodcock-Mitchell, J. (1983). Keratin Classes: molecular markers for different types of epithelial differentiation. *J. Invest. Dermatol.* **81:**109s–115s.

Takahashi, T., Nau, M. M., Chiba, I., Birrer, M. J., Rosenberg, R. K., Vinocour, M., Levitt, M., Pass, H., Gazdar, A. J., and Minna, J. D. (1989). p53: a frequent target for genetic abnormalities in lung cancer. *Science* **246:**491–494.

Taylor, S. M., and Jones, P. A. (1979). Multiple new phenotypes induced in 10T1/2 and 3T3 cells treated with 5-azacytidine. *Cell* **17:**771–779.

Thacher, S. M., and Rice, R. H. (1985). Keratinocyte-specific transglutaminase of cultured human epidermal cells: relation to cross-linked envelope formation and terminal differentiation. *Cell* **40:**685–695.

Thomassen, D. G., Saffiotti, U., and Kaighn, M. E. (1986). Clonal proliferation of rat tracheal epithelial cells in serum free-medium and their responses to hormones, growth factors and carcinogens. *Carcinogenesis* **7:**2033–2039.

Topping, D. C., and Nettesheim, P. (1980). Promotion-like enhancement of tracheal carcinogenesis in rats by 12-0-tetradecanoylphorbol-13-acetate. *Cancer Res.* **40:** 4352–5355.

Twardzik, D. R., Ranchalis, J. E., McPherson, J. M., Ogawa, Y., Gentry, L., Purchio, A., Plata, E., and Todaro, F. J. (1989). Inhibition and promotion of differentiated-like phenotype of a human lung carcinoma in athymic mice by natural and recombinant forms of transforming growth factor-b. *J. Natl. Cancer Inst.* **81:**1182–1185.

van Muyen A., G. N. P., Wagenaar, S., and Vooijs, G. P. (1988). Cytokeratins in different types of lung cancer as monitored by chain-specific monoclonal antibodies. *Cancer Res.* **48:**3221–3229.

Vennstrom, B., Fanshier, L., Moscovici, C., and Bishop, J. M. (1980). Molecular cloning of the avian erythroblastosis virus genome and recovery of oncogenic virus by transfection of chicken cells. *J. Virol.* **36:**575–585.

Vollberg, T. M., Nervi, C., George, M. A., and Jetten, A. M. (1990). Identification of multiple stages in the program of squamous differentiation in tracheobronchial epithelial cells. In *Biology, Toxicology and Carcinogenesis of Respiratory Epithelium*. Edited by D. G. Thomassen and P. Nettesheim. New York, Hemisphere Publishing, pp. 74–87.

Wakefield, L. M., Smith, D. M., Masui, T., Harris, C. C., and Sporn, M. B. (1987). Distribution and modulation of the cellular receptor for transforming growth factor-beta. *J. Cell Biol.* **105:**965–975.

Watt, F. M. (1988). Proliferation and terminal differentiation of human epidermal keratinocytes in culture. *Biochem. Soc. Trans.* **16:**666–668.

Wilhelm, D. L. (1954). Regeneration of the tracheal epithelium in the vitamin A-deficient rat. *J. Pathol.* **67:**361–365.

Willey, J. C., Moser, C. E., Lechner, J. F., and Harris, C. C. (1984). Differential effects of 12-0-tetradecanoylphorbol-13-acetate on cultured normal and neoplastic human bronchial epithelial cells. *Cancer Res.* **44:**5124–5126.

Wolbach, S. B., and Howe, P. R. (1926). Tissue changes following deprivation of fat-soluble A vitamin. *J. Exp. Med.* **42:**753–781.

Wong, Y-C., and Buck, R. C. (1971). An electronic microscopic study of metaplasia of the rat tracheal epithelium in vitamin A deficiency. *Lab. Invest.* **24:**55–66.

Woodworth, C. D., Mossman, B. T., and Craighead, J. E. (1983). Squamous metaplasia of the respiratory tract: possible pathogenic role in asbestos-associated bronchogenic carcinoma. *Lab. Invest.* **48:**578–584.

World Health Organization histological typing of lung tumors. 2d ed. (1982). *Am. J. Clin. Pathol.* **77:**123–136.

Wu, R. (1987). In vitro differentiation of airway epithelial cells. In *In Vitro Models of Respiratory Epithelium*. Edited by L. J. Schiff. Boca Raton, FL, CRC Press, pp. 1–26.

Wu, R., Groelke, J. W., Chang, L. Y., Porter, M. E., Smith, D., and Nettesheim, P. (1982). Effects of hormones on the multiplication and differentiation of tracheal epithelial cells in culture. In *Growth of Cells in Hormonally Defined Media*. Edited by D. Sirbasku, G. H. Sato, and A. Pardee. Cold Spring Harbor, NY, Cold Spring Laboratory, pp. 641–656.

Wu, R., and Wu, M. M. J. (1986). Effects of retinoids on human bronchial epithelial cells: differential regulation of hyaluronate synthesis and keratin protein synthesis. *J. Cell. Physiol.* **127:**73–82.

Yamamoto, S., Gotah, H., Aizu, E., and Kato, R. (1985). Failure of 1-oleoyl-2-acetylglycerol to mimic the cell-differentiating action of 12-0-tetradecanoylphorbol 13-acetate in HL 60 cells. *J. Biol. Chem.* **260:**14230–14234.

Yesner, R. (1978). Spectrum of lung cancer and ectopic hormone. *Pathol. Annu.* **13** (Part I)**:** 217–240.

Yokota, J., Akiyama, T., Fung, Y. T., Benedict, W. F., Namba, Y., Hanaoka, M., Terasaki, T., Shimosato, Y., Sigimura, T., and Terada, M. (1988). Altered expression of the retinoblastoma (RB) gene in small-cell carcinoma of the lung. *Oncogene* **3:**471–475.

Yost, R. W., Harrison, E. H., and Ross, A. C. (1988). Esterification by rat liver microsomes of retinol bound to cellular retinol-binding protein. *J. Biol. Chem.* **263:**18693–18699.

Zelent, A., Krust, A., Petkovich, M., Kastner, P., and Chambon, P. (1989). Cloning of murine α and β retinoic acid receptors and a novel receptor γ predominantly expressed in skin. *Nature* **339:**714–717.

2

Early Cancer and Preneoplastic Lesions of the Lung: Extracellular Matrix Components

A. FISSELER-ECKHOFF and K.-M. MÜLLER

Berufsgenossenschaftliche Krankenanstalten "Bergmannsheil"
University Clinic Bochum
Bochum, Germany

I. Introduction

The varying histologic features of malignant bronchogenic neoplasms and the frequent findings of cellular, stemline, and growth pattern heterogeneity within a given tumor, demonstrated by electron microscopy (McDowell et al., 1978; McDowell and Trump, 1983; Saba et al., 1983), cytophotometric (Höring et al., 1982), immunohistochemical (Schlegel and Blanks-Schlegel, 1980), and morphometric studies has raised the question of the histogenesis of lung tumor heterogeneity. A baseline for the explanation for these findings in fully developed carcinomas might be provided by studying preneoplastic lesions of the bronchial system. Preneoplastic lesions of the bronchial mucosa can be identified as intermediate conditions between regular mucosal structures and invasive carcinomas by means of light and electron microscopy (McCarter and Vasquez, 1966; Auerbach et al., 1975; Mullins and Rohrlich, 1983; Müller, 1985; Gonzales et al., 1986; McDowell 1987). Many observations of a varied spectrum of preneoplastic abnormalities and atypias in epithelial proliferation such as basal cell and goblet cell hyperplasia, squamous cell metaplasia, micropapillomatosis, as well as dysplasia up to carcinoma in situ have concurred in the concept of a histogenetic sequence for each of the different histologic types of lung cancer. Preneoplastic abnormalities are well defined (Nasiell et al., 1982; Müller and Müller, 1983; Gonzales et al., 1986) and can be compared with preneoplastic changes observed and defined in other organs such as portio uteri, larynx, breast, and stomach (Grundmann, 1980). Since hyperplasia and metaplasia are temporary regenerative changes, dysplasia and carcinoma in situ are associated with an increasing risk of the development of invasive carcinoma.

Until now, the characterization of preneoplastic lesions was mainly based on epithelial changes and the extracellular matrix was neglected. The penetration of epithelial cells through the basement membrane is a crucial event during the transition from carcinoma in situ to an invasive carcinoma. Basement membrane (BM) proteins are important components of the extracellular matrix of the normal bronchial wall. By immunoelectron microscopy it could be demonstrated that the basement membrane mainly consists of laminin and type IV collagen, whereas the presence of fibronectin is controversial (Laurie et al., 1982; Martinez-Hernandez and Amenta, 1983; Abrahamson, 1986). By light microscopic investigations only it is not possible to differentiate between matrix components of basement membrane and interstitial connective tissue. The ultrastructural investigations of Madri et al. (1980) have shown that the distance between the basement membrane and the underlying fibrillar connective tissue is less than 100 μm, and that fibronectin is often associated with type III collagen, indicating that the routinely stained BM of the bronchus seen by light microscopy might be a consolidation of collagen and BM components (Kefalides et al., 1979). In discussing whether tumor cell populations interact with extracellular matrix molecules during invasion and metastasis (Liotta et al., 1983, 1986; Bracke et al., 1988) point to the fact that changes of the extracellular matrix might already be observed in preneoplastic lesions of the bronchus. We were interested to find possible characteristic features in the composition of extracellular matrix in different types of preneoplastic lesions and in early lung cancer.

II. Immunofluorescence and Immunohistochemical Investigations

Tissue samples of 150 preneoplastic lesions (30 specimens from basal cell hyperplasia, 30 specimens from goblet cell hyperplasia, 30 specimens from squamous cell metaplasia up to mild dysplasia, 20 specimens from micropapillomatosis, 10 specimens of moderate dysplasia, 30 specimens of severe dysplasia and carcinoma in situ), 30 specimens of normal bronchial mucosa, and 10 cases of early squamous cell carcinoma (infiltrating not beyond the tunica fibrocartilaginea) were obtained from lung biopsies, lobectomies, or pneumonectomies. Immunofluorescent and immunohistochemical investigations were carried out to determine whether changes of the extracellular matrix may contribute to a classification of preneoplastic lesions due to their biological significance (Fisseler-Eckhoff et al., 1990). Tissue samples were either fixed in 5% neutral formalin and embedded in paraffin or snap frozen on carbon dioxide ice and stored at −70°C.

Paraffin sections were cut at 3–4 μm and dewaxed in xylene. Hematoxylin and eosin, elastic van Gieson, periodic acid–Schiff (PAS), and Gomori staining methods were used. To answer the question of basement membrane changes due to preneoplastic lesions, the thickness of the BM zone was investigated morphometrically using an ocular micrometer. In each specimen, 5 values were determined to give the mean value.

For the immunohistochemical typing of extracellular matrix, both paraffin and fresh frozen sections were investigated by an indirect immunofluorescence method using polyclonal monospecific antibodies directed against collagen type I and III. For the immunohistochemical typing of noncollagenous glycoproteins laminin and fibronectin, the indirect ABC peroxidase technique was used as well as immunofluorescence methods. The antigens of the collagen types I and III were isolated from human skin according to the method of Miller et al. (1971) (for details and method see Fisseler-Eckhoff et al., 1990).

The antibody to human fibronectin was obtained from Dako (Hamburg; rabbit fractionated antifibronectin antisera, AES 212) and to human laminin from Heyl (Berlin; rabbit fractionated antilaminin antisera, AES 212).

For the streptavidin-ABC-peroxidase technique, predigestion with 0.06% protease (bacterial protease, sigma type XXIV, 9.6 units/mg solid) in TRIS buffer (pH 7.6) was carried out for 10 min at 37°C and washing with TRIS buffer were followed by background blocking with 3% H_2O_2 for 20 min at room temperature. Slides for laminin and fibronectin staining were incubated with normal goat serum for 20 min at room temperature. Overnight incubation with primary antisera followed. After being washed with TRIS buffer, incubation with biotinylated goat-antirabbit antibody was performed. ABC-streptavidin and biotinylated peroxidase incubation for 30 min was done. The reaction was visualized with 3-amino-9-ethylcarbazol substrate with 0.3% H_2O_2 and acetate buffer. The preparation was then counterstained with hematoxylin and mounted with glycerin gelatin. Negative controls were made by omitting the primary antibody and replacing it with normal serum of the correspondent species.

III. Extracellular Matrix Changes

The median thickness of normal BM was found to be 5.3 μm. It remained during metaplasia and micropapillomatosis. However, it was enhanced to 7.5 and 6.5 μm in cases of basal cell hyperplasia and goblet cell hyperplasia, respectively. In dysplastic epithelium of grade II, the thickness of the basement membrane decreased to about 3.3 μm and in dysplasia grade III to about 1.7 μm. Standard deviations for each group remained under 50% of the mean values.

A. Normal Bronchial Mucosa

In the basement membrane zone, a linear intact, homogeneously stained, and argyrophilic zone directly beneath the surface epithelium could be differentiated from a homogeneous, less PAS-positive line at the border of the tunica propria (Fig. 1A). PAS staining revealed a small, clearly limited, intensely stained line close to the epithelium, whereas a strong specific reaction for laminin was observed immunohistochemically (Fig. 1B). Collagen type III and fibronectin were demonstrated in the homogeneous zone of the BM and in the tunica propria. Fibronectin was also found under the vascular endothelium, and around the mucous areas of bronchial glands as well as in the vicinity of goblet cells of bronchial mucosa. Collagen type I was restricted to fibers of the interstitial stroma in the tunica propria.

B. Basal and Goblet Cell Hyperplasia

The basement membrane was widened to a median diameter of about 7 μm, accompanied by intensive staining for collagen type III within the BM zone. Staining for laminin remained unchanged. A mild chronic inflammatory reaction was found.

C. Squamous Cell Metaplasia

With mild and moderate dysplasia, no pathologic alterations of the extracellular matrix were observed (Fig. 1C, D).

D. Micropapillomatosis

In micropapillomatosis characterized by hernialike protrusions of vascularized stromal papillae extending toward the surface (Fig. 1E), numerous laminin-positive capillaries were found both in connection with the BM zone and in the

Figure 1 Light microscopic and immunohistochemical findings in normal bronchial mucosa and preneoplastic lesions. (A) Normal bronchial mucosa with a small, clearly limited staining BM zone close to the epithelium, and dense, homogeneous, unstable PAS line at the border of the tunica propria (PAS, × 560). (B) Positive staining for collagen type III within the corresponding unstable PAS line (× 80). (C) Squamous cell metaplasia with moderate dysplasia (× 220). (D) Linear staining of the BM zone with collagen type III antibodies (× 220). (E) Micropapillomatosis with hernialike stroma protrusions with capillary proliferation (× 350). (F) Numerous capillaries stained by laminin antibodies in the BM zone and tunica propria. Proliferation of collagen fibers in the tunica propria (×

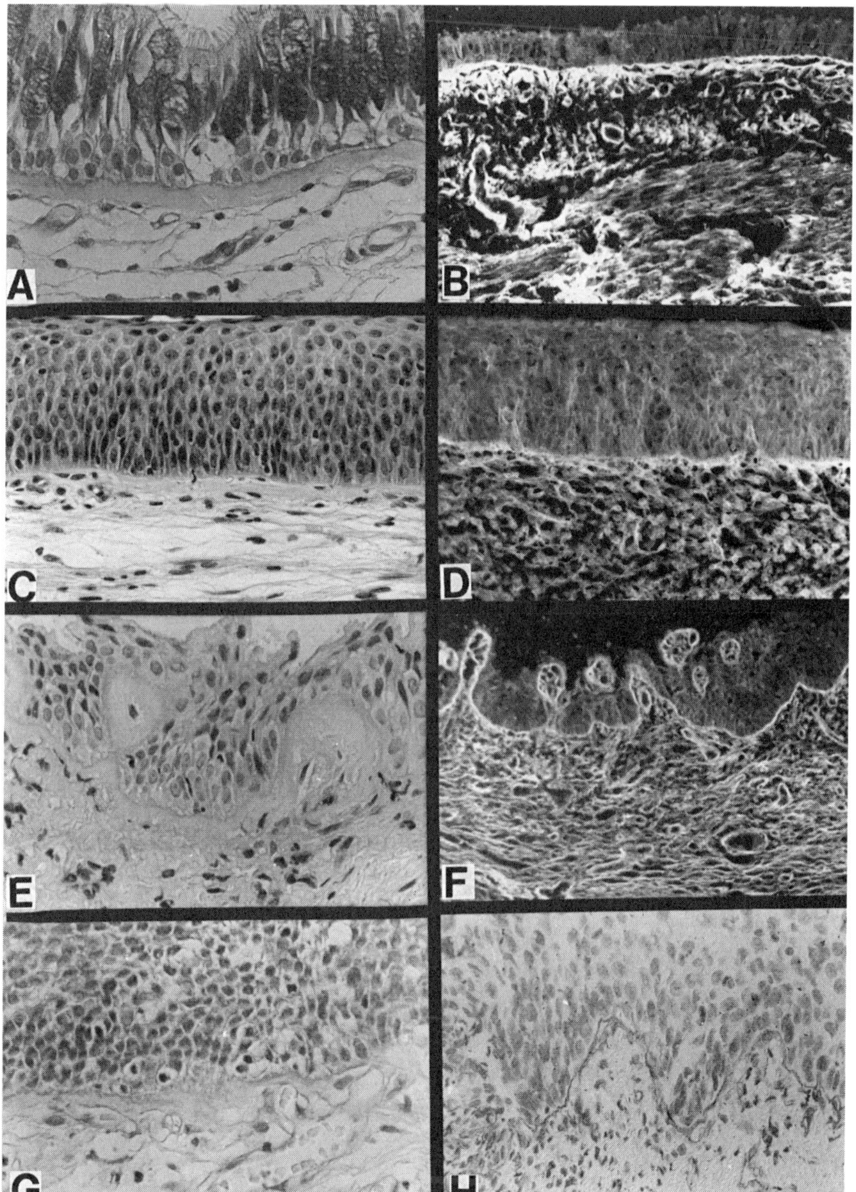

140). (G) Carcinoma in situ with discontinuity between the BM and the basal epithelial cells. The dysplastic cells have entered the loosened matrix (× 80). (H) Interrupted, unclear, limited BM stained with laminin antibodies; capillary proliferation is also visible (× 560).

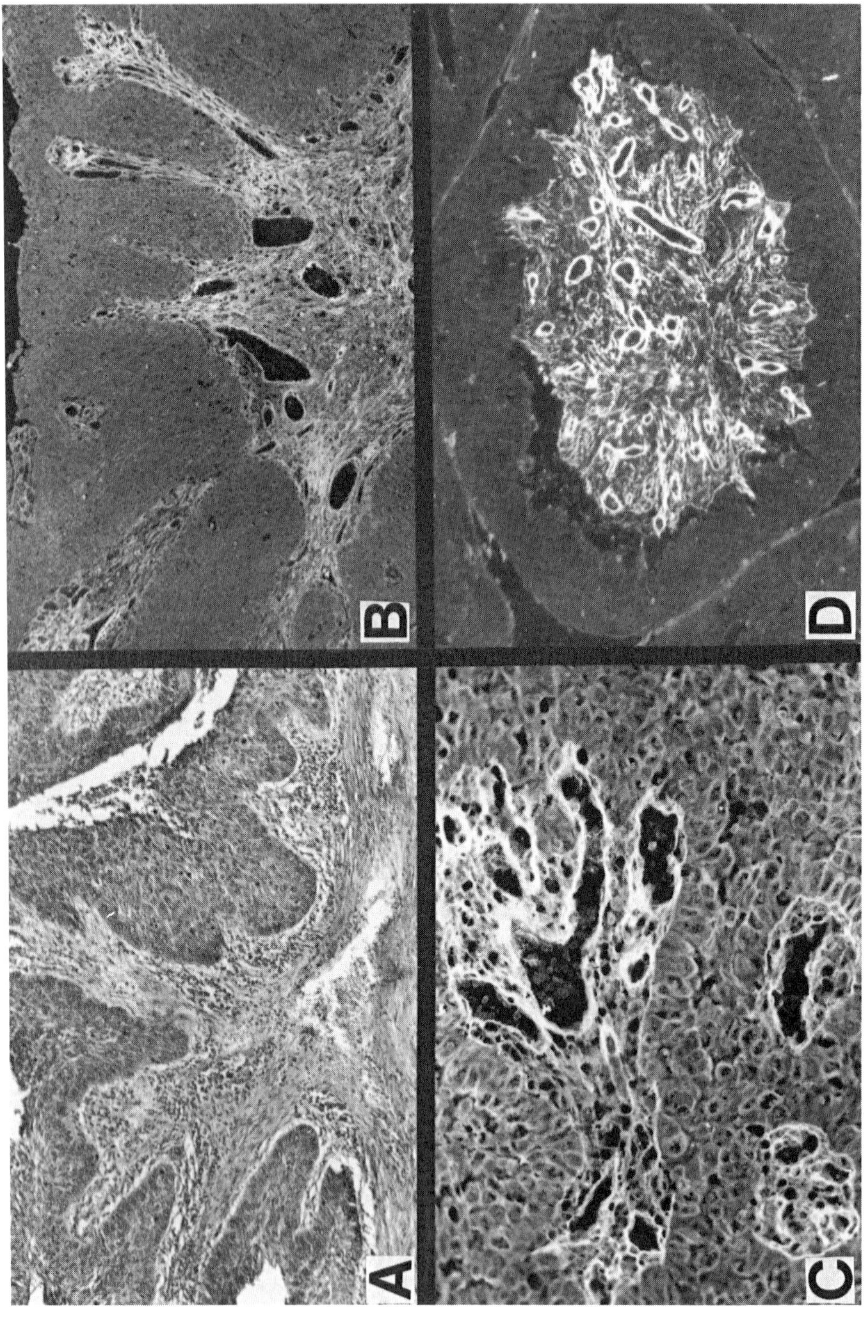

Figure 2

upper part of the tunica propria (Fig. 1F). A concomitant proliferation of fibroblasts and increased amount of collagens type I and III were observed in this site. The BM was continuously positively stained for FN, collagen type III, and laminin.

E. Severe Dysplasia

The BM is disintegrated, split, and thinned out to 2–3 μm in severe dysplasia with a continuous staining only for laminin. The staining for FN and type III collagen is weak below the dysplastic basal cell layer.

F. Carcinoma in Situ

The BM zone showed an even looser texture with detachment of basal epithelial cells that focally infiltrated the loosened BM. The BM, split and thinned out to about 1 μm (Fig. 1G) as an interrupted, inhomogeneous, indistinct limited line, revealed positive reaction only for laminin. Numerous capillary vessels oriented vertically to the BM were found right under the BM zone (Fig. 1H), revealing an intensive positive reaction for laminin. In the tunica propria a proliferation of connective tissue and an increased amount of collagen type I and III fibers were observed in both severe dysplasia and in carcinoma in situ accompanied by a strong inflammatory reaction.

G. Early Cancer

The bronchial wall is infiltrated by atypical epithelial cells not beyond the tunica fibrocartilaginea (Fig. 2A). The BM is always completely destroyed. In early stages of tumor development we found fine fiber structures, which were characterized as collagen type I and III fibers arranged in a coarse net structure surrounding tumor cell protrusions (Fig. 2B). A higher degree of immunofluorescence for collagen type I and III proved collagen neosynthesis. Many laminin-positive BM-like structures were found not only in the area of the original BM but also in deeper layers of the bronchial wall along atypical basal cell layers of tumor islets (Fig. 2C). Positive staining for laminin could be demonstrated around single tumor cells within tumor nodules accompanied by proliferation of capillaries (Fig. 2D).

Figure 2 Changes of extracellular matrix in early cancer of the lung. (A) Squamous cell carcinoma with early stromal invasion and inflammatory reaction (× 140). (B) Borderline of early squamous cell cancer surrounded by fiberlike structures of collagen type III (× 140). (C) Laminin-positive BM-like structures deposited along atypical basal cell layers of tumor cell arrangement (× 350). (D) Proliferation of numerous capillaries in tumor cell nodules with positive laminin staining (× 140).

IV. Discussion

The invasive growth of malignant tumors is always accompanied by inflammatory reactions as well as changes in the vascularization of the connective tissue. This was first described at the beginning of the 20th century (Russel, 1908; Ribbert, 1911; Böhmig, 1930). The pathogenetic significance of this phenomenon remained unclear. The modification of extracellular matrix as an expression of a disturbed cell–matrix interaction plays an important role in tumor growth (Van Den Hoof, 1984). As well as the destruction and solution of extracellular matrix components (Albrechtsen et al., 1981; Labat-Robert et al., 1981; Birembaut et al., 1985; Gay and Gay, 1985; Gabbert et al., 1987; Caselitz et al., 1988), neosynthesis of BM-like structures around tumor cell islets was demonstrated even in cases of invasion (Forster et al., 1984; Gusterson et al., 1984, 1986; Fisseler-Eckhoff et al., 1988). These observations, concentrated on invasive carcinomas of the lung, point to a correlation of the distribution of extracellular matrix components with different histologic growth pattern. The basement membrane glycoprotein laminin was prominent in small cell carcinomas, while in the extracellular matrix of squamous cell carcinomas and adenocarcinomas mainly collagen types I and III were found in different distribution in the central and peripheral tumor zones (Fisseler-Eckhoff et al., 1988). If a modification of the extracellular matrix is an expression of a rearranged cell–matrix interaction, one could expect to observe changes also in preneoplastic lesions (Meinl and Brunner, 1980). Although Barsky et al. (1983) demonstrated an intact linear basement membrane, which seemed to be thinned and fragmented in areas of microinvasion, separations of BM in preneoplastic lesions in areas without stroma invasion were found (Birembaut et al., 1985). The purpose of this paper was to give a qualitative evaluation of extracellular matrix composition in preneoplastic lesions of the bronchus. Characteristic changes of extracellular matrix components, such as loss of fibronectin, collagen type III, and laminin in the BM zone, correlated with an increasing degree of epithelial dysplasia, could be demonstrated.

In benign epithelial hyperplasia of basal and goblet cells a thickening of the BM due to increased production of collagen type III associated with chronic inflammatory processes was prominent. These findings are in good correlation with the results found on the bronchial mucosa of patients with asthma, where an increase of collagen type III production after inflammation of bronchial mucosa was observed (McCarter and Vasquez, 1966; Meinl and Brunner, 1980; Bateman et al., 1981).

The stromal changes in cases of micropapillomatosis start to show characteristics of definitive malignancies: no alterations in the BM zone but proliferation in the tunica propria characterized by increased collagen type I and III fibers and neovascularization. Although in mild dysplasia the basal cell layer is found to extend toward the ultrastructurally visible BM, we could not demonstrate changes in the BM zone or the tunica propria.

In severe dysplasia and carcinoma in situ the epithelial changes of bronchial mucosa present various degrees of atypia up to intraepithelial malignant transformation. Today we know that dysplastic cells can either release proteolytic enzymes including collagenases, which can digest extracellular matrix components (Liotta et al., 1980, 1983, 1986; Mullins and Rohrlich, 1983; Kao and Stern, 1986) or directly activate inflammatory cells (e.g., macrophages) to release lysosomal enzymes (Henry et al., 1983). On the other hand, the inflammatory cells release their own matrix-destroying enzymes at the site of tumor invasion after recognizing the atypical cells (Mullins and Rohrlich, 1983; Campbell et al., 1987).

A focal dissolution of BM in preneoplasias can mainly be observed in areas with a strong inflammatory reaction (Gusterson et al., 1984) indicating a loss of specific cell functions correlated with the pathologic capacity for proliferation. These results do correlate well with our observations of degradation of the BM zone parallel to an increased degree of dysplasia and a decreased staining for BM components such as laminin, fibronectin, and collagen type III. The process of BM degradation was accompanied by neosynthesis of capillary blood vessels in the tunica propria as well as close to the BM zone. In connection with the vascularization, collagen fibers and laminin were also produced. With an increasing degree of epithelial dysplasia, an increasing abnormality in the structure of the BM zone could be observed. As well as a disintegration of extracellular matrix components, neosynthesis of collagen type III and especially laminin in close association with neoangiogenesis could be demonstrated in cases of noninvasive lesions.

As we know, extracellular matrix components can be set up by epithelial basal cells (Martinez-Hernandez and Amenta, 1983; Abrahamson, 1986). The results indicate a partial loss of this function in preneoplastic cells. On the other hand, our findings in early stages of squamous cell carcinoma (neosynthesis of laminin in positive basement membranes around tumor islets) point to the fact that extracellular matrix components can be produced by tumor cells in invasive squamous cell cancer (Gusterson et al., 1984, 1986; Forster et al., 1984). Neosynthesis of extracellular matrix components might be induced by mesenchymal cells, macrophages, and tumor cells.

Acknowledgment

This work was completed with the financial support of the European Research Centre for Air Pollution Control Measures, Kernforschungszentrum Karlsruhe.

References

Abrahamson, D. R. (1986). Recent studies on the structure and pathology of basement membranes. *J. Pathol.* **149:**257–278.

Albrechtsen, R., Nielson, M., Wever, U., Engvall, E., and Ruoslahti, E. (1981). Basement membrane changes in breast cancer detected by immunohistochemical staining of laminin. *Cancer Res.* **41:**5076–5081.

Auerbach, O., Garfinkel, L., and Parks, V. R. (1975). Histologic types of lung cancer in relation to smoking habits. Year of diagnosis and sites of metastasis. *Chest* **67:**382–387.

Barsky, S. H., Siegal, G. P., Jannotta, F., and Liotta, L. A. (1983). Loss of basement membrane components by invasive tumours but not by their benign counterparts. *Lab. Invest.* **49:**140–147.

Bateman, E. D., Turner-Warwick, M., and Adelmann-Grill, B. C. (1981). Immunohistochemical study of collagen types in human foetal lung and fibrotic lung disease. *Thorax* **36:**645–653.

Birembaut, P., Caron, Y., Adnet, J. J., and Foidart, J. M. (1985). Usefulness of basement membrane markers in tumoral pathology. *J. Pathol.* **145:**283–296.

Böhmig, R. (1930). Das Krebsstroma und seine morphologischen Reaktionsformen. *Beitr. Pathol. Anat. Allg. Pathol.* **83:**333–382.

Bracke, M., Castronovo, V., De Bruyne, G., Coopman, P., Foidart, J. M., and Mareel, M. (1988). Interactions of invasive cells with native and modified extracellular matrix in vitro. In *Cancer Metastasis.* Edited by G. Prodi, L. A. Liotta, P.-L. Lollini, S. Garbisa, S. Gorini, and K. Hellmann. New York, Plenum, pp. 171–178.

Campbell, E. J., Senior, R. M., and Welgus, H. G. (1987). Extracellular matrix injury during lung inflammation. *Chest* **92:**161–167.

Caselitz, J., Schmitt, P., Seifert, G., Wustron, J., and Schuppan, D. (1988). Basal membrane associated substances in human salivary glands and salivary gland tumors. *Pathol. Res. Pract.* **183:**386–394.

Fisseler-Eckhoff, A., Voss, B., Kunze, W. P., and Müller, K. M. (1988). Differenzierung des Matrix-bildenden Bindegewebes in histologisch unterschiedlich differenzierten Lungentumoren. *Verh. Dtsch. Ges. Pathol.* **72:**272–277.

Fisseler-Eckhoff, A., Prebeg, M., Voss, B., and Müller, K. M. (1990). Extracellular matrix in preneoplastic lesions and early cancer of the lung. *Pathol. Res. Pract.* **186:**95–101.

Forster, S. J., Talbot, I. C., and Critchley, D. R. (1984). Laminin and fibronectin in rectal adenocarcinoma: relationship to tumour grade, stage and metastasis. *Br. J. Cancer* **50:**51–61.

Gabbert, H., Gerharz, C. D., Ramp, U. and Bohl, J. (1987). The nature of host tissue destruction in tumour invasion. An experimental investigation on carcinoma and sarcoma xenotransplants. *Virchows Arch. B (Cell. Pathol.)* **52:**513–527.

Gay, S., and Gay, R. E. (1985). Pathobiochemistry of connective tissue in breast cancer. *Verh. Dtsch. Ges. Pathol.* **69:**62–73.

Gonzales, S., Von Bassewitz, B. D., Grundmann, E., Nahkhosteen, J. A., and Müller, K. M. (1986). The ultrastructural heterogeneity of potentially preneoplastic lesions in the human bronchial mucosa. *Pathol. Res. Pract.* **181:**408–417.

Grundmann, E. (1980). Precancerous lesions and their clinical consequences. *Arch. Geschwulstforsch.* **50:**539–548.

Gusterson, B. A., Warburton, M. J., Mitchell, D., Kraft, N., and Hancock, W. W. (1984). Invading squamous cell carcinoma can retain a basal lamina. An immunohistochemical study using a monoclonal antibody to type IV collagen. *Lab. Invest.* **51:**82–87.

Gusterson, B. A., Clinton, S. S., and Gough, G. (1986). Studies of early invasive and intraepithelial squamous cell carcinomas using an antibody of type IV collagen. *Histopathology* **10:**161–169.

Henry, N., Eeckhout, Y., Van Lamsweerde, A. L., and Vaes, G. (1983a). Cooperation between metastatic tumour cells and macrophages in the degradation of basement membrane (Type IV) collagen. *FEBS* **161:**243–246.

Henry, N., Van Lamsweerde, A. L., and Vaes, G. (1983b). Collagen degradation by metastatic variants of Lewis lung carcinoma: cooperation between tumour cells and macrophages. *Cancer Res.* **43:**5321–5327.

Höring, E., Wörmann, B., Büchner, T., and Müller, K. M. (1982). Heterogeneity of tumor cells in human bronchial carcinoma. Histological and flow-cytomorphometrical analysis. *Verh. Dtsch. Krebs. Ges. Bd.* **4:**846.

Kao, R. T., and Stern, R. (1986a). Collagenases in human breast carcinoma cell lines. *Cancer Res.* **46:**1349–1354.

Kao, R. T., and Stern, R. (1986b). Elastases in human breast carcinoma cell lines. *Cancer Res.* **46:**1355–1358.

Kefalides, N. A., Alper, R., and Clark, C. C. (1979). Biochemistry and metabolism of basement membranes. *Int. Rev. Cytol.* **61:**167–228.

Labat-Robert, J., Birembaut, P., Robert, L., and Adnet, J. J. (1981). Modification of fibronectin distribution pattern in solid human tumours. *Diagn. Histopathol.* **4:** 299–306.

Laurie, G. W., Leblond, C. P., and Martin, G. R. (1982). Localization of type IV collagen, laminin, heparan sulfate proteoglycan and fibronectin to the basal lamina of basement membranes. *J. Cell. Biol.* **95:**340–344.

Liotta, L. A., Tryggvason, K., Garbisa, S., Hart, I., Foltz, C. M., and Shafie, S. (1980). Metastatic potential correlates with enzymatic degradation of basement membrane collagen. *Nature* **284:**67–70.

Liotta, L. A., Rao, C. N., and Barsky, S. H. (1983). Tumour invasion and the extracellular matrix. *Lab. Invest.* **49:**636–649.

Liotta, L. A., Rao, C. N., and Wever, U. M. (1986). Biochemical interactions of tumour cells with the basement membrane. *Annu. Rev. Biochem.* **55:**1037–1057.

Madri, J. A., Roll, F. J., Furthmayr, H., and Foidart, J. M. (1980). Ultrastructural localization of fibronectin and laminin in the basement membrane of the murine kidney. *J. Cell. Biol.* **86:**682–687.

Martinez-Hernandez, A., and Amenta, P. S. (1983). The basement membrane in pathology. *Lab. Invest.* **48:**656–677.

McCarter, J. H., and Vasquez, J. J. (1966). The bronchial basement membrane in asthma. *Arch. Pathol.* **82:**328–335.

McDowell, E. M., McLaughlin, J. S., Merenyi, D. K., Kieffer, R. F., Harris, C. C., and Trump, B. F. (1978). The respiratory epithelium. V. Histogenesis of lung carcinomas in the human. *J. Natl. Cancer Inst.* **61:**587–606.

McDowell, E. M., and Trump, B. F. (1983). Histogenesis of preneoplastic and neoplastic lesions in tracheobronchial epithelium. *Surv. Synth. Pathol. Res.* **2:**235–279.

McDowell, E. M. (1987). Bronchogenic carcinomas. In *Current Problems in Tumor*

Pathology: Lung Carcinomas. Edited by E. M. McDowell. New York, Churchill-Livingstone, pp. 255–285.

Meinl, M., and Brunner, P. (1980). Alterations in the structure of bronchial basement membrane in relation to textural changes of the bronchial mucosa. *Pathol. Res. Pract.* **169:**21–28.

Miller, E. J., Epstein, E. M., and Piez, K. A. (1971). Identification of three genetically distinct collagens by cyanogen bromide cleavage of insoluble human skin and cartilage collagen. *Biochem. Biophys. Res. Commun.* **42:**1029–1049.

Müller, K. M. (1985). Pathologie der Lungentumoren. In *Tumoren der Atmungsorgane und des Mediastinums (Handbuch der inneren Medizin*, vol. 4/4A). Edited by F. Trendelenburg. Berlin-Heidelberg-New York, Springer-Verlag, pp. 87–127.

Müller, K. M., and Müller, G. (1983). The ultrastructure of preneoplastic changes in the bronchial mucosa. In *Current Topics in Pathology*, vol. 73, *Pulmonary Diseases*. Edited by K. M. Müller. Berlin-Heidelberg-New York, Springer-Verlag, pp. 233–263.

Mullins, D. E., and Rohrlich, S. T. (1983). The role of proteinases in cellular invasiveness. *Biochim. Biophys. Acta* **695:**177–214.

Nasiell, M., Carlens, E., Auer, G., Hayata, Y., Kato, H., Konaka, C., Roger, V., Nasiell, K., and Enstad, I. (1982). Pathogenesis of bronchial carcinoma, with special reference to morphogenesis and the influence on the bronchial mucosa of 20-methylcholanthrene and cigarette smoking. *Cancer Res.* **82:**53–68.

Ribbert, H. (1911). *Das Karzinom des Menschen*. Bonn, Cohen-Verlag.

Russel, B. R. G. (1908). The nature of resistance to the inoculation of cancer. Third Scientific Report on the investigation of the Imperial Cancer Research Foundation 3:341–358.

Saba, S. R., Espinoza, C. G., Richman, A. V., and Azar, H. A. (1983). Carcinomas of the lung: an ultrastructural and immunocytochemical study. *Am. J. Clin. Pathol.* **80:** 6–13.

Schlegel, R., and Blanks-Schlegel, S. (1980). Immunohistochemical localization of keratin in normal human tissue. *Lab. Invest.* **42:**91–96.

Van Den Hooff, A. (1984). The part played by the stroma in carcinogenesis. *Perspect. Biol. Med.* **27:**498–509.

3

Differentiation of Lung Epithelial Cells and Lung Cancers in Relation to Adhesion and Drug Resistance

SAMUEL D. BERNAL, MIKA KAKEFUDA,* YUK-CHOR WONG, GODOFREDO URBANO, and MA-TERESA BARZAGA†

Boston University Medical Center
Boston, Massachusetts

I. Introduction

Lung cancer is an ideal model system for studies of the differentiation pathways of epithelial cancers because of the widely divergent differentiation properties exhibited by lung cells. Subpopulations of bronchial epithelium exhibit glandular, squamous, and neuroendocrine differentiation; however, the origin of the different histologic types of lung cancers remains unclear. A striking property of bronchial epithelium is the change in proportions of cell types in response to various types of injury (Reid and Coles, 1984). Metaplastic conversion of bronchial cells into differentiated squamous epithelium as a result of both chemical and mechanical injury has been well described (Trump et al., 1978; Auerbach et al., 1957). It was previously assumed that basal cells are the primary cells that hyperproliferate in response to injury and give rise to squamous cells in bronchial epithelium. Other investigators suggest that secretory cells play an important role as progenitor cells in fetal development, and that in response to injury the secretory cells proliferate and differentiate to give rise to squamous metaplastic cells (McDowell and Trump, 1983). Hyperplasia and dysplasia of bronchial neuroendocrine cells can also occur with lung injury (Gould et al., 1983). These cells, with amine precursor uptake and decarboxylation (APUD) characteristics and cytoplasmic electron dense membrane-

**Present affiliation*: Johns Hopkins Hospital, Baltimore, Maryland
†*Present affiliation*: Lung Center of the Philippines, Quezon City, Philippines

bound vesicles, were postulated to be derived from neural crest cells (Pearse, 1969), but are now thought to be derived from endodermal stem cells (Cutz, 1982). Based upon studies of the ultrastructure, histochemistry, and mitotic activity in tracheobronchial epithelium during fetal development and focal injury, it has been proposed that poorly differentiated columnar cells are the stem cells that give rise to basal cells, secretory cells, and ciliated cells during in utero development of the tracheobronchial epithelium (Saffiotti et al., 1985). Subsequently, basal cells are thought to replicate to propagate basal cells, whereas secretory cells replicate to produce both secretory cells and ciliated cells. After injury, most of the cells that hyperproliferate and change shape were found to be secretory cells, and the metaplastic squamous cells that arose contained mucous granules, consistent with their origin from secretory cells (Keenan et al., 1983).

With the advance in culturing techniques, it has been possible to grow normal bronchial epithelial cells (NBE) from bronchial explants in culture (Stoner et al., 1980). Secretory, mucin-containing cells and ciliated cells are observed early during culture. The addition of serum and calcium to the medium induces squamous differentiation of these bronchial epithelial cells (Lechner et al., 1983). Other factors have been found to modulate differentiation in these cells, such as retinoic acid, phorbol esters, and transforming growth factor-beta (TGF-β), but the effect of these factors on subpopulations of NBE cells remains unclear. The study of human bronchial epithelial differentiation is hindered by the lack of markers of differentiation, particularly at the early stages of differentiation. NBE cells induced to differentiate in vitro show changes in cell size, shape, and amounts of keratins and involucrin but these changes appear late during NBE differentiation. Little information is available on the biochemical changes that occur during commitment, the critical step of squamous differentiation. The differentiation state of lung epithelial cells and lung cancers is affected by cell–cell and cell–matrix adhesion, but there are limited data on the specific molecules that may mediate these interactions. The differentiation phenotypes of lung cancer differ in responsiveness to chemotherapy, but the cellular components that contribute to differences in drug sensitivity and drug transport have not been identified. In this chapter, we review some recent findings on membrane molecules associated with differentiation of human lung epithelial cells and lung cancers. We will also describe the molecular cloning and characterization of a new differentiation-related membrane protein that appears to play a role in cell adhesion and drug transport in lung epithelial cells and lung cancers.

II. Subpopulations of Normal Human Bronchial Epithelial Cells: Membrane Antigen Expression

Cultivation of primary cultures of normal human bronchial epithelium has been well established (Bernal et al., 1988; Willey et al., 1988; Stoner et al., 1980;

Lechner et al., 1981, 1982). Bronchial epithelial cells in culture are capable of differentiating in to both ciliated and squamous cells (Lechner et al., 1981). Secretory and mucin-containing cells are also observed in these cultures. However, the predominant response of these cells to differentiation-inducing agents is to undergo squamous differentiation similar to squamous metaplasia in response to chronic injury (Lechner et al., 1983, 1984; Trump et al., 1978; Auerbach et al., 1957; Reid and Coles 1984). NBE cells induced to differentiate with serum and calcium show changes in cell size, shape, and amount of cross-linked envelopes. In addition, specific intermediate filaments, involucrin, and other markers of differentiation increase with induction of differentiation, similar to what is seen in differentiation of epidermal cells. This in vitro system allows the identification of subpopulations of normal human bronchial epithelial cells and the biochemical changes in these cells associated with differentiation.

The NBE cells were cultivated from bronchial tissues obtained at surgery. The margins for the tissues were examined and only tissues deemed to contain normal epithelium were used. The surrounding lung parenchyma and connective tissue were trimmed away and the bronchi were cut into 2 × 2 cm sections. These sections were placed epithelial side up and covered with RPMI 1640 medium with 0.6 mM calcium and 10% fetal bovine serum (R/0.6/10), supplemented with 1 mM L-glutamine, 0.18 mg/ml streptomycin, 100 units/ml penicillin, and 50 μg/ml gentamycin [1]. The medium was changed every day for 4–6 days. The plates were incubated at 37°C in 5% CO_2 atmosphere.

Subsequently, the bronchial tissues were cut into 4 mm^2 sections, placed epithelial side down, and cultured in 60 mM tissue culture dishes containing 2 ml of RPMI 1640 medium with 0.6 mM calcium and 1% fetal bovine serum (R/0.6/1), with 1 mM glutamine, 20 mM HEPES buffer (pH 7.6), 20 ng/ml epidermal growth factor (Collaborative Research), 5×10^{-7} M hydrocortisone, 0.2 μg/ml insulin, 0.18 mg/ml streptomycin, 100 U/ml penicillin, and 50 μg/ml gentamycin. The following trace elements were also added: 3×10^{-8} M selenium oxide, 1×10^{-9} M molybdic acid, 5×10^{-10} M stannous chloride, and 5×10^{-10} M nickel sulfate.

When a perimeter of cells radiated 1 cm outward, the explant was removed and transferred to new culture plates. The initial cultures of NBE cells (uninduced NBE) were maintained for 4–7 days in medium MCDB 151 medium with 0.1 mM calcium and 0% serum (M/0.1/0), and supplements: 1 mM L-glutamine, 5 ng/ml epidermal growth factor, 5 μg/ml insulin, 10 μg/ml transferrin, 5×10^{-7} M ethanolamine, 5×10^{-7} M phosphoethanolamine, 1×10^{-9} M, 3,3′-5-triiodo-d-thyronine, 20 mM HEPES buffer (pH 7.6), 5×10^{-7} M hydrocortisone, 30 μg/ml pituitary extract (Collaborative Research), trace elements, and antibiotics. The plates were incubated at 37°C in 5% CO_2 atmosphere.

Subpopulations of normal human bronchial epithelial cells were identified in these primary cultures, based upon their reactivity with antibodies against lung epithelial membrane antigens. None of these antibodies reacted with lung fibroblasts or lymphocytes. The reactivities of these antibodies with bronchial epithelial cells and lung cancer cells are presented in Table 1. The antibodies with broad reactivity with cancers of the lung and other tissues, such as LAM 2 and LAM 6, also showed broad reactivity with normal bronchial epithelial (NBE) cells and tissues. LAM 7 had intermediate reactivity with various lung cancers and also showed intermediate reactivity with NBE cells whereas the antibodies with restricted reactivities, such as LAM 8 and SQM1, also showed narrow reactivities with NBE cells. LAM 2 stained 80% of NBE cells, with an intense, complete ring of surface fluorescence. LAM 6 reacted with 75% of NBE cells, showing an uneven, mottled membrane fluorescence. LAM 7 staining showed marked heterogeneity, showed significant staining in only 60% of cells with many cells showing a speckled membrane pattern. LAM 8 stained less than 5% of NBE cells, many of which were larger and elongated. Staining was often concentrated on one pole of the cells. SQM1 stained 5–10% of NBE cells, which were indistinguishable by phase microscopy from other NBE cells.

Subpopulations of cells in sections of normal human bronchial epithelial tissues (NBET) were also identified by immunoperoxidase staining. LAM 2 stained 80% of NBET cells. The most intense staining was seen with the membrane of ciliated cells. The ciliary filaments themselves were highly reactive. Many of the basal cells were unreactive with LAM 2. LAM 6 stained most of the basal cells but only 10% of the ciliated cells. The most intense staining with LAM 6 was seen with the basal bodies of cilia but the cilia themselves were unstained. Unlike LAM 2 and LAM 6, only the basal cells were stained with LAM 7, although the intensity of staining was heterogeneous. All the other cells, including ciliated and nonciliated columnar cells, were unreactive with LAM 7. LAM 8 stained only 1% of basal cells, which tended to be larger than other basal cells. SQM1 stained 5–10% of basal cells, but all other NBET cells were unreactive.

Table 1 Membrane Antigens of Subpopulations of Normal Bronchial Cells and Various Epithelial Cancers

Antibody	NBE culture (%)	NBE tissues (%)	Carcinoma cell lines and tissues
LAM 2	80	80	SCCL, SqCL, AdCL, LCCL, breast, colon, pancreas, ovary
LAM 6	75	65	SCCL, SqCL, AdCL, carcinoid, cervix
LAM 7	60	50	SCCL, SqCL, breast
LAM 8	1	1	SCCL
SQM1	5–10	10–15	SCCL, SqCL

SCCL, small cell carcinoma of the lung; SqCL, squamous carcinoma of the lung; AdCL, adenocarcinoma of the lung; LCCL, large cell carcinoma of the lung.

The breadth of reactivity of the different antibodies in NBE and NBET cells paralleled their breadth of reactivity with carcinomas of the lung and other tissues. The antibody with the broadest reactivity was LAM 2, which reacted with cell lines derived from small cell lung carcinoma, squamous carcinomas (lung, head and neck, cervix), and adenocarcinomas (breast, colon, pancreas, and ovary). LAM 6 showed more restricted staining, showing reactivity with small cell carcinoma, squamous carcinomas (lung, head and neck, cervix), and bronchial carcinoid. LAM 7 showed even more restricted staining, reacting primarily with small cell carcinoma, squamous carcinomas (lung, head and neck, cervix), and breast cancer. LAM 8 was highly restricted to small cell carcinoma of the lung and was much less reactive with non-small cell lung carcinoma and other cancers. SQM1 was reactive primarily with squamous carcinomas (lung, head and neck, cervix) and small cell carcinomas, and showed less reactivity with other cancers.

III. Differentiation of Normal Human Bronchial Epithelial Cells: Shifts in Expression of Epithelial Markers

To induce and observe squamous differentiation in the outgrowth epithelial cell layer, RPMI 1640 medium with 0.6 mM calcium, 5% fetal bovine serum and supplements, described above (R/0.6/5) was added after removal of the tissue. Keratin content was examined by immunofluorescence of permeabilized cells and by immunoblotting of cell extracts with antikeratin antibodies AE1 and AE3. The cells were examined for cornified envelopes and stained with antiinvolucrin antibody (Watt and Green, 1981). The NBE cells were allowed to attach to glass cover slips and induced to differentiate. The cells were fixed in 3.7% formaldehyde in PBS at room temperature for 8 min and then in methanol at −20°C for 5 min. After being incubated with rabbit antiserum to involucrin (provided by Dr. H. Green, Harvard Medical School, Boston MA), the slides were washed and incubated with FITC-antirabbit antibody.

The morphologic changes associated with terminal differentiation of these cells include flattening, an increase of cell surface area and cytoplasmic/nucleus ratio, and the formation of cross-linked envelopes (Lechner et al., 1983, 1984). Some biochemical markers of differentiation have been characterized in trachea and bronchial epithelial differentiation (Jetten 1989, Thacher and Rice, 1985; Jetten and Shirley, 1986; Banks-Schlegel and Green, 1981; Banks-Schlegel et al., 1985; Rearick et al., 1987). These include the specific keratins, involucrin, transglutaminase type I, and the accumulation of cholesterol sulfate (Jetten, 1989; Sun et al., 1983; Banks-Schlegel and Green, 1981; Jetten and Shirley, 1986; Thacher and Rice, 1985; Rearick et al., 1987). We have focused on using these markers to develop a model system to study normal differentiation in order to identify new markers of differentiation.

Before induction, the poorly differentiated NBE cells were small with high nuclear–cytoplasmic ratio and proliferated rapidly. For up to 48 hr after induction with serum and calcium, the cells continued to proliferate but did not show morphologic changes. Between 24 and 36 hr after treatment with serum and calcium, the cells were committed such that even after removal of serum and calcium, the cells continued to differentiate terminally. In these committed cells, morphologic and biochemical evidence of epithelial differentiation did not appear until later stages of differentiation. By 72 hr, cell size increased and cornified cells characteristic of terminal differentiation (Banks-Schlegel and Green, 1981) were evident. By day 8–10, most of the cells expressed membrane surface involucrin, a marker of differentiation and a component of cross-linked envelopes in epidermal cells (Fuchs and Green, 1980).

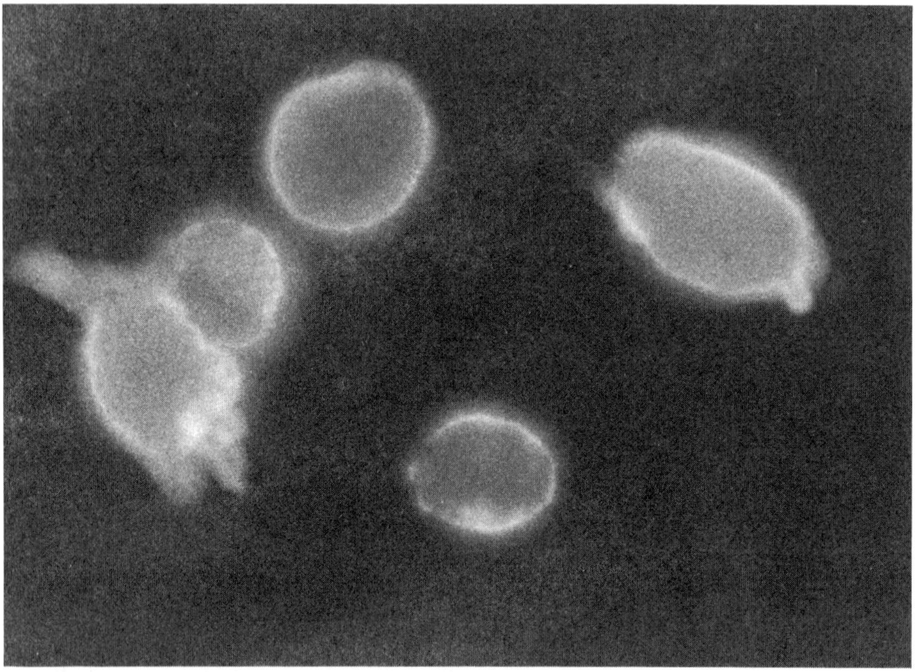

Figure 1 Immunofluorescence staining of NBE cells during early induction of differentiation with serum and calcium using anti-SQM1 antibody. During the early stages of differentiation these cells begin to express a large amount of SQM1 antigen on the membrane surface, peaking at 20–36 hr after induction to differentiation in culture.

The major change in antigenic characteristics of differentiating NBE cells was in membrane SQM1 content. Only minor changes were observed with LAM 2, LAM 6, LAM 7, and LAM 8. Although only 5–10% of NBE cells were reactive with anti-SQM1 antibody prior to induction, approximately 70% of these cells were highly reactive by 36 hr after induction, at the time of commitment. Anti-SQM1 immunofluorescence staining of NBE cells after induction of differentiation is shown in Figure 1. At later stages of differentiation, including the terminal stages at day 8–10, the level of membrane SQM1 declined. The peak of SQM1 expression was at the time of commitment when there were no significant changes in morphology or growth rate, although the cells were more strongly attached to the culture substratum.

IV. Relationship of SQM1 to Epithelial Differentiation

SQM1 was first identified in membranes of squamous carcinomas of the head and neck (SCCHN). Anti-SQM1 antibody showed little reactivity with most carcinomas of breast, colon, ovary, leukemias, and some lung carcinomas (Boeheim et al., 1985, 1986). A few cells in the smears of normal buccal mucosa, which contain mostly well-differentiated cells, were stained with SQM1 (Boeheim et al., 1985, 1986). Normal epidermal cells in the stratum spinosum layer (not completely differentiated) and most primary cultures of normal epidermal cells reacted with the antibody (Boeheim et al., 1985). In skin, reactivity was seen mainly in the stratum spinosum, but not in the surface epithelium (Boeheim et al., 1985). Well-differentiated SCCHN specimens by histologic grading stained much more heavily than the poorly differentiated carcinomas (Boeheim et al., 1986). In squamous carcinomas of the lung, SQM1 staining was strongest in cells surrounding keratin pearls, but the structures within the keratin pearls themselves were not reactive with anti-SQM1 antibody (Fig. 2). Some small cell carcinomas were also heavily stained with anti-SQM1 antibody (Fig. 3).

SQM1 appears to be a differentiation marker that is normally present in squamous cells and well-differentiated carcinomas, but not in undifferentiated cells or terminally differentiating cells. The antigen immunoprecipitated from ^{35}S methionine-labeled cell membrane extracts was a 48 kD protein on reducing sodium dodecyl sulfate-polyacrylamide gel electrophoresis (SDS-PAGE) (Boeheim et al., 1985).

The time course and tissue distribution of SQM1 antigen were also studied during mouse embryonic development. There was no expression of the antigen during the first and second trimesters. During the third trimester, SQM1 antigen appeared, during the time that squamous epithelia became stratified. In addition, the first tissues to express SQM1 antigen were the first tissues to stratify, such as in

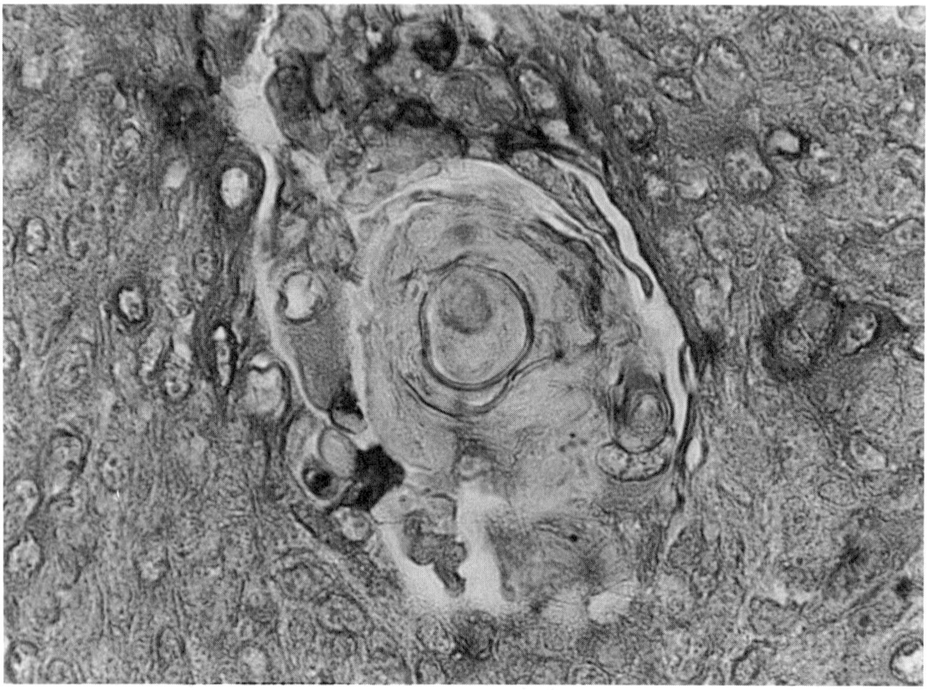

Figure 2 Well-differentiated squamous carcinoma of the lung with keratin pearl. Note the progression of SQM1 staining from the outer to inner parts of the tumor islet. Cells at the periphery were weakly stained. Cells surrounding the keratin pearl were strongly stained. Keratinized cells and the keratin pearl itself are weakly stained. This staining pattern is also found in epidermal cells where only the stratum spinosum (intermediate) layer was stained, but the basal and cornified layers were unstained.

the skin of the head and neck. SQM1 antigen also did not stain the entire stratified epithelium but was specific to the stratum spinosum, first seen in the epithelial of skin, oral, nasal, and tongue mucosa, and then later in the suprabasal layer of the oropharyngeal epithelium. There was no staining of the basal or cornified layers or other nonepithelial and nonsquamous tissues. Electron microscopy of SQM1-immunogold-stained stratified epithelium localizes the antigen on the membrane, at intercellular connections. SQM1 antigen was not associated with desmosomes (Tsao et al., 1989). These data suggest that SQM1 expression is highly regulated during embryonic development, is associated with early stages of differentiation, and is localized in the surface membrane at sites of intercellular connections.

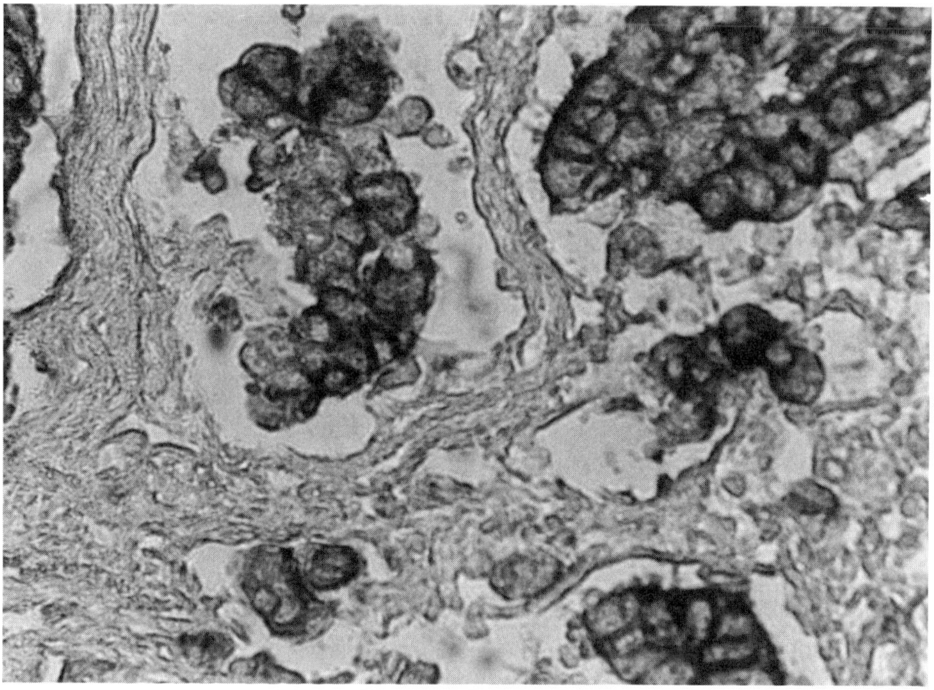

Figure 3 Small cell carcinoma of the lung with clumps of intra-alveolar tumor cells staining strongly for SQM1.

V. SQM1 and Cell Adhesion

The importance of the interaction between cells and extracellular matrix (ECM) adhesion proteins and its role in regulation of differentiation, as well as its contribution to neoplastic growth, have been well established (Juliano, 1987; Yamada, 1983; Poste and Fidler, 1980; Liotta, 1986). Fibronectin, vitronectin, and laminin are well-known extracellular matrix adhesion proteins involved in binding to collagen, proteoglycans, actin, and other specific molecules (Yamada, 1983; Juliano, 1987). Recently, a family of membrane glycoproteins (integrins) has been identified as the cell adhesion receptors in lymphoid and myeloid cells (reviewed by Hynes, 1987; Juliano, 1987). In addition, it was found that beta integrins may function in keratinocytes in cell–cell interactions, as well as in cell substrate adhesion dependent on calcium for expression (Larjava et al., 1990).

Since we observed that SQM1 was induced in the early stages of NBE differentiation, at the time when there was increased cell adhesion, we further examined the possible role of SQM1 in cell adhesion. The effect of anti-SQM1 monoclonal antibody on adhesion of intact cells to various extracellular matrix proteins and to other cells was tested. The test cells were preincubated with SQM1 antibody for 1 hr. As controls, normal serum, or an irrelevant antibody reactive with epithelial membrane, instead of SQM1 antibody was incubated with the cells. After being washed with medium, the cells were labeled with a fluorescent dye, Rh-123, for 30 min (Bernal et al., 1982) and then washed with medium. The labeled cells were added to round coverslips with cell monolayers or ECM proteins. After 2 hr, the coverslips were rinsed with medium and examined by fluorescence microscopy to count the total number of adherent cells.

SQM1 antibody interfered with epithelial and endothelial cell–cell adhesion (Table 2). The greatest inhibition by SQM1 antibody was observed in epithelial–endothelial adhesion; moderate inhibition was seen in endothelial–endothelial and epithelial–ECM adhesion. Epithelial–epithelial adhesion was also inhibited, although to a lesser degree. Anti-SQM1 antibody did not inhibit adhesion of lymphocytes or fibroblastic cells. A control antibody (SM1), which is known to bind epithelial and endothelial surface membranes, also did not interfere with adhesion. These results suggest that SQM1 antibody specifically blocked adhesion interactions of epithelial and endothelial cells. There was greater inhibition of epithelial–endothelial adhesion compared to epithelial–epithelial adhesion, which suggests that the contribution of SQM1 protein toward epithelial–endothelial adhesion was greater than in epithelial–epithelial adhesion. Between epithelial cells, there are likely to be many strong adhesion interactions, such as those mediated by desmosomal proteins (Jones et al., 1986), which are not affected by SQM1 antibody. SQM1 protein may be more important in mediating epithelial–

Table 2 Inhibition of Cell Adhesion by Anti-SQM1 Antibody

Cell type	Monolayer cell type or matrix	Adherent cells (% of control)
SCC25	HUVEC	18 ± 3
HUVEC	SCC25	20 ± 3
SCC25	Fibronectin	23 ± 4
SCC25	Collagen type IV	25 ± 5
HUVEC	HUVEC	28 ± 6
SCC25	SCC25	72 ± 5
SCC25	Fibroblast	94 ± 5
CEM	Fibronectin	102 ± 5

SCC25, human squamous carcinoma of the head and neck; HUVEC, human endothelial cell line; CEM, human lymphoblastic leukemia cell line.

endothelial and epithelial–ECM interactions, which may in turn be important in the metastatic behavior of epithelial tumors.

Other known cell–cell adhesion molecules include the cadherins and cadherinlike molecules, which are organized into subclasses based upon tissue distribution. These include liver L-CAM, neural N-CAM (described by Souhami and Walsh in Chap. 10), neural–glial Ng-CAM, uvomorulin, and others (Obrink, 1986; Volk et al., 1987; Hatta and Takeichi, 1986), some of which are calcium dependent (Hirano et al., 1987). SQM1 is distinct from these previously described molecules in both tissue distribution and temporal expression in embryonic development (Richa et al., 1985); however, the relationship between SQM1 and these molecules requires further investigation.

VI. Relationship between SQM1 and Drug Sensitivity

The reactivity of anti-SQM1 antibody with several methotrexate (MTX)-resistant carcinoma cell lines was compared by indirect immunofluorescence and radioimmunoassay (Table 3). The cell lines with the lowest SQM1 reactivity (SCC15R1, SCC15R2, and SCC15R3), with binding percentages of 9%, 2%, and 2%, also had the lowest rates of MTX transport influx rates (0.06, 0.03, and 0.07 pmol/min/mg protein). Although these three cell lines had similar SQM1 reactivity and MTX influx rates, they differed widely in dihydrofolate reductase (DHFR) relative levels (0.9, 4.3, and 73). The mean number of glutamate residues also varied (1.0, 2.2, and 1.0). Another MTX-resistant SCC15 cell line, SCC15R4 was 9000-fold resistant to MTX, showed high levels of DHFR enzyme (276x) and gene (10x), but retained MTX transport to 30% of control and also showed retention of SQM1 reactivity to 27% of control. These results suggest that marked reduction in SQM1 expression is most closely associated with defects in MTX transport and not with other mechanisms of resistance. The MTX-resistant SCC25R1, SCC68R1, and SCC78R1 sublines also show reduced binding of SQM1. SCC25R1 did not show reduced transport compared to the parent line but the SCC25S parent cell line was unusual in having low MTX influx rate at only 23% of control. SCC68R1 and SCC78R1, which showed moderate reduction in MTX influx (at 0.2 μM MTX), also showed moderate reduction of SQM1 binding. The DHFR levels of these cell lines varied greatly (3.5, 4.9, 1.5) and the mean number of glutamate residues was not significantly different from the parent cell lines. In these various cell lines, SQM1 reactivity correlated most closely with MTX transport and not with levels of DHFR or polyglutamylation (Bernal et al., 1990a,b).

MTX resistance is multifactorial and includes not only increased DHFR enzyme and gene amplification (Alt et al., 1978; Carman et al., 1984) but also altered forms of DHFR with decreased affinity for inhibitor (Flintoff and Essani, 1980), reduced polyglutamylation (Cowan and Jolivet, 1984; Frei et al., 1984) and

Table 3 SQM1 Membrane Antigen in MTX-Sensitive and Resistant Cells

Cell Line	SQM1	MTX transport	DHFR enzyme	DHFR gene	Poly (glu) (n)	IC_{50} (μM MTX)
SCC68S	100[a]	100[b]	1.0	1.0	2.5	0.019
SCC15S	87	51	1.0	1.0	2.9	0.030
SCC78S	81	36	1.0	1.0	3.5	0.011
SCC25S	35–65[c]	23	1.0	1.0	3.3	0.0075
SCC78R1	48	38	1.5	1.2	3.1	0.074
SCC68R1	30	45	4.9	2.0	2.2	0.24
SCC15R4	27	31	276	10.0	nd	270
SCC25R1	25–45	25	3.5	2.1	3.0	0.15
SCC15R1	9	8	0.9	1.0	1.0	0.50
SCC15R2	2	4	4.3	2.7	2.2	3.60
SCC15R3	2	9	73.0	4.4	1.0	22.0

The cell lines with the highest SQM1 reactivity (SCC68S, SCC15S, SCC78S) were all drug-sensitive cell lines, which also had the highest rates of MTX transport. The cell lines with the lowest SQM1 reactivity (SCC15R1, SCC15R2, SCC15R3) were all drug-resistant cell lines, which also had the lowest rates of MTX transport. SQM1 did not correlate with DHFR enyme, DHFR gene, polyglutamylation, or cell doubling times (Bernal et al. 1990a).

[a]SCC68S had the highest anti-SQM1 reactivity (RIA binding % = 1450) and was used as reference control (100%) for SQM1 reactivity.

[b]SCC68S had the highest rate of MTX transport (0.77 pmol/min/mg protein at 2.0μM) and was used as reference control (100%) for rates of MTX transport.

[c]The noncloned SCC25S cell line and sublines were unusual in having marked heterogeneity of SQM1 staining and variable radioimmunoassay results.

nd, Not determined.

diminished thymidylate synthesis with reduced requirement for tetrahydrofolate regeneration (White and Goldman, 1981; Moran et al., 1979). Recent studies, however, suggest that defects in MTX membrane transport appear early in the development of resistance (Ohnuma et al., 1985). Changes in levels of DHFR enzyme and gene amplification were observed between 200 and 10,000-fold levels of MTX resistance. In human squamous carcinomas that were 10–100-fold resistant to MTX, the major mechanism of resistance was decreased MTX transport (Frei et al., 1984). In our studies, multiple mechanisms, including increased DHFR enzyme and decreased polyglutamulation, were found at high (>100×) levels of MTX resistance, but the primary mechanism was decreased membrane transport at low levels, associated with membrane protein changes (Bernal et al., 1990a). Most interesting was the identification of SQM1, which was not only associated with differentiation but also appeared to be a protein involved in the regulation of MTX transport.

Comparisons were made between the expression of the 46 kD (SQM1) protein in cis-platinum (CDDP)-sensitive and revertant cells by indirect immunofluorescence and radioimmunoassays. SQM1 was reduced in CDDP-resistant carcinoma cells compared to CDDP-sensitive cells (Table 4). The SW2 and SCC25S cell lines were sensitive to CDDP with IC_{50} between 10 and 15 μM CDDP. The SW2-resistant cell line developed about fivefold resistance and the SCC25-resistant cell line was 12.5-fold resistant to CDDP, associated with a decrease in intracellular uptake responsible for differences in drug accumulation. No change in glutathione level was seen in the resistant cells. Although the CDDP resistance is more likely to be multifactorial, decreased CDDP transport appeared to be a major mechanism operating early in the development of CDDP resistance. SQM1 binding of the CDDP-resistant cell lines was found to be markedly reduced compared to the parent cell lines. These results indicate that reduced SQM1 membrane protein was also associated with CDDP resistance, and was primarily associated with reduced CDDP transport. Reversion to CDDP sensitivity was associated with increased SQM1 and increased MTX sensitivity (Table 4). In these sets of sensitive, resistant, and revertant cell lines, the level of SQM1 expression was associated with sensitivity to CDDP. There was overall congruence between SQM1 expression, CDDP sensitivity, and MTX sensitivity. Although the mechanism for this congruence is not fully understood, alterations of membrane transport for both MTX and CDDP were noted in these cell lines. Further investigation is needed to determine this relationship between both MTX and CDDP resistance. In contrast to the congruence between MTX and CDDP resistance, no cross-resistance was observed in these cell lines to Adriamycin or vincristine. No changes in SQM1 expression were observed in cells resistant to Adriamycin or VP-16 (Bernal et al., 1990a).

Table 4 Reduced SQM1 Membrane Antigen in Carcinoma Cells Resistant to Cis-Platinum

Cell line	SQM1 immunofluorescence	SQM1 radioimmunoassay (%)
SW2-sensitive	3+	100
SW2-CDDP resistant	1+	20
SW2-CDDP revertant	3+	85
SCC25-sensitive	4+	100
SCC25-CDDP resistant	1+	15
SCC25-CDDP revertant	3+	70

SW2, small cell carcinoma of the lung; SCC25, squamous carcinoma of the head and neck.

VII. cDNA Cloning and Molecular Characterization of SQM1

To determine if the antibody would recognize the epitope in an in-vitro-synthesized protein, in vitro translation of mRNA from SCC25 was performed and immunoblotted with SQM1 antibody. The antibody recognized two bands (15 and 14 kD) in the SCC25 mRNA translation products, where rabbit globin mRNA did not have these bands (Wong et al., 1991). Thus anti-SQM1 antibody recognized the core protein and was not dependent upon posttranslational processing.

Since SQM1 appeared to be related to differentiation and played a role in cell adhesion and drug resistance, further definition of its structure became important in elucidating its function. A lambda gt11 expression library from mRNA of SCC15 cells, a SCCHN cell line expressing large amounts of the protein, was constructed. Several separate candidate clones were isolated from this library after tertiary screening with anti-SQM1 antibody and sequenced by excision with EcoR1 and ligation into M13mp18. The DNA sequence was determined by the dideoxynucleotide chain termination method (Sanger et al., 1977).

The insert of the cDNA clones was sequenced and the sequence of one of the clones, Q12, is shown in Figure 4. A polyadenylation signal sequence AAATAAAA (Proudfoot and Brownlee, 1976), (base pairs [bps] 438–445) is located 14 bp upstream of the poly(dA), which suggests that clone Q12 probably contains the complete 3′ end of the gene. The sequence encompassing the first ATG, CAGC-CATGG, conforms to the eukaryotic initiation consensus, CA(A/G)CCAUGG (Kozak, 1984). The first AUG starts a 135 amino acid encoding open reading frame that ends at bp406, 32 bp upstream of the polyadenylation signal. The calculated molecular weight of the unmodified polypeptide is about 15 kD, which is in close agreement with the size of the in vitro translation products recognized by SQM1 antibody (15 and 14 kD). Three Ser-Gly dipeptides can form the minimal attachment sites of chondroitin sulfate glycosaminoglycan side chains via O-glycosyl linkage to serines, as in proteoglycans (Bourdon et al., 1985). Proteoglycans are known to interact with ECM and are thought to be involved in cellular adhesion (Laterra et al., 1983).

By comparing with the sequences in the data bases, regions were found in the SQM1 polypeptide that were similar to the cysteine repeats of human EGF receptor and to a group of related human adhesion molecules/ligands: beta subunit of the leukocyte adhesion proteins, endothelial GpIIIa, vWF, and complement C8 beta chain. The sequence similarity is mainly localized to a sequence motif containing cysteines and a positively charged residue, found near the C-terminal of the SQM1 polypeptide, overlapping two arginines of the heptadic repeat. Other than this sequence motif, SQM1 polypeptide has an additional region, on the N-terminal side of the heptadic repeat, that is similar to the beta chain of leukocyte adhesion proteins and von Willebrand's factor.

```
-35    -30           -20           -10           1                     15
CCCTC  GGTGCTGCAG   GGATCTGCAG   GACTGCAGCC    ATG GGG GCG CAC CTG GTC CGG
                                               Met Gly Ala His Leu Val Arg
                                               1

        30                   45                    60                  75
CGC TAC CTG GGC GAT GCT TCG GTG GAG CCC GAC CCC CTG CAG ATG CCA ACC TTC
Arg Tyr Leu Gly Asp Ala Ser Val Glu Pro Asp Pro Leu Gln Met Pro Thr Phe
        10                                         20

                90                  105                     120
CCG CCA GAC TAC GGC TTC CCC GAA CGC AAG GAG CGC GAG ATG GTG GCC ACA CAG
Pro Pro Asp Tyr Gly Phe Pro Glu Arg Lys Glu Arg Glu Met Val Ala Thr Gln
                30                                          40

    135                 150                     165                 180
CAG GAG ATG ATG GAC GCG AGT GAG GCT CAG CTG CGG GAC TAC TGC GCC CAC CAC
Gln Glu Met Met Asp Ala Ser Glu Ala Gln Leu Arg Asp Tyr Cys Ala His His
                        50                                          60

            195                 210                 225
CTC ATC CGG CTG CTC AAG TGC AAG CGT GAC AGC TTC CCA AGT TGC TGG CCT GCA
Leu Ile Arg Leu Leu Lys Cys Lys Arg Asp Ser Phe Pro Ser Cys Trp Pro Ala
                                70

240                     255                 270                 285
AGC AGG AAG CGG CAC GAC TCG GGA CTA CTG CGC ACC GCA AGC TAT GTG ATG CGC
Ser Arg Lys Arg His Asp Ser Gly Leu Leu Arg Thr Ala Ser Tyr Val Met Arg
 80  +   +   +  (+)                      +                           +

        300                 315                 330                 345
ATG AAG GAG TTT GAG CGG GAC GAG GGC TGC TCC AGC GGA AGA AGC GGC GGG AGA
Met Lys Glu Phe Glu Arg Asp Glu Gly Cys Ser Ser Gly Arg Ser Gly Gly Arg
     +  100          +                          110  +               +

                360                 375                 390
AGA AGG CGG CAA ATC TGC AAA GGC CAG GGA CCC GGG GAA GTG GAC CCC AAG GTG
Arg Arg Arg Gln Ile Cys Lys Gly Gln Gly Pro Gly Glu Val Asp Pro Lys Val
 +   +   +      120                                     130

    405                 420         430          440          450
GCC CTG TAG GG    GTGCACCCCC   CACCCTATGG   ACCAGTCAAA   TAAAACCTTC
Ala Leu  *
    135

       460          470          480        486
AGGCCCCTCA   AAAAAAAAAA   AAAAAAAAAA   AAAAAA
```

Figure 4 Gene and predicted amino acid sequence of SQM1 membrane protein.

The protein most closely similar to SQM1 polypeptide is the beta subunit of the human leukocyte adhesion proteins (Kishimoto et al., 1987), which are members of the integrin superfamily. The regions of similarity were located at one of the tandem repeats of the 8-cysteine motif and to the proximal extracellular region to the transmembrane domain of the leukocyte adhesion molecules. The region of endothelial GpIIIa, another member of the integrin superfamily, similar to SQM1 polypeptide is located at one of its cysteine-rich repeat (Fitzgerald et al., 1987).

GpIIIa is known to complex with GpIIb to form a Ca^{++}-dependent heterodimer that can bind fibronectin and vWF (Fitzgerald et al., 1987), and can form attachment sites for cytoskeletal proteins (Dejana et al., 1988). Two regions of the SQM1 polypeptide are similar to two regions abutting the N-terminus of two of the tandem triple repeats (Sadler et al., 1985) and promote endothelial cell adhesion (Dejana et al., 1988). The region of complement C8beta similar to SQM1 polypeptide is located near its C-terminus (Haefliger et al., 1987). This region is also repeated in its N-terminus as a duplicated sequence. The beta chain is known to mediate binding of C8 and C5b-7 during the formation of the membrane pore-forming complex (Monahan and Sodetz, 1981).

The evidence presented suggests that SQM1 polypeptide has several domains similar to those found in the beta subunit of integrins. However, the limited sequence similarity with the beta subunit of integrins, the smaller molecular weight, and the lack of transmembrane domain differentiate it from the integrins. Its presumptive role in cell adhesion of carcinoma cells, endothelial cells, and extracellular matrix (ECM) proteins, and its similarity with the leukocyte adhesion molecules and GpIIIa suggest that SQM1 polypeptide may play an important role in the metastasis of squamous carcinomas. It is possible that these SQM1 polypeptide-containing squamous carcinoma cells might detach from the primary site and be able to adhere to and penetrate the subendothelial matrix and the endothelium to establish secondary sites. The elevated expression of a lymphocyte adhesion protein, CDw44 in colon carcinomas, has recently been postulated to facilitate tumor cell adherence to EMC and promote tumor invasiveness (Stamenkovic et al., 1989).

The most striking feature of the deduced polypeptide is the presence of an almost perfect heptadic repeat of positively charged arginine residues over a range of 36 residues, near the C-terminal region. This heptadic repeat is found in the region of the polypeptide that can assume an alpha helical secondary structure (Chou and Fasman, 1978). Within a span of 11 turns of the alpha helix, the positively charged side chains of these 6 arginine residues are aligned on one side of the alpha helix. There are only a few sequences in the GenBank/Los Alamos translated sequence database (Release 58) and the National Biomedical Research Foundation (NBRF) protein sequence database (Release 18) containing a heptadic repeat of six or more positively charged residues. The protein with the highest number of arginines in heptadic repeat is the *Drosophila* glue protein, Sgs4C1 (Muskavitch and Hogness 1982), which is used for pupil attachment during metamorphosis. It is interesting that, aside from SQM1 polypeptide, another protein with a heptadic repeat of positively charged residues also has adhesive function. In addition, it was found that the DHFR gene also contains a similar motif of heptadic repeat of positive charges, which is of interest because of SQM1's possible role in the regulation of methotrexate transport.

Flanking these heptadic repeat are runs of four positively charged amino acid residues. Charged runs have been found to be important in protein transport, localization, and regulatory function (Karlin et al., 1989). In SQM1 polypeptide, these runs of positive charges are themselves flanked by cysteines. These flanking cysteines, through intermolecular or intramolecular disulfide bonds, may stabilize the positions of the runs of positively charged residues and align positive charges on one side of the helix. This stabilized alignment of positive charges may contribute to quaternary interaction of SQM1 polypeptide with negatively charged polypeptides. The deduced amino acid sequence of SQM1 polypeptide does not reveal any significant hydrophobic region suggestive of a transmembrane domain. However, in light of this possible quaternary interaction, SQM1 polypeptide may be stabilized on the surface membrane by its interaction with an integral membrane protein as part of a protein complex. Preliminary immunoprecipitation and immunoblotting studies suggest that SQM1 antigen forms complexes with at least two other proteins. Characterization of these other proteins will allow us to clarify the protein–protein interactions of SQM1 protein.

VIII. Conclusion

Parallel studies of the differentiation of normal human bronchial epithelial (NBE) cells and lung cancers are useful for investigations of the role of specific membrane molecules in differentiation-related functions. Subpopulations of NBE cells, which are indistinguishable by morphologic criteria, can be identified in culture and in tissues by characterization of epithelial membrane antigens expressed in these cells. During squamous differentiation of NBE cells in culture, a new membrane antigen (SQM1) is induced. The expression of SQM1 is associated with increased NBE cell adhesion. In carcinomas, SQM1 also appears to play a role in cell–cell adhesion and drug transport. These studies suggest that specific membrane molecules, such as SQM1, may provide links between differentiation, cell adhesion, and drug sensitivity.

References

Alt, F. W., Kellems, R. E., Bertino, J. R., and Schimke, R. T. (1978). Selective multiplication of dihydrofolate reductase genes in methotrexate-resistant variants of cultured murine cells. *J. Biol. Chem.* **253:**1357–1370.

Auerbach, O., Gere, J. B., and Forman, J. B. (1957). Changes in the bronchial epithelium in relation to smoking and cancer of the lung. *N. Engl. J. Med.* **256:**97–104.

Banks-Schlegel, S., and Green, H. (1981). Involucrin synthesis and tissue assembly by keratinocytes in natural and cultured human epithelia. *J. Cell. Biol.* **90:**732–737.

Banks-Schlegel, S., Gazdar, A. F., and Harris, C. C. (1985). Intermediate filament and cross-linked envelope expression in human lung tumor cell lines. *Cancer Res.* **45:** 1187–1197.

Bernal, S. D., Shapiro, H. M., and Chen, L. B. (1982). Monitoring the effect of anti-cancer drugs on L1012 cells by a mitochondrial probe, rhodamine-123. *Int. J. Cancer* **30:** 219–224.

Bernal, S. D., Weinberg, K., Kakefuda, M., Stahel, R., O'Hara, C., and Wong, Y.-C. (1988). Membrane antigens of human bronchial epithelial cells identified by monoclonal antibodies. *In Vitro* **24**(No.2)**:**February.

Bernal, S. D., Speak, J. A., Boeheim, K., Dreyfuss, A. I., Wright, J. E., Teicher, B. A., Rosowsky, A., Tsao, S. W., and Wong, Y. C. (1990a). *Mol. Cell. Biochem.* **95:**61–70.

Bernal, S. D., Wong, Y. C., and Kakefuda, M. (1990b). A new membrane protein antigen is associated with differentiation and drug sensitivity in respiratory carcinomas. In *Biology of Respiratory Cells*. Edited by S. D. Bernal and S. Baylin. New York, Marcel Dekker.

Boeheim, K., Speak, J. A., Frei, E. 3d, and Bernal, S. D. (1985). SQM1 antibody defines a surface in squamous carcinoma of the head and neck. *Int. J. Cancer* **36:**137–142.

Boeheim, K., Scwarzfurtner, H., Boeheim, C., Frei E. 3d, and Bernal, S. D. (1986). Immunohistochemical identification of squamous carcinoma of the head and neck with monoclonal antibody SQM1. *Acta Otolaryngol. (Stockh.)* **102:**333–340.

Bourdon, M. A., Oldberg, A., Pierschbacher, M., and Ruoslahti, E. (1985). *Proc. Natl. Acad. Sci. USA* **82:**1321–1325.

Carman, M. D., Schornagel, J. H., Rivest, R. S., Srimatkandada, S., Portlock, C. S., Duffy, T., and Bertino, J. R. (1984). Resistance to methotrexate due to gene amplification in a patient with acute leukemia. *J. Clin. Oncol.* **2:**16–20.

Chou, P. Y., and Fasman, G. D. (1978). Prediction of the secondary structure of proteins from their amino acid sequence. *Adv. Enzymol.* **47:**45–148.

Cowan, K. H., and Jolivet, J. (1984). A methotrexate-resistant human breast cancer cell line with multiple defects, including diminished formation of methotrexate polyglutamates. *J. Biol. Chem.* **259:**10793–10800.

Cutz, E. (1982). Neuroendocrine cells of the lung. An overview of morphologic characteristics and development. *Exp. Lung Res.* **3**(3–4)**:**185–208.

Dejana, E., Languino, L. R., Colella, S., Corbascio, G. C., Plow, E., Ginsberg, M., and Marchisio, P. C. (1988). The localization of a platelet GpIIb-IIa-related protein in endothelial cell adhesion structures. *Blood* **71:**566–572.

Fitzgerald, L. A., Steiner, B., Rall, S. C. Jr., and Phillips, D. R. (1987). Protein sequence of endothelial glycoprotein IIIa derived from a cDNA clone. Identity with platelet glycoprotein IIa and similarity to "integrin." *J. Biol. Chem.* **262:**3936–3939.

Flintoff, W. F., and Essani, K. (1980). Methotrexate-resistant chinese hamster ovary cells contain a dihydrofolate reductase with an altered affinity for methotrexate. *Biochemistry* **19:**4321–4327.

Frei, E. 3d, Rosowsky, A., Wright, J. E., Cucchi, C. A., Lippke, J. A., Ervin, T. J., Jolivet, J., and Haseltine, W. A. (1984). Development of methotrexate resistance in a human squamous cell carcinoma of the head and neck in culture. *Proc. Natl. Acad. Sci. USA* **81:**2873–2877.

Fuchs, E., and Green, H. (1980). Changes in keratin expression during terminal differentiation of the keratinocyte. *Cell* **19:**1033–1042.

Gould, V. E., Linnoila, I., Memoli, V. A., and Warren, W. H. (1983). The neuroendocrine component of the bronchopulmonary tree: hyperplasias, dysplasias and neoplasms. *Lab. Invest.* **49:**519.

Haefliger, J.-A., Tschopp, J., Nardelli, D., Wahli, W., Kocher, H.-P. Tosi, M., and Stanley, K. K. (1987). Complementary DNA cloning of complement C8 beta and its sequence homology to C9. *Biochemistry* **26:**3551–3556.

Hatta, K., and Takeichi, M. (1986). Expression of N-cadherin adhesion molecules associated with early morphogenetic events in chick development. *Nature* **320:**447–449.

Hirano, S., Nose, A., Hatta, K., Kawakami, A., and Takeichi, M. (1987). Calcium-dependent cell–cell adhesion molecules (cadherins): subclass specificities and possible involvement of actin bundles. *J. Cell Biol.* **105:**2501–2510.

Hynes, R. O. (1987). Integrins: a family of cell surface receptors. *Cell* **48:**549–554.

Jetten, A. M. (1989). Multistep process of squamous differentiation in tracheobronchial epithelial cells in vitro: analogy with epidermal differentiation. *Environ. Health Perspect.* **80:**149–160.

Jetten, A. M., and Shirley, J. E. (1986). Characterization of transglutamase activity in rabbit tracheal epithelial cells. Regulation by retinoids. *J. Biol. Chem.* **261:**15097–15101.

Jones, J. C., Yokoo, K. M., and Goldman, R. D. (1986). Further analysis of pemphigus autoantibodies and their use in studies on the heterogeneity, structure, and function of desmosomes. *J. Cell Biol.* **102:**1109–1117.

Juliano, R. L. (1987). Membrane receptors for extracellular matrix molecules: relationship to cell adhesion and tumor metastasis. *Biochim. Biophys. Acta* **907:**261–278.

Karlin, S., Blaisdell, B. E., Mocarski, E. S., and Brendel, V. (1989). *J. Mol. Biol.* **205:** 165–177.

Keenan, K. P., Wilson, T. S., and McDowell, E. M. (1983). Regeneration of hamster tracheal epithelium after mechanical injury. IV. Histochemical, immunocytochemical and ultrastructural studies. *Virchows Arch. [B].* **43**(3)**:**213–240.

Kishimoto, T. K., O'Connor, K., Lee, A., Roberts, T. M., and Springer, T. A. (1987). Cloning of the beta subunit of the leukocyte adhesion proteins: homology to an extracellular matrix receptor defines a novel supergene family. *Cell* **48:**681–690.

Kozak, M. (1984). Compilation and analysis of sequences upstream from the translational start site in eukaryotic mRNAs. *Nucl. Acids Res.* **12:**857–872.

Larjava, H., Peltonen, J., Akiyama, S. K., Yamada, S. S., Gralnick, J. U., and Yamada, K. M. (1990). Novel function for betal integrins in keratinocyte cell–cell interactions. *J. Cell Biol.* **110:**803–815.

Laterra, J., Silbert, J. E., and Culp, L. A. (1983). Cell surface heparan sulfate mediates some adhesive responses to glycosaminoglycan-binding matrices, including fibronectin. *J. Cell Biol.* **96**(1)**:**112–123.

Lechner, J. F., Haugen, A., Autrum, H., McClendon, I. A., Trump, B. F., and Harris, C C. (1981). Clonal growth of epithelial cells from normal adult human bronchus. *Cancer Res.* **41:**2294–2304.

Lechner, J. F., Haugen, A., McClendon, I. A., and Pettis, E. W. (1982). Clonal growth of normal adult human bronchial epithelial cells in a serum-free medium. *In Vitro* **18** (7)**:**633–642.

Lechner, J. F., McClendon, I. A., LaVeck, M. A., Shamsuddin, A. M., and Harris, C. C.

(1983). Differential control by platelet factors of squamous differentiation in normal and malignant human bronchial epithelial cells. *Cancer Res.* **43:**5915–5921.

Lechner, J. F., Haugen, A., McClendon, L. A., and Shamsuddin, A. M. (1984). Induction of squamous differentiation of normal human bronchial epithelial cells by small amounts of serum. *Differentiation* **25:**229–237.

Liotta, L. A. (1986). Tumor invasion and metastases—role of the extracellular matrix: Rhoads Memorial Award lecture. *Cancer Res.* **46:**1–7.

McDowell, E. M., and Trump, B. F. (1983). Histogenesis of preneoplastic and neoplastic lesions in tracheobronchial epithelium. *Surv. Synth. Pathol. Res.* **2:**235–279.

Monahan, J. B., and Sodetz, J. M. (1981). Role of the beta subunit in interaction of the eighth component of human complement with the membrane-bound cytolytic complex. *J. Biol. Chem.* **256:**3258–3262.

Moran, R. G., Mulkins, M., and Heidelberger, C. (1979). Role of thymidylate synthetase activity in development of methotrexate cytotoxicity. *Proc. Natl. Acad. Sci. USA* **76:** 5924–5928.

Muskavitch, M. A. T., and Hogness, D. S. (1982). An expandable gene that encodes a *Drosophila* glue protein is not expressed in variants lacking remote upstream sequences. *Cell* **29:**1041–1051.

Obrink, B. (1986). Epithelial cell adhesion molecules. *Exp. Cell. Res.* **163:**1–21.

Ohnuma, T., Lo, R. J., Scanlon, K. J., Kamen, B. A., Ohnoshi, T., Wolman, S. R., and Holland, J. F. (1985). Evolution of MTX resistance of human acute lymphoblastic leukemia cells in vitro. *Cancer Res.* **45:**1815–1822.

Pearse, A. G. (1969). The cytochemistry and ultrastructure of polypeptide hormone-producing cells of the APUD series and the embryologic, physiologic and pathologic implications of the concept. *J. Histochem. Cytochem.* **17**(5)**:**303–313.

Poste, G., and Fidler, I. J. (1980). The pathogenesis of cancer metastasis. *Nature* **283:**139–146.

Proudfoot, N. J., and Brownlee, G. G. (1976). 3′ Non-coding region sequences in eukaryotic messenger RNA. *Nature* **263:**211–214.

Rearick, J. I., Hesterberg, T. W., and Jetten, A. M. (1987). Human bronchial epithelial cells synthesize cholesterol sulfate during squamous differentiation in vitro. *J. Cell. Physiol.* **133:**573–578.

Reid, L. M., and Coles, S. J. (1984). The bronchial epithelium of humans. In *The Endocrine Lung*. Edited by K. L. Becker and A. F. Gazdar. Philadelphia, W. B. Saunders, pp. 56–78.

Richa, J., Damsky, C. H., Buck, C. A., Knowles, B. B., and Solter, D. (1985). Cell surface glycoproteins mediate compaction, trophoblast attachment, and endoderm formation during early mouse development. *Dev. Biol.* **108:**513–521.

Sadler, J. E., Shelton-Inloes, B. B., Sorace, J. M., Harlan, J. M., Titani, K., and Davie, E. W. (1985). Cloning and characterization of two cDNAs coding for human von Willebrand factor. *Proc. Natl. Acad. Sci. USA* **82**(19)**:**6394–6398.

Saffiotti, U., Stinson, S. F., Keenan, K. P., and McDowell, E. M. (1985). Tumor enhancement factors and mechanisms in the hamster respiratory tract carcinogenesis model. *Carcinogen. Compr. Surv.* **8:**63–92.

Sanger, F., Nicklen, S., and Coulson, A. R. (1977). DNA sequencing with chain-terminating inhibitors. *Proc. Natl. Acad. Sci. USA* **74:**5463–5467.

Stamenkovic, I., Amiot, M., Pesando, J. M., and Seed, B. (1989). A lymphocyte molecule implicated in lymph node homing is a member of the cartilage link protein family. *Cell* **56:**1057–1062.

Stoner, G. D., Harris, C. C., Myers, G. A., Trump, B. F., and Connor, R. D. (1980). Putrescine stimulates growth of human bronchial epithelial cells in primary culture. *In Vitro* **51:**399–406.

Sun, T.-T., Eichner, R., Nelson, W. G., Tseng, S. C. G., Weiss, R. A., Jarvinen, M., and Woodcock-Mitchell, J. (1983). Keratin classes: molecular markers for different types of epithelial differentiation. *J. Invest. Dermatol.* **81:**109s–115s.

Thacher, S. M., and Rice, R. H. (1985). Keratinocyte-specific transglutamase of culture human epidermal cells: relation to cross-linked envelope formation and terminal differentiation. *Cell* **40:**685–695.

Trump, B. F., McDowell, E. M., Glavin, F., Battet, L. A., Becci, P. J., Schurch, W., Kaiser, H. E., and Harris, C. C. (1978). The respiratory epithelium III. Histogenesis of epidermoid metaplasia and carcinoma in situ in the human. *J. Natl. Cancer Inst.* **61:** 563–575.

Tsao, S.-W., Chew, E. C., Yam, H. F., and Bernal, S. D. (1989). Ultrastructural localization of a new surface membrane antigen (SQM1) related to squamous differentiation. *In Vivo* **3:**367–374.

Volk, T., Cohen, O., and Geiger, B. (1987). Formation of heterotypic adherens-type junctions between L-CAM containing lens cells. *Cell* **50:**897–894.

Watt, F. M., and Green, H. (1981). Involucrin synthesis is correlated with cell size in human epidermal cultures. *J. Cell. Biol.* **90:**738–742.

White, J. C., and Goldman, I. D. (1981). MTX resistance in an L1210 cell line resulting from increased dihydrofolate reductase, decreased thymidylate synthetase activity, and normal membrane transport. Computer simulations based on network thermodynamics. *J. Biol. Chem.* **256:**5722–5727.

Willey, J. C., LaVeck, M. A., McClendon, I. A. et al., (1988). Relationship of ornithine decarboxylase activity and cAMP metabolism to proliferation of normal human bronchial epithelial cells. *J. Cell. Physiol.* **124:**207–212.

Wong, Y.-C., Tsao, S.-W, Kakefuda, M., and Bernal, S. D. (1990). cDNA cloning of a novel cell adhesion protein expressed in human squamous carcinoma cells. *Biochem. Biophys. Res. Commun.* **166**(2)**:**984–992.

Yamada, K. M. (1983) Cell surface interactions with extracellular materials. *Annu. Rev. Biochem.* **52:**761–799.

4

Transcriptional Enhancers Associated with Differentiation of Lung Carcinoma Cells

YUK-CHOR WONG and SAMUEL D. BERNAL

Boston University Medical Center
Boston, Massachusetts

I. Introduction

The human bronchial epithelium is a complex structure made up of many different cell types (Gail and Lenfant, 1983; Reid and Coles, 1984). Experimental evidence suggests that the various bronchial mucosal cells and their corresponding tumors are likely to be derived from a common stem cell (see review by Yesner, 1979). Progenitor cells derived from the stem cells undergo progressive differentiation into various differentiated cell types. Along the differentiation pathway are critical landmarks where the progenitor cells embark on more specialized and restricted differentiation pathways. Dependent on where tumorigenesis takes place with respect to these landmarks, the resultant tumor will assume a particular histologic characteristic and a particular level of differentiation. It is assumed that the switching occurring at these landmarks is affected by the expression of specific subsets of genes, which in turn are regulated by their enhancers and the corresponding transcription regulatory factors in the cell. We discuss here the use of heterologous enhancers in characterizing the differentiation of lung carcinoma cell lines.

II. Enhancers and Gene Expression

Enhancers are *cis*-regulatory elements of gene transcription and are known to consist of multiple and sometimes overlapping DNA sequence motifs, which are binding sites for specific *trans*-acting transcription factors (Schirm et al., 1987; Ondek et al., 1988; Dynan, 1989). Whether an enhancer functions in a particular cell type is ultimately dependent upon the repertoire of transcription factors present in that cell type. Enhancer cell-type specificity has been observed in many systems, including the SV40, polyoma, and immunoglobulin enhancers (de Villiers et al., 1982; Davidson et al., 1986; Gillies et al., 1983).

III. Differentiation and Enhancers

Cellular differentiation is affected by the expression of specific subsets of genes. The differentiation state of a cell is assumed to be maintained by the coordinate regulation of transcription of a specific subset of genes, mediated through transcription factors that bind to the enhancers of these genes. It is known that the differentiation state of the host cell can determine whether a particular virus can express its genome via its enhancer. Many viruses, such as SV40, polyoma virus, and Moloney murine leukemia virus, are able to express their genomes in differentiated cells but not in undifferentiated cells (Linenbach et al., 1980; Swartzendruber and Lehman, 1975; Stewart et al., 1982). One possible explanation is that the cellular transcription factors required for essential viral function are induced during host cell differentiation. Since these factors are likely to be involved in the regulation of important cellular functions in the host cell, they must be tightly regulated during differentiation.

Enhancer activity is known to be modulated by the differentiation state of the cell. Using transient transfection assays, Nakshatri et al. (1990) found that the enhancer of the human papovavirus, JCV, was active in differentiated but not in undifferentiated embryonic carcinoma cells. In human embryonic carcinoma cells, activities of SV40, BKV, adenovirus, and RSV enhancer are greatly induced in differentiated cells (Hasegawa et al., 1990). On the other hand, the SV40 enhancer is highly active in a preadipose cell line, but is suppressed when the cells are induced to differentiate into adipose cells (Djian et al., 1988). This suppression of enhancer activity can be due to a loss of a transcription activator or the gain of a transcription repressor in differentiated cells. A *trans*-acting negative factor has been implicated previously in the suppression of enhancer activity in embryonic carcinoma cells (Gorman et al., 1985). Based on these observations, and coupled with the fact that enhancer-binding factors are required at the establishment but not the maintenance step of enhancer-dependent transcriptional activation (Wang and Calame, 1986), it is reasonable to assume that the difference in repertoire of transcription factors can be exploited to probe the differentiation state of cells by using a panel of heterologous enhancers.

IV. SV40 Enhancer

SV40 enhancer, one of the best characterized enhancers, is known to function in a wide variety of cell types. It is made up of hierarchically organized subunits called enhansons, which bind different cellular transcription factors (Ondek et al., 1988). The function of the SV40 enhancer is ultimately dependent on the summation of the interactions between these transcription factors and their corresponding enhansons. Transcription factors including AP-1, AP-2, and AP-3, and their binding sites, have been studied extensively (Lee et al., 1987a; Mitchell et al., 1987). The AP-2 site, together with the adjacent AP-3 site, form the SV40 enhancer core domain. Transcription factor AP-1 has been observed in the activation of many cellular genes including the metallothionein gene and the collagenase gene (Lee et al., 1987b). The product of *c-jun*, a major component of AP-1, can form dimers with the product of *c-fos*. These complexes can then either activate or repress transcription activity of genes containing an AP-1 site. Murine embryonic carcinoma cells studied so far lack *c-jun*/AP-1 activity, while differentiation of these cells induces a great increase in *c-jun*/AP-1 activity (de Groot et al., 1990).

V. SV40 Enhancer and Lung Carcinomas

A. SV40 Enhancer Utilization

In transient expression experiments using a reporter gene encoding bacterial chloramphenicol acetyltransferase, we found that non-small-cell lung carcinoma cells, especially adenocarcinomas and squamous carcinomas were 2–3 orders of magnitude more efficient than small cell lung carcinoma cells in utilizing the SV40 enhancer (Wong and Bernal, 1990). Among the small cell carcinomas, variant small cell carcinomas used the SV40 enhancer more efficiently than the classic small cell carcinomas (Fig. 1). We also found that an attached variant small cell carcinoma cell line had an intermediate level of utilization of the SV40 enhancer between the parent suspension small cell carcinoma cell line and non-small-cell carcinoma cell lines. These observations are consistent with the previously described cell-type-specific and differentiation-regulated expression of the SV40 enhancer.

B. Differential Expression of Enhancer-Binding Proteins

To correlate the differential utilization of the SV40 enhancer in the various types of lung carcinoma with the expression of functional transcription factors in these

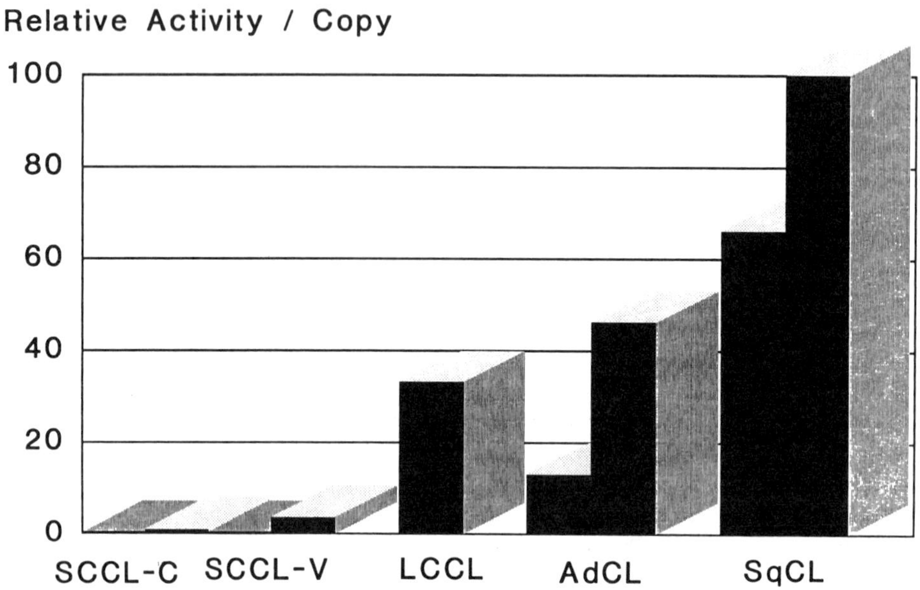

Figure 1 SV40 enhancer activity in transfected lung carcinoma cell lines. Squamous carcinoma (SqCL), adenocarcinoma (AdCL), large cell carcinoma (LCCL), classic small cell carcinoma (SCCL-C), and variant small cell carcinoma (SCCL-V) cells of the lung were transfected with pSV2*cat*, a plasmid containing the bacterial chloramphenicol acetyltransferase (CAT) gene under the control of the SV40 enhancer. CAT activity was measured and expressed as relative CAT activity per CAT gene copy. (Gorman et al., 1982).

carcinoma cells, gel mobility shift experiments were performed. The Sph I 72 bp fragment containing AP-1, AP-2, and AP-3 sites was used as the target sequence for incubation with nuclear extracts from the various lung carcinoma cells. Complex formation between transcription factors and the target DNA sequence was then detected by the altered electrophoretic mobility in polyacrylamide gels. As shown in Figure 2, large cell carcinoma cells (lane 3) and classic small cell carcinoma cells (lane 4) contained very little DNA-binding activity to the 72 bp fragment. On the other hand, squamous carcinoma cells (lane 1) and adenocarcinoma cells (lane 2) showed a much higher DNA-binding activity. However, the species of DNA-protein complexes were different between the squamous carcinoma cells (indicated by arrows b and c) and the adenocarcinoma cells (indicated by arrows d, e, and f). This difference could be due to the presence of different DNA-binding proteins and/or different DNA–protein stoichiometry in these carcinoma cells. Variant small cell carcinoma cells were found to show a DNA–protein pattern resembling that of adenocarcinoma cells.

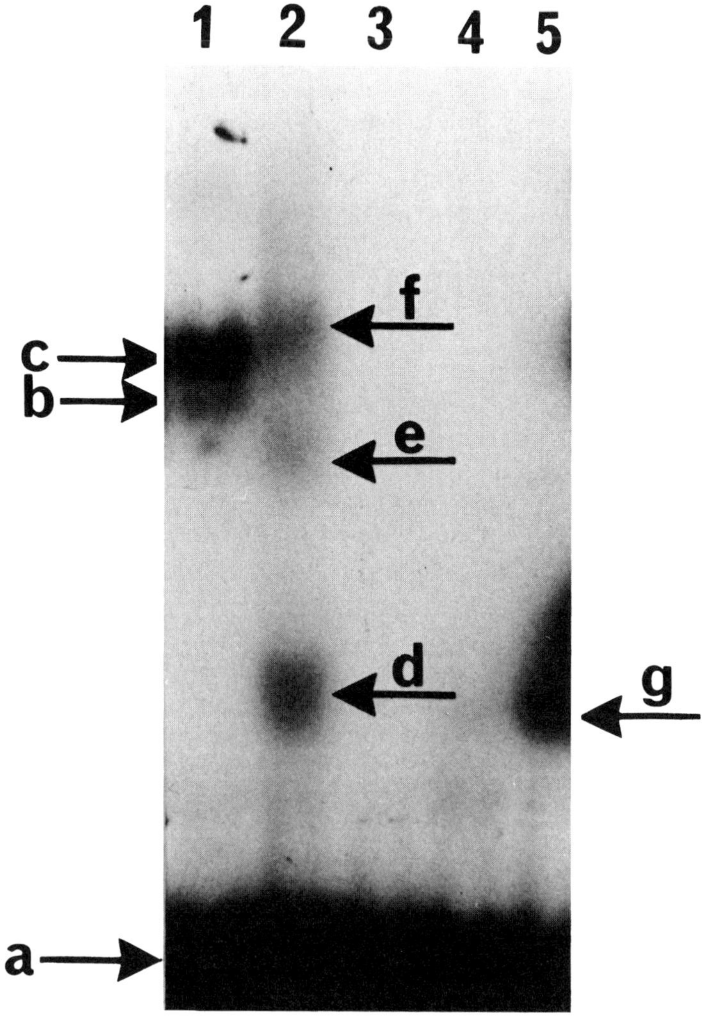

Figure 2 Electrophoretic mobility shift experiments. 2 ng of ^{32}P-labeled 72 bp SphI-SphI DNA fragment of the SV40 enhancer was incubated with 1 μg of nuclear protein extract from squamous carcinoma (lane 1), adenocarcinoma (lane 2), large cell carcinoma (lane 3), classic small cell carcinoma (lane 4), or variant small cell carcinoma (lane 5) cells in the presence of 100 ng of poly(I)poly(C) at 22°C for 15 min before electrophoresis in an 8% low ionic strength polyacrylamide gel. The different species of DNA-protein complex are indicated by arrows (a–g). Arrow a indicates the free 72 bp fragment.

VI. Conclusions

The different histologic types of lung carcinomas, although sharing a likely common cellular origin, differ in their biological and biochemical characteristics (Carney et al., 1984). Different subsets of genes regulated by different repertoires of transcription factors are assumed to be operating in these various types of lung carcinomas. We have demonstrated that a heterologous enhancer such as the SV40 enhancer can be used to probe the histologic type and the differentiation state of lung carcinoma cells. Small cell carcinoma cells were found likely to be lacking the transcription factors AP-1, AP-2, and AP-3 required for functioning of the SV40 enhancer, whereas adenocarcinoma cells and squamous carcinoma cells expressed large amounts of these factors. A rat pituitary cell line with neurosecretory characteristics similar to that of small cell lung carcinoma cells was found to be incapable of using the SV40 enhancer (Schirm et al., 1987). AP-2 and AP-3 sites were found to be essential for SV40 enhancer function in HeLa cells, a squamous carcinoma, and in MCF-7, an adenocarcinoma (Schirm et al., 1987). Thus, a panel of enhanson elements might be useful tools in the study of differentiation-related transcription regulation in lung carcinomas.

References

Carney, D. N., Gazdar, A. F., Cuttitta, F., and Minna, J. D. (1984). In vitro studies of the biology of lung cancer. In *Lung Cancer: Causes and Prevention*. Edited by M. Mizell and P. Correa. Deerfield Beach, FL, Verlag Chemie, pp. 247–261.

Davidson, I., Fromental C., Augereau, P., Wilderman, A., Zenke, M., and Chambon, P. (1986). Cell-type specific protein binding to the enhancer of simian virus 40 in nuclear extract. *Nature* **323**:544–548.

de Groot, R. P., Kruyt, F. A. E., Van der Saag, P. T., and Kruijer, W. (1990). Ectopic expression of c-jun leads to differentiation of P19 embryonic carcinoma cells. *EMBO J.* **9**:1831–1837.

de Villiers, J., Olson, L., Tyndall, C., and Schaffner, W. (1982). Transcriptional "enhancers" from SV40 and polyoma virus show a cell type preference. *Nucl. Acids Res.* **10**:7965–7976.

Djian, P., Phillips, M., and Green, H. (1988). Suppression of SV40-promoted gene expression by differentiation of preadipose cells. *Genes Dev.* **2**:1251–1257.

Dynan, W. S. (1989). Modularity in promoters and enhancers. *Cell* **58**:1–4.

Gail, D. B., and Lenfant C. J. M. (1983). Cells of the lung: biology and clinical implications. *Am. Rev. Respir. Dis.* **127**:366–387.

Gillies, S. D., Morrison, S. L., Oi, V. T., and Tonegawa, S. (1983). A tissue-specific transcription enhancer element is located in the major intron of a rearranged immunoglobulin heavy chain gene. *Cell* **33**:717–728.

Gorman, C. M., Moffat, L. F., and Howard, B. H. (1982). Recombinant genomes which express chloramphenicol acetyltransferase in mammalian cells. *Mol. Cell. Biol.* **2:** 1044–1051.

Gorman, C. M., Rigby, P. W. J., and Lane, D. P. (1985). Negative regulation of viral enhancers in undifferentiated embryonic stem cells. *Cell* **42:**519–526.

Hasegawa, T., Nakada, S., Nakajima, T., Oda, K., Kawata, M., Kimura, H., and Sekiya, S. (1990). Expression of various viral and cellular enhancer-promoters during differentiation of human embryonal carcinoma cells. *Differentiation* **42:**191–198.

Lee, W., Haslinger, A., Karin, M., and Tjian, R. (1987a). Activation of transcription by two factors that bind promoter and enhancer sequences of the human metallothionein gene and SV40. *Nature* **325:**368–372.

Lee, W., Mitchell, P., and Tjian, R. (1987b). Purified transcription factors AP-1 interacts with TPA-inducible enhancer elements. *Cell* **49:**741–752.

Linenbach, A., Huebner, K., and Croce, C. M. (1980). DNA transformed murine teratocarcinoma cells: regulation of expression of Simian virus 40 tumor antigens in stem versus differentiated cells. *Proc. Natl. Acad. Sci. USA* **77:**4875–4879.

Mitchell, P. J., Wang, C., and Tjian, R. (1987). Positive and negative regulation of transcription in vitro: enhancer-binding protein AP-2 is inhibited by SV40 T antigen. *Cell* **50:**847–861.

Nakshatri, H., Pater, A., and Pater, M. M. (1990). Activity and enhancer binding factors for JC virus regulatory elements in differentiating embryonic carcinoma cells. *Virology* **177:**784–789.

Ondek, B., Gloss, L., and Winship, H. (1988). The SV40 enhancer contains two distinct levels of organization. *Nature* **333:**40–45.

Reid, L. M., and Coles, S. J. (1984). The bronchial epithelium of humans. In *The Endocrine Lung in Health and Disease*. Edited by K. L. Becker and A. F. Gazdar. Philadelphia, WB Saunders, pp. 56–78.

Schirm, S., Jiricny, J., and Schaffner, W. (1987). The SV40 enhancer can be dissected into multiple segments each with a different cell type specificity. *Genes Devel.* **1:**65–74.

Stewart, C. L., Stuhlmann, H., Jahner, D., and Jaenisch, R. (1982). De novo methylation, expression and infectivity of retroviral genomes introduced into embryonal carcinoma cells. *Proc. Natl. Acad. Sci. USA* **79:**4098–4102.

Swartzendruber, D. E., and Lehman, J. M. (1975). Neoplastic differentiation: interaction of Simian virus 40 and polyoma virus with murine teratocarcinoma cell in vitro. *J. Cell Physiol.* **85:**179–188.

Wang, X.-F., and Calame, K. (1986). SV40 enhancer-binding factors are required at the establishment but not the maintenance step of enhancer-dependent transcriptional activation. *Cell* **47:**241–247.

Wong, Y.-C., and Bernal, S. D. (1990). Differential utilization of the SV40 enhancer and early promoter in various human lung carcinoma cell lines. *Int. J. Cancer* **45:** 911–915.

Yesner, R. (1979). Spectrum of lung cancer and ectopic hormones. In *Pathology Annual*, part I. Edited by S. C. Somers and P. P. Rosen. New York, Appleton-Century-Crofts, pp. 217–240.

5

A Cellular 68,000 MW Protein as a Differentiation Marker in Human Lung Cancer

JAMES A. RADOSEVICH, G. KENNETH HAINES, GHANASHYAM GHADGE, and BAYAR THIMMAPAYA

Northwestern University
VA Lakeside Medical Center
Chicago, Illinois

I. Introduction

The need to further our basic understanding about the biology of neoplasms arising in the lungs has recently been reinforced by reports that outline the lack of progress in treating these tumors (Humphrey et al., 1990; Brambilla et al., 1991). While considerable effort over the past two decades has greatly changed the way we view these neoplasms, there still remains a great deal to be clarified regarding their biology (Rosen et al., 1988; Gruhn et al., 1990). For a variety of reasons, problems arise in the design of new and effective treatment strategies. In part, this is because we lack a sufficient understanding of the biological properties that govern this diverse group of tumors. We also lack markers that will allow the consistent classification of these neoplasms. In addition, many other factors influence how these tumors behave in vivo, including their degree of differentiation, location, expression of various biological characteristics, as well as other factors. While great effort, and some progress, has been made using monoclonal antibodies (MCAs) and other biological probes to classify these neoplasms, much remains to be done. Reviews of the MCAs directed against pulmonary neoplasms, as well as those with selective activity against these tumors, have been reported elsewhere (Radosevich et al., 1988). The majority of these MCAs have been directed at providing a selective and sensitive way to differentiate one histologic subtype from another.

In general, patients with well-differentiated tumors have a more indolent course, and therefore do better than patients with less well-differentiated tumors. Various histologic features such as keratin pearl formation in squamous cell carcinomas, and glandular structures in adenocarcinomas, have been used as indicators of the degree of differentiation being expressed by a particular tumor. The use of light microscopic evaluation and routine hematoxylin and eosin-stained tissue sections have limitations that have been outlined elsewhere (Radosevich et al., Chapter 11, this volume). The use of immunoperoxidase staining with MCAs can greatly reduce the subjective elements of evaluation, provided that the MCA is specific. This approach can also provide an assessment of the biological potential of the tissue in question. Any biological component that correlates with differentiation, which could be measured easily, would therefore be a valuable addition to the assessment of neoplastic tissue. In light of these considerations, we have produced a MCA that is directed against a fraction that contains p68 activity. We hypothesized that this normal cellular component could be important in cellular differentiation and cell growth potential. This chapter will review the current knowledge about the cellular enzyme, double-stranded RNA (dsRNA)-dependent protein kinase, p68 (also known as DAI, dsI, and P1) as it relates to differentiation and cell growth potential in lung cancer.

II. Functional Roles of p68

A. Biochemical and Molecular Properties

The cytoplasmic protein, p68, is constitutively expressed and has a molecular weight of 65–72 kD. In human cells it has a molecular weight of 68–70 kD, and 65–67 kD in other species (Farrel et al., 1977; Levin and London, 1978; Hovanessian, 1980; Krust et al., 1984; Buffet-Janvresse et al., 1986). Both monoclonal and polyclonal antisera have been made against p68 (Laurent et al., 1985; Galabru and Hovanessian, 1987). These immunoreagents have been used to select lambda phage constructs encoding the cDNA for this enzyme (Meurs et al., 1990). This protein has two activities: one is autophosphorylation, which is dependent on double-stranded RNA; the other is phosphorylation of protein synthesis initiation factor 2 (eIF-2). It is also activated by heparin and possibly by other unknown factors (Galabru and Hovanessian, 1985; Hovanessian and Galabru, 1987; Szyszka et al., 1989; Galabru et al., 1989). The activation of this enzyme is stimulated by Mn^{2+}. During activation p68 is phosphorylated at serine and threonine residues. The activation is independent of cyclic AMP and GMP (Samuel, 1979; Krust et al., 1984; Lasky et al., 1982; Galabru and Hovanessian, 1985). Autophosphorylation of p68, in part, results in the molecular weight differences observed upon separation by sodium dodecyl sulfate-polyacrylamide gel electrophoresis (SDS-PAGE). Once activated by autophosphorylation, p68 phosphorylates exogenous substrates.

B. Function During Protein Synthesis

One of the exogenous substrates that p68 phosphorylates is the alpha-subunit of eIF-2 (Galabru and Hovanessian, 1985). During the normal protein synthesis cycle, eIF-2 is activated in a GTP-coupled form. This reaction is carried out by guanine nucleotide exchange factor (GEF). GTP-eIF-2 forms a ternary complex with met-$tRNA_F$. This ternary complex then binds to the 40S ribosome subunit, which in turn binds to mRNA. These events further lead to the initiation of protein synthesis. During the initiation, the bound GTP is hydrolyzed to GDP. For the next cycle of initiation, GDP needs to be exchanged to GTP by GEF. When activated, p68 phosphorylates the alpha subunit of eIF-2, which results in the trapping of GEF with GDP-eIF-2. The inactive phosphorylated form of eIF-2 thereby blocks the initiation of protein synthesis by a reduction in the free pool of GEF. This activity can be monitored in a cell-free in vitro protein synthesis system, after separation on standard polyacrylamide gel electrophoresis. This assay system requires the use of fresh viable cells or tissue, and is relatively laborious.

C. Function During Viral Infection

During viral infection of cells by reovirus or encephalomyocarditis virus, p68 is activated and subsequently phosphorylates eIF-2 (Golgher et al., 1980; Gupta et al., 1982; Nilsen et al., 1982; Samuel et al., 1984; Rice et al., 1985; Hovanessian and Galabru, 1987). Studies using cells infected with adenovirus have shown that the p68 plays an important role in the control of both viral and host protein synthesis. However, the "small" RNAs synthesized by adenovirus at late times of infection prevent the activation of p68 (Reichel et al., 1985) and facilitate the protein synthesis required for replication of the virus. During the replication cycle of the virus, comparatively large amounts of "small" viral RNAs are produced. In this way, the virus may overwhelm the host defense system to allow viral protein synthesis.

Interferon is known to induce the expression of this enzyme (Hovanessian, 1989). This would seem appropriate in that cells infected by virus produce interferon, which in turn induces the expression of p68. This interferon induction would enhance the cell's ability to resist viral replication, in part, by increasing the host's p68 reserve.

D. Potential Role in Differentiation

The current understanding of the function of p68 in the absence of viral infection is limited. It has been speculated that it may play a role in the control of translation, which could influence both cell growth and differentiation (De Benedetti and

Baglioni, 1984, 1985; Pain, 1986; Petryshyn et al., 1988). In brief, if p68 were responsible, at least in part, for the slowing of cell growth, it might trigger events that would cause differentiation. As an alternative, as the cell becomes more differentiated, it could possibly express higher levels of p68. This would result in the inhibition of translation of other cell replication gene products, thereby holding the cell in a more differentiated state. If this hypothesis is correct, it would be reasonable that in normal tissues that are comparatively more differentiated there would be significantly more p68 expression. Likewise, in tissues that are continuously regenerating at a moderate rate (e.g., skin), there would be a spectrum of p68 expression, whereby the actively replicating basal layer would express less p68 than the more differentiated stratified epithelial layers. As a corollary to this, it might be postulated that neoplastic tissues may also express p68 to various degrees, depending on their degree of differentiation. However, in these "nonnormal" cells, it would be anticipated that there would be tumors that could bypass this regulatory element, and express p68 while retaining a modest growth rate. Likewise, other neoplastic cells may not express enhanced levels of p68 and have only marginal growth rates.

III. Expression of p68 in Lung Cancer

A. TJ4C4 as a Probe for p68

Using the now routine technique for producing MCAs directed against selected antigens, we produced the anti-p68 MCA, TJ4C4 (Gefter et al., 1977; Radosevich et al., 1985). In brief, pure soluble p68 from a human cervical carcinoma cell line (HeLa) was isolated essentially as previously reported. The enriched p68 preparation showed a single band at the expected position on standard silver-stained SDS polyacrylamide gels. Balb/c mice were immunized and their immune response was monitored using a standard radioimmunoassay to detect specifically the mouse antibody response directed against p68. The spleen was harvested 3 days after challenge and fused to SP2/O cells. Anti-p68 antibody-secreting hybrids were selected by testing the culture supernatant from those hypoxanthine aminopterin thymidine (HAT)-positive clones in a radioimmunoassay against crude preparations of p68. Hybrids that reacted positively were subsequently screened for reactivity against pure p68. Hybrids were cloned on soft agar three times, and only one clone was subsequently chosen from the initial plating wells (clone TJ4C4). Although all of the evidence to date suggests that this MCA is directed against p68, it is possible that this MCA detected another 68 Kd protein similar to p68 described herein. Experiments now underway are directed at defining further the specificity of TJ4C4.

Large-scale growth of TJ4C4 resulted in culture supernatants having 1–10 μg/ml of mouse monoclonal antibody. Ascitic fluid from pristane-primed Balb/c mice resulted in high-titer, reactive fluid (1–2 mg/ml of antibody). Isotyping of TJ4C4 revealed that it was of the IgM subclass. This MCA was able to precipitate a 68 Kd protein; the phosphorylation of this protein was dependent on double-stranded RNA.

Others have produced MCAs and polyclonal antisera against p68 as reported previously, and TJ4C4 reactivity was similar to these reported agents (Laurent et al., 1985; Galabru and Hovanessian, 1987). However, it is not clear whether these other reagents react with formalin-fixed paraffin-embedded tissues.

B. Human Tissues and Detection Methods

Two hundred and eleven surgically resected primary pulmonary neoplasms were obtained as formalin-fixed paraffin-embedded tissues. After standard deparaffinization and rehydration, the 6μm thick sections were immunostained using the avidin–biotin–complex (ABC) method (Hsu et al., 1981; Radosevich et al., 1985). 3,3′-diaminobenzidine tetrahydrochloride (DAB) was used to visualize the antigen (p68)–antibody (TJ4C4)–ABC complexes, and the tissues were counterstained using hematoxylin. All of the tissue samples were immunostained at the same time, using identical conditions. Serial sections of each of the tissues were analyzed after being stained with no primary antibody, as well as with an irrelevant isotypic antibody. In addition, this panel of tumors has been studied using a variety of other mouse MCAs. The expression of p68 within each tissue was assessed using a semiquantitative scoring system of no (0), weak (1+), moderate (2+), or strong (3+) staining, and is reported herein as the average of each group tumor subtype studied. The frequency of p68 expression was based on the percentage of tumor cells within each tissue section that showed immunolocation for p68, regardless of the intensity of staining. All of the immunostained tissues were studied before the reviewing pathologist knew the final diagnosis.

C. Pattern and Frequency of Expression

The expression of p68 as it is detected by TJ4C4 in these pulmonary neoplasms is outlined in Table 1.

Control studies documented that the no primary immunostained tissues, as well as the irrelevant antibody-stained tissues, failed to show any nonspecific reactivity. The frequency, pattern, and apparent subcellular localization of p68 was found to be unique when compared to other MCAs used to study this same panel of pulmonary neoplasms. In studies such as this, it is important to consider that there is some selection bias on the tissue being analyzed, based on the surgical and gross pathologic dissection of the tissue. In addition, the assessment of the expression for any marker is further influenced by the fact that only a 6 μm thick section of the tumor is being studied. The heterogeneous expression of other biological markers in solid tumors has been well documented. In addition, the

Table 1 Expression of p68 in Human Pulmonary Neoplasms

Tumor type	Average % staining	Average intensity	Number of cases studied	
SCC	55	1.1	37	
Grade I	85	1.8		11
Grade II	43	0.9		16
Grade III	40	0.6		10
AD	48	1.1	64	
Acinar	54	1.4		50
Grade I	69	1.8		18
Grade II	52	1.2		16
Grade III	39	1.1		16
PAC	35	0.6		14
BAC	41	0.9	26	
LCC	50	0.9	29	
SCNC	31	0.7	21	
ICNC	48	1.1	17	
WDNC	18	0.3	6	
CRCD	30	0.7	11	
Total			211	

SCC, squamous cell carcinoma; AD, adenocarcinoma; PAC, papillary carcinoma; BAC, bronchioloalveolar carcinoma; LCC, large cell carcinoma; SCNC, small cell neuroendocrine carcinoma; ICNC, intermediate cell neuroendocrine carcinoma; WDNC, well-differentiated neuroendocrine carcinoma; CRCD, carcinoid.

staining results are reported on tumors that have been grouped and selected, based on histologic features seen using light microscopic evaluation. This fact, in part, results in the apparently broad expression pattern of many markers within subclasses of tumors arising in pulmonary tissues, and the expression of any one biological feature in several subgroups. In light of these constraints, the study of relatively large groups of human tumors does allow a practical assessment of potentially relevant biological properties as markers for human neoplasms.

The detection of p68 with TJ4C4 in cases that were immunopositive showed staining consistent with the subcellular localization to p68 to the cytoplasm. No staining was seen outside of cells, nor was any apparent increase in staining observed in the nucleus or at the cell membrane. These findings are consistent with the biochemical localization of p68; however, electron microscopic evaluation remains to be completed to verify the localization using TJ4C4 as a probe for p68.

A broad spectrum in the intensity of immunostaining for all of the subgroups of pulmonary tumors studied was noted, and ranged from 0 to 3, except for the grade I SCCs, which ranged from 1 to 3. The percentage of tumors within each subgroup also showed a similar broad spectrum of staining, except for the SCCs (grade III) and the well-differentiated neuroendocrine carcinomas which ranged from 30 to 100 and 0–60%, respectively. This spectrum of expression was not unexpected, since it has long been appreciated that tumors frequently show a comparatively wide range of expression for any given biological property.

A graphic representation of the relationships between the frequency and intensity of p68 expression is shown in Figure 1 for the various subtypes of lung cancer studied. In general, the non-small-cell carcinomas expressed more p68 than the small cell carcinomas. It is of interest that there is very good correlation in SCCs with the degree and frequency of expression with the grade of the tumor. The staining pattern within these SCCs was remarkable in that the central areas of cell nests and pearls showed a greater expression of p68 than did the peripheral regions fo the lesion. The areas of keratinization within the pearls did not immunostain (Fig. 2).

This general trend is also seen for the various grades within the acinar adenocarcinomas (AD), and in the ADs as a group. Mucin vacuoles were clearly negative, as were central luminal spaces, as would be expected (Fig. 3). Comparatively weak cytoplasmic staining was noted for both the papillary carcinoma (PAC) and bronchioloalveolar carcinoma (BAC) (Fig. 4). This finding supports the

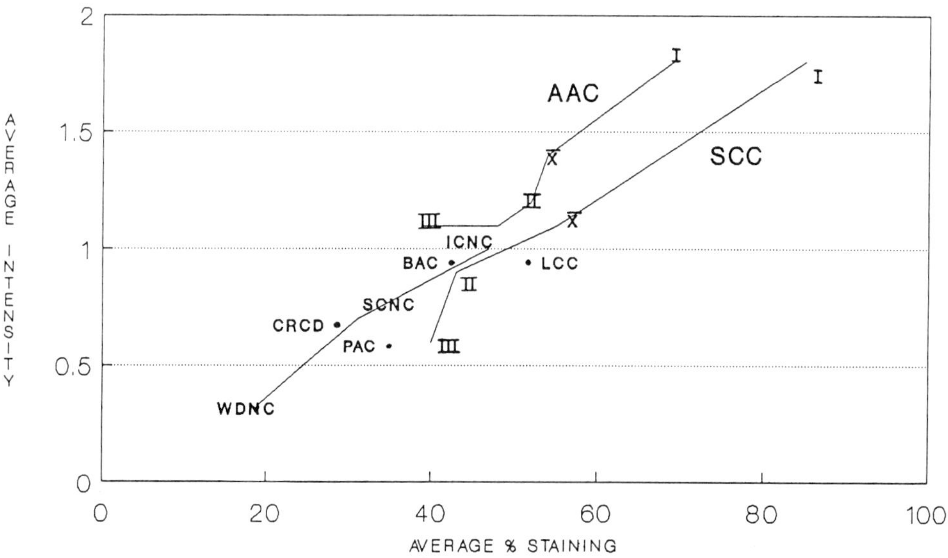

Figure 1 The mean values of the reactivity for the expression of p68 are shown for each subtype. $\overline{\mathrm{X}}$, average.

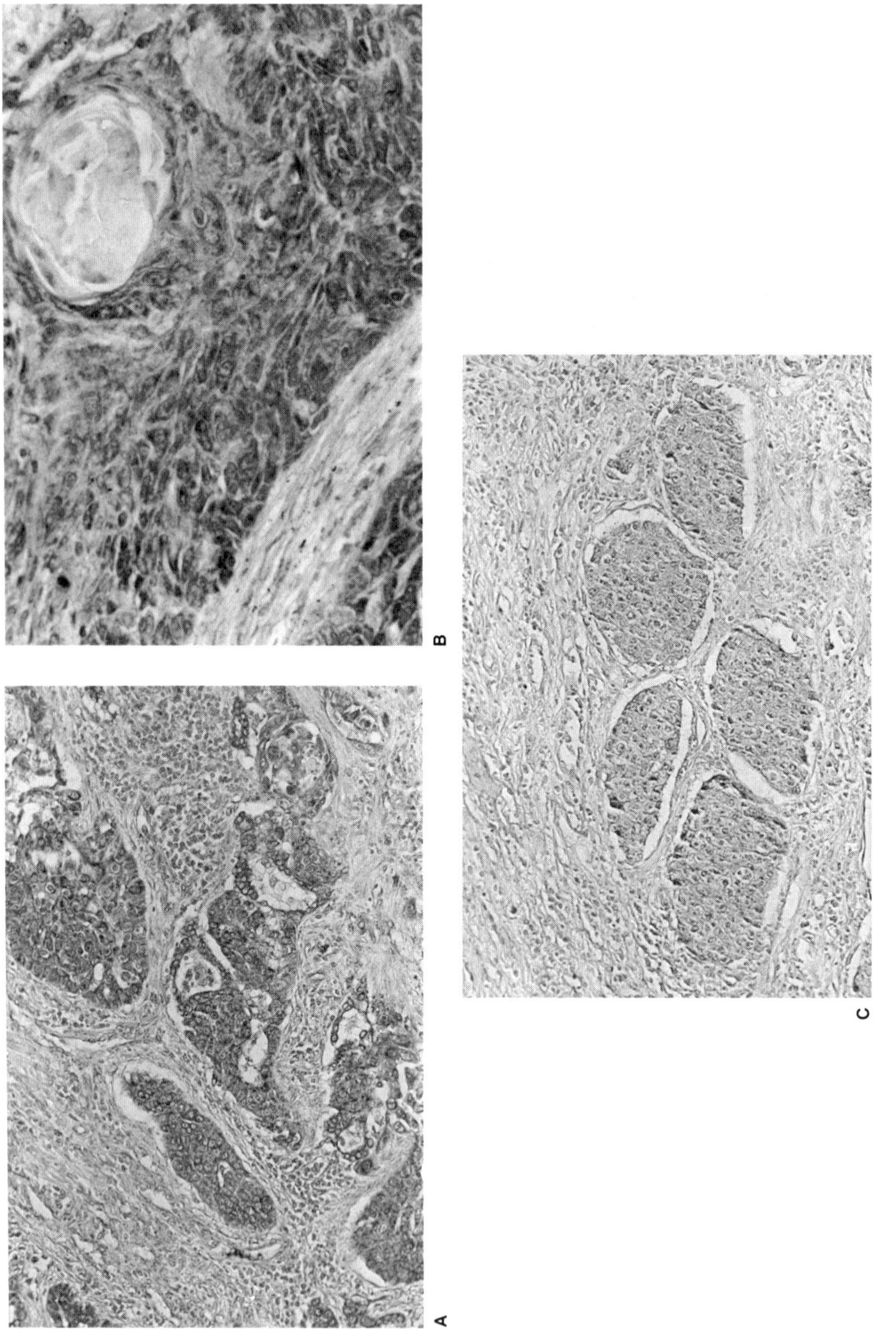

Figure 2 (A) Grade I SCC shows intense staining in neoplastic cells (×40). (B) Grade I SCC shows intense cytoplasmic staining (×72). (C) Grade III SCC shows weak expression of p68 seen in isolated tumor cells (×40).

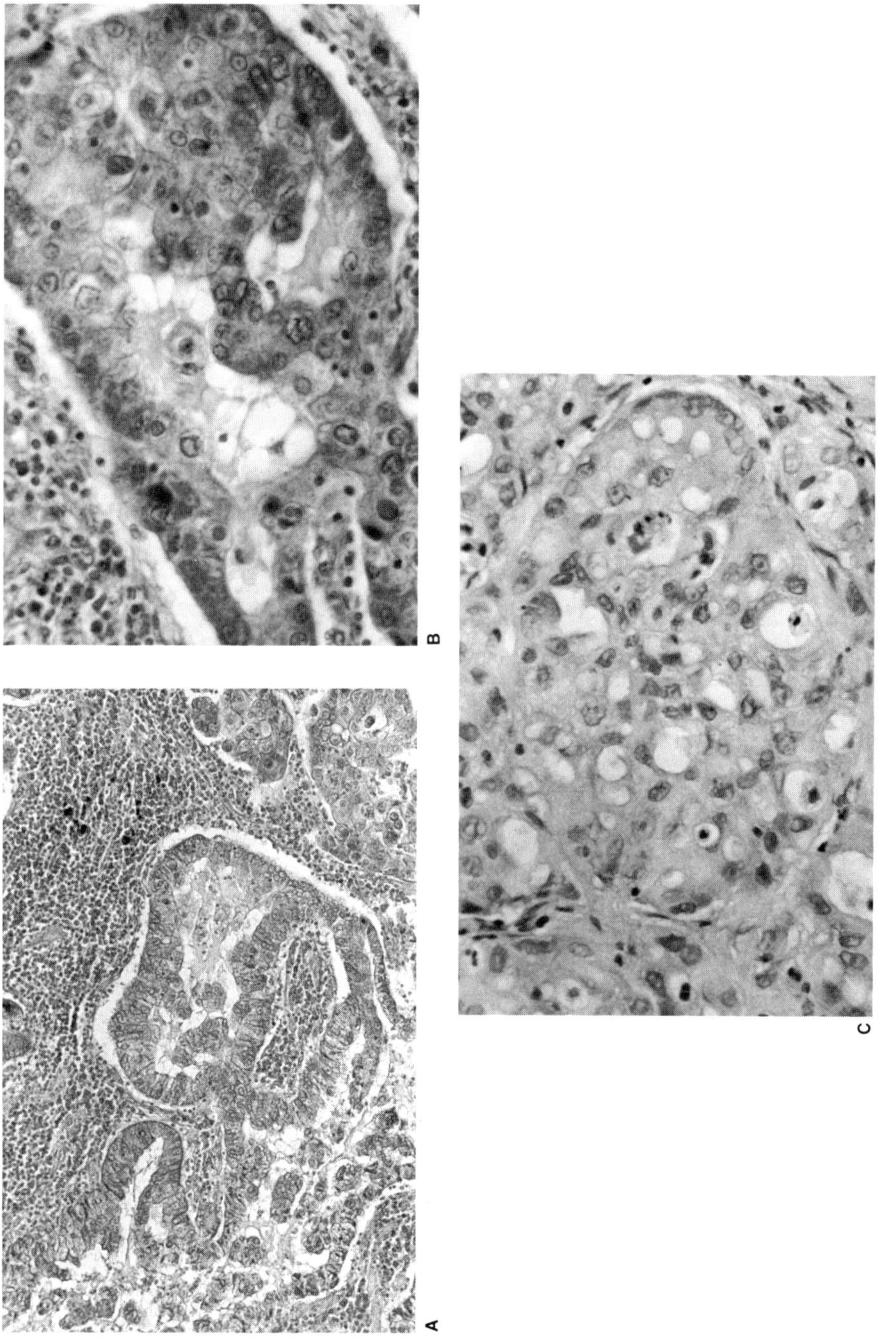

Figure 3 (A) Grade I acinar AC shows intense staining of tumor cells (×40). (B) Grade I acinar AC shows strong cytoplasmic immunoreactivity with no staining of mucin (×72). (C) Grade III acinar AC shows weak cytoplasmic expression of p68 (×72).

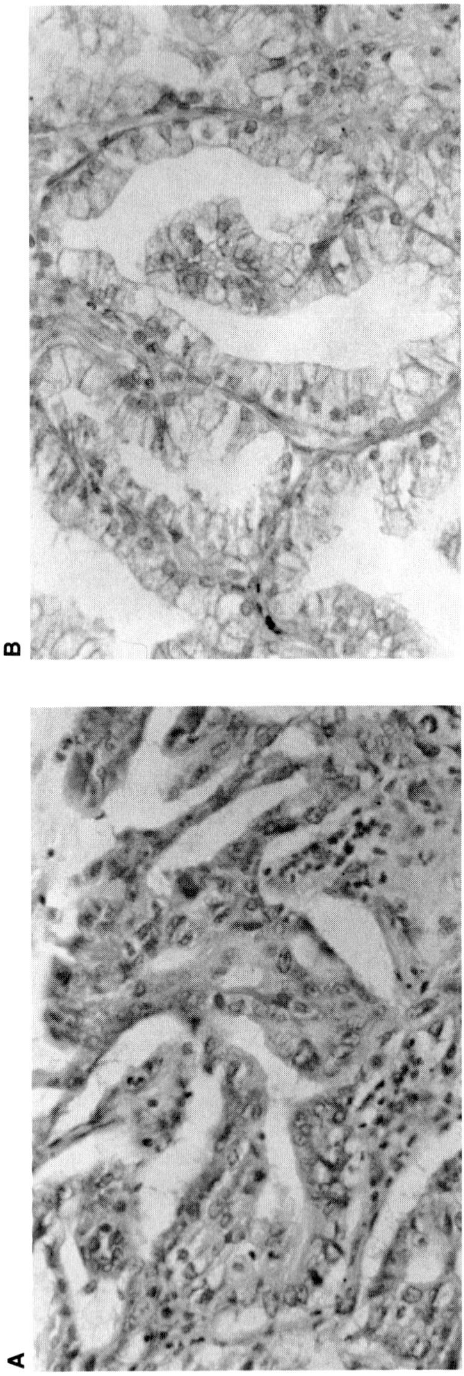

Figure 4 (A) PAC shows weak cytoplasmic staining for p68 (×72). (B) BAC of the goblet cell type shows weak expression of p68 with the absence of staining in mucin vacuoles (×72).

hypothesis that at least the BACs express distinct biological features, as previously reported (Radosevich et al., 1990). It is interesting to note that the LCCs express a spectrum of immunoreactivity that overlaps the higher-grade SCCs and ADs, as well as the small cell carcinomas (Fig. 5). The LCCs, by definition, are a group of neoplasms arising in the lung that lack the salient features of the other subtypes. It is, therefore, not surprising that there is significant overlap by this group of neoplasms with both the small cell and the non-small-cell carcinomas. Various reports have suggested that these tumors are comprised of poorly differentiated neoplasms (WHO, 1982). The possibility that there are some small cell carcinomas in the group is supported by the finding that some of these neoplasms express neuroendocrine features, similar to small cell carcinomas.

Within the small cell carcinoma subgroup (small cell carcinoma [SCNC], intermediate cell neuroendocrine carcinoma [ICNC], and well differentiated neuroendocrine carcinoma [WDNC]), the expression of p68 did not follow the predicted pattern of expression: the ICNC expressed more p68 than the SCNC and the WDNC (Fig. 6). The carcinoid (CRCD) tumors also expressed a comparatively large amount of p68, although they were significantly lower than any of the non-small-cell carcinomas. It is unclear at this time why the small cell group does not express p68 as expected. One possible explanation is that these tumors may have growth patterns independent of p68. Another possibility is that the number of cases studied in each of these groups is too small to represent accurately the true spectrum of expression within each group.

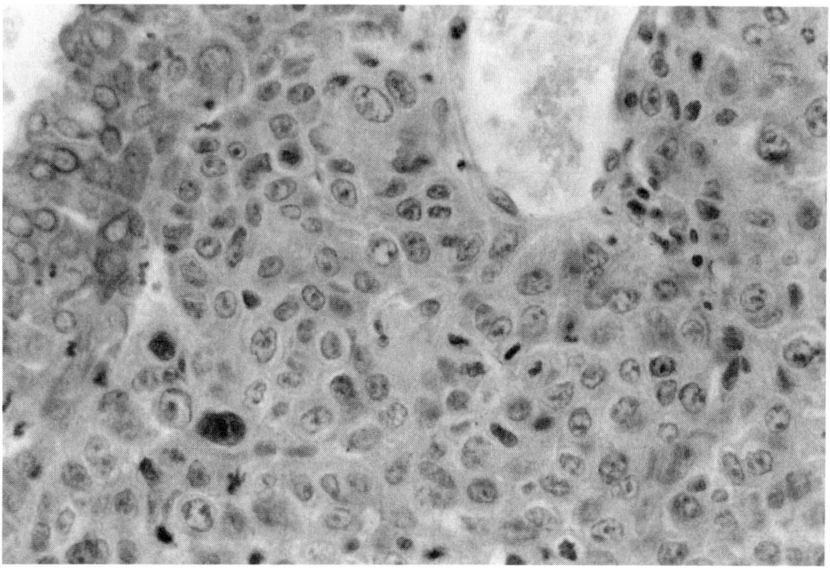

Figure 5 LCC shows diffuse moderate staining of tumor cells with strong staining of metaplastic squamous mucosa (×72).

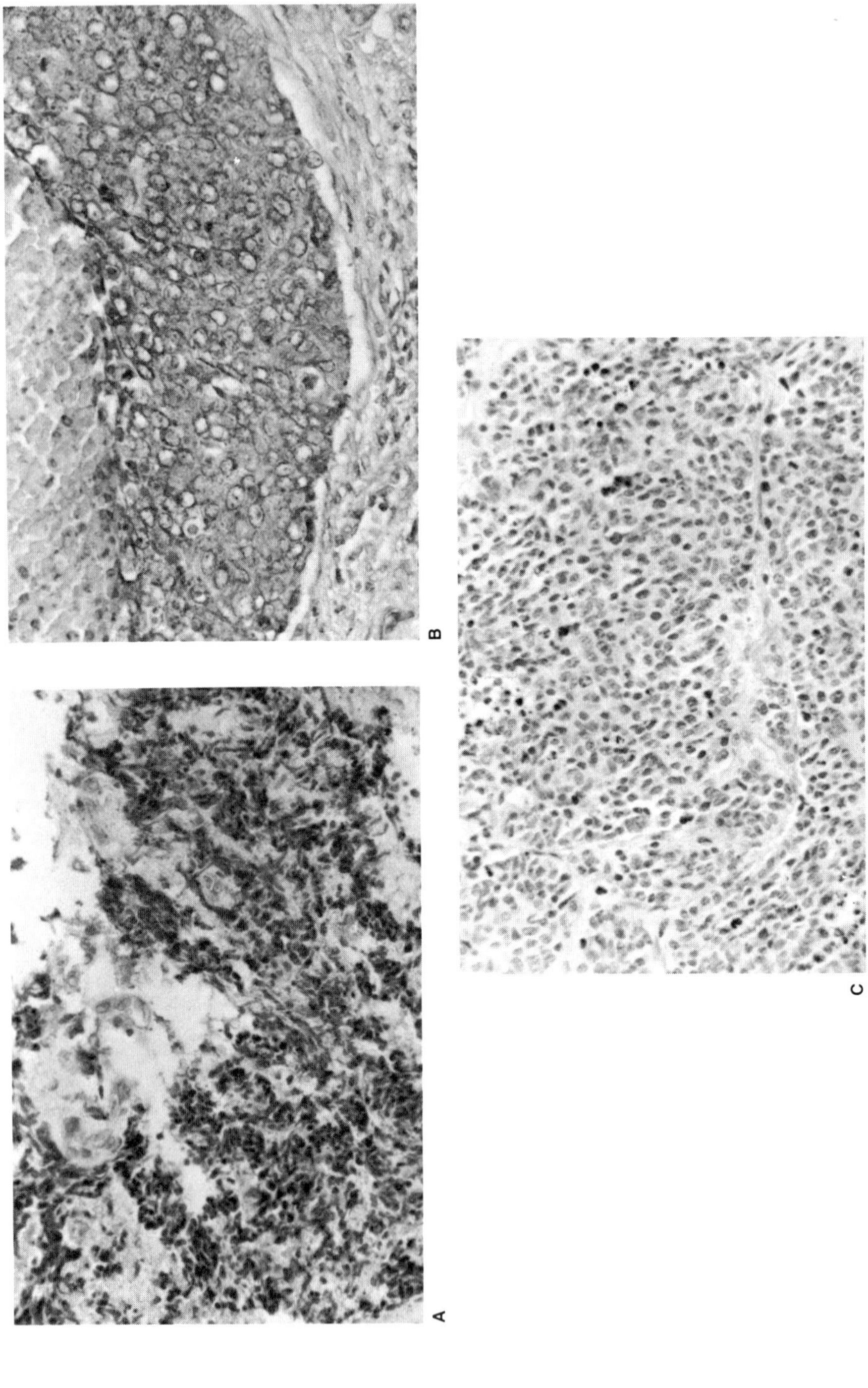

Figure 6 (A) SCNC shows no immuoreactivity for p68 (×100). (B) ICNC shows moderate immunoreactivity (×100). (C) WDNC shows very low levels of immunoreactivity for p68 (×72).

An additional observation consistent for SCCs was that, at the peripheral regions of the tumors, the expression of p68 was lower than at the central areas. This is consistent with the presence of more slowly growing cells in the center, which are potentially deprived of oxygen and nutrients, compared to cells adjoining normal tissue. As an alternative, these centrally located cells are more differentiated and express higher levels of p68. Well-differentiated cell types within each tissue section served as a good internal control for p68 expression (Fig. 6b).

D. Relationship to Other Pulmonary Differentiation Markers

The relationships and spectra of expression for other pulmonary tumor-associated antigens have been outlined in this volume and elsewhere (Radosevich et al., 1988). It is important to note that comparatively few antigens are useful in assessing the degree of differentiation, although keratin expression is frequently studied. The expression pattern of p68 in human pulmonary neoplasms is unique in that it does not appear to select a histologic subtype preferentially, as is seen with other MCAs. In addition, it does not appear to be a marker primarily expressed by non-small-cell or small cell tumors as are other tumor-associated antigens. Although the expression of oncogene products has been associated with the growth potential of these neoplasms, their increased expression is usually associated with more rapidly growing tissues (Kaul, 1988). The ability to assess p68 expression, which appears to be one regulation point of cellular proliferation, provides an antithesis to these positive growth-related markers. Like these markers, the expression of p68 is not restricted exclusively to any one subtype, nor is it always expressed by one subtype. The possible use of p68 expression and a "positive" growth marker may provide a valuable biological assessment of the proliferative growth state of the tumor.

IV. Conclusions

Viewed from the perspective of our growing understanding of the biology of pulmonary neoplasms, and the evolving ability to classify these diverse tumors into biologically related groups, future efforts must address which biological feature(s) have true prognostic, diagnostic, and monitoring values. The use of p68 as a differentiation marker, and possibly a growth rate indicator, appears to have good potential; however, much remains to be done. Efforts underway are directed at quantitating the expression levels of p68 in both fresh tissue and fixed tissue sections to support and confirm immunohistologic evaluations. The findings reported herein suggest that p68 expression, at least in the SCCs and ACs, does correlate well with the degree of cellular differentiation. This is important since there are few easy and reliable markers that can be used, especially in SCCs. In addition, since p68 can be modulated by interferon, and potentially other biological response modifiers and/or chemopreventive agents, it may provide an easy way to assess the biological effectiveness of these agents in vivo.

Note added in proof: TJ4C4 has been shown to be specific for p68 by inhibition of immunohistochemical staining using recombinantly derived p68 kinase protein.

Acknowledgment

This work was supported in part by a Veterans Administration Merit Review grant to J.A.R.

References

Brambilla, E., Moro, D., Gazzeri, S., Brichon, P. Y., Nagy-Mignotte, H., Morel, F., Jacrot, M., and Brambilla, C. (1991). Cytotoxic chemotherapy induces cell differentiation in small cell carcinoma. *J. Clin. Oncol.* **9:**50–61.

Buffet-Janvresse, C., Vannier, J. P., Laurent, A. G., Robert, N., and Hovanessian, A. G. (1986). Enhanced level of double-stranded RNA dependent protein kinase in peripheral blood mononuclear cells of patients with viral infections. *J. Interferon Res.* **6:** 85–96.

De Benedetti, A., and Baglioni, C. (1984). Inhibition of mRNA binding to ribosomes by localized activation of the dsRNA dependent protein kinase. *Nature* **311:**79–81.

De Benedetti, A., and Baglioni, C. (1985). Kinetics of dephosphorylation of eIF2 (P) and mRNA. *J. Biol. Chem.* **260:**3135–3139.

Farrel, P. J., Balkow, K., Hunt, T., Jackson, R. J., and Trachsel, H. (1977). Phosphorylation of initiation factor eIF2 and the control of reticulocyte protein synthesis. *Cell* **11:** 187–200.

Galabru, J., and Hovanessian, A. G. (1985). Two interferon-induced proteins are involved in the protein kinase complex dependent on double-stranded RNA. *Cell* **43:**685–694.

Galabru, J., and Hovanessian, A. G. (1987). Autophosphorylation of the protein kinase dependent on double-stranded RNA. *J. Biol. Chem.* **262:**15538–15544.

Galabru, J., Katze, M. G., Robert, N., and Hovanessian, A. G. (1989). The binding of double-stranded RNA and adenovirus VAI RNA to interferon induced protein kinase. *Eur. J. Biochem.* **178:**581–589.

Gefter, M. L., Margulies, D. H., and Scharff, M. D. (1977). A simple method for polyethylene glycol promoted hybridization of mouse myeloma cells. *Somatic Cell Genet.* **3:**231–236.

Golgher, R. R., Williams, B. R. G., Gilbert, C. S., Brown, R. E., and Kerr, I. M. (1980). Protein kinase activity and the natural occurrence of 2-5A in interferon-treated EMC virus-infected L-cells. *Ann. N.Y. Acad. Sci.* **350:**448–458.

Gruhn, J., Koukoulis, G., Radosevich, J. A., and Rosen, S. T. (1990). Lung cancer: changing concepts. In *Advances in Pathology*. Edited by C. Fenoglio-Preiser. Chicago, Mosby Year Book, vol. 3.

Gupta, S. L., Holmes, S. L., and Mehra, L. L. (1982). Interferon action against reovirus: activation of interferon-induced protein kinase in mouse L-(2) cells upon reovirus infection. *Virology* **120:**495–499.

Hovanessian, A. G. (1980). Double-stranded RNA dependent protein kinase(s) in rabbit reticulocyte lysates analogous to that from interferon-treated cells. *Biochimie* **62:** 775–778.

Hovanessian, A. G. (1989). The double-stranded RNA-activated protein kinase induced by interferon: dsRNA-PK. *J. Interferon Res.* **9:**641–647.

Hovanessian, A. G., and Galabru, J. (1987). The double-stranded RNA-dependent protein kinase is also activated by heparin. *Eur. J. Biochem.* **167:**467–473.

Hsu, S. M., Raine, L., and Fanger, H. (1981). The use of avidin–biotin–peroxidase complex (ABC) in immunoperoxidase techniques: a comparison between ABC and unlabeled antibody (PAP) procedures. *J. Histochem. Cytochem.* **29:**577–581.

Humphrey, E. W., Smart, C. R., Winchester, D. P., Steel, G. D., Yarbro, J. W., Chu, K. C., and Triolo, H. H. (1990). National survey of the pattern of care for carcinoma of the lung. *J. Thorac. Cardiovas. Surg.* **100:**837–843.

Kaul, K. (1988) Oncogenes in human lung cancer. In *Biology of Lung Cancer: Diagnosis and Treatment.* Edited by S. T. Rosen, J. L. Mulshine, F. Cuttitta, and P. G. Abrams. New York, Marcel Dekker, vol. 37.

Kostura, M., and Mathews, M. B. (1989). Purification and activation of the double-stranded RNA-dependent eIF-2 kinase DAI. *Mol. Cell. Biol.* **9:**1576–1586.

Krust, B., Galabru, J., and Hovanessian, A. G. (1984). Further characterization of the protein kinase activity mediated by interferon in mouse and human cells. *J. Biol. Chem.* **259:**8494–8498.

Lasky, S. R., Jacobs, B. L., and Samuel, C. E. (1982). Characterization of sites of phosphorylation in the interferon induced phosphoprotein P1 from mouse fibroblasts: evidence for two forms of P1. *J. Biol. Chem.* **257:**11087–11093.

Laurent, A. G., Krust, B., Galabru, J., Svab, J., and Hovanessian, A. G. (1985). Monoclonal antibodies to interferon induced 68,000 Mr protein and their use for the detection of double-stranded RNA dependent protein kinase in human cells. *Proc. Natl. Acad. Sci. (USA)* **82:**4341–4345.

Levin, D. H., and London, I. M. (1978). Regulation of protein synthesis: activation by double-stranded RNA of a protein kinase that phosphorylates eukaryotic initiation factor 2. *Proc. Natl. Acad. Sci. (USA)* **75:**1121–1125.

Meurs, E., Chong, K., Galabru, J., Thomas, N. S. B., Kerr, I. M., Williams, B. R. G., and Hovanessian, A. G. (1990). Molecular cloning and characterization of the human double-stranded RNA-activated protein kinase induced by interferon. *Cell* **62:**379–390.

Nilsen, T. W., Maroney, P. A., and Baglioni, C. (1982). Inhibition of protein synthesis in reovirus-infected HeLa cells with elevated levels of interferon-induced protein kinase activity. *J. Biol. Chem.* **257:**14593–14596.

Pain, V. M. (1986). Initiation of protein synthesis in mammalian cells. *Biochem. J.* **235:** 625–637.

Petryshyn, R., Chen, J. J., and London, I. M. (1988). Detection of activated double-stranded RNA-dependent protein kinase in 3T3-F442a cells. *Proc. Natl. Acad. Sci. USA* **85:**1427–1431.

Radosevich, J. A., Ma, Y., Lee, I, Salwen, H. R., Gould, V. E., and Rosen, S. T. (1985). Monoclonal antibody 44-3A6 as a probe for a novel antigen found on human lung carcinomas with glandular differentiation. *Cancer Res.* **45:**5808–5812.

Radosevich, J. A., Lee, I., Rosen, S. T., and Gould, V. E. (1988). Monoclonal antibody assays for lung cancer. In *Cancer Diagnosis In Vitro Using Monoclonal Antibodies*. Edited by H. Z. Kupchik. New York, Marcel Dekker.

Radosevich, J. A., Noguchi, M., Rosen, S. T., and Shimosato, Y. (1990). Immunohistochemical analysis of human adenocarcinomas of the lung using the monoclonal antibody 44–3A6. *Tumor Biology* **11:**181–188.

Reichel, P. A., Merrick, W. C., Siekierka, J., Mathews, M. B. (1985). Regulation of a protein synthesis initiation factor by adenovirus virus-associated RNAI. *Nature* **313:** 196–200.

analysis of differentiation markers for non-small-cell lung cancer. In *Lung Cancer Differentiation*. Edited by C. L'Enfant, S. Bernal, and S. Baylin. New York, Marcel Dekker.

Rice, A., Duncan, R., Hearshy, J. W. B., and Kerr, I. M. (1985). Double stranded RNA-dependent protein kinase and 2-5A system are both activated in interferon-treated, encephalomyocarditis virus-infected HeLa cells. *J. Virol.* **50:**229–236.

Rosen, S. T., Mulshine, J. L., Cuttitta, F., and Abrams, P. G. (eds). (1988). *Biology of Lung Cancer: Diagnosis and Treatment*. New York, Marcel Dekker.

Samuel, E. C., Duncan, R., Knutson, G. S., and Hearshy, J. W. B. (1984). Mechanism of interferon action: increased phosphorylation of protein syntheses initiation factor eIF2 in interferon-treated reovirus infected mouse 1-929 fibroblasts in vitro and in vivo. *Proc. Natl. Acad. Sci. USA* **76:**515–526.

Szyska, R., Kudlicki, W., Kramer, G., Hardesty, B., Galabru, J., and Hovanessian, A. G. (1989). A type 1 phosphoprotein phosphatase active with phosphorylated Mr 68,000 initiation factor 2 kinase. *J. Biol. Chem.* **264:**3827–3831.

World Health Organization (1982). The World Health Organization histological typing of lung tumours, second edition. *Am. J. Clin. Pathol.* **77:**123–136.

PART II

ONCOGENES AND GROWTH FACTORS IN LUNG CANCER

6

Induction of Non-Small-Cell Lung Cancer Phenotypic Features by Oncogenic Transformation of Small Cell Lung Cancer Cells

L. AUSTIN DOYLE

University of Maryland Cancer Center
Baltimore, Maryland

FRANK CUTTITTA

National Navy Medical Center
Bethesda, Maryland

MACK MABRY

Johns Hopkins Oncology Center
Baltimore, Maryland

I. Modulation of Small Cell Lung Cancer Antigens by Oncogenic Transformation

A. Transfection of Small Cell Lung Cancer Cells with c-myc

Amplification and overexpression of members of the myc proto-oncogene family have been seen frequently in tumor cells from human small cell lung cancer (SCLC) (Little et al., 1983). Overexpression of c-myc, N-myc, and L-myc have been demonstrated both in SCLC cell lines and in biopsy samples from patients with SCLC. Amplification of the c-myc proto-oncogene has always been associated with the variant subtype of SCLC. Compared with classic SCLC lines, variant lines have altered large cell morphology, shorter doubling times, higher cloning efficiencies in soft agarose, and very low levels of L-dopa decarboxylase production and bombesinlike immunoreactivity, which are key markers of neuroendocrine differentiation (Carney et al., 1985). The variant subtype of SCLC has cellular phenotypic features that appear to be intermediate between that of classic SCLC and large cell undifferentiated lung cancer (Goodwin et al., 1983).

To investigate if c-myc amplification and expression are responsible for the variant SCLC phenotype, copies of the c-myc proto-oncogene were transfected into a cloned classic SCLC line, NCI-H209, not expressing detectable c-myc messenger RNA (Johnson et al., 1986). The c-myc gene was covalently linked to the neomycin resistance gene, aminoglycoside 3′ phosphotransferase. Transformants expressing the transfected DNA were selected using the aminoglycoside antibiotic G-418. Clones were isolated with up to six copies of c-myc stably integrated into DNA with proportional overexpression of c-myc mRNA.

The expression of the c-myc proto-oncogene, in the transfected SCLC line, was associated with an altered large cell morphology similar to variant SCLC, a shorter doubling time, and an increased cloning efficiency. However, no decreases in L-dopa decarboxylase levels or bombesinlike immunoreactivity were noted in the transfectants. The levels of c-myc amplification and overexpression in the transfectants did not reach those seen in many spontaneously occurring variant SCLC lines.

B. Transformation of SCLC Cells with v-Ha-ras

Mutations of members of the RAS gene family have not been demonstrated in SCLC cells. Activating mutations of the Kras gene have been seen frequently in biopsy specimens from non-small-cell lung cancer (NSCLC), particularly in the adenocarcinoma subclass of NSCLC (Rodenhuis et al., 1987). Furthermore, an abnormal c-Ha-ras allele distribution has been found in patients with NSCLC, which suggests a possible linkage of a chromosome 11p haplotype to NSCLC (Heighway et al., 1986). Complementation of transformation is known to occur between MYC oncogenes, which code for nuclear proteins, and RAS family genes, whose products are involved in ligand signal transduction (Land et al., 1983).

To examine the interaction of RAS and MYC gene expression in human lung cancer, representative classic and variant SCLC cell lines were infected with the Harvey murine sarcoma virus (Ha-MSV). For viral infection, the cells were exposed for 3 days to conditioned medium from infected NIH3T3 cells, which produce high titers of Ha-MSV and 1504 amphotropic murine leukemia helper virus (Mabry et al., 1988). DNA from the infected SCLC cells, when hybridized to an SstI-PstI restriction fragment containing only the v-Ha-ras coding region, showed the predicted 880-base pair v-Ha-ras internal HindIII fragment, demonstrating the presence of proviral DNA. The integrated Ha-MSV sequences were highly expressed in the infected SCLC cells.

The classic and variant SCLC subtypes had markedly different phenotypic responses to similar levels of expression of v-Ha-ras RNA (Mabry et al., 1988). No biochemical or morphologic changes were observed in classic SCLC cells. In contrast, in variant SCLC cells, v-Ha-ras expression induced features typical of large cell undifferentiated lung carcinoma, including adherent monolayer growth patterns, increased cloning efficiency, a reduction in the neuroendocrine marker creatine kinase BB, the appearance of primitive desmosomes, and an acquired resistance to polyamine depletion typical of NSCLC, but not SCLC, in vitro. The introduction of v-Ha-ras into variant SCLC cells also caused the induction of mRNA for the NSCLC growth factors transforming growth factor (TGF)-alpha and PDGF, as well as the epidermal growth factor (EGF) receptor (Falco et al., 1989). Transformation of variant SCLC cells by v-Ha-ras also caused a decrease in both gastrin releasing peptide (GRP), an important SCLC mitogen, and the GRP receptor. The induction of NSCLC features in variant SCLC cells by v-Ha-ras infection directly demonstrates that important transitions can occur between phenotypes of human lung cancer cells that may play an important role in tumor progression and differentiation.

To demonstrate that the c-myc amplification of variant SCLC cells complemented the v-Ha-ras phenotypic changes, the NCI-H209 cells previously transfected with six copies of the c-myc proto-oncogene (clone E) were infected with Ha-MSV (Doyle et al., in press). The infected cells developed a NSCLC morphology similar to that of variant SCLC cells transformed with v-Ha-ras, suggesting that overexpression of c-myc and v-Ha-ras is sufficient to transform classic SCLC cells into an NSCLC phenotype. The L-myc proto-oncogene, which is expressed in NCI-H209 and some other classic SCLC lines, does not appear to complement v-Ha-ras functionally in this system (Mabry et al., 1988).

C. Surface Cluster Antigens on Lung Cancer Cells

We were interested in whether cotransformation of classic SCLC cells by c-myc and v-Ha-ras oncogenes would alter the expression of characteristic SCLC surface antigens, particularly the antigens that link SCLC to other neuroendocrine tumors, but differentiate the tumor from NSCLC. Many monoclonal antibodies reactive with SCLC cells have been generated by various laboratories. The tissue distribution patterns and immunoprecipitation data of over 50 monoclonal antibodies reactive with SCLC cells were analyzed extensively at the First International Workshop on Small Cell Lung Cancer (Beverly et al., 1988). Most of these antibodies were found to react with a small group of dominant SCLC antigens (Souhami et al., 1987). Clusters of monoclonal antibodies reactive against six such antigens have been labeled SC-1–SC-6.

Although the function of most of the SCLC cluster antigen proteins is unknown, the SC-1 protein on SCLC has been recently demonstrated to be closely related to the neural cell adhesion molecule (NCAM). Monoclonal antibodies that recognize the SCLC SC-1 antigen were compared with a specific polyclonal antisera generated against purified NCAM (Moolenaar et al., 1990). Immunoinhibition, immunoprecipitation, and *Staphylococcus aureus* V8 digestion studies indicated that the SCLC SC-1 protein and NCAM were identical. Long polysialic acid units composed of alpha-(2.8)-linked N-acetylneuraminic acid units, which in mammals are found exclusively on NCAM, were present on the SC-1 antigen of SCLC. A striking feature of the SC-1 antigen is its association with neural tissues and tumors, and the antigen does not appear to be present on NSCLC tumors.

D. Modulation of SCLC Surface Antigens by Oncogenic Transformation

We have used classic SCLC cells transfected with c-myc, or cotransformed with c-myc and v-Ha-ras, to examine the expression of SC-1 and other characteristic SCLC cluster antigens. Flow cytometric assays reveal that SCLC cells cotransformed with c-myc and v-Ha-ras oncogenes downmodulate SC-1, SC-2, and SC-5A surface antigens to levels approaching, in some cases, those seen with NSCLC cells (Doyle et al., in press). The SC-4 surface antigen is not modulated by activation of these oncogenes.

The antigen defined by SC-2 monoclonal antibodies is not specific for SCLC, but can be found on some NSCLC tumors as well as other epithelial cancers (Souhami et al., 1987). Thyroid, prostate, and bronchial epithelia are also positive. The SC-2 antibodies precipitate a single band of 35–40 kDa. A cDNA corresponding to this protein has been recently cloned and sequenced, revealing a transmembrane domain and several potential N-glycosylation sites (Strnad et al., 1989). The SC-2 antigen appears to be more heavily expressed in classic than in variant SCLC cells (Reeve et al., 1988). The decreased expression of the Sc-2 antigen in oncogene-transformed classic SCLC cells may mimic the levels seen in the variant subtype of SCLC.

SC-5A monoclonal antibodies define a SCLC surface sialoglycoprotein with little or no reactivity with NSCLC, most epithelial tumors, or normal tissues, including cells of epithelial and neural origin or leukocytes (Stahel et al., 1988). The SC-5A antigen is more heavily expressed on classic than on variant SCLC cells (Reeve et al., 1988). Immunoblotting experiments with SC-5A monoclonal antibodies demonstrate specific bands with approximate molecular weights of 40,000, 100,000, and 180,000 daltons. The SC-5A antigen is only present on a subset of SCLC cells, and does not appear to be downmodulated by c-myc transfection alone. However, cotransformation of classic SCLC cells by c-myc and v-Ha-ras oncogenes appears to reduce the surface expression of the SC-5A antigen to NSCLC levels in indirect immunofluorescence assays (Doyle et al., in press).

E. Relation of Cluster I Expression to Lung Cancer Adhesive Properties

A striking difference between SCLC and NSCLC cells in vitro is that SCLC cells generally grow in spheroid aggregates and NSCLC cells grow as surface-adherent monolayers. Classic SCLC cells tend to grow in tight spheroids with central necrosis, whereas variant SCLC cells grow in looser branching chains. A small number of variant SCLC lines have been noted to grow as adherent monolayers in vitro (Carney et al., 1985). These adherent variant cells, referred to as having type 4 SCLC morphology, are clearly SCLC based on other morphologic, cytogenetic, and biochemical features. One SCLC line, NCI-H446, is unique in that it grows long-term with coexisting floating and surface-adherent populations.

We were interested in whether expression of the neural cell adhesion molecule (NCAM) might be related to the adherent properties of SCLC cells in culture. As noted, the c-myc and v-Ha-ras cotransformed SCLC cells adopted a NSCLC-like surface-adherent growth pattern in association with low NCAM expression. NCAM has an important role in homophilic (self–self) binding between neural cells, and might have a role in the tight adhesion of SCLC cells in spheroids.

The variant SCLC line, NCI-H446, was divided into surface-adherent and floating sublines by physical segregation of these two populations over many generations in vitro (Doyle et al., 1990a). No differences in c-myc expression, keratin pattern, or cytogenetic appearance were found between the monolayer and floating sublines. However, expression of the neuroendocrine marker neuron-specific enolase in the floating cells was three times that found in the surface-adherent cells. The floating subline also had much greater surface expression of NCAM, as detected by monoclonal antibody UJ13A. Two other surface-adherent (type 4) variant SCLC lines were also found to be unreactive with UJ13A, which generalized the association between NCAM expression and the growth of most SCLC cultures as floating aggregates (Doyle et al., 1990a).

The association between NCAM-related determinants and homophilic cell–cell adhesion between SCLC cells is strengthened by other findings we have reported with variant SCLC cells incubated with retinoic acid (Doyle et al., 1989). These retinoid-treated cells have a marked phenotypic change, with the loosely aggregated variant cells becoming much more tightly clustered spheroids. This increased cell–cell adhesion is associated with a marked increase in NCAM immunoreactivity among the retinoid-treated cells compared with untreated control cells.

Other factors besides the total amount of NCAM protein may be responsible for the different adhesive properties of floating and surface-adherent lung cancer cells. Polysialylation of NCAM has been demonstrated to reduce markedly the homophilic binding of neural cells (Hoffman and Edelman, 1983). Differential sialylation could explain variations in the adhesive phenotypes of SCLC lines, and could be important in explaining the early metastases characteristic of this tumor. SCLC lines have been found to be deficient relative to NSCLC cells in producing fibronectin and laminin, which may partly explain why most SCLC lines do not grow in monolayers in vitro (Scarpa et al., 1988).

II. Induction of NSCLC-Secreted Proteins by Oncogenic Transformation of SCLC Cells

A. Adaptation of Lung Cancer Cells to Serum-Free Medium

Recent studies have shown that human cancer cell lines can be adapted to grow in serum-free, unsupplemented RPMI-1640 (R0) medium. We have developed techniques to grow both NSCLC and SCLC cells long-term under basal serum-free conditions (Doyle et al., 1990b). SCLC cells have been previously grown in serum-free conditions using HITES medium, which contains hydrocortisone, insulin, transferrin, estradiol and sodium selenite (Simms et al., 1980). SCLC cells are known to secrete a number of peptide hormones, some of which serve as autocrine growth factors for these tumor cells. If the cells are adapted to hormone-free conditions at a high density, some of these secreted autocrine factors might take the place of exogenous hormones.

We have found that both SCLC and NSCLC cells can be adapted to basal R0 medium, as long as the initial seeding density of the cells is kept over 5×10^5 cells/ml, and the cells are adapted over a period of several weeks. The RPMI medium used was phenol-red-free, both because phenol red interferes with subsequent chromatographic analysis and because the dye has weak estrogenic effects. The only additions to the RPMI medium were 2 mM glutamine and 30 nM sodium selenite. The floating spheroid colonies of viable tumor cells were allowed to settle by gravity and 75% of the medium was replaced by fresh R0 medium every 4–7 days. The conditioned medium from the R-adapted lung cancer cell lines has been found to facilitate the rapid adaptation of other lung cancer lines, of the same subtype, to serum-free conditions. Bombesinlike immunoreactivity has been detected in fractions of conditioned medium (CM) separated by high-pressure liquid chromatography.

B. Chromatographic Analysis of Lung Cancer CM Proteins

After a minimum of five passages in R0 medium over several weeks of culture, the CM was serially removed for chromatographic analysis. This CM is advantageous for protein and peptide analysis because contaminating serum proteins have been removed, and any proteins detected in the CM can be assumed to be secreted or shed from the lung cancer cells themselves. Changes in the pattern of secreted proteins between lung cancer subtypes, or by oncogenic transformation, can be examined. The CM was clarified by centrifugation and filtration. Protease inhibitors were added, as well as the detergent CHAPS (0.1%) to stabilize the proteins. Liter volumes of CM were concentrated 10–20-fold with a Minisette tangential flow unit (Pharmacia), which was also useful for buffer exchange before chromatography.

Equivalent amounts of CM protein from classic and variant SCLC lines, from NSCLC lines, and from sublines of SCLC transformed with c-myc, or co-transformed with c-myc and v-Ha-ras, were separated by anion exchange, using a Pharmacia filter paper liquid chromatographic (FPLC) unit. The proteins in each fraction of the separation could be easily displayed by SDS-PAGE using the automated PHAST system from Pharmacia and silver staining. Reproducible chromatograms and gel protein patterns were obtainable from each cell line. The phenotype of secreted proteins was found to differentiate SCLC CM from that of NSCLC, and to discriminate between classic and variant subtypes of SCLC. Proteins of interest could be further purified, often to apparent homogeneity, by subsequent reversed-phase separations on the FPLC. These purified proteins were amenable to further analysis by protein microsequencing. One protein, which was found prominently in the CM of classic but not variant SCLC cell lines, was identified by microsequencing as human histone H2B (Doyle et al., 1990b). We believe that these rapid automated techniques have general use in the rapid identification of CM proteins associated with the differentiation or progression of many types of neoplastic cells that can be adapted to growth in serum-free medium.

C. Purification of NSCLC Proteins Induced by Oncogenic Transformation of SCLC Cells

We use similar cell culture and chromatographic techniques to analyze and purify serum-free CM proteins from SCLC sublines transformed with oncogenes to assume NSCLC phenotypic features. The classic SCLC cell line NCI-H209, its c-myc-transfected subline, and its c-myc and v-Ha-ras cotransformed subline were all adapted to growth in R0 medium, as was the NSCLC line NCI-H157. CM was collected from all four lines and processed for chromatographic analysis. Separation of the CM proteins by anion exchange on a NaCl gradient, with display on silver-stained gels, demonstrated a 55 kD protein found in CM from the H209-myc-ras subline and the H157 NSCLC cells, but not in the CM of the parental H209 classic SCLC line or in the subline transfected with c-myc alone (Fig. 1). This protein eluted off of the Mono Q anion exchange column at 0.3 M NaCl. Another protein eluted at 0.7 M NaCl, which was also found in the NSCLC CM and the H209-myc-ras CM, but not in CM from the H209 or H209-myc lines (Fig. 2). This second protein had a molecular weight of 50 kD. We believe that these two proteins are naturally secreted by NSCLC cells, but are induced in SCLC cells cotransformed by c-myc and v-Ha-ras oncogenes. This induction is consistent with the many other NSCLC phenotypic features described in the cotransformed NSCLC cells by Mabry and collaborators (1988).

The 55 and 50 kD proteins have been subsequently further purified using other chromatographic techniques. The proteins cannot be identified in fractions

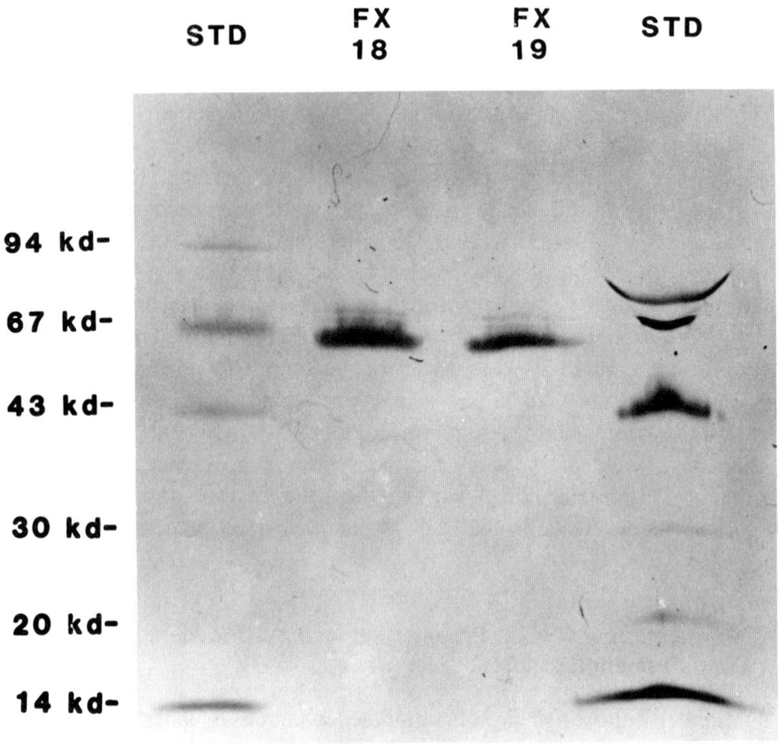

Figure 1 Silver stain detection of a 55 kD protein eluting at 0.3 M NaCl of anion exchange separations of CM from SCLC and NSCLC cell lines. Equivalent fractions from each separation were concentrated, and 1 μl samples were loaded onto lanes of 8–25% SDS-PAGE gradient minigels. Electrophoretic separations were performed at 65 volt-hours on a PHAST system.

coming off a Phenyl Superose reversed-phase column, and may be irreversibly bound to it. The 55 kD protein has been further purified to homogeneity using hydrophobic interaction chromatography (Fig. 3). The purified protein was subjected to amino acid analysis and microsequencing. The limited sequence data suggest a homology to the integrin superfamily of proteins, but is insufficient to identify the 55 kD protein. Further efforts at purification and microsequencing of both proteins are currently in progress.

In conclusion, classic human SCLC cells can be cotransformed by c-myc and v-Ha-ras oncogenes to assume many phenotypic features of NSCLC cells. The oncogene-transformed SCLC cells decrease expression of several characteristic

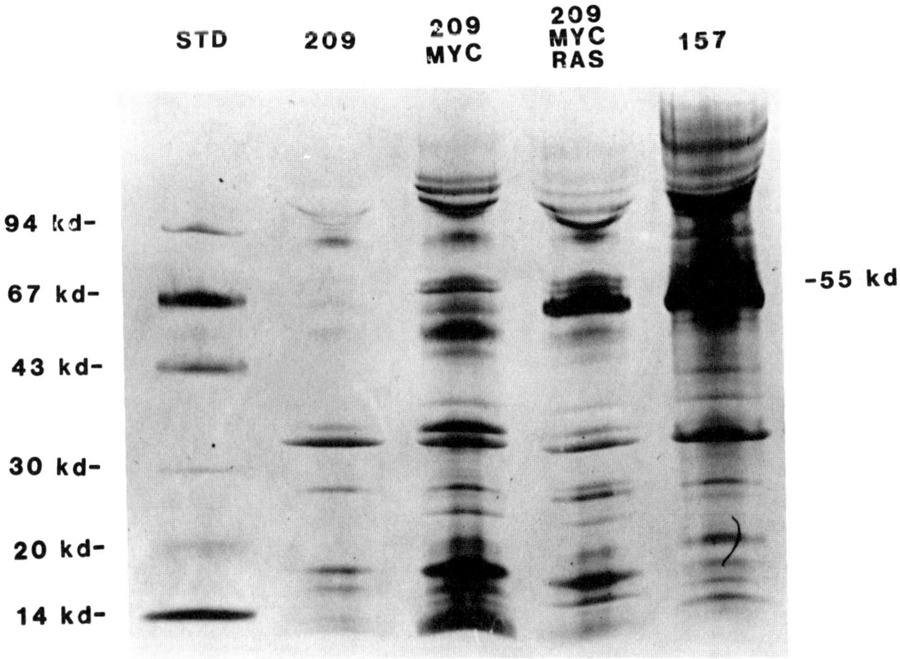

Figure 2 Silver stain detection of a 50 kD protein eluting at 0.7 M NaCl of anion exchange separations of CM from SCLC and NSCLC cell lines. Concentration and electrophoresis of the proteins in these fractions were identical with the procedures in Figure 1.

markers, including two surface antigens that link SCLC to other neuroendocrine tumors and differentiate it from NSCLC. The downmodulation of neural cell adhesion molecule on the oncogene-transformed SCLC cells may be related to the change in their colony morphology to monolayer growth. The ability to examine CM from lung cancer cells adapted to serum-free conditions has permitted the identification of two secreted NSCLC proteins induced in c-myc and v-Ha-ras cotransformed SCLC cells. We believe that changes in surface and CM proteins by oncogene activation support other evidence demonstrating plasticity between SCLC and NSCLC cell types, and may argue for a common cell of origin for all human bronchogenic carcinoma.

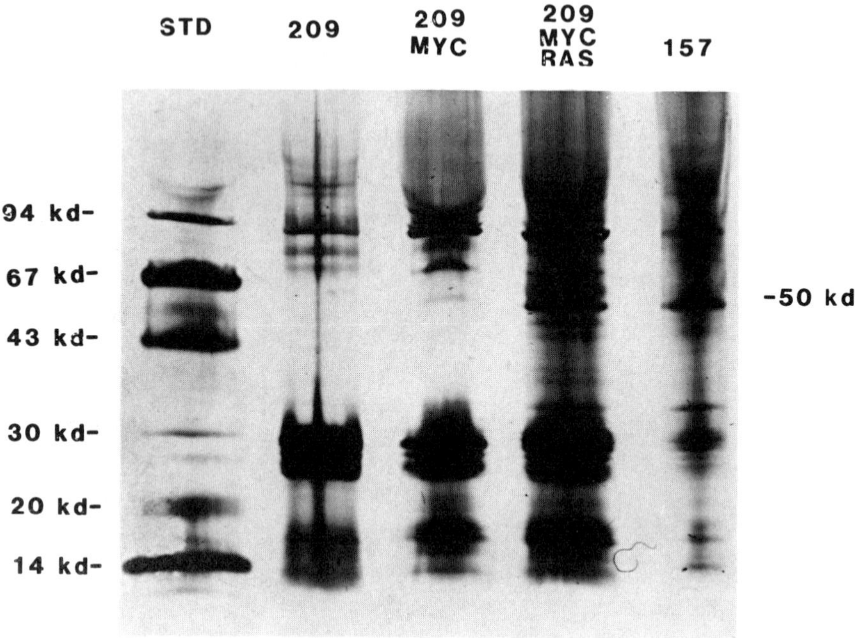

Figure 3 Silver stain detection of the 55 kD protein from the NCI-H209 subline transformed with c-myc and v-Ha-ras oncogenes after further purification by hydrophobic interaction chromatography. Fractions containing the 55 kD protein after initial anion exchange chromatography were loaded onto a Pharmacia Phenyl Superose column and eluted on a decreasing gradient of $(NH_4)_2SO_4$. The 55 kDa protein eluted in fractions 18 and 19 at approximately 0.1 M $(NH_4)_2SO_4$. Concentration and electrophoresis of the proteins in these fractions were identical with the procedures in Figure 1.

References

Beverly, P. C. L., Souhami, R. L., and Bobrow, L. G. (1988). Results of the central data analysis. *Lung Cancer* **4:**15–36.

Carney, D. N., Gazdar, A. F., Bepler, G., Guccion, J. G., Marangos, P. J., Moody, T. W., Zweig, M. H., and Minna, J. D. (1985). Establishment and identification of small-cell lung cancer cell lines having classic and variant features. *Cancer Res.* **45:**2913–2923.

Doyle, L. A., Giangiulio, D., Hussain, A., Park, H.-J., Yen, R.-W. C., and Borges, M. (1989). Differentiation of variant small cell lung cancer to a classic morphology by retinoic acid. *Cancer Res.* **49:**6745–6751.

Doyle, L. A., Borges, M., Hussain, A., Elias, A., and Tomiyasu, T. (1990a). An adherent subline of a unique small-cell lung cancer cell line down-regulates antigens of the neural cell adhesion molecule. *J. Clin. Invest.* **86:**1848–1854.

Doyle, L. A., Goldstein, L. H., Clingroth, C. J., and Cuttitta, F. (1990b). Identification of conditioned medium proteins from human cancer cells adapted to serum-free conditions. *Anal. Biochem.* **190:**238–243.

Doyle, L. A., Mabry, M., Stahel, R. A., Waibel, R., and Goldstein, L. H. Modulation of neuroendocrine surface antigens in oncogene-activated small cell lung cancer lines. *Br. J. Cancer* (in press).

Falco, J., Baylin, S., Lupu, R., Borges, M., Jasti, R., Nelkin, B., Davidson, N., and Mabry, M. (1989). Appearance of epidermal growth factor receptors and transforming growth factor-alpha accompanies viral Harvey ras-induced conversion of small cell lung cancer to non-small cell lung cancer in vitro. *Proc. Am. Assoc. Cancer Res.* **30:**438(abstract).

Goodwin, G., Shaper, J. H., Abeloff, M. D., Mendelsohn, G., and Baylin, S. B. (1983). Analysis of cell surface proteins delineates a differentiation pathway linking endocrine and nonendocrine human lung cancers. *Proc. Natl. Acad. Sci. USA* **80:**3807–3811.

Heighway, J., Thatcher, N., Cerny, T., and Hasleton, P. (1986). Genetic predisposition to human lung cancer. *Br. J. Cancer* **54:**453–457.

Hoffman, S., and Edelman, G. M. (1983). Kinetics of homophilic binding of embryonic and adult forms of the neural cell adhesion molecule. *Proc. Natl. Acad. Sci. USA* **80:** 5762–5766.

Johnson, B. E., Battey, J., Linnoila, I., Becker, K. L., Makuch, R. W., Snider, R. H., Carney, D. N., and Minna, J. D. (1986). Changes in the phenotype of human small cell lung cancer cell lines after transfection and expression of the c-myc proto-oncogene. *J. Clin. Invest.* **78:**525–532.

Land, H., Parada, L. F., and Weinberg, R. A. (1983). Tumorigenic conversion of primary embryo fibroblasts requires at least two cooperating oncogenes. *Nature (Lond.)* **304:** 596–602.

Little, C. D., Nau, M. M., Carney, D. N., Gazdar, A. F., and Minna, J. D. (1983). Amplification and expression of the c-myc oncogene in human lung cancer cell lines. *Nature* **306:**194–196.

Mabry, M., Nakagawa, T., Nelkin, B. D., McDowell, E., Gesell, M., Eggleston, J. C., Casero, R. A., Jr., and Baylin, S. B. (1988). v-Ha-ras oncogene insertion: a model for tumor progression of human small cell lung cancer. *Proc. Natl. Acad. Sci. USA* **85:**6523–6527.

Moolenaar, C. E. C., Muller, E. J., Schol, D. J., Figdor, C. G., Bock, E., Bitter-Suermann, D., and Michalides, R. J. A. M. (1990). Expression of an NCAM related sialoglycoprotein in small cell lung cancer and neuroblastoma. *Cancer Res.* **50:**1102–1106.

Reeve, J. G., Shaw, J. J., Twentyman, P. R., and Bleehen, N. M. (1988). Identification of antigenic phenotypes characterizing lung tumour cell lines in vitro. *Lung Cancer* **4:** 65–66.

Rodenhuis, S., van de Wetring, M. L. Mooi, W. J., Evers, S. G. Zandwijk, N., and Bos,

J. L. (1987). Mutational activation of the K-ras oncogene: a possible pathogenetic factor in adenocarcinoma of the lung. *N. Engl. J. Med.* **317**:929–935.

Scarpa, S., Morstyn, G., Carney, D. N., Modesti, A., and Triche, T. J. (1988). Small cell lung cancer cell lines: pure and variant types can be distinguished by their extracellular matrix synthesis. *Eur. Respir. J.* **1**:639–644.

Simms, E., Gazdar, A. F., Abrams, P. G., and Minna, J. D. (1980). Growth of human small-cell (oat cell) carcinoma of the lung in serum-free growth factor-supplemented medium. *Cancer Res.* **40**:4356–4363.

Souhami, R. L., Beverly, P. C. L., Bobrow, L. G. (1987). Antigens of small-cell lung cancer. *Lancet* **2**:325–326.

Stahel, R. A., O'Hara, C. J., Mabry, M., Waibel, R., Sabbath, K., Speak, J. A., Bernal, S. D. (1986). Cytotoxic murine monoclonal antibody LAM8 with specificity for human small cell lung carcinoma of the lung. *Cancer Res.* **45**:2077–2084.

Strnad, J., Hamilton, A. E., Beavers, L. S., Gamboa, G. C., Apelgren, L. D., Taber, L. D., Sportsman, J. R., Bumol, T. F., Sharp, J. D., and Gadski, R. A. (1989). Molecular cloning and characterization of a human adenocarcinoma/epithelial cell surface antigen complementary DNA. *Cancer Res.* **49**:314–317.

7

Production of Growth Factors by Non-Small-Cell Lung Carcinomas

JILL M. SIEGFRIED

University of Pittsburgh
Pittsburgh, Pennsylvania

PHYLLIS G. ANDREWS, SUZANNE K. HANSEN,* and SARA E. OWENS

Environmental Health Research and Testing, Inc.
Research Triangle Park, North Carolina

I. Introduction

Uncontrolled cell proliferation in tumors may result from aberrations in response to or production of peptide growth factors (for review, see Sporn and Roberts, 1985; Goustin et al., 1986). Secretion of growth factors has been postulated by Sporn and Todaro to produce an autocrine or paracrine loop by which tumor cells direct their growth autonomously (Sporn and Todaro, 1980; Todaro et al., 1980). Production of one such growth factor, transforming growth factor-α (TGF-α), has been described in solid tumors and cultured tumor cells from many tissues (Roberts et al., 1980; Moses et al., 1981; Todaro et al., 1980; Derynck et al., 1987). TGF-α, which acts by binding to the epidermal growth factor (EGF) receptor (Todaro et al., 1980), can also be found in the urine of patients with advanced cancer (Sherwin et al., 1983) and is expressed during fetal development (Lee et al., 1985). TGF-α has also recently been found in normal adult keratinocytes (Coffey et al., 1987) and in normal mammary epithelial cells (Salmon et al., 1988), and so may have more general in vivo effects than was originally thought.

**Present affiliation*: Sphinx Biotechnologies Corporation, Durham, North Carolina

Peptides resembling another potential autocrine factor, insulin-like growth factor I (IGF-I) are produced by breast carcinoma cells (Huff et al., 1986) and small cell lung tumors (Macauly et al., 1988). This secretion may contribute to autonomous growth of tumors, since IGF-I is the principal growth-stimulator present in serum, and plasma levels are controlled by growth hormone in vivo (for review, see Froesch et al., 1985). IGF-I has growth-promoting effects on cells of epithelial and mesenchymal origin, mediated through its own high-affinity receptor. Other potential autocrine factors that have been described in small cell carcinoma include bombesin (Cuttitta et al., 1985) and its analog gastrin-releasing hormone (Carney et al., 1987), which are secreted by small cell tumors displaying neuroendocrine properties.

Our laboratory has undertaken to identify potential autocrine growth factors secreted by non-small-cell lung tumors in culture (Siegfried, 1987; Siegfried et al., 1988). Non-small-cell lung tumors, which are comprised mainly of squamous and adenocarcinomas, account for the majority of all lung tumors. We have also investigated the growth-modulating effects of secreted peptides on primary tumor cells obtained from patients with lung cancer (Siegfried and Owens, 1988). This chapter summarizes our findings and presents additional evidence of growth factor messenger RNA production in cultured lung tumors.

II. Methods

A. Analysis of Conditioned Medium

Collection of serum-free conditioned medium (CM) and analysis for growth-promoting properties was done as described (Siegfried, 1987). Culture of primary lung carcinomas has also been described (Siegfried and Owens, 1988). For biochemical analysis, serum-free CM was concentrated by dialysis against 0.1 M acetic acid followed by lyophilization, or by application to a Seppak C18 preparatory column (Waters) followed by elution with 40% acetonitrile/60% water, and lyophilization. Concentrated material was resuspended in the appropriate buffer for each assay.

TGF-α in cell extracts and conditioned medium was measured in an EGF receptor-binding radioassay in which EGF receptor-rich membranes were prepared from A431 cells by hypotonic lysis and immobilized onto polypropylene tubes, adapted from the method described by Kimball and Warren (1984). EGF and IGF-I were determined by radioimmunoassays using commercially supplied kits (Biomedical Technologies, Stoughton, MA, and Amersham, respectively). IGF-I was also measured by radioreceptor assay using whole MCF7 cells.

Experiments with monoclonal antibody 225 (generously supplied by Dr. John Mendelsohn of Memorial–Sloan Kettering Cancer Center) were performed in 24-well plates. A549-1 cells were plated at 1000 cells/well in basal medium

Eagles' with 0.5% fetal bovine serum. Serial dilutions of antibody were added to each well, four wells per condition. After 10 days, cells were fixed and stained and the average number of cells per colony determined in 25 colonies per well. Doubling time was calculated from the formula $2^n = X$, where X is average number of cells per colony.

B. RNA Isolation and Northern Analysis

RNA from growing cells was extracted using the acid guanidinium thiocyanate–phenol–chloroform method according to procedures described by Chomczynski and Sacchi (1987). Polyadenylated messenger RNA (PA+) was selected using an oligo-dT column (Aviv and Leder, 1972). One to 21 μg of PA+ RNA from each of the cell lines was size fractionated on 1% agarose denaturing gels containing 2.2 M formaldehyde (Maniatis et al., 1982). Marker lanes of DNA and RNA were cut off the gels, stained in 0.5 μg/ml ethidium bromide, and photographed using ultraviolet (UV) excitation for sizing of bands. RNA in the gels was subjected to Northern transfer without pretreatment by placing the gels against nitrocellulose filters in the standard configuration for Southern transfers (Southern, 1975). The nitrocellulose filters (Schleicher and Schuell, Inc.) were baked 2 h at 80°C.

C. Hybridization to ^{32}P-labeled DNA Probes

All filters were prehybridized in 50% formamide, 5X SSC, 0.1% sodium dodecyl sulfate (SDS), 10 X Denhardt's solution (Maniatis et al., 1982), and 0.2 mg/ml sheared salmon sperm DNA overnight at 42°C. The filters were then hybridized in 50% formamide, 5X SSC, 1 X Denhardt's solution, 0.04 mg/ml sheared denatured salmon sperm DNA, and labeled probe ($1–5 \times 10^9$ cpm/μg DNA). ^{32}P-labeled cDNA fragments were isolated from plasmids or used as uncut plasmids. Hybridization was performed overnight at 40°C. The filters were washed in 2X SSC, 0.1% SDS, and then washed for 2 h at 55°C in 0.1X SSC, 0.1% SDS. These procedures are essentially as described by Maniatis et al., 1982. Autoradiography was for 1–18 days against Kodak XOMAT XAR film at −80°C using intensifier screens. The cDNA fragments were labeled using the Amersham Multiprime Labeling kit according to the manufacturer's instructions.

D. Colony-Forming Assays Testing Peptide Growth Factors

The effects of the various peptide growth factors were tested on normal bronchial epithelial cells and early passage lung tumor cells in colony-forming assays. Cells were plated onto mouse 3T3 fibroblast feeder layers (Siegfried and Nesnow, 1984) and allowed to grow in the presence of the growth factor for approximately 1 week, after which colonies were fixed, stained, and counted. Interleukin 1 and 2, platelet-derived growth factor (PDGF), and multiplication stimulating factor (MSA) were purchased form Collaborative Research (Bedford, MA). ACTH, bombesin, gastrin-releasing peptide (GRP), and prolactin were purchased from Sigma (St. Louis, MO).

III. Results and Discussion

A. Growth-Promoting Activity of CM

In initial experiments to identify lung carcinoma cell lines that might produce autocrine growth factors, filtered serum-free medium conditioned for 72 h was screened for growth-stimulating activity using colony-forming assays. Several cell types were used as the recipients of conditioned medium (CM), which was added in a 1:1 ratio with the corresponding basal medium required for growth of each cell type (Siegfried, 1987). Colony-forming efficiency (CFE) was used as an endpoint because it is an indicator of actual cell replication and requires that each parent cell undergo several divisions to from a colony. A549-1 cells, which were derived from the parent A549 bronchioloalveolar carcinoma cell line (Giard et al., 1973) by selection at low density, produced CM that was a potent stimulator of colony formation (Table 1). CM added to A549-1 cells themselves, to normal human bronchial epithelial cells, or to primary carcinoma cells derived from two solid lung tumors increased colony formation over fivefold. CM harvested from Calu 1, a cell line derived from an epidermoid carcinoma of lung, was less effective, as were CM from SK-MES-1, a squamous lung carcinoma, and from H128, a small cell carcinoma that secretes high levels of bombesin (Cuttitta et al., 1985).

Table 1 Growth Stimulation of Conditioned Medium

	Source of conditioned medium				
Responding cell	A549-1	Calu 1	SK-MES 1	H128	W138
A549-1	5.1[a]	1.5	2.0	—	3.3
Calu 1	1.7	1.0	1.0	—	3.1
Human bronchial epithelial cells	8.5	1.6	0.9	0.6	1.4
81-86T, primary undifferentiated lung carcinoma	5.9	—	—	—	—
82-86T, primary adenosquamous lung carcinoma	6.1	—	—	—	0.2

Filtered, unconcentrated conditioned medium was added at a final volume of 50% to wells containing cells used as responders. Colonies were enumerated after 7–10 days and response determined as percentage of control colony-forming efficiency. Five wells were used per condition and maximum response was used to compare conditioned medium from different sources.

[a]Fold increase in colony-forming efficiency over control.

This suggests that bombesin may not be an autocrine factor for lung tumors other than small cell. CM from W138, human embryonic lung fibroblasts, was only growth-enhancing toward the two established tumor cell lines tested. Embryonic cells may express growth factors in limited amounts.

It is possible that the differentiated state of the tumor determines the extent of active growth factor secretion. A549-1 cells were derived from a tumor with characteristics of adenocarcinoma. Cells cultured from this tumor may retain some of the secretory ability of the original tumor. CM from A549-1 cells was used to promote growth of primary tumor cells from solid lung tumors. These assays were performed using carcinoma cells that attached to flasks of irradiated Swiss 3T3 cells after tumor tissue was minced. Carcinoma cells were harvested from flasks after mild treatment with EDTA to remove feeder cells and used in colony-forming assays (Siegfried and Owens, 1988). As shown in Table 2, the extent of stimulation of CM (1:1 mixture of medium conditioned by A549-1 cells and fresh medium) varied from 1.9- to 11.8-fold over basal medium with different tumor specimens. Addition of A549-1 CM to cultures of solid lung tumors has resulted in viable primary colonies in 20 of 22 cases and subcultures in 18 of 22 (Siegfried and Owens, 1988). This success rate demonstrates that the growth factors found in CM may be involved in tumor growth in vivo. Responsiveness of primary tumor cells was higher in the adenocarcinomas and large cell carcinomas tested than in the squamous cell carcinomas. This may indicate that the state of differentiation of the responding cell is important in determining the growth-promoting effect. Analysis of more tumor types will be needed to verify this observation.

B. Biochemical Assays for Growth Factor Production

We have demonstrated that both normal and neoplastic lung epithelial cells are stimulated by TGF-α and IGF-1 (Siegfried, 1987; Siegfried and Owens, 1988). We therefore assayed CM and cell pellets for the presence of these peptides. A competitive EGF radioreceptor assay in A431 cell membranes was used to determine if TGF-α-like products, which bind to the EGF receptor, were present in

Table 2 Effect of A549-1 CM on Colony Formation of Primary Tumor Cells

Specimen no.	Histologic type	No. cells seeded per well	No. colonies/well basal medium	No. colonies/well CM
82-86T	Adenosquamous	4000	13.2 ± 1.7	58.0 ± 3.6
91-86T	Adenosquamous	2500	23.5 ± 7.5	276.7 ± 87.6
101-87T	Squamous cell	5000	213.3 ± 47.3	409.7 ± 109.2
105-87T	Large cell	5000	76.0 ± 30.0	504.3 ± 120.7
109-87T	Squamous cell	5000	11.0 ± 2.2	21.3 ± 6.2

CM and cell pellets from four lung cell lines (Table 3). Such activity was found both in cell extracts and secreted into medium in A549-1, Calu 1, and W138 cells. Calu 6, an adenocarcinoma of the lung, showed little activity. The competing activity was found not to be due to EGF by radioimmunoassay using an EGF-specific antibody (data not shown). IGF-I-like activity was measured by both radioreceptor assay using intact MCF7 cells and radioimmunoassay. Competing activity in these assays was found in A549-1 and Calu 1 cells, both in CM and cell extracts (Table 3). The superior growth-enhancing activity of A549-1 CM compared to Calu 1 CM is not due simply to the amount of these two growth factors and is probably accounted for by the exact form in which the proteins are secreted. The prohormone form of a growth factor may be produced and detected by a radioimmunoassay but will show little biological activity unless the cell producing it is capable of converting it to the mature peptide form by appropriate proteolytic cleavage. Another possibility is that other peptides, either growth-promoting or growth-inhibiting, are present in the CM, accounting for differences in biological activity. We have observed an activity in the CM of A549-1 cells that promotes anchorage-independent growth of primary lung tumor cells (Siegfried and Owens, 1988). This factor may be an additional growth-promoting peptide, similar to transforming growth factor E, which has been described by Halper and Moses (1987).

The IGF-I-related activity could be due to IGF-I binding protein, which might interfere with competitive assays by acting as a sink for radiolabeled IGF-I. The binding protein itself has been reported to enhance the activity of IGF-I, and to have biological activity of its own (Elgin et al., 1987). However, Western blot analysis showed a 21 kd protein present in A549-1 cell extracts that is immunoreactive to an antibody raised to the carboxy terminal of the IGF-I precursor (data not

Table 3 Growth Factor Activity in Cultured Lung Cells

Cell type	Secreted into medium (ng/ml/10^7 cells)	Present in cell extract (ng/mg protein)
TGF-α-like		
A549-1	0.23	9.9
Calu 1	0.13	21.6
Calu 6	0.03	0.46
W138	0.22	14.1
IGF-I-like		
A549-1	14.5	22.5
Calu 1	17.1	4.40
Calu 6	0	0.78
W138	0	0

shown). Since this is the expected size of the precursor, either IGF-I or a very similar protein is produced by A549-1 cells.

C. Blockage of EGF Receptors Suppresses Growth of A549-1 Cells

If secreted growth factors act through an autocrine mechanism, it should be possible to alter growth of cells that secrete the peptide by blocking receptors for it in the absence of exogenous peptide. This was attempted by colony assays performed with A549-1 cells in the presence of mAb225, a monoclonal antibody that blocks the EGF receptor and acts as an EGF antagonist (Gill et al., 1984; H. Masui et al, 1986). A549-1 cells were plated in medium containing 0.5% fetal bovine serum, the lowest amount of serum in which colonies will form, at a density of 1000 cells/9.6 cm^2 well and grown for 10 days in the presence of mAb225 or control IgGs in the absence or presence of exogenous growth factor (Fig. 1). Doubling time was calculated from average size of colonies formed.

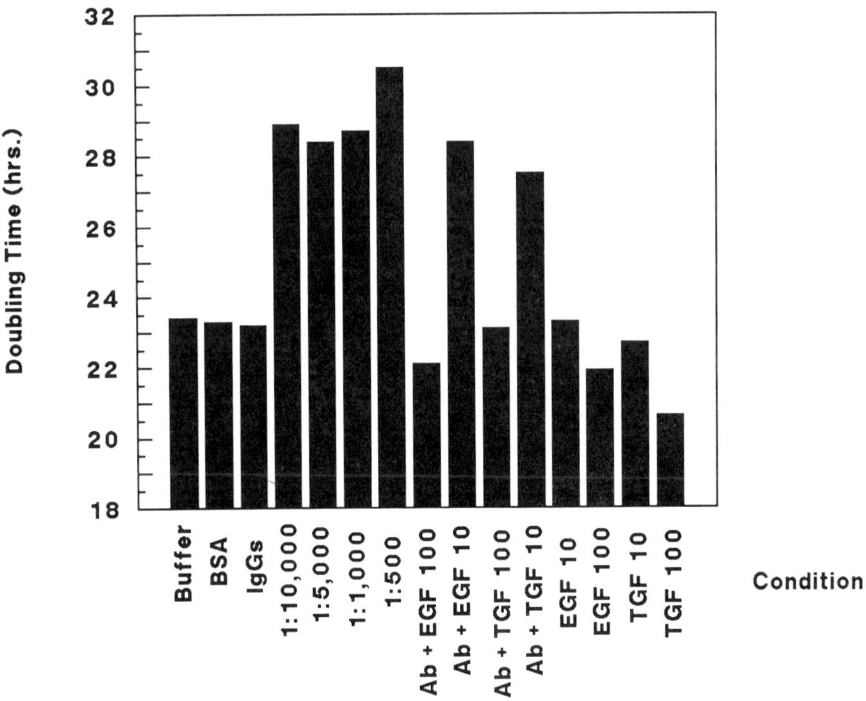

Figure 1 Effect of monoclonal antibody (mAb) 225 on doubling time of A549-1 cells. Buffer, control; BSA, bovine serum albumin control. Dilutions shown are made from an antibody stock solution of 10 mg/ml. EGF or TGF_α was added as 10 or 100 ng per well.

Doubling time increased from 23.5 to 29 h with as little as a 1:10,000 dilution of antibody (1 μg/ml in wells). Cells could be rescued from effects of antibody by addition of excess EGF or TGF-α (100 ng/well). These results demonstrate that by blocking the EGF receptor, cells that secrete TGF-α are growth-inhibited, implying that the secreted peptide does act on the secreting cell.

D. Demonstration of Growth Factor mRNA

Production of mRNA of the growth factors TGF-α and IGF-I was monitored in the human lung tumor cell lines A549-1 and Calu 6 by Northern analysis of polyadenylated RNA. Figure 2 shows the autoradiograph of polyadenylated RNA probed with [^{32}P]TGF-α cDNA. The cell line A549-1 shows a distinct band at 4.8 kb, which is the size expected for TGF-α mRNA (Derynck et al., 1984). Calu 6 also expresses TGF-α mRNA. The control, total mRNA from normal human lung tissue, does not express the TGF-α mRNA.

In Figure 2, [^{32}P]IGF-I cDNA was used to probe the polyadenylated mRNA from A549-1 and Calu 6, and total RNA from normal human lung tissue. Only the cell line A549-1 showed any evidence of expression of IGF-I. IGF-I, a multigene family with apparent tissue specific expression, has many different sizes reported for mRNA length (Huff et al., 1986; Hoppener et al., 1987). In our hands, the probe detects a smear from 4.7 kb up to greater than 20 kb and one distinct band at 2.5 kb. The cell line Calu 6 and the normal human lung control showed no hybridization to the IGF-I probe.

The expression of TGF-β, as shown in Figure 3, is apparent in all the lung tumor cell lines we tested. The expected 2.5 kb band (Derynck et al., 1985) for the TGF-β mRNA is seen in polyadenylated mRNA from the cell lines A549, A549-1, Calu 6, Calu 1, and WI38, a human embryonic cell line. Total RNA from normal human lung tissue did not show any detectable amounts of TGF-β RNA even after prolonged autoradiography.

E. Activity of Other Purified Growth Factors

Colony-forming assays were used to determine whether other known peptides are candidates for autocrine factors in the lung. Normal bronchial epithelial cells and newly cultured tumor cells were used in these assays. The peptides ACTH and prolactin were examined because they have been reported to be aberrantly expressed in lung tumors (Gerwitz and Yalow, 1974; Davis et al., 1979) and it is possible that they have some function in lung cancer. Bombesin has been reported by Willey et al. (1984) to enhance growth of bronchial epithelial cells and is stimulatory in small cell carcinoma of the lung (Cuttitta et al., 1985). Other peptides assayed were MSA (the mouse equivalent of IGF-2), TGF-β, gastrin-releasing peptide (GRP), platelet-derived growth factor (PDGF), and interleukin-1 and -2 (IL-1 and IL-2). Results are shown in Figures 4 through 9.

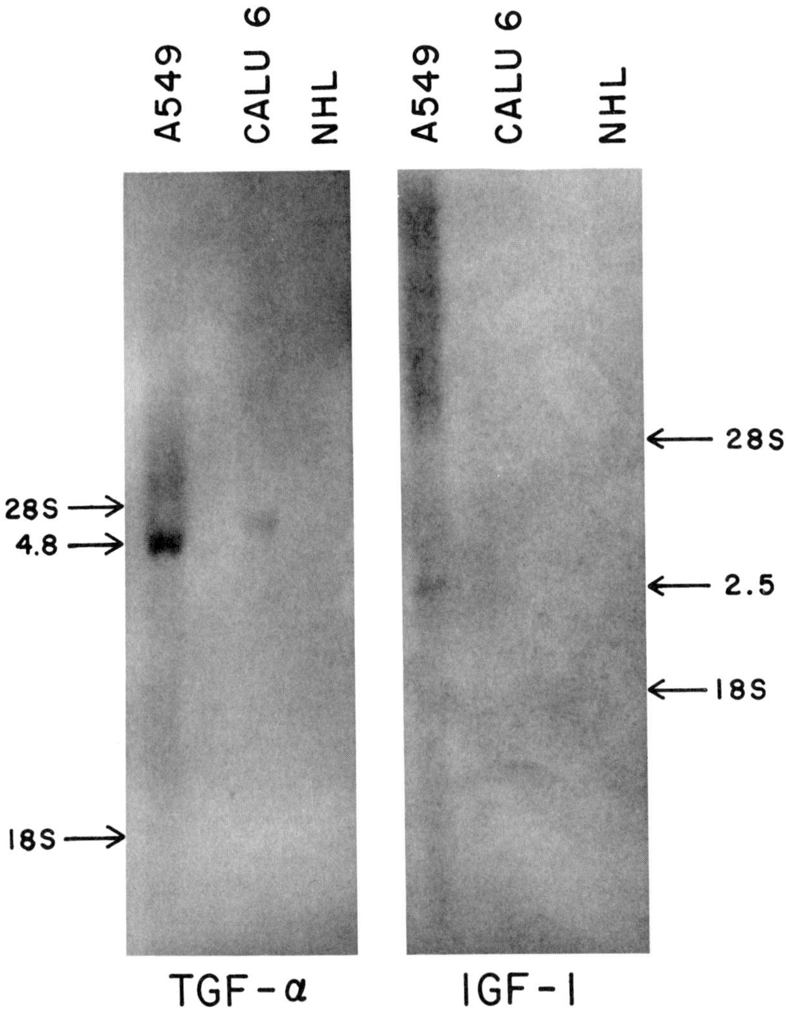

Figure 2 Polyadenylated RNA isolated from human lung tumor cell lines and total RNA from normal human lung tissue were size fractionated on a denaturing agarose gel, transferred to nitrocellulose, and hybridized to a ^{32}P-labeled 1.35 Kbp EcoRI fragment of the plasmid pSP65C17N3 (Derynck et al., 1984) containing the cDNA of the human TGF-α gene or to a ^{32}P-labeled 3.5 Kbp EcoRI fragment of the plasmid phIGF-I/RI-6 (Ullrich et al., 1984) containing the cDNA of the human IGF-I gene. Sizes of the bands were determined by the size markers λ Hind III/ΦX Hae III and by 28s and 18s rRNA standards.

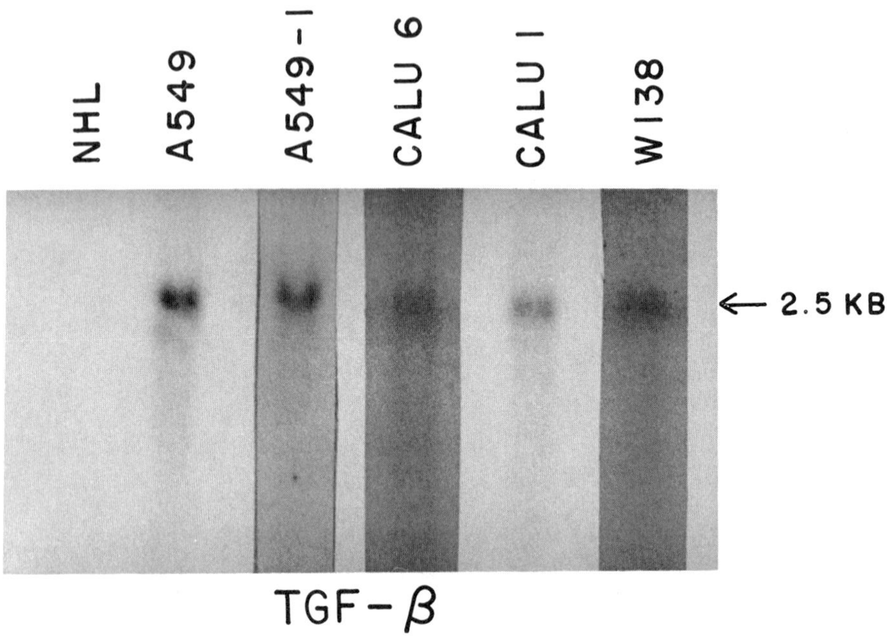

Figure 3 Polyadenylated RNA isolated from human lung tumor cell lines and total RNA from normal human lung tissue were size fractionated on a denaturing agarose gel, transferred to nitrocellulose, and hybridized to a ^{32}P-labeled 1.0 Kbp EcoRI fragment of the plasmid pβas (Derynck et al., 1985) containing the cDNA of the human TGF-β gene. Sizes of the bands were determined as in Figure 2.

TGF-β (Fig. 4) showed an overall inhibitory effect on both normal and neoplastic cells, but normal bronchial cells in one case were more sensitive. Inhibitory effects were observed as low as 0.015 ng/ml in normal cells from case 134-88, but in tumor cells inhibition was only observed at 1.5 ng/ml or higher. T. Masui et al. (1986) have reported that established lung carcinoma cell lines are resistant to inhibition by TGF-β. This may be due to the fact that established lines were selected to grow in high serum, which contains TGF-β, and may not be indicative of the lung tumor cell population in general.

Little or no effect on colony formation was seen with bombesin (Fig. 5) or GRP (data not shown), except in the case of tumor cells form one donor, 113-87, derived from an undifferentiated large cell carcinoma. This indicates that effects of bombesin may be limited to small cell carcinoma. Bombesin in our hands had no effect on bronchial epithelial cells. Prolactin and ACTH also had no effect, except in the case of 113-87 tumor cells (Figs. 6, 7). A stimulation of 85% and

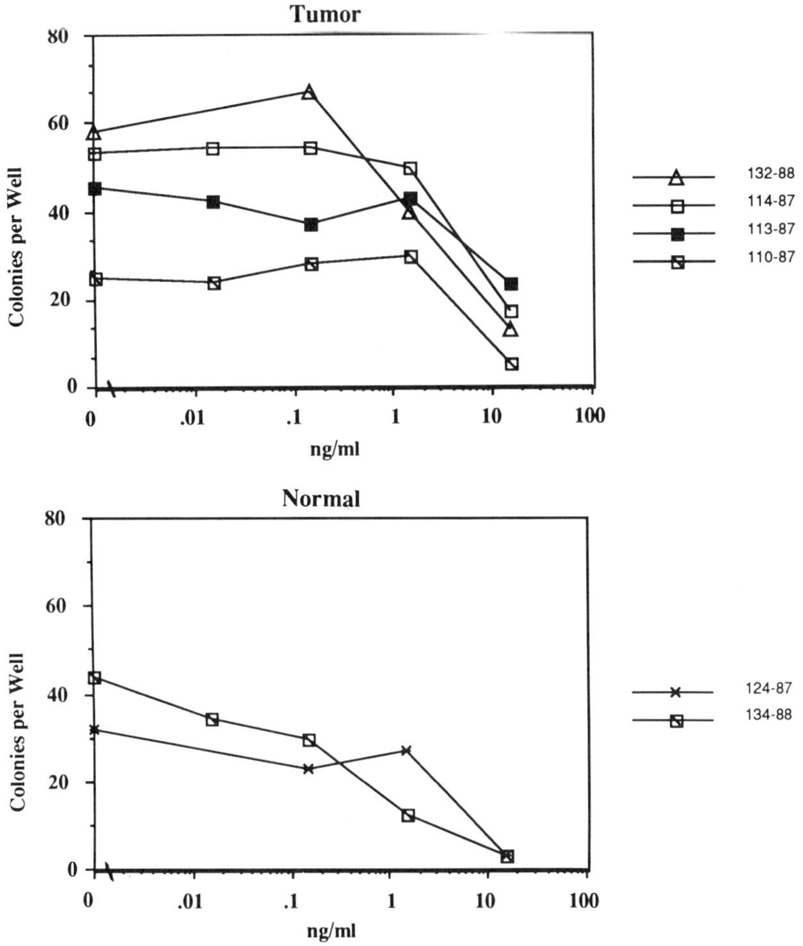

Figure 4 Effect of TGF-β on colony formation of normal bronchial cells and newly cultured lung carcinoma cells from different human donors. Each specimen is graphed separately, as indicated. Data are expressed as number of colonies per well per 4000 cells seeded (specimen 113-87); per 2000 cells seeded (specimen 110-87); per 200 cells seeded (specimen 114-87); per 20,000 cells seeded (specimen 132-88); per 5000 cells seeded (specimen 124-87); and per 800 cells seeded (specimen 134-88). Number of cells seeded was determined by the expected colony-forming efficiency of each specimen.

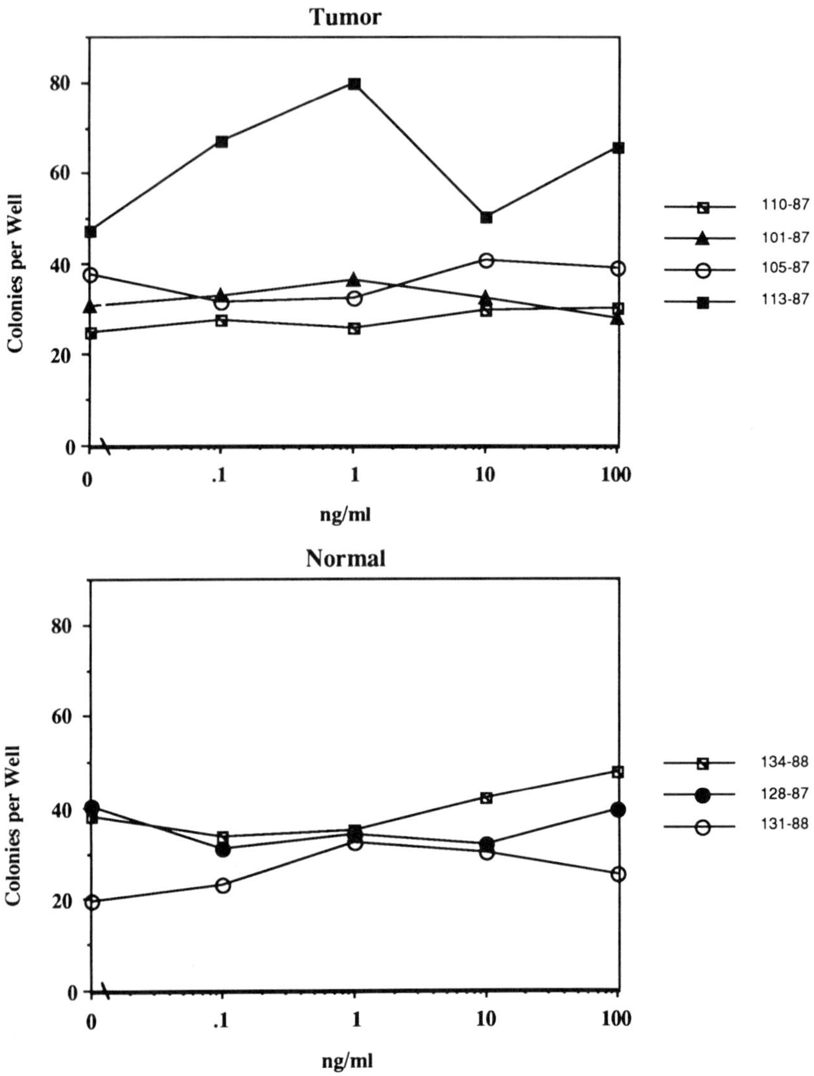

Figure 5 Effect of bombesin on colony formation. Data are expressed as described in Figure 4, with the additions of number of colonies per 200 cells seeded (specimen 101-87); per 250 cells seeded (specimens 105-87 and 128-87); and per 1000 cells seeded (specimen 131-88).

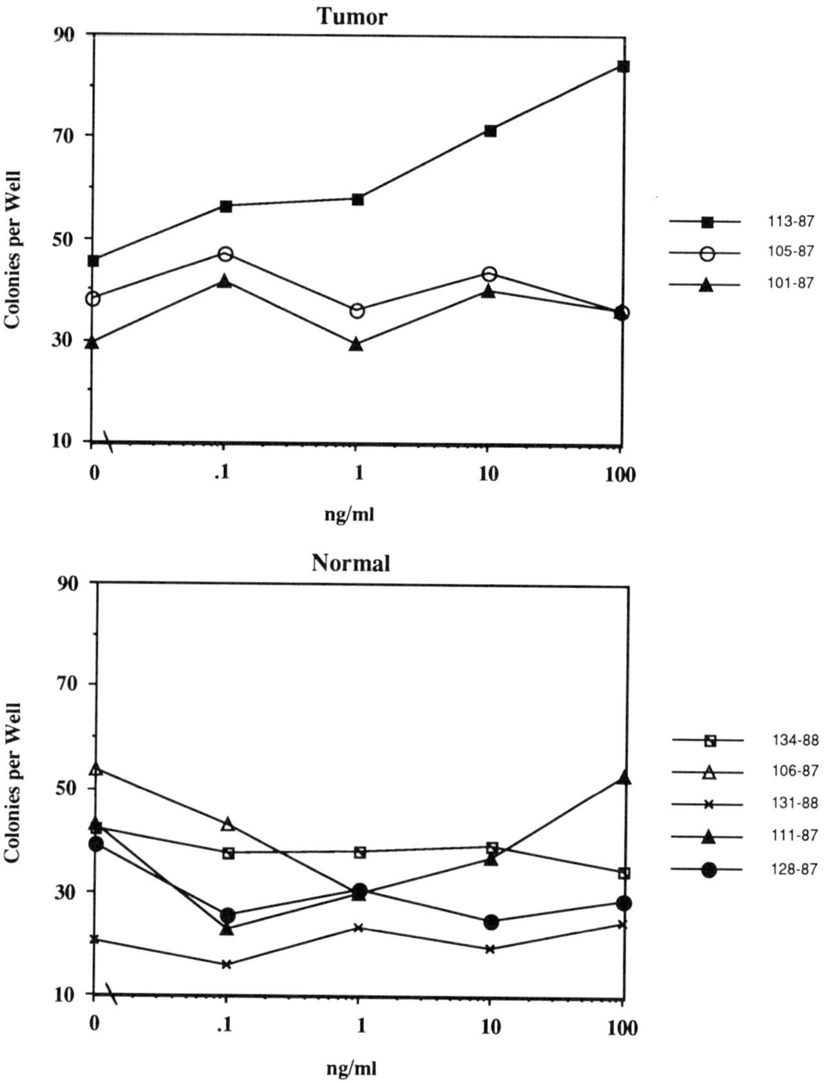

Figure 6 Effect of prolactin on colony formation. Data are expressed as described in Figures 4 and 5, with the addition of number of colonies per 2500 cells seeded (specimens 106-87 and 111-87).

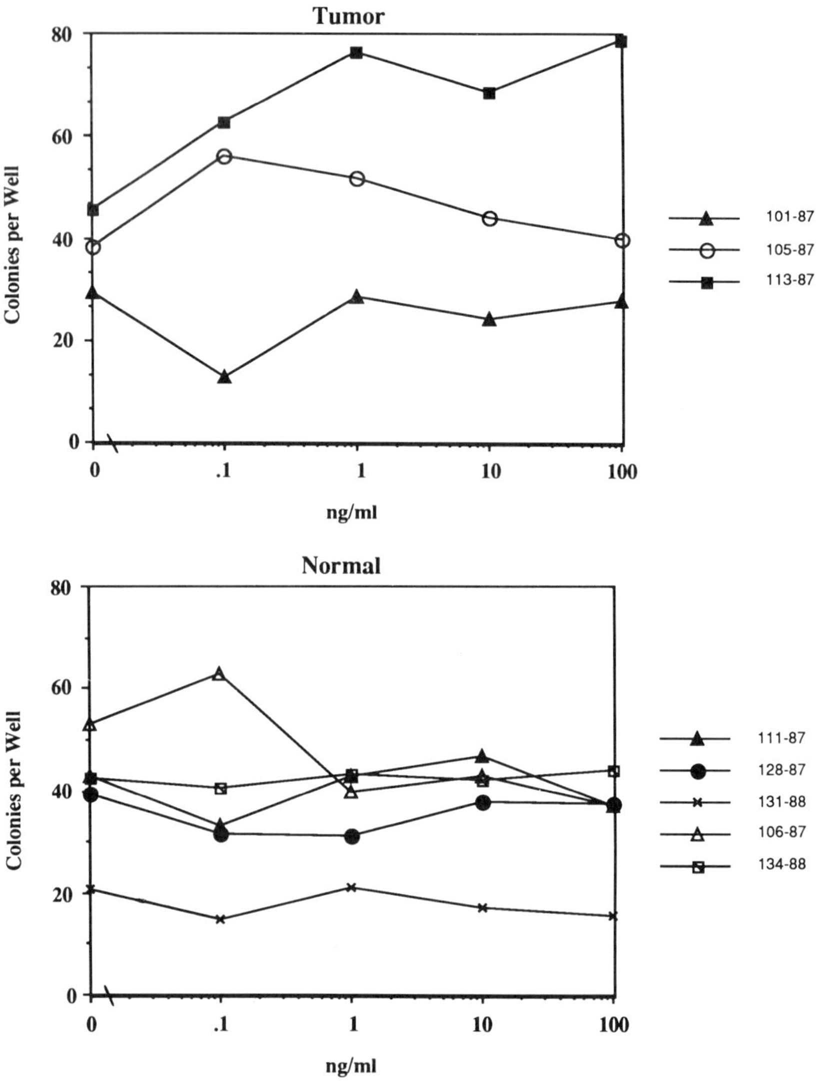

Figure 7 Effect of ACTH on colony formation. Data are expressed as described in Figures 4–6.

73%, respectively, was observed for these two compounds. No effect of PDGF was observed (data not shown), as expected for epithelial cells.

IL-1 has been reported to stimulate anchorage-independent growth of human adrenal carcinoma cells (Hamburger et al., 1987). Sporn and Roberts (1986) have suggested that peptides released by inflammatory cells may help to maintain neoplastic cells in vivo. Other laboratories have reported inhibitory effects of IL-1 in breast tumor cells (Gaffney and Tsai, 1986) and melanoma (Onozaki et al., 1985). As seen in Figure 8, we observed a growth stimulation of IL-1 in one tumor (a large cell carcinoma, 105-87). In one case, 101-87, a squamous cell carcinoma, 60% inhibition was observed. Similar results were seen in assays using bronchial cells; depending on the individual case, a slight inhibition or stimulation was observed.

Two tumor specimens were stimulated by IL-2, and IL-2 also stimulated bronchial cells from two individuals (Fig. 9). These individual variations may be due to expression of receptor or to state of differentiation of the cells. MSA showed no effect on either normal or neoplastic cells (data not shown).

IV. Future Directions

Much experimental evidence supports the hypothesis that autocrine growth factors contribute to the neoplastic state in tumor cell lines. The importance of this process in maintaining tumor growth in vivo remains to be demonstrated. Our laboratory will focus in the future on measuring the production of growth factors in solid tumors and the response of primary cells to such factors. Another avenue of investigation is the development of a defined, serum-free medium that can be used to culture primary solid tumors and to investigate the effects of secreted factors on primary solid lung tumor cells. Propagation of A549-1 cells in completely serum-free medium will also simplify identification of the peptide that stimulates anchorage-independent growth of primary tumor cells.

V. Conclusions

Production of messenger RNA that hybridizes to probes for the TGF-α and IGF-I genes and of proteins with the characteristics of TGF-α and IGF-I by non-small-cell lung carcinoma cell lines has been demonstrated. These growth factors probably account at least in part for the growth-enhancing activity of conditioned medium from A549-1 cells. Blocking the EGF receptor in A549-1 cells causes growth inhibition in the absence of exogenous growth factor, indicating an autocrine function for secreted growth factor in these cells. Primary cells isolated from solid non-small-cell lung tumors are responsive to the secreted growth factor activity produced by A549-1 cells, indicating that the autocrine or paracrine

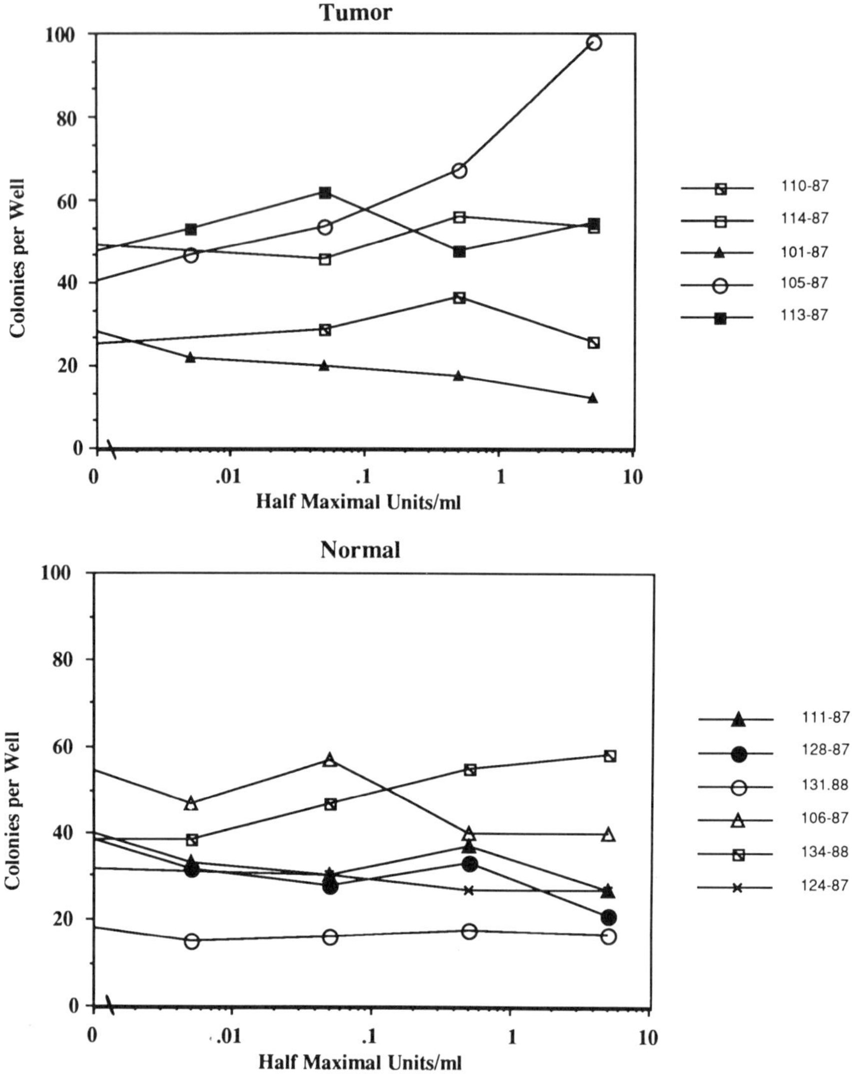

Figure 8 Effect of interleukin-1 on colony formation. Data are expressed as described in Figures 4–6.

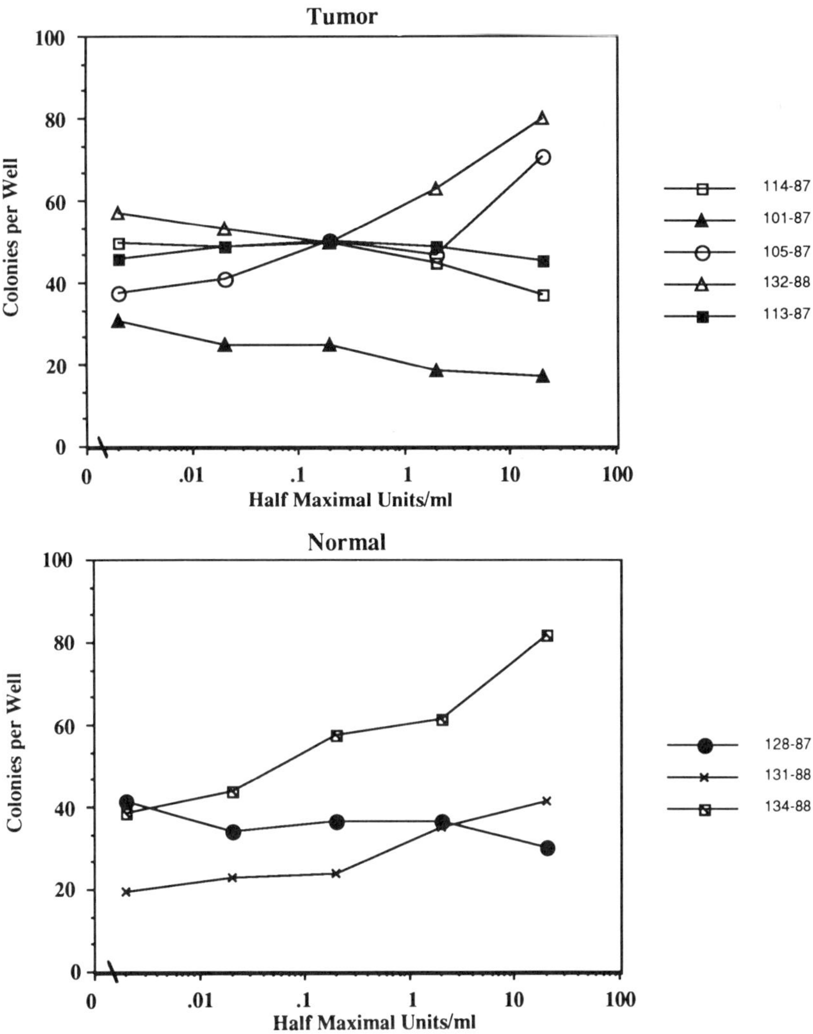

Figure 9 Effect of interleukin-2 on colony formation. Data are expressed as described in Figures 4–6.

process may operate in vivo. Response in tumors to other potential autocrine or paracrine factors may depend on expression of receptors or other factors that vary among individual cases, such as the state of differentiation. Some evidence was found indicating that IL-1 and IL-2 may modulate lung tumor growth. Additional work needs to focus on primary tumor cells as producers of and responders to secreted growth factors. Knowledge of growth factor status may aid in better defining lung cancer subtypes and in identifying targets for therapy of non-small-cell lung cancer. Antibodies to growth-promoting peptides or their receptors may be active as chemotherapeutic agents in non-small-cell tumors that secrete autocrine factors.

Acknowledgments

The authors thank Marcy Fetter and Mary Beth Tyndall for technical assistance. This research was conducted in part under contract No. 68-02-4456 from the U.S. Environmental Protection Agency. This research was supported in part by a Research Starter Grant from the Pharmaceutical Manufacturers' Association Foundation, by an institutional award, IN-58-28, from the American Cancer Society, and by a grant from NIH, CA50694. Jill M. Siegfried is the recipient of an American Cancer Society Junior Faculty Research Award.

References

Aviv, H., and Leder, P. (1972). Purification of biologically active globin messenger RNA by chromatography on oligothymidylic acid-cellulose. *Proc. Natl. Acad. Sci. USA* **69:**1408–1412.

Carney, D. N., Cuttitta, F., Moody, T. W., and Minna, J. D. (1987). Selective stimulation of small cell lung cancer clonal growth by bombesin and gastrin-releasing peptide. *Cancer Res.* **47:**821–825.

Chomczynski, P., and Sacchi, N. (1987). Single-step method of RNA isolation by acid guanidinium thiocyanate–phenol–chloroform extraction. *Anal. Biochem.* **162:** 156–159.

Coffey, R. J., Derynck, R., Wilcox, J. N., Bringman, T. S., Goustin, A. S., Moses, H. L., and Pittelkow, M. R. (1987). Production and auto-induction of transforming growth factor-α in human keratinocytes. *Nature (Lond.)* **328:**817–820.

Cuttitta, F., Carney, D. N., Mulshine, J., Moody, T. W., Fedorko, J., Fischler, A., and Minna, J. D. (1985). Bombesin-like peptides can function as autocrine growth factors in human small-cell lung cancer. *Nature (Lond.)* **316:**823–826.

Davis, S., Proper, S., May, P. B., and Ertel, N. H. (1979). Elevated prolactin levels in bronchogenic carcinoma. *Cancer* **44:**676–679.

Derynck, R., Roberts, A. B., Winkler, M. E., Chen, E. Y., and Goeddel, D. V. (1984). Human transforming growth factor-α: precursor structure and expression in *E. coli*. *Cell* **38:**287–297.

Derynck, R., Jarrett, J. A., Chen, E. Y., Eaton, D. H., Bell, J. R., Assoian, R. K., Roberts, A. B., Sporn, M. B., and Goeddel, D. V. (1985). Human transforming growth factor-β complementary DNA sequence and expression in normal and transformed cells. *Nature* **316:**701–705.

Derynck, R., Goeddel, D. V., Ullrich, A., Gutterman, J. U., William, R. D., Bringman, T. S., and Berger, W. H. (1987). Synthesis of messenger RNAs for transforming growth factors α and β and the epidermal growth factor receptor by human tumors. *Cancer Res.* **47**:707–712.

Elgin, R. G., Busby, W. H. Jr., and Clemmons, D. R. (1987). An insulin-like growth factor (IGF) binding protein enhances the biological response to IGF-I. *Proc. Natl. Acad. Sci. USA* **84**:3254–3258.

Froesch, E. R., Schmid, C., Schwander, J., and Zapf, J. (1985). Actions of insulin-like growth factors. *Annu. Rev. Physiol.* **47**:443–467.

Gaffney, E. V., and Tsai, S. C. (1986). Inhibition of cell proliferation by interleukin-1 derived from monocytic leukemia cells. *Cancer Res.* **46**:1471–1477.

Gerwirtz, G., and Yalow, R. S. (1974). Ectopic ACTH production in carcinoma of the lung. *J. Clin. Invest.* **53**:1022–1032.

Giard, D. J., Aaronson, S. A., Todaro, G. J., and Arnstain, P., Kersey, J. H., Dasik, H., and Parks, W. P. (1973). *In vitro* cultivation of human tumors: establishment of cell lines derived form a series of solid tumors. *J. Natl. Cancer Inst.* **51**:1417–1423.

Gill, G. N., Kawamoto, T., Cochet, C., Le, A., Sato, J. D., Masui, H., McLeod, C., and Mendelsohn, J. (1984). Monoclonal anti-epidermal growth factor binding and antagonists of epidermal growth-factor-stimulated tyrosine protein kinase activity. *J. Biol. Chem.* **259**:7755–7760.

Goustin, A. S., Leof, E. B., Shipley, G. D., and Moses, H. L. (1986). Growth factors and cancer. *Cancer Res.* **46**:1015–1029.

Halper, J., and Moses, H. L. (1987). Purification and characterization of a novel transforming growth factor. *Cancer Res.* **47**:4552–4559.

Hamburger, A. W., Lurie, K. A., and Condon, M. E. (1987). Stimulation of anchorage-independent growth of human tumor cells by interleukin 1. *Cancer Res.* **47**:5612–5615.

Huff, K. K., Kaufman, D., Gabbay, K. H., Spencer, E. M., Lippman, M. E., and Dickson, R. B. (1986). Secretion of an insulin-like growth factor-I-related protein by human breast cancer cells. *Cancer Res.* **46**:4613–4619.

Höppener, J. W. M., Steenbergh, P. H., Slebos, R. J. C., de Pogter-Holthuigen, P., and 6 others (1987). Expression of insulin-like growth factor-I and II genes in rat medullary thyroid carcinoma. *FEBS Letts.* **215**:122–126.

Kimball, E. S., and Warren, T. C. (1984). Epidermal growth factor (EGF) binding to membranes immobilized in microtiter wells and estimation of EGF-related transforming growth factor activity. *Biochim. Biophys. Acta* **771**:82–88.

Lee, D. C., Rochford, R. M., Todaro, G. J., and Villareal, L. P. (1985). Developmental expression of rat transforming growth factor-α mRNA. *Mol. Cell Biol.* **5**:3644–3646.

Macauly, V. M., Teale, J. D., Everard, M. J., Joshi, G. P., and Smith, I. E., Millar, J. L. (1988). Somatomedin C/insulin-like growth factor-I is a mitogen for human small cell lung cancer. *Br. J. Cancer* **57**:91–93.

Maniatis, T., Fritsch, E. F., and Sambrook, J. (1982). *Handbook of Molecular Cloning*. Cold Spring Harbor, NY, Cold Spring Harbor Laboratory.

Masui, H., Moroyama, T., and Mendelsohn, J. (1986). Mechanism of antitumor activity in mice for anti-epidermal growth factor receptor monoclonal antibodies with different isotypes. *Cancer Res.* **46**:5592–5598.

Masui, T., Wakefield, L. M., Lechner, J. F., LaVeck, M. A., Sporn, M. B., and Harris, C. C. (1986). Type beta transforming growth factor is the primary differentiation-inducing serum factor for normal human bronchial epithelial cells. *Proc. Natl. Acad. Sci. USA* **83:**2438–2442.

Moses, H. L., Branum, E. L., Proper, J. A., and Robinson, R. A. (1981). Transforming growth factor production by chemically transformed cells. *Cancer Res.* **41:**2842–2848.

Onozaki, K., Matsushima, K., Aggarwal, B., and Oppenheim, J. J. (1985). Human interleukin 1 is a cytocidal factor for several tumor cell lines. *J. Immunol.* **135:**3962–3968.

Roberts, A. B., Lamb, L. C., Newton, D. L., Sporn, M. B., DeLarco, J. E., and Todaro, G. J. (1980). Transforming growth factors: isolation of polypeptides from virally and chemically transformed cells by acid/ethanol extraction. *Proc. Natl. Acad. Sci. USA* **77:**3494–3498.

Salomon, D. S., Kim, N., Ciardiello, F., Bates, S., Valverius, E., Dickson, R., Kidwell, W. R., Callahan, R., Ali, I., Merlo, G., Liscia, D., and Lippman, M. (1988). Expression of transforming growth factor alpha in human mammary epithelial cells. *Proc. Am. Assoc. Cancer Res.* **29:**235.

Sherwin, S. A., Twardzik, D. R., Bohn, W. H., Cockley, K. D., and Todaro, G. J. (1983). High-molecular-weight transforming growth factor activity in the urine of patients with disseminated cancer. *Cancer Res.* **43:**403–407.

Siegfried, J. M., and Nesnaw, S. (1984). Cytotoxicity of chemical carcinogens toward human bronchial epithelial cells evaluated in a clonal assay. *Carcinogenesis* **5:**1317–1322.

Siegfried, J. M. (1987). Detection of human lung epithelial cell growth factors produced by a lung carcinoma cell line: use in culture of primary solid lung tumors. *Cancer Res.* **47:**2903–2910.

Siegfried, J. M., and Owens, S. E. (1988). Response of primary human lung carcinomas to autocrine growth factors produced by a lung carcinoma cell line. *Cancer Res.* **48:** 4976–4981.

Siegfried, J. M., Hansen, S. K., Lawrence, V. L., and Owens, S. E. (1988). Secretion of autocrine growth factors by cultured human lung tumors: effects on neoplastic lung epithelial cells. *Lung Cancer* **4:**205–209.

Southern, E. M. (1975). Detection of specific sequences among DNA fragments separated by gel electrophoresis. *J. Mol. Biol.* **98:**503–517.

Sporn, M. B., and Roberts, A. B. (1985). Autocrine growth factors and cancer. *Nature (Lond.)* **313:**747–751.

Sporn, M. B., and Roberts, A. B. (1986). Peptide growth factors and inflammatory tissue repair and cancer. *J. Clin. Invest.* **78:**329–333.

Sporn, M. B., and Todaro, G. J. (1980). Autocrine secretion and malignant transformation of cells. *N. Engl. J. Med.* **303:**878–880.

Todaro, G. J., Fryling, C., and DeLarco, J. E. (1980). Transforming growth factors produced by certain human tumor cells: polypeptides that interact with epidermal growth factor receptors. *Proc. Natl. Acad. Sci. USA* **77:**5258–5262.

Ullrich, A., Berman, C. H., Dull, T. J., Gray, A., and Lee, J. M. (1984). Isolation of the human insulin-like growth factor I gene using a single synthetic DNA probe. *EMBO J.* **3:**361–364.

Willey, J. C., Lechner, J. F., and Harris, C. C. (1984). Bombesin and the C-terminal tetradecapeptide of gastrin-releasing peptide are growth factors for normal human bronchial epithelial cells. *Exp. Cell Res.* **153:**245–248.

8

Epidermal Growth Factor Receptors in Lung Cancer

NOBUYOSHI SHIMIZU

Keio University School of Medicine
Tokyo, Japan

I. Introduction

Since the discovery of epidermal growth factor (EGF) (Cohen, 1962, 1986), its physiological role has been widely studied, especially in rodents, in the development of intestine (Malo and Menard, 1982; Oka et al., 1983), oocyte (Downs et al., 1988), and lung (Catterton et al., 1979), as well as in eyelid opening and tooth growth (Cohen, 1962, 1986). These results, utilizing the binding of ligand, suggested that the receptor is localized on the epithelial cell surface. Using monoclonal antibodies, localization of the EGF receptor in human normal and cancerous tissues (Adamson and Rees, 1981; Damjanov et al., 1986; Gullick et al., 1986; Nanney et al., 1984; Ozawa et al., 1987a,b) has been examined to elucidate the possible role of the EGF–EGF receptor system in these physiological states. EGF receptor expression is, in general, restricted to proliferating cells and its expression ceases when the cells differentiate and stop proliferating (Fukuyama and Shimizu, 1991). EGF expression occurs after proliferating cells differentiated into glandular cells and some cells express both EGF and the EGF receptor (Fukuyama and Shimizu, 1991).

EGF stimulates the growth of a variety of cell types in vitro and in vivo through interaction with a specific cell surface receptor (Carpenter and Cohen,

1979). This receptor is a 170,000 dalton transmembrane glycoprotein consisting of 1,186 amino acids with intrinsic protein tyrosine kinase activity (Cohen et al., 1980; Hunter, 1984). The tyrosine kinase domain of the EGF receptor is found to be homologous to the product of avian erythroblastosis virus oncogene v-*erb*B (Downward et al., 1984b), and the v-*erb*B oncogene product has been suggested to be a truncated form of the EGF receptor, which is derived from the host cell proto-oncogene c-*erb*B (Ullrich et al., 1984). Thus, the relation between the EGF receptor and cancer has been studied in a variety of systems.

In this chapter, I will summarize the molecular and cellular aspects of the EGF receptor system and review recent studies on EGF receptor expression in various types of lung cancer. Molecular pathologies and possible use of the EGF receptor system for targeting therapy will be discussed.

II. EGF Receptor

A. Structure and Function

The EGF receptor is a membrane-spanning glycoprotein with a molecular weight of 170,000 daltons (Fig. 1). The EGF receptor cDNA has been cloned from human placenta and the epidermoid carcinoma cell line A431, and sequence analysis revealed that the human EGF receptor has three functional domains (Ullrich et al., 1984; Lin et al., 1984; Merlino et al., 1984): an extracellular EGF binding domain, a membrane-spanning domain, and a cytoplasmic tyrosine kinase domain. The extracellular domain is characterized by two structural features: 2 cysteine-rich regions and 10 N-linked oligosaccharide acceptor sites. The transmembrane domain is highly hydrophobic. The tyrosine kinase domain contains an autophosphorylation site (Downward et al., 1984a), a protein kinase C phosphorylation site (Davis and Czech, 1985), and an ATP binding site (Russo et al., 1985), and it is homologous to the product of avian erythroblastosis virus oncogene v-*erb*B (Downward et al., 1984b). In response to EGF binding, the EGF receptor tyrosine kinase is activated through autophosphorylation and phosphorylates a number of intracellular target proteins to transmit the signal. These target (substrate) proteins include PLC-γl, PI-3 kinase, GAP, MAP kinase, *raf* kinase, lipocortin I, and c-*erb*B-2 (Carpenter and Cohen, 1990; Carpenter, 1987). However, the exact mechanism that generates mitogenic signals via tyrosine phosphorylation is not yet completely understood. The EGF receptor is downregulated by threonine phosphorylation by protein kinase C (Davis and Czech, 1985). The receptor/ligand complex is internalized into cells and processed through lysosomes or lysosome-like organelles, termed mitosomes (Miskimins and Shimizu, 1984).

B. Biosynthesis Pathway

Previous work (Mayes and Waterfield, 1984; Stoscheck and Carpenter, 1984; Gamou and Shimizu, 1987; Gamou et al., 1988a) using the glycosylation inhibitor

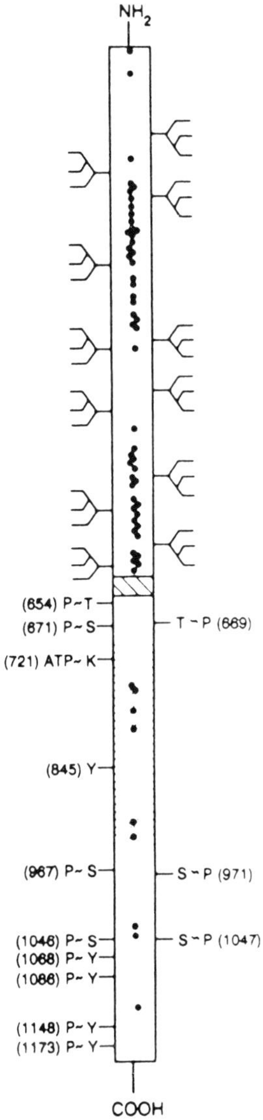

Figure 1 Known features of the EGF receptor. Cross-hatched area, single membrane anchor sequence; ⋑—, potential sites for N-linked glycosylation; filled dots, cysteine residues; striped area, *src*-like tyrosine kinase sequences; P-Y, tyrosine autophosphorylation sites; P-T and P-S, phosphothreonine and phosphoserine residues, respectively; ATP-K, a lysine residue critical for ATP binding. (From Carpenter and Cohen, 1990.)

tunicamycin demonstrated that an unglycosylated EGF receptor of molecular weight (Mr) 130K is synthesized from mRNA and is cotranslationally glycosylated to a 160K form that further matures to the 170k form through monensin- and swainsonine-sensitive processes (Fig. 2). The mature receptor of Mr 170K contains both complex- and high-mannose-type N-linked oligosaccharides but no O-linked oligosaccharide, whereas the precursor of Mr 160K contains only the high-mannose type. The complex-type chains in the mature receptor are tri- or tetra-antennary species and contain fucose but only a few sialic acid moieties (Cummings et al., 1985).

Intracellular transport of the newly synthesized EGF receptor and processing for acquisition of ligand binding ability have recently been elucidated (Gamou

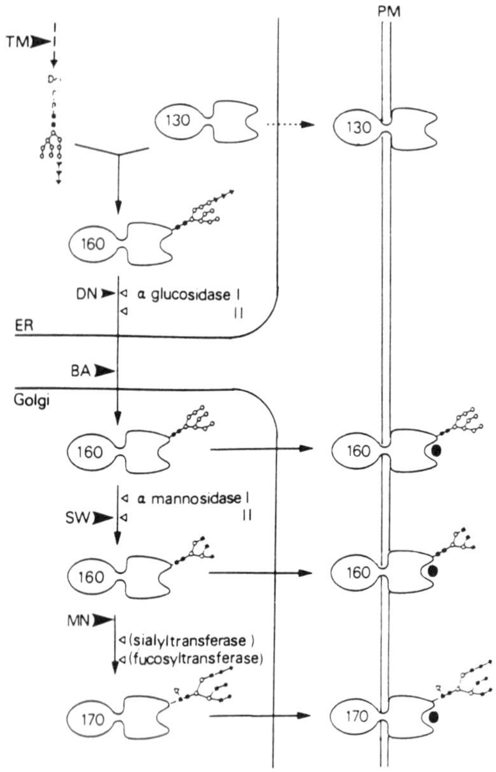

Figure 2 Schema for the biosynthesis pathway of the EGF receptors. Possible processes of glycosylation, membrane transport and ligand binding are shown. TM, tunicamycin; DN, 1-deoxynojirimycin; BA, brefeldin A; SW, swainsonine; MN, monensin. Closed circles, EGF as a ligand. Large arrowheads, inhibition of the processing enzymes and transport. Small arrowheads, incomplete inhibition. (From Gamou and Shimizu, 1988.)

et al., 1989). The unglycosylated Mr 130K receptor and the Mr 160K receptor seen soon after synthesis at the endoplasmic reticulum had no EGF-binding activity, whereas the Mr 160K receptor seen at later time in the Golgi region and the Mr 170K receptor had binding activity. Thus, not only glycosylation but also some oligosaccharide processing is necessary for EGF binding. Treatment with processing inhibitors, such as monensin, swainsonine, and 1-deoxynojirimycin, affected neither receptor transport to the plasma membrane nor binding activity. The EGF receptor appears to acquire ligand binding activity after the brefeldin A-sensitive process but prior to the swainsonine-sensitive mannose removal.

C. Gene Structure and Regulation

The EGF receptor (EGFR) gene is located in the p12–p11 region of human chromosome 7 (Shimizu et al., 1980; Kondo and Shimizu, 1983; Merlino et al., 1985). The EGFR gene is approximately 100 kilobase pairs (kb) and consists of at least 25 exons (Wakunaga, unpublished data) and a promoter region (Ishii et al., 1985). Analysis using chimeric plasmids containing the chloramphenicol acetyltransferase (CAT) gene and various deletions of the EGFR gene promoter revealed that the 5′CpG-rich region plays an important role in the regulation of gene expression. Furthermore, Sp1 and a *trans*-acting factor specific for the EGFR gene (ETF) bind to the 5′CpG-rich region and are required for maximal expression (Kageyama et al., 1988). More recently a negative regulatory factor (GCF) and its binding sites have been identified (Kageyama and Pastan, 1990). Thus, the EGFR gene expression is apparently regulated by a group of *trans*-acting factors that interact with several unique *cis*-elements within the promoter region.

The EGFR gene appears to be highly polymorphic in human populations. These polymorphic sites include *Hin*dIII fragments (4.9/5.2 and 9.8/11/12kb) (Lee et al., 1988).

III. EGF Receptor Expression in Lung Cancer

EGF receptor levels of cells and tissues have been measured by radioreceptor assay or immunohistochemical staining. We examined EGF-binding activity using homogenates of lung cancer tissue specimens (Kaseda et al., 1989). The EGF-binding activity of 68 tissue samples from 4 histologic cell types of lung cancer including squamous cell carcinoma, adenocarcinoma, large cell carcinoma, and small cell carcinoma is shown in Figure 3. Lung squamous cell carcinoma possesses substantially higher EGF-binding activities than other types of lung cancer. Two of these squamous cell carcinoma tissues exhibited EGF-binding values as high as A431 tumors. Small cell carcinoma showed almost no EGF-binding activity. Adenocarcinoma showed intermediate levels, but are definitively elevated from the normal tissue levels, of EGF receptors. An elevated level of EGF

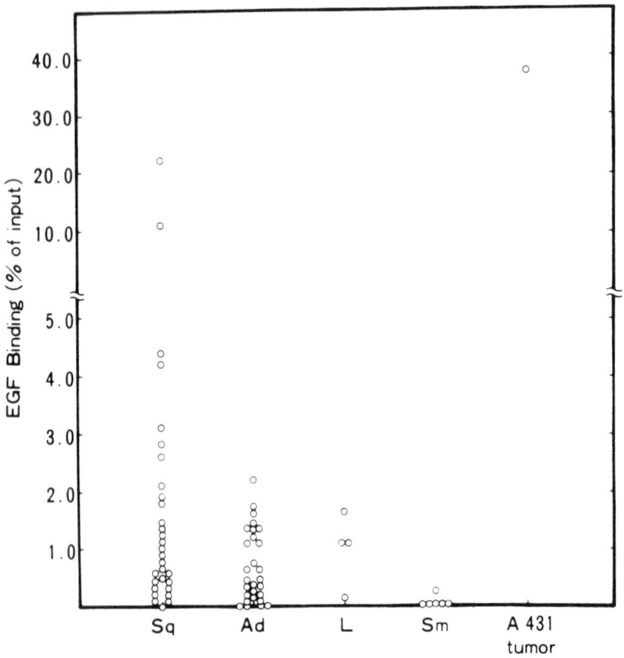

Figure 3 EGF binding activity of four major histologic types of lung cancer. Sq, squamous cell carcinoma; Ad, adenocarcinoma; L, large cell carcinoma; Sm, small cell carcinoma; A431 tumors, tumor obtained from nude mice inoculated with A431 tumor cells. (From Kaseda et al., 1989.)

receptors has been observed in an established cell line (UCVA-1) from a pancreatic tumor (Gamou and Shimizu, 1987). Several adenocarcinoma cell lines overproduce EGF receptors through gene amplification (Sakiyama et al., 1986). Furthermore, immunohistochemical staining revealed the expression of EGF receptors in a substantial fraction of lung adenocarcinoma (Sobol et al., 1987). Thus, elevated levels of EGF receptors appear to be involved in the development of adenocarcinomas as well as squamous cell carcinomas.

EGF receptor distribution in lung and esophageal squamous cell carcinomas was examined by immunohistochemical staining with a monoclonal anti-EGF receptor antibody (Ozawa et al., 1987a). EGF receptors were found to be localized on the membranes of all cancer cells and the number of EGF receptors gradually decreased towards the center of cancer pearls. Bromodeoxyuridine incorporation analysis revealed that peripheral cells of cancer pearls are active for DNA synthesis and rapidly proliferate. Thus, there is a direct correlation between EGF receptor expression and malignant growth of tumor cells.

IV. Elevated EGF Receptor Levels

A. Squamous Cell Carcinomas of Different Origin

As well as in lung squamous cell carcinoma, extremely high levels of EGF receptors have been demonstrated in a number of squamous carcinoma cell lines from different origins (Yamamoto et al., 1986) and in squamous cell carcinoma tissues of the head, neck, skin, cervix, and esophagus (Hendler and Ozanne, 1984; Ozanne et al., 1985; Ozawa et al., 1988). Elevated levels of EGF receptors are also reported in some gliomas (Libermann et al., 1984), breast tumors (Fitzpatrick et al., 1984; Sainsbury et al., 1985a,b), bladder tumors (Neal et al., 1985), thyroid tumors (Duh et al., 1985), sarcomas (Gusterson et al., 1985), gynecologic tumors (Gullick et al., 1986), and gastrointestinal tumors (Yasui et al., 1988).

B. Mechanisms for EGF Receptor Hyperproduction

Elevated levels of EGF receptor are caused by at least three different mechanisms: enhanced transcription of the receptor gene (Rao et al., 1985; Hunts et al., 1986a), reduced metabolic turnover rate of surface receptors (Gamou et al., 1988a), and amplification of the receptor gene (Libermann et al., 1985; Lin et al., 1984; Hunts et al., 1985b). EGF receptor hyperproduction is most often associated with the gene amplification and is readily detected by Southern blot hybridization of tumor DNAs with a radiolabeled EGF receptor cDNA probe. A 5- to 15-fold amplification of the EGF receptor gene was detected in lung squamous cell carcinomas (Kaseda et al., 1989).

C. Receptor Gene Amplification and Amplicon Structure

A megabase scale physical map of the 5′- and 3′-flanking regions of the EGF receptor gene has been established using CpG-recognition rare-cutting restriction enzymes and pulsed field gel electrophoresis (Fig. 4) (Kawasaki et al., 1988). In this map, a methylation-free CpG island (HTF island) is located within an 8 kilobase pair (Kb) *Eco*RI fragment that includes exon 1 of the EGF receptor gene. From this HTF island, a 390 kb *Not*I fragment was identified as the longest 5′-flanking region and a 540 kb *Mlu*I fragment as the longest 3′-flanking region. Utilizing this map information, the structure of the flanking regions of amplified EGF receptor genes found in various squamous cell carcinomas has been determined. Among 7 cell lines tested, 4 cell lines carrying EGF receptor genes in amounts more than 20 times that of normal cells showed amplification together with large 5′- and 3′-flanking regions. The amplified 5′-flanking regions were arranged in different forms but were distinct in each cell line. The amplified 3′-flanking regions were at least 540 kb and common to all the cell lines except one. Thus, the size of amplification units (amplicons) appears to be large (>1 Mb). It was postulated that the as yet unveiled genes coamplified with EGF receptor

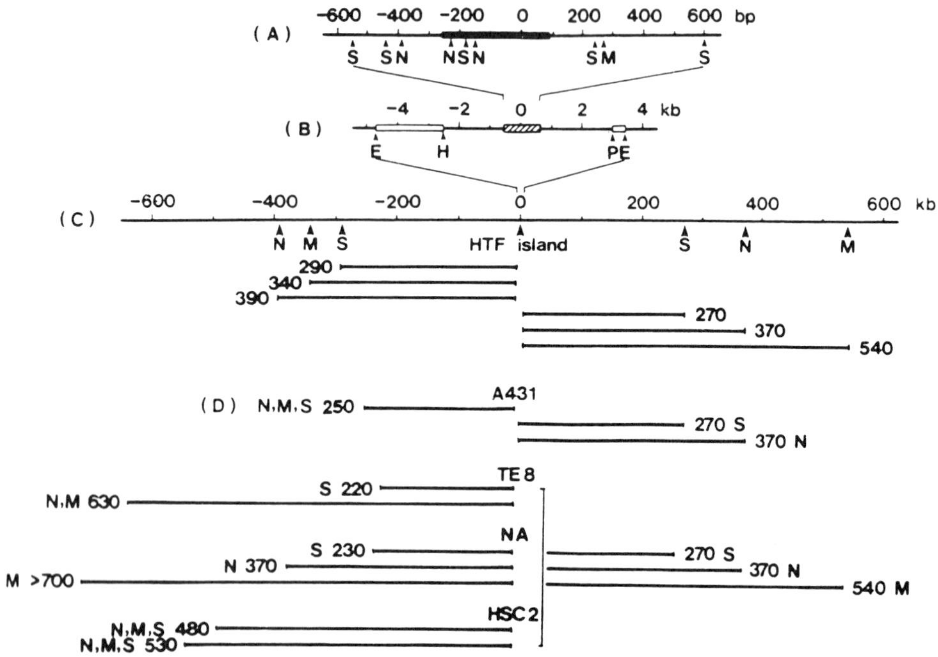

Figure 4 Physical map of the EGF receptor gene promoter regions and flanking regions. (A) Restriction map of the HTF island. The closed box represents exon 1 of the EGF receptor gene. (B) Restriction map of the pERP8 insert. The shaded box represents the HTF island and the open boxes represent the location of probes A and B. (C) Physical map of the 5′- and 3′-flanking regions of EGF receptor gene in GM130B cells. Horizontal lines represent the length and location of restriction fragments detected by pulsed field gel electrophoresis. (D) Size and location of restriction fragments seen in squamous cell carcinoma lines. Restriction enzymes used were *Sac*II (S), *Mlu*I (M), *Not*I (N), *Eco*RI (E), *Hind*III (H), and *Pvu*II (P). Each triangle represents a recognition site of a restriction enzyme. (From Kawasaki et al., 1988.)

gene may have important roles in determining the malignant phenotype of the tumors (Kawasaki et al., 1988).

D. Chromosomal Abnormality

In the A431 epidermoid carcinoma cell line, the amplified EGF receptor gene was correlated with marker chromosome M4 (Shimizu et al., 1984; Gill et al., 1985), in which an unknown chromosomal segment was translocated to the short arm of chromosome 7 (Hunts et al., 1985b; Merlino et al., 1985). Amplification of the EGF receptor gene in a breast cancer cell line MDA-468 was localized in an abnormal banding region (ABR) of the aberrant chromosome 7 (Filmus et al., 1985). Thus, amplification of the EGF receptor gene was often associated with structural alterations in the short arm of chromosome 7. However, in the squamous cell carcinoma line NA of tongue origin, the amplified EGF receptor gene was localized in the ABR of one of the aberrant chromosomes, MH1, which has no structural homology to chromosome 7 (Gamou et al., 1988b). The amplification units in NA cells are over 1200 kb, and are 30 times amplified (Kawasaki et al., 1988); therefore they are sufficient to account for the ABR on the MH1 chromosome. Unlike the *myc* family genes, double-minute chromosomes (DMs) have not been reported for EGFR gene amplification.

E. Stimulation of Tumor Formation by EGF in Nude Mice

Growth of EGF receptor-hyperproducing cells in nude mice has been examined and found to be stimulated by EGF when constantly delivered through an Alzet miniosmotic pump (Ozawa et al., 1987b). Stimulation of tumor development was correlated with the number of EGF receptors present in the tumor cell lines used. Thus, EGF plays an important role in promoting growth of squamous cell carcinoma in vivo. Lung cancer cells with high numbers of EGF receptors may be advantageous for growth during tumor development.

F. Pathologic Correlations and Prognostic Values

A correlation between EGF receptor level and biological behavior has been reported for some types of cancer. In breast cancer, there is a significant inverse relationship between EGF receptor and estrogen receptor status, and a significant association between metastatic potential and poor prognosis (Fitzpatrick et al., 1984; Sainsbury et al., 1985a,b). In bladder cancer, the presence of EGF receptors is associated with poor differentiation and active invasion (Neal et al., 1985). In the case of esophageal cancer, no definite correlation was found between elevated EGF receptor levels and pathologic findings (Ozawa et al., 1989a). However, an elevated level of EGF receptors was definitely associated with poor prognosis (Ozawa et al., 1989a). EGF-binding activities in lung squamous cell carcinoma were examined for possible correlation with clinical and pathologic characteristics. These criteria included clinical stage (pTNM), degree of differentiation, diameter of tumor, and lymph node metastasis. However, no significant correlation was found (Kaseda et al., 1989). Similar comparison was made for lung adenocarcinomas, but no obvious correlation was found (Kaseda et al., 1989). Thus, the elevated EGF receptor levels are not simply correlated with the progression of lung cancer.

V. Lack of EGF Receptor Expression in Small Cell Lung Carcinoma

A. Molecular Evidence

Many types of tumor cells are known to produce and release polypeptide growth factors into the culture medium (Todaro et al., 1980; Marquardt and Todaro, 1982), and these same cells often possess functional receptors for these factors. TGF-α is one such autocrine growth factor and is structurally related to EGF. The EGF receptor is assumed to be the functional receptor for TGF-α, through which all effects are mediated. Therefore, we examined several SCLC cell lines for the possibility that they may have the EGF receptors but that the receptors are masked by an EGF-like protein factor(s), which may be produced by an autocrine mechanism. However, we clearly demonstrated that SCLC cells neither produce nor release an EGF-competing TGF-α-like factor (Gamou et al., 1987).

We then used an EGF receptor cDNA to determine the state of the EGF receptor gene by Southern blot analysis. The receptor gene appears to be present in these cells in an intact, unrearranged form (Gamou et al., 1987). These cells, however, were found to lack detectable levels of EGF receptor mRNA, suggesting a possible reason for the absence of EGF receptors on the cell surface. SCLC is known to exhibit many properties common to neural crest-derived cells or amine precursor uptake and decarboxylation cells (Baylin et al., 1980; Gazdar et al., 1980). Some melanoma cells, which have a distinct embryonal origin in the neural crest, are also known to lack EGF receptors (Fabricant et al., 1977). Kudlow et al. (1984) found no EGF receptors in TGF-α-secreting melanoma cells, even under conditions that prevent the downregulation and degradation of the receptor, suggesting that the lack of EGF receptors on the cell surface is independent of TGF-α secretion. Our study also showed the absence of TGF-α-like growth factors and the complete lack of EGF receptors on the cell surface of SCLC. Therefore, a negative regulatory mechanism for EGF receptor gene expression in both SCLC and melanoma was postulated (Gamou et al., 1987). It is possible that this negative regulation may be caused by a paucity or modification of some of the *trans*-acting regulatory factor(s). As an alternative, it may be regulated at the *cis*-acting elements by DNA methylation. Nonetheless, the lack of EGF receptors, as frequently found in both SCLC cell lines and fresh SCLC tissues, appears to be characteristic of SCLC among various types of the lung cancer and may be used for a unique marker.

B. Methylation Events

The methylation status of the EGF receptor gene was compared in cell lines from four major types of lung carcinoma to examine whether DNA methylation is responsible for the suppression of EGFR gene expression in SCLC cells. Southern blot analysis revealed that the structural region of the EGFR gene is methylated to various degrees regardless of the expression of EGF receptor on the surface (Gamou et al., 1988c). An 8-kb *Eco*RI fragment that contains the EGFR gene promoter region (see Fig. 4) is readily digested with various methylation-sensitive restriction enzymes in all types of cells, indicating that the EGFR gene 5′ region is barely methylated. Although the methylation status in the tumor tissues remain to be investigated, the regulatory mechanism for the EGFR gene in SCLC may be independent of DNA methylation.

C. Chromosomal Abnormality

Karyotype analysis (Gamou et al., 1987) revealed that SCLC cell lines Lu134 and H69 contained a morphologically normal chromosome 7, which carries the EGF receptor gene. Although studies are very limited, there appears to be no association with abnormal chromosome 7 in SCLC.

D. Morphologic Variants

Most cell lines derived from SCLC grow in an anchorage-independent manner; they neither possess EGF binding activity nor express EGF receptor mRNA. A variant, AD320, which grew in an anchorage-dependent manner with altered morphology, was isolated from the SCLC cell line Lu134 by treatment with the demethylating agent 5-azacytidine (Gamou et al., 1990). The analysis using methylation sensitive-restriction enzymes revealed that the methylation pattern was altered only in the structural region of the EGFR gene and not in the promoter region, but that EGFR mRNA and EGF-binding activity could be detected in the variant. In addition, drastic changes in gene expression, including a decrease of creatine kinase B mRNA and an increase of c-*myc* mRNA, were observed in the variant. The EGF receptor in the variant appeared to be an active part of the transmembrane signaling machinery, since c-*fos* and c-*jun* mRNA accumulated after EGF treatment, followed by EGFR and c-*myc* mRNA accumulation. A potent tumor promoter, 12-O-tetradecanoyl-phorbol-13-acetate (TPA), also induced EGFR mRNA in the variant. Thus, the inducible regulatory mechanism for the EGFR gene was activated in the variant even though the EGFR gene was constitutively expressed. The exact molecular mechanism for restoring EGF receptor gene expression in SCLC cell variants and its physiological significance remain to be elucidated.

VI. EGF Receptors as a Target for Therapy

A. Immunotoxin Approach

The need for precisely targeted cancer chemotherapy has recently become critical (Frankel et al., 1986). To date, a variety of monoclonal antibodies against colorectal cancer cells (Gilliland et al., 1980), ovarian cancer cells (Pirker et al., 1985), breast cancer cells (Bojorn et al., 1985; Coombes et al., 1986; Monaco et al., 1986; LeMaistre et al., 1987), prostate cancer cells (Webb et al., 1986), colon cancer cells (Gallagher and Burk, 1986), and laryngeal cancer cells (Zenner, 1986), as well as transferrin receptor (Pirker et al., 1985; Akiyama et al., 1985; Zovickian et al., 1987) and nerve growth factor receptor (Disrefano et al., 1985) have been utilized for immunotoxins conjugated to various protein toxins. The EGF receptor was thought to be an excellent target for therapy against squamous cell carcinoma because these cells hyperproduce EGF receptors (Cowley et al., 1984; Hunts et al., 1985a; Ozawa et al., 1988), EGF promotes the growth of EGF receptor-hyperproducing cells in vivo (Ozawa et al., 1987b), and EGF receptors on the cell surface are known to be internalized upon ligand or antibody binding (Das and Fox, 1978; Das et al., 1977).

Our murine monoclonal antibody (B4G7) against the human EGF receptor immunoreacts mainly with the low-affinity type EGF receptor (Behzadian and Shimizu, 1985a), which is predominantly overproduced in EGF receptor-hyperproducing cells of squamous cell carcinoma. Thus, we conjugated it to gelonin, a 60S ribosome inactivating protein (Fig. 5). The B4G7–gelonin conjugate bound to the cell surface in proportion to the number of EGF receptors and competed with B4G7 antibody for binding to EGF receptors (Ozawa et al., 1989b). The conjugate inhibited protein synthesis and killed EGF receptor-hyperproducing tumor cells. It was slightly cytotoxic to normal human fibroblasts but did not kill EGF receptor-deficient SCLC cells and mouse fibroblasts. Free B4G7, gelonin, or a mixture of these did not kill EGF receptor-hyperproducing cells. The number of EGF receptors was correlated to the degree of cytotoxicity at 10^{-8} M of the conjugate.

A more recent study indicated that these conjugates are effective in suppressing the development of tumors from EGF receptor-hyperproducing cells in nude mice (Hirota et al., 1989). The suppression of tumor growth depended on the dose of conjugate administered. Nude mice bearing an A431 cell tumor that were injected for 5 consecutive days intraperitoneally with at least 10 μg of the conjugate showed significant suppression of tumor growth for about 7 days. The growth of an EGF receptor-deficient SCLC tumor was not suppressed by injection of the conjugate. No toxic effects were observed in histologic examination of nontumor tissues of mice treated with at least 250 μg of conjugate per mouse. These results suggest that the B4G7–gelonin conjugate may be useful for targeting therapy to EGF receptor-hyperproducing squamous cell carcinomas.

B. Use of Antisense-Expression Vector

By reversing the orientation of the gene of interest relative to an upstream promoter, the opposite strand of DNA will be transcribed, generating an antisense

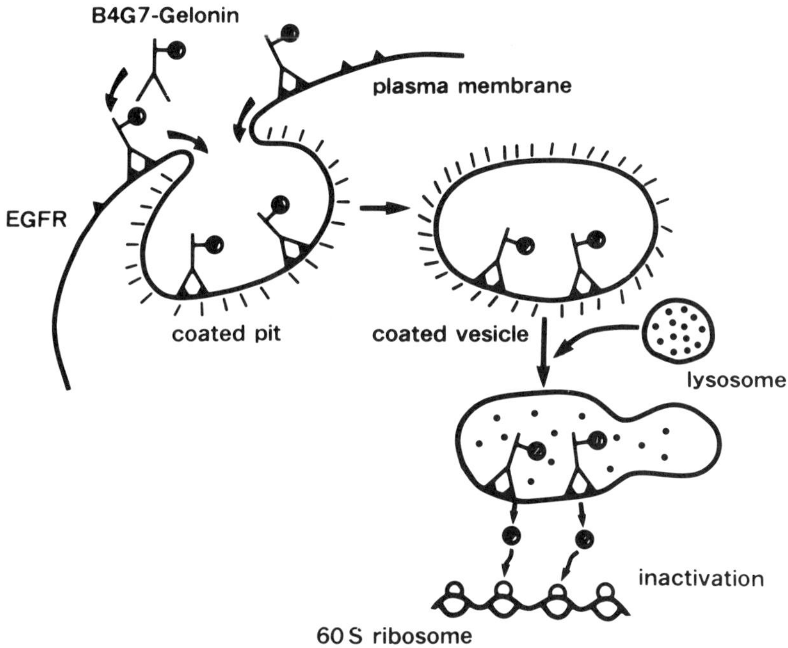

Figure 5 Schema for the cytotoxic effects of the immunotoxin conjugate of gelonin and a monoclonal anti-EGF receptor antibody B4G7.

RNA complementary to the natural mRNA (Hunts et al., 1986b). Antisense RNA, when injected into cells, can hybridize with sense mRNA and apparently blocks the translation of sense mRNA into protein. When the antisense RNA is generated in the nucleus, the hybridization is thought to prevent precursor mRNA transport out of the nucleus (Kim and Wold, 1985).

An expression vector was constructed from part of pSV2neo with the 3′*Cla*I fragment of the EGFR cDNA inserted in an inverted orientation downstream from the human metallothionein IIa (hMTIIa) promoter (Yamada et al., 1989). The human squamous carcinoma cell line NA was transfected with this vector and selected for resistance to the neomycin derivative G418. One of the stable transfectants had a 90% reduction in cell surface receptor in response to $ZnSO_4$. Nascent polypeptide of EGF receptor was also decreased with concurrent induction of MT mRNA from endogenous MT genes. Thus, the transfection with the antisense vector provides a technique to reduce the number of EGF receptors on the surface of tumor cells.

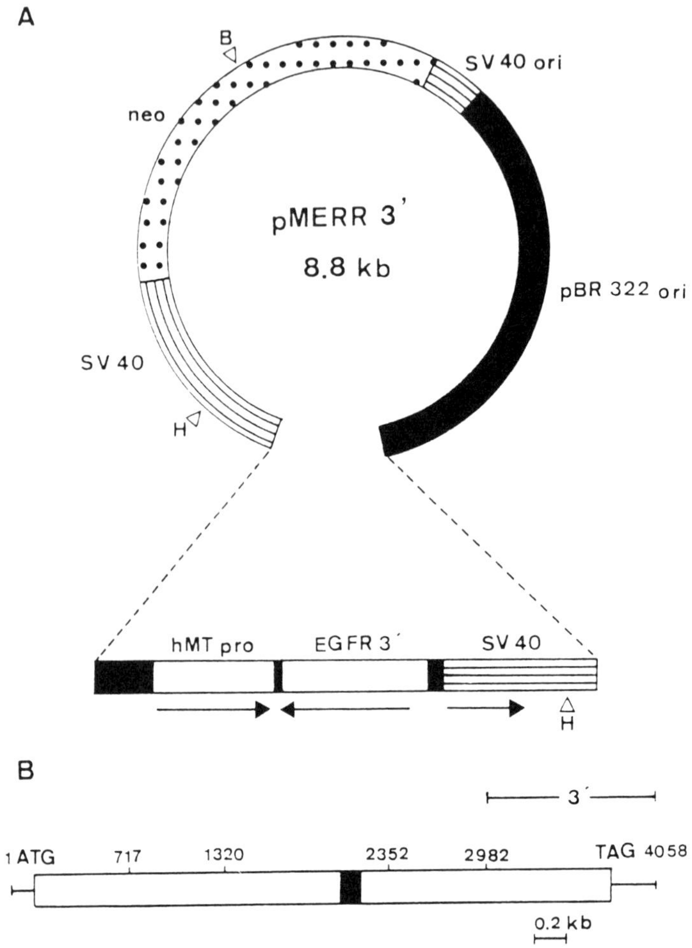

Figure 6 Antisense EGF receptor mRNA expression vector pMERR3′. (A) The vector was constructed with the 3′-fragment of EGF receptor cDNA oriented in the opposite polarity to human MTIIa promoter. The arrows indicate the polarity of the genes. B, *Bgl*II site; H, *Hpa*I site. (B) the 3′-*Cla*I fragment of the EGF receptor cDNA used for constructing the vector. The dark region shows the transmembrane domain. (From Yamada et al., 1989.)

VII. Prospects

The EGF receptor overproduction is frequently observed in squamous cell carcinoma of lung and is often associated with gene amplification. Prognostic values of this finding are not yet clear, but evidence suggests that the EGF receptor, a product of the proto-oncogene c-*erb*B, is involved in malignant tumor formation. Since the amplified DNA segments (amplicons) include several genes up- and downstream of the EGF receptor gene, the significance of these coamplified genes must be exploited. The exact mechanisms of gene amplification during tumor development remain to be investigated.

Small cell lung carcinoma is unique because of the lack of EGF receptor expression and the morphologic variants with restored expression. These cell lines will be extremely useful for further investigation of the molecular mechanisms of EGF receptor gene regulation.

The ability to suppress EGF receptor expression with an antisense-expression vector suggests that strategies for experimentally manipulating oncogenic gene expression in human tumor cells may be possible and further exploited.

The immunotoxin approach to killing EGF receptor-overproducing tumor cells has been successful using in vitro cell culture and nude mouse tumors. This approach may have great potential for clinical application. The EGF/EGF receptor system was the first growth factor system for extensive studies, but there are many more to be investigated. The exact role(s) the EGF receptor plays in the normal developmental process as well as the malignant cell transformation process remains to be determined.

Acknowledgments

Thanks are extended to the following individuals who participated in the research projects cited here for their hard work and valuable discussions: Shinobu Gamou, Masamichi Hirai, Shinsei Minoshima, Jun Kudoh, Ryuichi Fukuyama, Kazuhiko Kawasaki, Hirotomo Yamada (Dept. of Molecular Biology, Keio University), Masakazu Ueda, Soji Ozawa, Tsuneo Ishihara, Osahiko Abe (Dept. of Surgery and Cancer Center, Keio University), Shizuka Kaseda (Tokyo Metropolitan Institute of Medicine), Yukio Shimosato (National Cancer Center Research Institute), Keiichi Omoto (Tokyo University), Yoshiko Shimizu, Keith Miskimins, Ikuko Kondo, Ali Behzadian, Fumiaki Ito, John Hunts, Scott Samuels, Grace Pavlath, Ingrid Stuiver and David Gardner (Dept. of Cellular and Molecular Biology, University of Arizona).

References

Adamson, E. D., and Rees, A. R. (1981). Epidermal growth factor receptors. *Mol. Cell. Biochem.* **34:**129–152.

Akiyama, S., Seth, P., Pirker, R., Fitzgerald, D., Gottesman, M. M., and Pastan, I. (1985). Potentiation of cytotoxic activity of immunotoxins on cultured human cells. *Cancer Res.* **45:**1005–1007.

Baylin, S. B., Abeloff, M. D., Goodwin, G., Carney, D. N., and Gazdar, A. F. (1980). Activities of l-dopa decarboxylase and diamine oxidase (histaminase) in human lung cancers and decarboxylase as a marker for small (oat) cell cancer in culture. *Cancer Res.* **40:**1190–1194.

Behzadian, M. A., and Shimizu, N. (1985a). Monoclonal antibody that immunoreacts with a subclass of human subclass of human receptors for epidermal growth factor. *Cell Struct. Funct.* **10:**219–232.

Behzadian, M. A., and Shimizu, N. (1985b). Variant of A431 cells isolated by ricin A-conjugated monoclonal antibody directed to EGF receptor: phosphorylation of EGF receptor and phosphatidylinositol. *Somat. Cell Mol. Genet.* **11:**579–591.

Bojorn, M. J., Ring, D., and Frankel, A. (1985). Evaluation of monoclonal antibodies for the development of breast cancer immunotoxins. *Cancer Res.* **45:**1214–1221.

Carpenter, G. (1987). Receptors for epidermal growth factor and other polypeptide mitogens. *Annu. Rev. Biochem.* **56:**881–914.

Carpenter, G., and Cohen, S. (1979). Epidermal growth factor. *Annu. Rev. Biochem.* **48:**193–216.

Carpenter, G., and Cohen, S. (1990). Epidermal growth factor. *J. Biol. Chem.* **265:**7709–7712.

Catterton, W. Z., Escobedo, M. B., and Sexson, W. R. (1979). Effect of EGF on lung maturation in fetal rabbits. *Pediatr. Res.* **13:**104–108.

Cohen, S. (1962). Isolation of a mouse submaxillary gland protein accelerating incisor eruption and eyelid opening in the newborn animal. *J. Biol. Chem.* **237:**1555–1562.

Cohen, S. (1986). Epidermal growth factor. *Biosci. Rep.* **6:**1017–1028.

Cohen, S., Carpenter, G., and King, L. Jr. (1980). Epidermal growth factor-receptor-protein kinase interactions. *J. Biol. Chem.* **255:**4834–4842.

Coombes, R. C., Buckman, R., Forrester, J. A., Shepherd, V., O'Hare, M. J., Vincent, M., Powles, T. J., and Neville, A. M., (1986). In vitro and in vivo effects of a monoclonal antibody–toxin conjugate for use in autologous bone marrow transplantation for patients with breast cancer. *Cancer Res.* **46:**4217–4220.

Cowley, G., Smith, J. A., Gusterson, B., Hendler, F., and Ozanne, B. (1984). The amount of EGF receptor is elevated on squamous cell carcinomas. In *Cancer Cells*, vol. 1. Edited by Levine and Van de Woude. New York, Cold Spring Harbor Laboratory, pp. 5–10.

Cummings, R. D., Soderquist, A. M., and Carpenter, G. (1985). The oligosaccharide moieties of the epidermal growth factor receptor in A-431 cells. *J. Biol. Chem.* **260:** 11944–11952.

Damjanov, I., Midner, B., and Knowles, B. B. (1986). Immunohistochemical localization of the epidermal growth factor receptor in normal human tissue. *Lab. Invest.* **55:** 588–592.

Das, M., Miyakawa, T., Fox, C. F., Pruss, R. M., Aharonov, A., and Herschman, H. R. (1977). Specific radiolabeling of a cell surface receptor for epidermal growth factor. *Proc. Natl. Acad. Sci. USA* **74:**2790–2794.

Das, M., and Fox, F. (1978). Molecular mechanism of mitogen action: processing of receptor induced by epidermal growth factor. *Proc. Natl. Acad. Sci. USA* **75:**2644–2648.

Davis, R. J., and Czech, M. P. (1985). Tumor-promoting phorbol diesters cause the phosphorylation of epidermal growth factor receptors in normal human fibroblasts at threonine-654. *Proc. Natl. Acad. Sci. USA* **82:**1974–1978.

Disrefano, P. S., Schweitzer, J. B., Taniuchi, M., and Johnson, E. M. (1985) Selective destruction of nerve growth factor receptor-bearing cells in vitro using a hybrid toxin composed of ricin A chain and a monoclonal antibody against the nerve growth factor receptor. *J. Cell Biol.* **101:**1107–1114.

Downs, S. M., Daniel, S. A. J., and Eppig, J. (1988). Induction of maturation in cumulus cell enclosed mouse oocyte by follicle-stimulating hormone and epidermal growth factor: evidence for a positive stimulus of somatic cell origin. *J. Exp. Zool.* **245:** 86–96.

Downward, J., Parker, P., and Waterfield, M. D. (1984a). Autophosphorylation sites on the epidermal growth factor receptor. *Nature* **311:**483–485.

Downward, J., Yarden, Y., Mayes, E., Scrace, G., Totty, N., Stockwell, P., Ullrich, A., Schlessinger, J., and Waterfield, M. D. (1984b). Close similarity of epidermal growth factor receptor and v-erb-B oncogene protein sequences. *Nature* **307:**521–527.

Duh, Q. Y., Gum, E. T., Gerend, P. L., Raper, S. E. and Clark, O. H. (1985). Epidermal growth factor receptors in normal and neoplastic thyroid tissue. *Surgery* **98:**1000–1007.

Fabricant, R. N., DeLarco, J. E., and Todaro, G. J. (1977). Nerve growth factor receptors on human melanoma cells in culture. *Proc. Natl. Acad. Sci. USA* **74:**565–569.

Filmus, J., Pollak, M. N., Cailleau, R., and Buick, R. N. (1985). A human breast cancer cell line with a high number of epidermal growth factor (EGF) receptors, has an amplified EGF receptor gene and is growth inhibited by EGF. *Biochem. Biophys. Res. Commun.* **128:**898–905.

Fitzpatrick, S. L., Brightwell, J., Wittliff, J. L., Barrows, G. H., and Schultz, G. S. (1984). Epidermal growth factor binding by breast tumor biopsies and relationship to estrogen receptor and progestin receptor levels. *Cancer Res.* **44:**3448–3453.

Frankel, A. E., Houston, L. L., Issell, B. F., and Fathman, G. (1986). Prospects for immunotoxin therapy in cancer. *Annu. Rev. Med.* **37:**127–142.

Fukuyama, R., and Shimizu, N. (1991). Expression of epidermal growth factor (EGF) and EGF receptor in human tissues. *J. Exp. Zool.* **258:**336–343.

Gallagher, W. J., and Burk, M. W. (1986). Monoclonal antibody-ricin A chain conjugates (immunotoxins): potential therapeutic agents for human colon carcinoma. *J. Surg. Res.* **40:**159–166.

Gamou, S., and Shimizu, N. (1987). Change in metabolic turnover is an alternate mechanism increasing cell surface EGF receptor levels in tumor cells. *J. Biol. Chem.* **262:**6708–6713.

Gamou, S., and Shimizu, N. (1988). Glycosylation of the epidermal growth factor receptor and its relationship to membrane transport and ligand binding. *J. Biochem.* **104:** 388–396.

Gamou, S., Hunts, J., Harigai, H., Hirohashi, S., Shimosato, Y., Pastan, I., and Shimizu, N. (1987). Molecular evidence for the lack of epidermal growth factor receptor gene expression in small cell lung carcinoma cells. *Cancer Res.* **47:**2668–2673.

Gamou, S., Hirai, M., Rikimaru, K., Enomoto, S., and Shimizu, N. (1988a). Biosynthesis of the epidermal growth factor receptor in human squamous cell carcinoma lines: secretion of the truncated receptor is not common to EGF receptor-hyperproducing cells. *Cell Struct. Funct.* **13:**25–38.

Gamou, S., Kobayashi, M., Furusho, T., and Shimizu, N. (1988b). Unique chromosome location of amplified EGF receptor genes in EGF receptor-hyperproducing tumor cell line NA. *Somat. Cell Mol. Genet.* **15:**179–184.

Gamou, S., Shimosato, Y., Merlino, G. T., and Shimizu, N. (1988c). Methylation status of epidermal growth factor receptor gene in lung carcinoma cell. *Jpn. J. Cancer Res.* **79:** 989–995.

Gamou, S., Shimagaki, M., Minoshima, S., Kobayashi, S., and Shimizu, N. (1989). Subcellular localization of the EGF receptor maturation process. *Exp. Cell Res.* **183:** 197–206.

Gamou, S., Shimosato, Y., and Shimizu, N. (1990). Regulation of the epidermal growth factor (EGF) receptor gene expression in a morphological variant isolated from an EGF receptor-deficient SCLC cell line. *Cell Growth and Differentiation* **1:**351–359.

Gazder, A. F., Carney, D. N., Russell, E. K., Sims, H. L., Baylin, S. B., Bunn, P. A., Jr., Guccion, J. G., and Minna, J. D. (1980). Establishment of continuous clonable cultures of small-cell carcinoma of the lung which have amine precursor uptake and decarboxylation cell properties. *Cancer Res.* **40:**3502–3507.

Gill, G. N., Weber, W., Thompson, D. M., Lin, C., Evans, R. M. Rosenfeld, M. G., Gamou, S., and Shimizu, N. (1985). Relationship between production of epidermal growth factor receptors, gene amplification, and chromosome 7 translocation in variant A431 cells. *Somat. Cell Mol. Genet.* **11:**309–318.

Gilliland, D. G., Steplewski, Z., Collier, R. J., Mitchell, K. F., Chang, T. H., and Koprowski, H. (1980). Antibody-directed cytotoxic agents: use of monoclonal antibody to direct the action of toxin A chains to colorectal carcinoma cells. *Proc. Natl. Acad. Sci. USA* **77:**4539–4543.

Gullick, W. J., Marsden, J. J., Whittle, N., Ward, B., Bobrow, L., and Waterfield, M. D. (1986). Expression of epidermal growth factor receptors in human cervical, ovarian, and vulval carcinomas. *Cancer Res.* **46:**285–292.

Gusterson, B., Cowley, G., McIlhinney, J., Ozanne, B., Fisher, C., and Reeves, B. (1985). Evidence for increased epidermal growth factor receptors in human sarcomas. *Int. J. Cancer* **36:**686–693.

Hendler, F. J., and Ozanne, B. W. (1984). Human squamous cell lung cancer express increased epidermal growth factor receptors. *J. Clin. Invest.* **74:**647–651.

Hirota, N., Ueda, M., Ozawa, S., Abe, O., and Shimizu, N. (1989). Suppression of an EGF receptor-hyperproducing tumor by an immunotoxin conjugate of gelonin and a monoclonal anti-EGF receptor antibody. *Cancer Res.* **49:**7106–7109.

Hunter, T. (1984). Growth factors: the epidermal growth factor receptor gene and its product. *Nature* **311:**414–416.

Hunts, J., Ueda, M., Ozawa, S., Abe, O., Pastan, I., and Shimizu, N. (1985a) Hyper-production and gene amplification of the epidermal growth factor in squamous cell carcinomas. *Jpn. J. Cancer Res.* **76:**663–666.

Hunts, J., Shimizu, N., Yamamoto, T., Toyoshima, K., Merlino, G. T., Xu, Y.-H., and Pastan, I. (1985b). Translocation chromosome 7 of A431 cells contains amplification and rearrangement of EGF receptor gene responsible for production of variant mRNA. *Somat. Cell Mol. Genet.* **11:**477–484.

Hunts, J., Gamou, S., Hirai, M., and Shimizu, N. (1986a). Molecular mechanisms involved in increasing epidermal growth factor receptor levels on the cell surface. *Jpn. J. Cancer Res.* **77:**423–427.

Hunts, J., Merlino, G., Pastan, I., and Shimizu, N. (1986b). Reduction of EGF receptor synthesis by antisense RNA vectors. *FEBS Lett.* **206:**319–322.

Ishii, S., Xu, Y.-H., Stratton, R. H., Roc, B. A., Merlino, G. T., and Pastan, I. (1985). Characterization and sequence of the promoter region of the human epidermal growth factor receptor gene. *Proc. Natl. Acad. Sci. USA* **82:**4920–4924.

Kageyama, R., Merlino, G. T., and Pastan, I. (1988). Epidermal growth factor (EGF) receptor gene transcription: requirement for SP1 and EGF receptor-specific factor. *J. Biol. Chem.* **263:**6329–6336.

Kageyama, R., and Pastan, I. (1989). Molecular cloning and characterization of a human DNA binding factor that represses transcription. *Cell* **59:**815–825.

Kaseda, S., Ueda, M., Ozawa, S., Ishihara, T., Abe, O., and Shimizu, N. (1989). Expression of epidermal growth factor receptors in four histologic cell types of lung cancer. *J. Surg. Oncol.* **42:**16–20.

Kawasaki, K., Kudoh, J., Omoto, K., and Shimizu, N. (1988). Mega base map of the epidermal growth factor (EGF) receptor gene flanking regions and structure of the amplification units in EGF receptor-hyperproducing squamous carcinoma cells. *Jpn. J. Cancer Res.* **79:**1174–1183.

Kim, S. K., and Wold, B. J. (1985). Stable reduction of thymidine kinase activity in cells expressing high levels of anti-serine RNA. *Cell* **42:**127–138.

Kondo, I., and Shimizu, N. (1983). Mapping of the human gene for epidermal growth factor receptor (EGFR) on the p13-q22 region of chromosome 7. *Cytogenet. Cell Genet.* **35:** 9–14.

Kudlow, J. E., Khosravi, M. J., Kobrin, M. S., and Mak, W. W. (1984). Inability of anti-epidermal growth factor receptor monoclonal antibody to block "autocrine" growth stimulation in transforming growth factor-secreting melanoma cells. *J. Biol. Chem.* **259:**11895–11900.

Lee, J. S., Ro, J. S., Eisbruch, A., Shtalrid, M., Ferrell, R. E., Gutterman, J. U., and Blick, M. (1988). Multiple restriction fragment length polymorphisms of the human epidermal growth factor receptor gene. *Cancer Res.* **48:**4045–4048.

LeMaistre, C. F., Edwards, D. P., Krolick, K. A., and McGuire, W. L. (1987). An immunotoxin cytotoxic for breast cancer cells in vivo. *Cancer Res.* **47:**730–734.

Libermann, T. A., Razon, N., Bartal, A. D., Yarden, Y., Schlessinger, J., and Soreq, H. (1984). Expression of epidermal growth factor receptors in human brain tumors. *Cancer Res.* **44:**753–760.

Libermann, T. A., Nusbaum, H. R., Razon, N., Kris, R., Lax, I., Soreq, H., Whittle, N., Waterfield, M. D., Ullrich, A., and Schlessinger, J. (1985). Amplification, enhanced expression and possible rearrangement of EGF receptor gene in primary human brain tumours of glial origin. *Nature* **313:**144–147.

Lin, C. R., Chen, W. S., Kruiger, W., Stolarsky, L. S., Weber, W., Evans, R. M., Verma, I. M., Gill, G. N., and Rosenfeld, M. G. (1984). Expression cloning of human EGF receptor complementary DNA: gene amplification and three related messenger RNA products in A431 cells. *Science* **224:**843–848.

Maekawa, T., Imamoto, F., Merlino, G. T., Pastan, I., and Ishii, S. (1989). Cooperative function of two separate enhancers of the human epidermal growth factor receptor proto-oncogene. *J. Biol. Chem.* **264:**5488–5494.

Malo, C., and Menard, D. (1982). Influence of epidermal growth factor on the development of suckling mouse intestinal mucosa. *Gastroenterology* **83:**28–35.

Marquardt, H., and Todaro, G. J. (1982). Human transforming growth factor: production by a melanoma cell line, purification and initial characterization. *J. Biol. Chem.* **257:** 5220–5225.

Mayes, E. L. V., and Waterfield, M. D. (1984). Biosynthesis of the epidermal growth factor receptor in A431 cells. *EMBO J.* **3:**531–537.

Merlino, G. T., Xu, Y.-H., Ishii, S., Clark, A. J. L., Semba, K., Toyoshima, T., Yamamoto, T., and Pastan, I. (1984). Amplification and enhanced expression of the epidermal growth factor receptor gene in A431 human carcinoma cells. *Science* **224:**417–419.

Merlino, G. T., Ishii, S., Whang-Peng, J., Knutsen, T., Xu, Y.-H., Clark, A. J. L., Stratton, R. H., Wilson, R. K., Ma, D. P., Roe, B. A., Hunts, J. H., Shimizu, N., and Pastan, I. (1985). Structure and localization of genes encoding aberrant and normal epidermal growth factor receptor RNAs from A431 human carcinoma cells. *Mol. Cell. Biol.* **5:**1722–1734.

Miskimins, W. K., and Shimizu, N. (1984). Uptake of epidermal growth factor into a lysosomal enzyme-deficient organelle: correlation with cell's mitogenic response and evidence for ubiquitous existence in fibroblasts. *J. Cell Physiol.* **118:**305–316.

Monaco, M. E., Mack, J., Dugan, M. D., and Ceriani, R. (1986). An antibody–toxin conjugate directed against human mammary cancer antigen. *Ann. N.Y. Acad. Sci.* **464:**389–399.

Nanney, L. B., Mckanna, J. A., Stoscheck, C. M., Carpenter, G., and King, L. E. (1984). Visualization of epidermal growth factor receptors in human epidermis. *J. Invest. Dermatol.* **82:**165–169.

Neal, D. E., Marsh, C., Bennett, M. K., Abel, P. D., Hall, R. R., Sainsbury, J. R. C., and Harris, A. L. (1985). Epidermal-growth-factor receptors in human bladder cancer: comparison of invasive and superficial tumors. *Lancet* **1:**366–368.

Oka, Y., Ghishan, F. K., Greene, H. L., and Orth, D. N. (1983). Effect of mouse epidermal growth factor/urogastrone on the functional maturation of rat intestine. *Endocrinology* **112:**940–944.

Ozanne, B., Shum, A., Richards, C. S., Cassells, D., Grossman, D., Trent, J., Gusterson, B., and Hendler, F. (1985). Evidence for an increase of EGF receptors in epidermoid malignancies. In *Cancer Cells*. Edited by Feramisco, Ozanne, and Stiles. New York, Cold Spring Harbor Laboratory, pp. 41–49.

Ozawa, S., Ueda, M., Ando, N., Abe, O., and Shimizu, N. (1987a). High incidence of EGF receptor hyperproduction in esophageal squamous cell carcinomas. *Int. J. Cancer* **39:**333–337.

Ozawa, S., Ueda, M., Ando, N., Abe, O., Hirai, M., and Shimizu, N. (1987b). Stimulation by EGF of the growth of EGF receptor-hyperproducing tumor cells in athymic mice. *Int. J. Cancer* **40:**706–710.

Ozawa, S., Ueda, M., Ando, N., Abe, O., and Shimizu, N. (1988). Epidermal growth factor receptors in cancer tissues of esophagus, lung, pancreas, colorectum, breast and stomach. *Jpn. J. Cancer Res.* **79:**1201–1207.

Ozawa, S., Ueda, M., Ando, N., Shimizu, N., and Abe, O. (1989a). Prognostic significance of epidermal growth factor receptor in esophageal squamous cell carcinomas. *Cancer* **63:**2169–2173.

Ozawa, S., Ueda, M., Ando, N., Abe, O., Minoshima, S., and Shimizu, N. (1989b). Selective killing of squamous carcinoma cells by immunotoxin that recognizes the EGF receptor. *Int. J. Cancer* **43:**152–157.

Pirker, R., Fitzgerald, D. J. P., Hamilton, T. C., Ozols, R. F., Laird, W., Frankel, A. E., Willingham, M. C., and Pastan, I. (1985). Characterization of immunotoxins active against ovarian cancer cell lines. *J. Clin. Invest.* **76:**1261–1267.

Rao, C. V., Ramani, N., Chegin, N., Stadig, B., Carman, F. R., Woost, P. G., Schultz, G. S., and Cook, C. L. (1985). Topography of human placental receptors for epidermal growth factor. *J. Biol. Chem.* **260:**1705–1710.

Russo, M. W., Lukas, T. J., Cohen, S., and Staros, J. V. (1985). Identification of residues in the nucleotide binding site of the epidermal growth factor receptor/kinase. *J. Biol. Chem.* **260:**5205–5208.

Sainsbury, J. R. C., Farndon, J. R., Sherbet, G. V., and Harris, A. L. (1985a). Epidermal-growth-factor receptors and estrogen receptors in human breast cancer. *Lancet* **1:** 364–366.

Sainsbury, J. R. C., Malcolm, A. J., Appleton, D. R., Farndon, J. R., and Harris, A. L. (1985b). Presence of epidermal growth factor receptors as an indicator of poor prognosis in patients with breast cancer. *J. Clin. Pathol.* **38:**1225–1228.

Sakiyama, S., Nakamura, Y., and Yasuda, S. (1986). Expression of epidermal growth factor receptor gene in cultured human lung cancer cells. *Jpn. J. Cancer Res.* **77:**965–969.

Shimizu, N., Behzadian, M. A., and Shimizu, Y. (1980). Genetics of cell surface receptors for bioactive polypeptides: binding of epidermal growth factor is associated with the presence of human chromosome 7 in human-mouse cell hybrids. *Proc. Natl. Acad. Sci. USA* **77:**3600–3604.

Shimizu, N., Kondo, I., Gamou, S., Behzadian, M. A., and Shimizu, Y. (1984). Genetic analysis of hyperproduction of epidermal growth factor receptors in human epidermoid carcinoma A431 cells. *Somat. Cell Mol. Genet.* **10:**45–53.

Sobol, R. E., Astarita, R. W., Hofedits, C., Masui, H., Fairshter, R., Roston, I, and Mendelsohn, J. (1987). Epidermal growth factor receptor expression in human lung carcinomas defined by a monoclonal antibody. *J. Natl. Cancer Inst.* **79:**403–407.

Stoscheck, C. M., and Carpenter, G. (1984). Characterization of the metabolic turnover of epidermal growth factor receptor protein in A-431 cells. *J. Cell. Physiol.* **120:** 296–302.

Todaro, G. J., Fryling, C., and DeLarco, J. E. (1980). Transforming growth factor receptors produced by certain human tumor cells: polypeptides that interact with epidermal growth factor receptors. *Proc. Natl. Acad. Sci. USA* **77:**5258–5262.

Ullrich, A., Coussens, L., Hayflick, J. S., Dull, T. J., Gray, A., Tam, A. W., Lee, J., Yarden, Y., Libermann, T. A., Schlessinger, J., Downward, J., Mayes, E., Whittle, N., Waterfield, M. D., and Seeberg, P. H. (1984). Human epidermal growth factor receptor cDNA sequence and aberrant expression of the amplified gene in A431 epidermoid carcinoma cells. *Nature* **309:**418–425.

Webb, K. S., Liberman, S. N., Ware, J. L., and Walther, P. J. (1986). In vitro synergism between hybrid immunotoxins and chemotherapeutic drugs: relevance to immunotherapy of prostate carcinoma. *Cancer Immunol. Immunother.* **21:**100–106.

Yamada, H., Koizumi, S., Kimura, M., and Shimizu, N. (1989). Reduction of EGF receptor levels in human tumor cells transfected with an antisense RNA expression vector. *Exp. Cell Res.* **184:**90–98.

Yamamoto, T., Kamata, N., Kawano, H., Shimizu, S., Kuroki, T., Toyoshima, K., Rikimaru, K., Nomura, N., Ishizaki, R., Pastan, I., Gamou, S., and Shimizu, N. (1986). High incidence of amplification of the epidermal growth factor receptor gene in human squamous carcinoma cell lines. *Cancer Res.* **46:**414–416.

Yasui, W., Sumiyoshi, H., Hata, J., Kameda, T., Ochiai, A., Ito, H., and Tahara, E. (1988). Expression of epidermal growth factor receptor in human gastric and colonic carcinomas. (1988). *Cancer Res.* **48:**137–141.

Zenner, H.-P. (1986). Selective killing of laryngeal carcinoma cells by a monoclonal immunotoxin. *Ann. Oto. Rhinol. Laryngol.* **95:**115–120.

Zovickian, J., Johnson, V. G., and Youle, R. J. (1987). Potent and specific killing of human malignant brain-tumor cells by an anti-transferrin receptor antibody-ricin immunotoxin. *J. Neurosurg.* **66:**850–861.

9

Lymphokines and Lung Cancer

JAMES J. VREDENBURGH and EDWARD D. BALL

Dartmouth Medical School
Hanover, New Hampshire

I. Introduction

The molecular cloning of the genes for cytokines in the last few years has facilitated a tremendous burst of knowledge concerning cellular communication and proliferation. In particular, the interferons (IFN-alpha [α],-beta [β], and -gamma [γ]), the interleukins-1 through -8 (IL-1–IL-8), the colony-stimulating factors (G-CSF, M-CSF, IL-3, and GM-CSF), and tumor necrosis factor (TNF) are now all available in large quantities for studies that can measure precisely their activities in various cellular systems. It is becoming clear that there is a complicated network of communication between cells in the lymphoreticular system, and between these cells and other tissues, involving the secretion and binding of cytokines to their receptors on target cells. Precise characterization and molecular cloning of most of the cytokine receptors have lagged behind characterization of the cytokines themselves. It does appear that one or more cell surface receptors exist that specifically bind to each cytokine and that mediate intracellular signaling, thus effecting changes in the behavior of the target cell.

The majority of studies with cytokines have focused on cells of the immune system, for obvious reasons. However, because of the intense interest in immunologically based approaches to the study and treatment of cancer, investigators have begun to examine the role of cytokines in lung cancer and other cancers. The interferons in particular have been of interest in this regard for many years since they have been found to be antiproliferative to many tumors. More recently, some lung tumors, especially from patients with small cell carcinoma of the lung (SCCL), or cell lines from patients with SCCL, have been found to express cell surface molecules characteristic of the lymphoreticular system. Thus, SCCL, which has exhibited numerous pleiotrophic phenotypic characteristics (Ball et al., 1986a; Bunn, et al., 1985; Ruff and Pert, 1984), also has come to be viewed as a potential lymphokine-responsive target cell due to its similarity to cells of the monocyte/macrophage lineage. In view of the recent clinical interest in the use of hematopoietic growth factors to abrogate the deleterious effects of chemotherapy on the bone marrow, it is even more important to consider the effect of the growth factors on tumor cells themselves (Baldwin et al., 1989; Saalmon and Lui, 1989; Yamashita et al., 1989; Berdel et al., 1989; Munker et al., 1987). This chapter will review the effects in vitro of the various cytokines on lung cancer cells, and the preliminary results of protocols incorporating the cytokines into the treatment of lung cancer.

II. Interferons

It has been known for many years that the interferons (IFNs) have an antiproliferative effect on selected cell populations, including certain tumors. These effects are potentially mediated through activation of other cell populations that in turn mediate cell lysis, such as natural killer cells (NK), monocytes, or T lymphocytes. As an alternative, the interferon molecule itself may mediate a direct antiproliferative effect on the tumor cell population. Such studies usually reveal that there is heterogeneity in lung cancer, especially SCCL, in responsiveness to the interferons (Munker et al., 1987; Twentyman et al., 1985; Beaupain et al., 1986; Krishnamurti et al., 1987). Some studies have shown an antiproliferative effect of the interferons on both SCCL and non-SCCL, while others have shown no effect, or even growth stimulation.

The interferons differ with regard to their effect on SCCL. Using tritiated thymidine ([^{3}H]thymidine) incorporation and nude mice xenografts, Twentyman et al. (1985) demonstrated that IFN-α had no effect on in vitro growth or clonogenic growth. However, IFN-γ inhibited the growth of the SCCL cell lines in the same system. In contrast, an assay utilizing colony formation in soft agar failed to detect a significant inhibition of clonal growth of six SCCL cell lines as a result of incubation with the IFNs (Munker et al., 1987).

The growth of human non-SCCL nodules maintained in continuous organotypic cultures demonstrated the antiproliferative effects of recombinant human IFN-α and -γ on a human non-SCCL cell line, A549 (Beaupain et al., 1986).

IFN-β had no inhibitory effect on the A549 cells. The growth inhibition occurred only at the highest dosage levels (10^3 and 10^4 IU/ml). An interesting finding was that all three IFNs stimulated growth at the lower dosage levels (10^1 and 10^2 IU/ml). The combination of IFN-α and -γ resulted in a synergistic growth inhibition of the non-SCCL cells (Martyre et al., 1987). A 35-day treatment with IFN-α and -γ 1000 IU/ml of each, led to a complete growth inhibition and necrosis of the tumor nodules.

Recombinant IFN-α, -β, and -γ inhibited ≥30% clonal growth from the majority of the non-SCCL lines using colony formation in soft agar (Munker et al., 1987). IFN-α inhibited seven of nine non-SCCL lines, and both IFNs-β and -γ inhibited five of nine non-SCCL lines.

The effects of IFN-γ on cell surface antigen expression have also been studied in lung cancer. In particular, the effects of IFN-γ on class I HLA have been studied, stimulated in part by the observation that class I HLA has been found to be absent or weakly expressed on some cell lines from patients with SCCL (Doyle et al., 1985). IFN-γ is a potent stimulator of class I HLA, the mechanism believed to be mediated through increased transcription of the class I HLA genes. Doyle found that class I HLA could be induced manyfold by both IFN-α and IFN-γ on a panel of SCCL cell lines. Ball et al. (1986a) confirmed that class I HLA was inducible on another panel of SCCL lines. However, most of the cell lines examined in this study were not deficient in class I HLA. This study revealed also that the monocyte-associated antigen CD14 (gp55) was also inducible on some lines by IFN-γ.

Studies of NK-cell-mediated lysis of lung cancer have employed each IFN used separately as an activator of NK cells. In vitro experimental systems usually involve preactivation of NK cells from the peripheral blood of normal donors. Chromium-labeled tumor cells are then exposed to these activated NK cells and chromium release is measured as an indicator of cell lysis. These studies have revealed that NK cells can be activated to mediate increased tumor cell killing against lung cancer. It is interesting that the target tumor cells, especially from SCCL, may have paradoxical responses to IFN-γ. Ball and colleagues (1986b) studied the effect of IFN-γ exposure on SCCL cells before incubating these cells with IFN-γ-activated peripheral blood mononuclear cells. Cells from some SCCL cell lines became resistant to IFN-γ-activated effector cells as a result of their short-term exposure to IFN-γ. Thus, potential in vivo use of the IFNs must consider the possibility that the tumor may become resistant to natural killing mechanisms.

The IFNs also enhance NK cell lysis of non-SCCL cells, although IFN-α and -β are superior compared to IFN-γ (Krishnamurti et al., 1987). A similar experimental design was used with the three non-SCCL cell lines, A-425, A-549, and SK-MES-1, and a chromium release assay. In response to IFN-α or -β, effector cells previously unable to lyse non-SCCL cells matured into fully functional killer cells capable of lysing lung cancer cells. IFN-γ did not produce tumor cell lysis by the effector cells.

The clinical experience with the use of the interferons for the treatment of SCCL and non-SCCL is limited. In one trial, 15 patients with untreated SCCL were treated with IFN-α: 6 patients with 5×10^6 IU intramuscularly three times per week and the other 9 patients with 1060×10^6 IU intravenously as a continuous infusion over 24 h for 5 days, followed by 6×10^6 IU intramuscularly three times per week (Mattson et al., 1985). Thoracic radiation therapy was given to the patients for local/regional control and whole brain radiation therapy to 3 patients for treatment of central nervous system (CNS) metastases. The mean duration of response to IFN-α was 16 weeks. The results suggested that IFN-α delayed metastases, since 6 of the 9 patients who received the high-dosage IFN-α had disease that progressed locoregionally only, and two had CNS metastases with no evidence of other metastases. The combination of IFN-α and radiation therapy did synergistically interact to produce fatal radiation pneumonitis in 3 of the 15 patients.

In a phase II study of patients with untreated SCCL or squamous cell carcinoma of the lung, IFN-α was administered at a dosage of 50×10^6 IU/m^2 intramuscularly three times weekly (Olesen et al., 1987). All 15 patients with SCCL showed progressive disease. Of the 13 patients with squamous cell carcinoma of the lung, 1 had a partial remission for 14 months, 6 had stable disease, and the remaining 6 had progressive disease. In another phase II study, 10 patients with SCCL were treated with 400×10^6 IU/m^2 of human lymphoblastoid interferon by intravenous infusion over 5 days and then 3×10^6 IU/m^2 intramuscularly three times weekly. None of the patients responded (Jones et al., 1983).

There have been few phase II trials of IFN-γ for patients with SCCL. In one trial of 12 patients with untreated SCCL, the patients received 28×10^6 IU/m^2 intravenously daily for 5 days, followed by 14×10^6 IU/m^2 intravenously 3 times weekly for 3 weeks, or until progression. There were no responses to the IFN-γ treatment (Newman et al., 1987).

The in vitro effects of IFN-γ suggested that the lymphokine may be useful as an adjunct to chemotherapy for patients with SCCL. After 76 patients responded to initial chemotherapy, they were randomized to receive γ-IFN, maintenance chemotherapy, or no further therapy (Mattson et al., 1989). The group receiving IFN-γ had significantly more patients alive at 2, 3, and 4 years. The IFN-γ may increase the expression of HLA class I and II, and myeloid surface antigens on any residual SCCL cells, thereby increasing NK-cell-mediated lysis. Cancer and leukemia group B (CALGB) is treating patients with extensive SCCL disease with aggressive chemotherapy, followed by IFN-γ, in an attempt to confirm the above promising results. The CALGB trial is in too early a phase to determine the effects of the IFN-γ.

The effects of the IFNs on non-SCCL tumors are heterogeneous. In a phase

II study of IFN-α at a dosage of 50×10^6 IU/m^2 intramuscularly 3 times weekly, 16 patients with non-SCCL showed no major responses, 1 minor response, and 6 patients had stable disease (Grunberg et al., 1985). Of the remaining 9 patients, 4 were unevaluable: 1 had a myocardial infarction, 1 developed ventricular arrhythmias, 1 stopped therapy due to severe fatigue, and 1 developed cellulitis at a biopsy site. The other 5 patients had progressive disease.

Recombinant IFN-β was administered to 18 patients with advanced non-SCCL in a phase II study (Ettinger and Harwood, 1988). The patients received 90×10^6 IU intravenously 3 times weekly. No responses were seen, although 5 patients had stable disease for up to 9 months. CALGB recently completed a phase II trial of IFN-β for patients with non-SCCL and the results are preliminary.

CALGB reported a phase II trial of IFN-γ for 69 patients with non-SCCL (Ringenberg et al., 1989). There was only one partial response, despite five dose levels, ranging from 0.01 to 0.5 mg/m^2, and moderate toxicity, consisting of fever without infection, neutropenia, mucositis, nausea, and allergic reaction.

III. Colony-Stimulating Factors

Cell lines from patients with SCCL express numerous antigens characteristic of the myeloid cell lineage (Ball et al., 1986a; Ruff and Pert, 1984). This observation has led to studies of the responsiveness of SCCL cell lines to myeloid colony-stimulating factors. The in vitro and in vivo effects of one of the colony-stimulating factors, GM-CSF, on SCCL and non-SCCL have been studied, but there is less literature on the effects of G-CSF, M-CSF, or IL-3 on lung cancer cells. Ruff and colleagues (1986) studied the effects of GM-CSF on tritiated thymidine ([^{3}H]thymidine) incorporation and clonal growth in agar. These studies revealed that GM-CSF inhibited the growth, as measured by [^{3}H]thymidine incorporation and clonal growth in agar, of several SCCL tumor cell lines. In addition, these studies showed that GM-CSF could induce increased expression of the leu-7 antigen (CD 57) on four SCCL cell lines. In contrast, studies by Munker and coworkers (1987) failed to reveal an effect of GM-CSF on clonal proliferation of six SCCL cell lines. Two of the cell lines were identical to those used by Ruff. Baldwin et al. (1989) demonstrated that GM-CSF can enhance proliferation of two SCCL cell lines, as shown by [^{3}H]thymidine incorporation and clonal growth in agar. One of the cell lines, NCI-H69, was used by Baldwin and Ruff. It is difficult to compare these results because the source of GM-CSF was different and the amounts of GM-CSF used may have been different. Given the disparate results, one can conclude that there is no one effect of GM-CSF on SCCL cells, and clinical trials are necessary to determine the significance of the in vitro results.

Many of the variant SCCL cell lines exhibit increased myeloid or monocytoid markers compared to the classic SCCL lines (Yamashita et al., 1989).

Yamashita studied the effect of three hematopoietic growth factors on the SCCL cell line, GKT3-1.3 and its variant cell line, GKT3-1.3V. GM-CSF inhibited the growth of the variant line, GKT3-1.3V, as demonstrated by clonogenic assay and suspension culture. This antiproliferative effect was abolished by an antihuman GM-CSF antibody. The addition of GM-CSF to the GKT3-1.3V cells resulted in increased expression of the surface marker, Mo1, normally found on monocytes, which suggested that the growth factor affected differentiation. GM-CSF did not affect the native cell line GKT3-1.3 and the other two growth factors, G-CSF and M-CSF, had no effect on either cell line.

Baldwin and colleagues (1984) have also shown that cells from SCCL cell lines have high-affinity receptors for GM-CSF. Biochemical cross-linking of ligand and receptor has shown that the GM-CSF receptor has a molecular weight of 84,000 daltons, in keeping with receptor size on neutrophils and myeloid leukemia cells. Few data are presently available concerning the presence of GM-CSF receptors on non-SCCL tumors to make the significance of this finding more clear.

The effects of GM-CSF on in vitro growth of human solid tumors were quite variable. Salmon used solid tumor biopsies from 33 patients and [^{3}H]thymidine uptake in the human tumor colony assay (Saalmon and Lui, 1989). GM-CSF had no effect on 58% of the tumor, inhibited the growth of 30%, and stimulated the growth of 12% of the tumors tested. Only 5 of the 33 tumor samples were lung cancers, and the authors do not classify the lung cancers into SCCL or non-SCCL. Furthermore, the growth stimulation observed with one of the five lung cancer specimens may have represented growth stimulation of granulocyte–macrophage progenitors within the biopsy specimen. Given the small sample size and methodology, it is impossible to discern the true effect of GM-CSF on human lung cancers.

In a phase I trial of GM-CSF for patients with advanced cancer, there were no antitumor responses or tumor growth promotion in 30 patients with advanced cancer (Hermann et al., 1989). There was only one patient with lung cancer, which was a SCCL, and he was withdrawn from study on day 9 of the continuous infusion because of increased bone pain in areas of bone metastases.

The diverse effects of GM-CSF on SCCL cell lines make the clinical use of GM-CSF for SCCL patients controversial. On the one hand, GM-CSF may limit the myelosuppression and improve the function of the phagocytes, thus allowing higher dosages of chemotherapy to be given. However, if GM-CSF stimulates SCCL cells to proliferate, the cytokine may adversely affect treatment results, and if GM-CSF inhibits SCCL cell proliferation, the cytokine may interfere with cytotoxic therapy. Preliminary clinical trials with GM-CSF and chemotherapy for patients with SCCL have not shown increased tumor growth or inferior responses to chemotherapy, although the results are early. GM-CSF has allowed increased dose-intensity and decreased myelotoxicity. Of 11 patients with SCCL treated with carboplatinum and etoposide, followed by GM-CSF, only 1 developed grade IV myelocytoxicity (polymorphonuclear leukocytes <500/mm³), compared to 31% of 89 patients previously treated with the same regimen (Morstyn et al., 1989). In another trial investigating intensive weekly chemotherapy and GM-CSF when the patients developed leukopenia (white blood cell count <1000/mm³), 5 patients with SCCL received an alternating regimen of cyclophosphamide, doxorubicin, and vincristine with etoposide and cisplatin in half the time that the regimen can usually be administered safely without the GM-CSF (Ardizzoni et al., 1989). GM-CSF resulted in approximately a doubling of the bone marrow and peripheral blood CFU-GMs and BFU-Es. In both of these small series, the response rates were similar to historical controls. There was significant toxicity from the GM-CSF, causing pain in the bone and abdomen, rash, headache, and lethargy in about half of the patients.

Recombinant G-CSF has also been used effectively to abrogate chemotherapy-induced myelosuppression in patients with SCCL. Twelve patients with extensive SCCL were treated with G-CSF at five dosage levels, and the patients received G-CSF with alternate cycles of chemotherapy, thus serving as their own control (Bronchud et al., 1987). In the cycles that patients received G-CSF, there was a median reduction in the period of absolute neutropenia by 80%. The shortened period of neutropenia was important clinically, since there were six episodes of severe infection during the cycles of chemotherapy that did not include G-CSF, and none during the cycles that did include G-CSF. There was no appreciable effect of the G-CSF on the SCCL tumors; the response rates were similar to historical controls. One patient who had extensive marrow involvement showing clearing of his marrow of SCCL after chemotherapy and G-CSF, and there was no in vitro effect of G-CSF on SCCL cells from a patient's cells grown in culture (Bronchud et al., 1988).

Another clinical trial using recombinant G-CSF and chemotherapy for patients with lung cancer included those with both SCCL and non-SCCL (Efuchi et al., 1989). The duration of neutropenia was shortened at all dose levels compared to patients treated with the same regimens and without the G-CSF. This trial determined that an effective biological response could be obtained at one-third the dosage of G-CSF by a subcutaneous route compared to the intravenous route, and no intolerable side effects were reported. There was no comment regarding the response rates in this phase I–II trial.

There are no profound growth inhibitory or growth stimulatory effects of the colony-stimulating factors on either SCCL or non-SCCL. We believe that the in vitro effects of the different colony-stimulating factors alone and in combination on lung cancer should be studied more thoroughly before widespread use of the colony-stimulating factors in the treatment of patients with lung cancer. The stimulation of clonal growth of colon adenocarcinoma cell lines by GM-CSF, G-CSF, and IL-3 (Berdel et al., 1989) points out the need for a better understanding of the growth factors and caution as we proceed in clinical trials.

IV. Tumor Necrosis Factor

Munker et al. (1987) failed to find any effect of tumor necrosis factor (TNF) on clonal growth of six SCCL cell lines. These investigators were able to correlate this lack of responsiveness with a lack of detectable TNF receptors on SCCL cells. However, TNF inhibited the proliferation of all nine non-SCCL cell lines, with a ⩾58% inhibition of clonal growth. Other investigators found no effect of TNF on three other non-SCCL cell lines using a crystal violet staining procedure (Sugarman et al., 1985). The clinical trials with TNF have all been phase I studies, with the purpose of determining the maximum tolerated dosage and toxicity. The patients had advanced, refractory malignancies; thus response rates were not an endpoint. Now that many phase I studies have been completed, it is appropriate to begin phase II studies. Because of the many diverse effects of TNF, the maximum potential benefit may result from a combination of TNF with other cytokines or chemotherapy. Pharmacologic doses of TNF induce the secretion of other cytokines, GM-CSF, IL-1 and IL-6 (Broudy et al., 1986; Le et al., 1987; Defilippi et al., 1987). TNF and IFN-γ together inhibit tumor cell growth in vitro significantly more than either agent alone (Munker et al., 1987). It appears that the cytokines, GM-CSF and IL-3 induce monocyte killing through TNF (Cannistra et al., 1988; Wing et al., 1989). Several chemotherapeutic drugs enhance the in vitro cytotoxicity of TNF. Topoisomerase II inhibitors, like the anthracyclines and mitoxantrone, as well as inhibitors of RNA synthesis, like dactinomycin, markedly increase the effect of TNF (Kirstein et al., 1986; Alexander et al., 1987). Different classes of chemotherapy also act synergistically with TNF. Many of the cell-cycle-specific agents, for example, 5-fluorouracil and etoposide, have produced exciting results when combined with TNF (Alexander et al., 1987; Regenass et al., 1987). Rather than proposing a series of phase II studies, ideally we should learn how TNF kills tumor cells and interacts with the other cytokines and chemotherapeutic agents, so that more focused and beneficial studies can be accomplished.

V. Interleukins

There are few published data on the in vitro or in vivo effects of the interleukins, with the exception of IL-2, on lung cancer. A soft agar clonogenic assay was used to determine the effect of IL-1 and IL-2 on 6 SCCL and 9 non-SCCL cell lines (Munker et al., 1987). Neither lymphokine had an effect on the clonal growth of any of the lung cancer lines. A number of investigators have studied NK and lymphokine-activated killer (LAK) lysis of lung cancer cells. In general, solid tumor cells are resistant to NK lysis, whereas lymphoid and myeloid tumor cells are sensitive. After isolating the large granular lymphocytes (LGLs) from peripheral blood, it was determined that two SCCL and three non-SCCL cell lines were resistant to NK lysis (Robinson and Morstyn, 1987). After incubation of the LGLs with IL-2, there was a three- to sixfold increase in lysis of the lung cancer cells, with the two SCCL cell lines demonstrating the most augmentation of lysis.

There are complex interactions between the different cytokines, growth factors, and effector cells in vivo that may be utilized in vitro to maximize tumor-cell killing. Yang et al. (1989) incubated peripheral blood mononuclear cells (PBMs) with IL-2 and, using a standard chromium release assay, demonstrated moderate LAK lysis of 7 non-SCCL cell lines and cells from 32 fresh non-SCCL tumors. The addition of TNF to the PBMs 2–6 h before IL-2 increased LAK-mediated cytotoxicity by a mean of four times.

Another possible mechanism to increase LAK cytotoxicity of lung cancer cells is by incubating the lung cancer cells with tumor-reactive monoclonal antibodies (mAb) before the addition of LAK cells. The LAK cells alone showed significant cytotoxicity against two SCCL cell lines: 69% against H69 and 97% against H128 (Tong et al., 1989). Preincubation of the SCCL cells with two SCCL-reactive mAb, 1096 and 5023, increased LAK cytotoxicity up to 270% compared to LAK cells alone. Pretreatment of the LAK cells with an anti-Fc receptor III mAb, Leu 11, blocked the mAb augmentation, but not LAK cytotoxicity, suggesting the LAK/mAb interaction is mediated by Fc binding. There is potential in vivo use of the mAb augmentation of LAK cytotoxicity. It has been demonstrated that mAb can be safely administered in vivo (Ball et al., 1983; Dillman, 1989), so infusion of the antitumor mAb followed by LAK cells may offer a therapeutic advantage over LAK cells alone.

The combination of LAK cells and chemotherapy may act synergistically to kill lung cancer cells, even drug-resistant tumor cells. LAK cells and cisplatin had a synergistic effect on a non-SCCL cell line, and its cisplatin resistant subclone (Ohtsu et al., 1989). Chemotherapy-resistant tumor cells may be more susceptible to LAK lysis than the chemotherapy-sensitive tumor cells. Another non-SCCL cell line was relatively resistant to LAK cells, but the cisplatin-resistant subclone demonstrated substantial LAK cytotoxicity (Ohtsu et al., 1989). Either the concurrent administration of chemotherapy and LAK cells or chemotherapy followed 1–4 days later by LAK cells may improve the response rates seen with chemotherapy in non-SCCL (Ohtsu et al., 1989; Kedar et al., 1989).

Tumor-infiltrating lymphocytes (TILs) may offer some advantages and be more specific against a patient's tumor than peripheral blood lymphocytes (PBLs). In a study of 16 patients with non-SCCL, TILs and autologous PBLs were cultured in IL-2 (Yano et al., 1989). The TILs proliferated in response to IL-2, as did PBLs, but the induced cytolytic activity of TILs was significantly lower than PBLs against autologous tumor and two human tumor cell lines. IL-2-mediated IFN-γ production by TILs was also lower than PBLs. The in vitro addition of anti-CD3 antibody to IL-2-treated TILs significantly increased their cytotoxicity against fresh autologous non-SCCL tumors, but not against the NK-sensitive cell line, K562, or NK-resistant cell lines, M14 (Pisani et al., 1989).

A clinical trial reported by the National Cancer Institute studied IL-2 alone or IL-2 and LAK cells (Rosenberg et al., 1987). Six patients with adenocarcinoma of the lung were treated, and one showed a minor response. In another trial, IL-2 was given as a constant infusion along with LAK cells and, similarly, there was one partial response among the 5 patients with lung cancer treated (West et al., 1987). In a trial of TILs and IL-2, 8 patients with non-SCCL were treated; the disease was stabilized in 3, while disease in the other 5 progressed (Kradin et al., 1989).

VI. Conclusion

Our understanding of lymphokines and lung cancer is only beginning. The preclinical studies will add to our knowledge of the biology of lung cancer. The many lymphokines and their complex interactions will require in depth study before their place in the treatment of lung cancer becomes known. However, lymphokines hold great promise, and may significantly change our treatment and its success for patients with lung cancer.

References

Alexander, R. B., Nelson, W. G., and Coffey, D. S. (1987). Synergistic enhancement by tumor necrosis factor of in vitro cytotoxicity from chemotherapeutic drugs targeted at DNA topoisomerase II. *Cancer Res.* **47**:2403–2406.

Andizzoni, A., Sertoli, M. R., Corcione, A., Pistoia, V., Madhavan, A., Pennucci, C., Serrano, J., Mazzanti, P., Ferrarini, M. K., and Rosso, R. (1989). Recombinant (r) GM-CSF in patients (PTS) with extensive disease (ED) small cell lung cancer (SCLC) treated with intensive weekly chemotherapy (CT). *Proc. ASCO* **8**:226, No 879.

Baldwin, G. C., Gasson, J. C., Kaufman, S. E., Quan, S. G., Williams, R. E., Avalos, B. R., Gazdar, A. F., Golde, D. W., and DiPersio, J. F. (1989). Nonhematopoietic tumor cells express functional GM-CSF receptors. *Blood* **73**:1033–1037.

Ball, E. D., Bernier, G. M., Cornwell, G. C. III, McIntyre, O. R., O'Donnell, J. F., and Fanger, M. W. (1983). Monoclonal antibodies to myeloid differentiation antigens: in vivo studies of three patients with acute myelogenous leukemia. *Blood* **62**:1203–1210.

Ball, E. D., Sorenson, D., and Pettengill, O. S. (1986a). Expression of myeloid and major histocompatibility antigens on small cell carcinoma of the lung cell lines analyzed by cytofluorography: modulation by γ-interferon. *Cancer Res.* **46**:2335–2339.

Ball, E. D., Nichols, K. E., Pettengill, O. S., Sorenson, G. D., and Fanger, M. W. (1986b). Lysis of small cell carcinoma of the lung tumor cell lines by gamma interferon-activated allogeneic peripheral blood mononuclear cells: abrogation of killing by pretreatment of tumor cells with gamma interferon. *Cancer Immunol. Immunother.* **22**:211–216.

Beaupain, R., Billard, C., and Falcoff, E. (1986). Effects of recombinant interferons alpha-2, beta, and gamma on growth and survival of human cancer nodules maintained in continuous organotypic culture. *Eur. J. Cancer Clin. Oncol.* **22:** 141–149.

Berdel, W. E., Danhauser-Riedl, S., Steinhauser, G., and Winton, E. F. (1989). Various human hematopoietic growth factors (interleukin-3, GM-CSF, G-CSF) stimulate clonal growth of nonhematopoietic tumor cells. *Blood* **73:**80–83.

Bronchud, M. H., Potter, M. R., Morgenstern, G., Blasco, M. J., Scarffe, J. H., Thatcher, N., Crowther, D., Souza, L. M., Alton, N. K., Testa, N. G., and Dexter, T. M. (1987). Phase I/II study of recombinant human granulocyte colony-stimulating factor in patients receiving intensive chemotherapy for small cell lung cancer. *Br. J. Cancer* **56:**809–812.

Bronchud, M. H., Potter, M. R., Morgenstern, G., Blasco, M. J., Scarffe, J. H., Thatcher, N., Crowther, D., Souza, L. M., Alton, N. K., Testa, N. G., and Dexter, T. M. (1988). In vitro and in vivo analysis of the effects of recombinant human granulocyte colony-stimulating factor in patients. *Br. J. Cancer* **58:**64–69.

Broudy, V. C., Kaushansky, K., Segal, G. M., Harlan, J. M., and Adamson, J. W. (1986). Tumor necrosis factor type α stimulates human endothelial cells to produce granulocyte/macrophage colony-stimulating factor. *Proc. Natl. Acad. Sci. USA* **83:** 7467–7471.

Bunn, P. A. Jr., Linnoila, I., Minna, J. D., Carney, D., and Gazdar, A. F. (1985). Small cell lung cancer, endocrine cells of the fetal bronchus, and other neuroendocrine cells express the Leu-7 antigenic determinant present on natural killer cells. *Blood* **65:** 764–768.

Cannistra, S. A., Vellenga, E., Groshek, P., Rambaldi, A., and Griffin, J. D. (1988). Human granulocyte–monocyte colony-stimulating factor and interleukin 3 stimulate monocyte cytoxicity through a tumor necrosis factor-dependent mechanism. *Blood* **72:** 672–676.

Defilippi, P., Poupart, P., Tavernier, J., Fiers, W., and Content, J. (1987). Induction and regulation of mRNA encoding 26-kDa protein in human cell lines treated with recombinant human tumor necrosis factor. *Proc. Natl. Acad. Sci. USA* **84:**4557–4561.

Dillman, R. O. (1989). Monoclonal antibodies for treating cancer. *Ann. Intern. Med.* **111:** 592–603.

Doyle, A., Martin, W. J., Funa, K., Gazdar, A., Carney, D., Martin, S. E., Linnoila, I., Cuttitta, F., Mulshine, J., Bunn, P., and Minna, J. (1985). Markedly decreased expression of class I histocompatibility antigens, protein, and mRNA in human small-cell lung cancer. *J. Exp. Med.* **161:**1135–1151.

Efuchi, K., Sasaki, S., Kunitou, H., Tamura, T., Sasaki, Y., Shinkai, T., Fukuda, M., Yamada, K., Soejima, Y., Fujiwara, Y., Tobinai, K., Suemasu, K., Takaku, F., and Saijo, N. (1989). Phase I/II study of recombinant human granulocyte colony stimulating factor (rh G-CSF) in patients with lung cancer. *Proc. ASCO* **8:**239, No 932.

Ettinger, D. S., and Harwood, K. (1988). Phase II study of recombinant beta interferon in patients with advanced non-small-cell lung carcinoma. *Med. Pediatr. Oncol.* **16:**30–32.

Grunberg, S. M., Kempf, R. A., Itri, L. M., Venturi, C. L., Boswell, W. D. Jr., and Mitchell, M. S. (1985). Phase II study of recombinant alpha interferon in the treatment of advanced non-small cell lung carcinoma. *Cancer Treat. Rep.* **69:**1031–1032.

Hermann, F., Schulz, G., Lindemann, A., Meyenburg, W., Oster, W., Krumwieh, D., and Mertelsmann, R. (1989). Hematopoietic responses in patients with advanced malignancy treated with recombinant human granulocyte–macrophage colony-stimulating factor. *J. Clin. Oncol.* **7:**159–167.

Jones, D. H., Bleehen, N. M., Slater, A. J., George, P. J. M., Walker, J. R., and Dixon, A. D. (1983). Human lymphoblastoid interferon in the treatment of small cell lung cancer. *Br. J. Cancer* **47:**361–366.

Kedar, E., Ben-Aziz, R., Epstein, E., and Leshem, B. (1989). Chemoimmunotherapy of murine tumors using interleukin-2 (IL2) and cyclophosphamide. *Cancer Immunol. Immunother.* **29:**74–78.

Kirstein, M., Fiers, W., and Baglioni, C. (1986). Growth inhibition and cytoxicity of tumor necrosis factor in L929 cells is enhanced by high cell density and inhibition of mRNA synthesis. *J. Immunol.* **137:**2277–2280.

Kradin, R. L., Lazarus, D. S., Dubinett, S. M., Gifford, J., Grove, B., Kurnick, J. T., Preffer, F. I., Pinto, C. E., Davidson, E. Callahan, R. J., and Strauss, H. W. (1989). Tumour-infiltrating lymphocytes and interleukin-2 in treatment of advanced cancer. *Lancet* **1:**577–580.

Krishnamurti, C., Ahrens, P., and Ankel, H. (1987). Differential effects of β and γ-interferons on natural killer cell-mediated lysis of lung carcinoma cells. *Immunobiology* **174:** 221–232.

Le, J., Weinstein, D., Gubler, U., and Vilcek, J. (1987). Induction of membrane-associated interleukin 1 by tumor necrosis factor in human fibroblasts. *J. Immunol.* **138:**2137–2142.

Martyre, M. C., Beaupain, R., and Falcoff, E. (1987). Potentiation of antiproliferative activity by mixtures of human recombinant IFN-α2 and -γ on growth of human cancer nodules maintained in continuous organotypic culture. *Eur. J. Cancer Clin. Oncol.* **23:**917–922.

Mattson, K., Holsti, L. R., Miiranen, A., Kivisaari, L., Iivanainen, M., Sovijarvi, A., and Cantell, K. (1985). Human leukocyte interferon as part of a combined treatment for previously untreated small cell lung cancer. *J. Biol. Response Modif.* **4:**8–17.

Mattson, K., Niiraned, A., Holsti, L., Pyrhonen, S., and Cantell, K. (1989). Low-dose natural α-interferon as maintenance therapy for small cell lung cancer (SCLC). A phase III study. *Proc. ASCO* **8:**227, No 883.

Morstyn, G., Stuart-Harris, R., Bishop, J., Raghavan, D., Kefford, R., Lieschke, G., Bonnem, E., Olver, I., Green, M., Rallings, M., and Fox, R. (1989). Optimal scheduling of granulocyte macrophage colony stimulating factor (GM-CSF) for the abrogation of chemotherapy induced neutropenia in small cell lung cancer (SCLC). *Proc. ASCO* **8:**219, No 850.

Munker, M., Munker, R., Saxton, R. E., and Koeffler, H. P. (1987). Effect of recombinant monokines, lymphokines, and other agents on clonal proliferation of human lung cancer cell lines. *Cancer Res.* **47:**4081–4085.

Newman, H. F., Bleehen, N. M., Galazka, A., and Scott, E. (1987). Small cell lung carcinoma: a phase II evaluation of r-interferon-γ. *Cancer* **60:**2938–2940.

Ohtsu, A., Sasaki, Y., Tamura, T., Fujiwara, Y., Ohe, Y., Minato, K., Nakagawa, K., Bungo, M., and Saijo, N. (1989). Inhibition of colony formation of drug-resistant human tumor cell lines by combinations of interleukin-2-activated killer cells and antitumor drugs. *Jpn. J. Cancer Res.* **80:**265–270.

Olesen, K., Ernst, P., Nissen, M. H., and Hansen, H. H. (1987). Recombinant interferon A (IFL-rA) therapy of small cell and squamous cell carcinoma of the lung. A phase II study. *Eur. J. Cancer Clin. Oncol.* **23:**987–989.

Pisani, R. J., Leibson, P. J., and McKean, D. J. (1989). In vitro activation of lymphocytes from nonsmall cell cancer patients by interleukin 2 and anti-CD3 antibody. *Clin. Immunol. Immunopathol.* **50:**348–363.

Regenass, U., Muller, M., Curschellas, E., and Matter, A. (1987). Anti-tumor effects of tumor necrosis factor in combination with chemotherapeutic agents. *Int. J. Cancer* **39:**266–273.

Ringenberg, Q. S., Propert, K., Crawford, L., Glenn, L., Modeas, M., and Green, M. (1989). Recombinant IFN-gamma in extensive non-small cell lung cancer (NSCLC): CALGB 8734. *Proc. ASCO* **8:**230, No 897.

Robinson, B. W. S., and Morstyn, G. (1987). Natural killer (NK)-resistant human lung cancer cells are lysed by recombinant interleukin-2-activated NK cells. *Cell. Immunol.* **106:**215–222.

Rosenberg, S. A., Lotze, M. T., Muul, L. M., Chang, A. E., Avis, F. P., Leitman, S., Linehan, W. M., Robertson, C. N., Lee, R. E., Rubin, J. T., Seipp, C. A., Simpson, C. G., and White, D. E. (1987). A progress report on the treatment of 157 patients with advanced cancer using lymphokine-activated killer cells and interleukin-2 or high-dose interleukin-2 alone. *N. Engl. J. Med.* **316:**889–897.

Ruff, M. R., and Pert, C. B. (1984). Small cell carcinoma of the lung: macrophage-specific antigens suggest hemopoietic stem cell origin. *Science* **225:**1034–1036.

Ruff, M. R., Farrar, W. L., and Pert, C. B. (1986). Interferon γ and granulocyte/macrophage colony-stimulating factor inhibit growth and induce antigens characteristic of myeloid differentiation in small-cell lung cancer cell lines. *Proc. Natl. Acad. Sci. USA* **83:**6613–6617.

Saalmon, S. E., and Lui, R. (1989). Effects of granulocyte–macrophage colony-stimulating factor on in vitro growth of human solid tumors. *J. Clin. Oncol.* **7:**1346–1350.

Sugarman, B. J., Aggarwal, B. B., Hass, P. E., Figari, I. S., Palladino, M. A. Jr., and Shepard, H. M. (1985). Recombinant human tumor necrosis factor-α: effects on proliferation of normal and transformed cells in vitro. *Science* **230:**943–945.

Tong, A. W., Lee, J. C., Wang, R. M., Ordonez, G., and Stone, M. J. (1989). Augmentation of lymphokine-activated killer cell cytotoxicity by monoclonal antibodies against human small cell lung carcinoma. *Cancer Res.* **49:**4103–4197.

Twentyman, P. R., Workman, P., Wright, K. A., and Bleehen, N. M. (1985). The effects of α and γ interferons on human lung cancer cells grown in vitro or as xenografts in nude mice. *Br. J. Cancer* **52:**21–29.

West, W. H., Tauer, K. W., Yannelli, J. R., Marshall, G. D., Orr, D. W., Thurman, G. B., and Oldham, R. K. (1987). Constant-infusion recombinant interleukin-2 in adoptive immunotherapy of advanced cancer. *N. Engl. J. Med.* **316:**898–905.

Wing, E. J., Magee, D. M., Whiteside, T. L., Kaplan, S. S., and Shadduck, R. K. (1989). Recombinant human granulocyte–monocyte colony-stimulating factor enhances monocyte cytotoxicity and secretion of tumor necrosis factor α and interferon in cancer patients. *Blood* **73:**643–646.

Yamashita, Y., Nata, N., and Aoki, N. (1989). Antiproliferative and differentiative effect of granulocyte–macrophage colony-stimulating factor on a variant human small cell lung cancer cell ine. *Cancer Res.* **49:**5334–5338.

Yang, S. C., Owen-Schaub, L., Grimm, E. A., and Roth, J. A. (1989). Inducton of lymphokine-activated killer cytotoxicity with interleukin-2 and tumor necrosis factor-α against primary lung cancer targets. *Cancer Immunol. Immunother.* **29:** 193–198.

Yano, T., Yasumoto, K., Togami, M., Ishida, T., Kumura, G., Sugimachi, K., and Nomoto, K. (1989). Properties of recombinant interleukin 2-cultured tumor-infiltrating lymphocytes in human lung cancer. *Int. J. Cancer* **43:**619–623.

PART III

BIOCHEMICAL MARKERS IN LUNG CANCER

10

Neural Cell Adhesion Molecule and Other Antigens Defined in the Small Cell Lung Cancer Antigen Workshops

ROBERT L. SOUHAMI

University College
and
Middlesex School of Medicine
London, England

FRANK S. WALSH

UMDS Guy's Hospital
London, England

I. Introduction

Small cell lung cancer (SCLC) cells express membrane antigens shared by cells of nervous tissue. These molecules, which are not found on most other tissues, are of great interest because of the light they shed on the histogenesis of SCLC, because they are potential targets for antibody directed therapy, and because it is now clear that some of the neurologic paraneoplastic syndromes that accompany SCLC are mediated by, or associated with, circulating autoantibodies to neural antigens.

As a result of the international workshops held in the years 1986–1987 and 1988–1990, several molecules were defined and one was subsequently shown to be the neural cell adhesion molecule (N-CAM). In this chapter we review what is known about membrane neural antigens in SCLC, discuss the approach of the 1987 and 1990 antigen workshops, and review the structure and function of N-CAM.

II. Background

In 1981, Cuttita et al. reported that they had prepared monoclonal antibodies that reacted with lung cancer. They used a binding assay to determine whether these reagents recognized antigens present on cell lines other than lung cancer. They showed that three antibodies had high binding ratios to cell lines of SCLC and neuroblastoma, and in an adenocarcinoma line, and two of them to the MCF-7 breast cancer line. In a note added in proof they state that they did not observe binding to brain. This paper was the first to document an affinity between SCLC and neuroblastoma (some lung adenocarcinomas are now known to show neural differentiation). The nature of the antigen and its detailed relationship to nervous tissue remained unknown. Allan et al. (1983) developed monoclonal antibodies to neuroblastoma (a small round cell tumor of childhood with many similarities to SCLC). In the screening of one of these, UJ13A, they noted over 90% binding to two SCLC lines as well as to a wide variety of neural tissue. They also noted that the luminal border of thyroid epithelium was stained, as were tubules of the fetal kidney, and a subset of fetal thymic cells and submucosal cells in the fetal gut. The antigen was also expressed on Wilms' tumor and rhabdomyosarcoma. These authors concluded that the antigen was a "neuroectodermal" antigen also expressed on fetal kidney. SCLC had been known to show other "neuroectodermal" features such as neurosecretory granules, L-dopa decarboxylase, and the neuropeptide bombesin. Lehto et al. (1983) reported that the tumors also expressed neural intermediate filaments, identified by polyclonal antisera, but not other intermediate filaments. This contrasted with other lung cancers, which showed no neurofilament expression (but stained strongly with antikeratin antibodies). Neurofilaments are part of the cytoskeleton of the neuron and are present in neuroectodermal cells early in embryogenesis (Tapscott et al., 1981).

Other investigators confirmed the findings of neural-related antigens on the SCLC surface. Okabe et al. (1984) made four monoclonal antibodies to SCLC, two of which showed panepithelial reactivity and two (TFS-3 and TFS-4) showed staining of SCLC and neuroblastoma. These latter antibodies did not bind to cell lines of adenocarcinoma, squamous, and large cell carcinoma of the lung. The M_r of the TFS-3 antigen was 110,000 and TFS-4 was 124,000. De Leij et al. (1985) developed MOC-1, an antibody that stained 26 of 27 SCLC specimens, 3 of 7 lung adenocarcinomas, and was also expressed on neuroblastoma, pheochromocytoma, insulinoma, and brain and Schwann's cells. In the normal lung, cells with an appearance "consistent with APUD cells" were stained. The major component of the antigen appeared to have a molecular weight of 60,000. Takahashi and coworkers (1986) defined a surface antigen, recognized by antibody NE-25, which corresponded to neuroendocrine differentiation, being present on neuroblastoma, carcinoid, thyroid, and adrenal glands, islet cells, and nervous tissue. It was also present on renal carcinoma cell lines and glioma. Unlike the antigens identified in previous studies, this molecule gave a single band of MW 25,000 kda on sodium dodecyl sulfate (SDS) polyacrylamide gel electrophoresis. Subsequently this same group (Watanabe et al., 1988) developed another antibody NE-150, which recognized an antigen of 150,000 kda that appeared to have the same reactivity as NE-25 and it seemed more likely that the true molecular weight of the neural-related antigen was 150,000 kda.

A variety of neurologic paraneoplastic syndromes may, rarely, accompany SCLC. Some of these appear to be mediated by antibody to antigens that cross-react on SCLC and neural tissue. SCLC is the tumor most frequently associated with these syndromes. Neural antigens on SCLC may be the source of the immunization and subsequent pathologic findings. The myasthenic syndrome described by Lambert and colleagues (1956) is often caused by SCLC and is known to be due to an IgG autoantibody that localizes at the motor endplate (Engel et al., 1987) and impairs acetylcholine release. The antibodies also bind to SCLC lines and inhibit depolarization-induced calcium flux in these lines (Roberts et al., 1985). Antibodies to cerebellum have been found in a patient with cerebellar degeneration accompanying SCLC (Greenlee and Lipton, 1986); the retinopathy associated with SCLC (Thurkill et al., 1987) and sensory neuropathy have been shown to be associated with antibodies to retina and dorsal root ganglia cells, respectively.

One explanation for the occurrence of these antibody-associated syndromes is that neural antigens are expressed on SCLC in a form in which they are immunogenic, leading to the clinical features. If true, this would have considerable importance in understanding the immunologically based paraneoplastic disorders.

Chromogranin is a constituent of the dense core granules found in the cytoplasm of the tumor cells and in other neuroendocrine tissues such as adrenal medulla, islet cells of the pancreas, and thyroid C cells. Antibodies to chromogranin stain SCLC (Linnoila et al., 1988). Leu-7 antigen is expressed on both SCLC and peripheral nerve as well as on natural killer cells (Bunn et al., 1985). Other neural antigens expressed in SCLC are the molecule recognized on nerve and neuroendocrine tissue to the antibody PGP 9.5 (Rode et al., 1985).

By 1986 it was therefore clear that many laboratories had made monoclonal antibodies to SCLC and had claimed varying degrees of specificity for the tumor. Some of these reagents were recognizing antigens also present on "neuroectodermal" and nervous tissue and appeared to be a marker of the neuroendocrine differentiation of the tumor. Other reagents had a more general epithelial reactivity and others appeared to be blood-group-related antigens. The first International Workshop on SCLC Antigens was undertaken to facilitate exchange of information and to introduce a common nomenclature for these antigens. This workshop proved successful and has led to a partial identification and classification of neural-related and other antigens on SCLC, which was extended by the second workshop.

III. Antibody Clusters Identified by the SCLC Workshops (1987–1990)

The workshops have used the methodology of the leukocyte antigen workshops in an attempt to codify the antigens being recognized in the numerous reports. At the time of the first workshop it was uncertain whether data derived from immunohistochemistry could be used for the statistical analysis (in the leukocyte workshops the data comes mostly from FACS analysis). The aims of the workshops were therefore:

1. to determine if clusters of antibodies could be defined that were reacting with the same or closely related antigens;
2. to determine the specificity of these clusters to SCLC and (conversely) the reactivity with neural and epithelial tissue and related cancers;
3. to develop methods that would allow immunohistochemistry to be used for cluster analysis;
4. to encourage collaboration between laboratories and to produce a generally accepted framework for future reporting and experiments.

The first workshop panel of 59 antibodies contained control reagents and duplicates by which the quality and variation of the data could be checked. In the second workshop 87 antibodies were submitted. The details of the first workshop are described in the symposium publication (Souhami et al., 1988). The number of laboratories and experiments are shown in Table 1 and the total numbers of results in Table 2. Table 3 shows the reproducibility using immunohistochemistry in the first workshop.

The method of performing the cluster analysis is shown in Figures 1 and 2. The completed dendrogram of the first workshop is shown in Figure 3 and the second in Figure 4. Five clusters of reactivity were found (cluster 0 were the

Table 1 Number of Laboratories and Experiments Performed[a]

	Laboratories	Experiments[b]
FACS	4	24
Immunocytochemistry	8	54
Immunohistology	11	337
Total	17[c]	415

[a]Excludes a small number of experiments in which there was clearly a technical failure.
[b]An experiment consists of the results from all monoclonal antibodies tested on one sample at the same time.
[c]Some laboratories performed more than one type of experiment.

Table 2 Number of Experiments Excluded and Numbers of Results Remaining

	Experiments		Results[a]	
	Excluded	Remaining	Remaining	Missing (%)[b]
FACS	2	22	1074	19
Immunocytochemistry	4	50	2579	14
Immunohistology	8	329	17,135	13
Total	14	401	20,460	15

[a]A result consists of the data from one monoclonal antibody applied to a sample.
[b]Amount, reactivity, or strength of reactivity not reported.

negative controls) and 20 antibodies could not be clustered (either because they were not recognizing the same antigens or because there were insufficient data). Of the six clusters, two had only two reagents. These were clusters 3 and 4. These were designated w3 and w4 (the "w" indicating "workshop") to emphasize the tentative nature of the clustering. The w3 cluster of two antibodies (Ki67 and B10) was designated because both identified an antigen in the nucleus that was also expressed in the cytoplasm of dividing cells. There was no other indication that the two antibodies were recognizing the same antigen and this grouping was dropped from the second workshop.

A. Cluster 1

Cluster 1 was the dominant cluster. Strong clustering was seen in both workshops. The antigen was clearly present on neural tissue as well as SCLC and was lost on

Table 3 Reproducibility in Immunohistologic Experiments (after Exclusions)

		Amount of staining: first antibody of duplicate pair			
		0	1	2	3
Amount of staining: second antibody of duplicate pair	3	9	0	2	96
	2	2	1	5	3
	1	5	0	0	0
	0	399	1	6	23

Each entry in the table is the number of times a duplicate pairs (antibodies 13 and 23, both S-L 11-14; or antibodies 16 and 25, both 704A1) were recorded with a particular combination of reactivities.

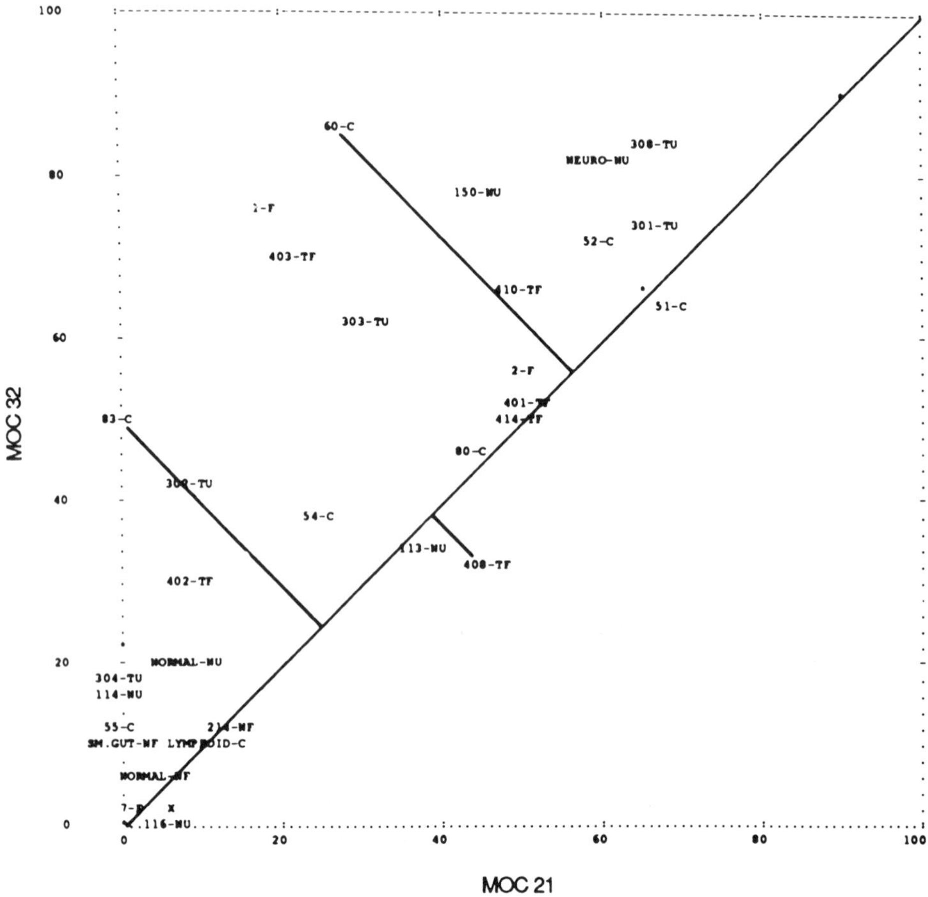

Figure 1 In this scatter-plot, two antibodies are compared for intensity of staining on various tissues. The vertical axis shows the percentage reactivity of antibody 2-MOC 32 and the horizontal axis shows MOC 21. If the antibodies stained all tissues to an equal degree, the points would lie along a line at 45 degrees. The extent to which they differ from this agreement is measured for each data point by constructing the vertical line as shown and computing the mean distance from the line of identity. This procedure is referred to as "euclidian distance." As an alternative, a compensation can be made for differing affinities of antibodies with the same specificity by constructing curves (which represent different affinity instead of the 45 degree line). This is referred to as "workshop distance." In practice, the cluster analysis was not substantially changed by the use of either method.

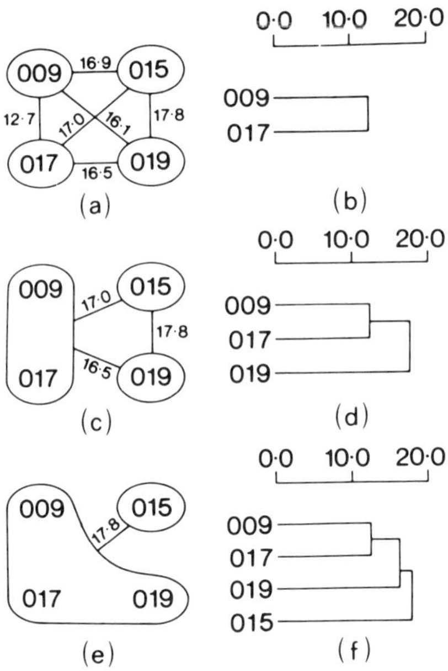

Figure 2 How the dendrogram is constructed. Four antibodies (9, 15, 17, 19) are shown with the distances (derived as in Fig. 1) between them. Antibodies 9 and 17 are the closest and the dendrogram is drawn at a distance of 12.7. Antibodies 9 and 17 are then combined and the distances of 15 and 19 are recalculated from these combined data. Antibody 19 is then the nearest at 16.5 and a further addition to the dendrogram is made. Antibodies 9, 17, and 19 are then combined to give a distance of 17.8 from antibody 15. This process is repeated for all antibodies.

formalin fixation (but one antibody—MOC 21—was able to stain formalin-fixed material). Several laboratories had suggested a molecular weight of about 120 kda. The antigen was also expressed on renal carcinoma lines, thyroid epithelium, and Leydig cells of the testis. It had very little expression on other normal or malignant epithelia including other types of lung cancer. By the time of the second workshop, the antigen was known to be the neural cell adhesion molecule (N-CAM, see below) and the human gene had been cloned and transfected into murine fibroblasts, allowing antibodies to be screened for reactivity.

B. Cluster 2

At the first workshop cluster 2 consists of four antibodies (AUA 1, S-L 4-20, MOC 31, LCA2/LC45) that recognized a 40 kda antigen. It was expressed on SCLC, other lung cancers, and on cancers of the breast, ovary, and kidney. It was found on

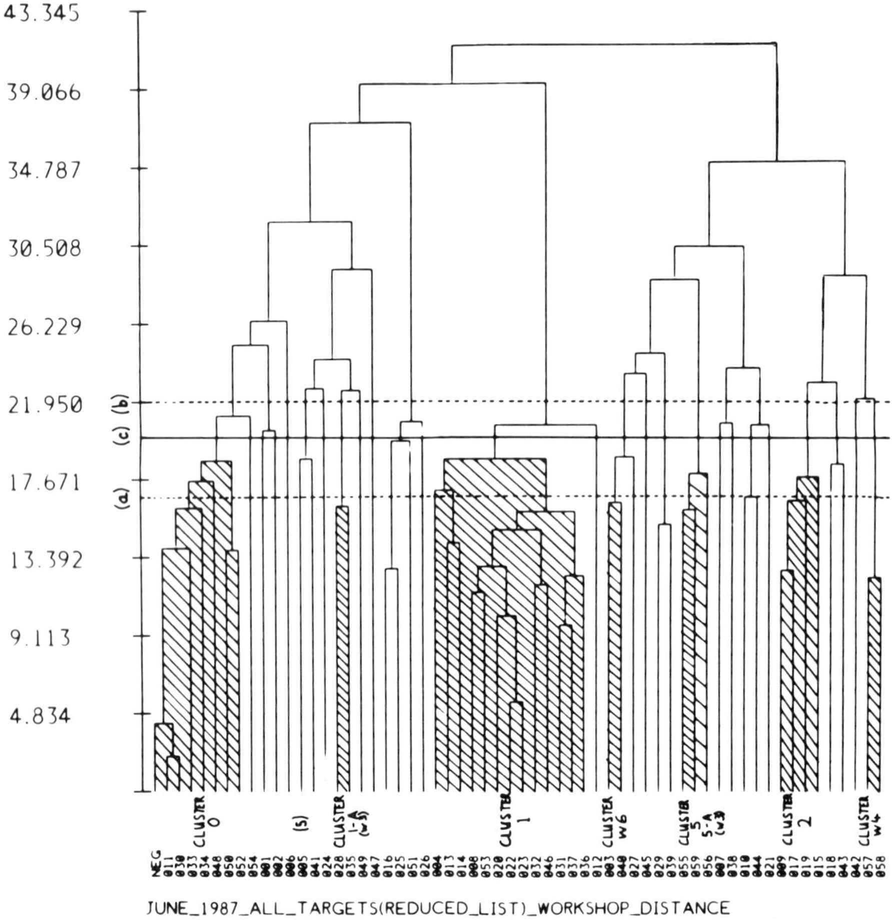

Figure 3 Completed dendrogram of the first workshop and clusters. Line (a) represents a line drawn at the distance level of the duplicates and triplicates (which are, of course identical). Line (b) is drawn at the level of the most generous interpretation of identity. Line (c), the level used, is drawn on the basis of additional helpful information (such as identical molecular weight or staining specificities). The antibodies below line (c) are considered clusters.

bronchial, thyroid, and prostate epithelium. It was to present on nerve. It does not cluster with antibodies to epithelial membrane antigen or human milk fat globule. By the time of the second workshop a gene product had been cloned (Strnad, 1989) to which some of the members of the cluster AUA1 showed sequence identity. The second workshop again identified AUA1 and MOC31 as members of the cluster and added MOC58, MOC151, MOC181, and S-L.2.21. Although LCA2/LCLC45 were not clustered on the second workshop, data derived from immunotoxin experiments indicates that this antibody is a probable member of the cluster. S-L.4.20 is a possible member (because of the first workshop clustering) and so is PE-35 (because of its molecular weight and immunotoxin data).

Cluster w4 (SWA 21 and SWA 22) antibodies were prepared by Stahel. The antigen is strongly expressed on SCLC, neuroblastoma, carcinoid, renal tubules, some granulocytes, and adeno- and squamous cell carcinoma of lung (but to a lesser degree than SCLC). It does not react with nerve. The antibodies also react with carcinoma of the breast, ovary, and kidney, and with normal glandular epithelia. Since the first workshop Stahel has published further data on SWA 11 (Smith et al., 1989), which appears to belong to the same cluster (SWA 21 and 22 competitively inhibit its binding). The molecular weight is 45 kda and the antigen is highly glycosylated (17 kda without sugars).

Cluster 5 antibodies (SWA 4, LAM 8, SWA 23) were closely associated with SWA 20 (designated 5A) at the first workshop. In the workshops they showed weak reactivity with neural and epithelial antigens. The antigen was expressed on a variety of tumors, including neuroblastoma carcinoid and breast cancer. Biochemistry suggests sialoglycoproteins of molecular weight 90–135 and 200 kda. LAM 8 has a tendency to stain membrane alone and SWA 4 and 24 may stain intracellular antigen.

C. Cluster 5A

Cluster 5A consisted of SWA 20 alone following the first workshop but at the second it was clear that SEN 3 and SEN 31 were probable members. Although not associated with SWA 20 in the cluster analysis, biochemical analysis of the antigen showed 3 bands of 40, 100, and 180 kda. The antigen is neuraminidase and periodate sensitive, and resistant to trypsin and mixed glycosidases. It appears, therefore, to be a sialoglycoprotein. Two other possible members of this cluster (not submitted to the second workshop) are SEN 11 and SEN 12. These data confirm the findings of Waibel et al. (1988), who showed SWA 20 to be a sialoglycoprotein. Maier et al. (1989) have carried out more detailed examination of tissue reactivity. This has shown that the antigen is strongly expressed on SCLC but not on other tumors (except some carcinoids). 5A appears to be separate from, but closely associated with, 5.

D. Cluster w6

At the first workshop cluster w6 consisted of two antibodies (MMC LU 152 and MOV 15) reactive with many normal epithelia but not nerve. The antigen was thought to be the y hapten. At the second workshop MOV 15 clustered with NCC-ST-433 but biochemical data showed that all three reagents recognized Le^y and they are considered to be clustered.

Second Workshop Cluster	Antigen and/or First Workshop Cluster	MAb Name	Donor	Isotype	WS No
		RNL 1	Broers	IgG1	004
	Cl 1	MOC-1*	de Leij	IgG1	012
		MOC-191	de Leij	IgG2a	021
	Cl 1	NCC-LU-243*	Shimosato	IgG2a	048
	Cl 1	NCC-LU-246*	Shimosato	IgG1	031
	Cl 1	NCC-LU-246*	Shimosato	IgG1	041
Cluster 1		SEN6	Stahel	IgG1	060
NCAM		SEN36	Stahel	IgG1	061
		NE-150	Ueda	IgG1	074
	Cl 1	NCC-LU-246*	Shimosato	IgG1	058
	Cl 1	NCC-LU-246*	Shimosato	IgG1	082
	Cl 1	S-L11.14*	Laurent	IgG2a	034
	Cl 1	NE-25*	Ueda	IgG1	077
		RNL 2	Broers	IgG1	005
	ras p 21	NCC-RA-001	Shimosato	IgG1	094
	GM3	MACG1	Johnson	IgG2a	088
		1D1	ICRF	IgM	084
	Cl 2	S-L4.20*	Laurent	?	085
		B5	Hay	IgM	087
Cluster w7	High MW	NCC-ST-439	Shimosato	IgM	097
	mucins	NCC-CO-450	Shimosato	IgM	098
		10B7-C8	Chan	IgG	010
		2A6	ICRF	IgM	083
		MLuC3	Menard	IgM	043
		NCC-ST-421	Shimosato	IgG3	093
	Mucin	BrE3	Ceriano	IgG1	049
	Mucin	HMFG1*	ICRF	IgG1	081
Cluster 5	Cl 5	SWA4*	Stahel	IgM	068
		SWA23*	Stahel	IgM	069
Cluster 5A	Cl5-A	SWA20*	Stahel	IgG	070
	Mucin	CID-4/KC4*	Ceriano	IgG3	050
	Mucin	Mc5	Ceriano	IgG1	079
		BS150	Ernst	?	022
		BS153	Ernst	?	024
		HBA71	Hamilton	IgG2b	026
		443A6	Radosevich	IgG	046
		OE-130	Ueda	IgG1	076
		703D4*	Manderino	IgG2a	039
	Cl 2 (rat)	LCA2/LC45*	Symann	IgG2b	073
	(rat)	LCA3/LC18*	Symann	IgG2a	096
	(rat)	LCA1/LC38	Symann	IgM	095

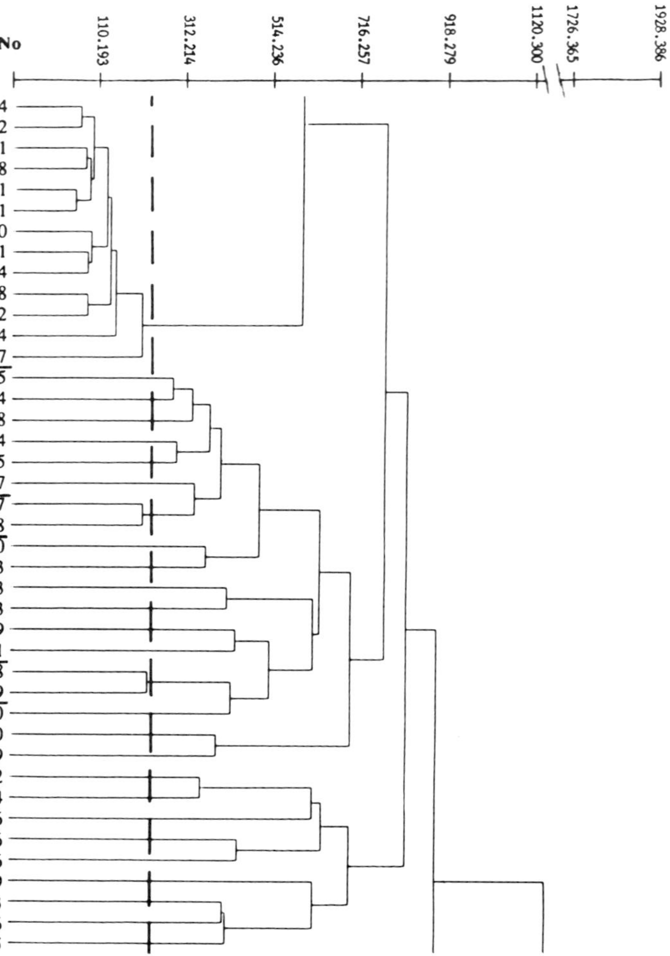

Second Workshop Cluster	Antigen and/or First Workshop Cluster	MAb Name	Donor	Isotype	WS No
	Cytokeratin	CAM 5.2*	ICRF	IgG2a	003
	control	CAM 5.2*	ICRF	IgG2a	056
	duplicates	CAM 5.2*	ICRF	IgG2a	028
		CAM 5.2*	ICRF	IgG2a	071
	Cl 2	MOC-31*	de Leij	IgG1	011
		MOC-58	de Leij	?	014
	Cl 2	MOC-31*	de Leij	IgG1	053
Cluster 2	Cl 2	AUA1*	ICRF	IgG1	080
		S-L2.21	Laurent	IgG2a	090
		MOC-151	de Leij	IgG1	016
		MOC-181	de Leij	?	020
		PE-35	Ueda	IgG1	075
		MOC-171	de Leij	IgG1	018
		SWA11	Stahel	IgG2a	059
Cluster w4	Cl w4	SWA21*	Stahel	IgG3	066
		SWA22*	Stahel	IgG3	067
		SM1*	Bernal	IgM	027
Cluster w6	Cl w6 Y-hapten	MOv15*	Menard	IgG2a	045
	Y-hapten	NCC-ST-433	Shimosato	IgM	054
		1A9-D4	Chan	IgM	008
		Fib75	Wawrzynczak	IgG2a	078

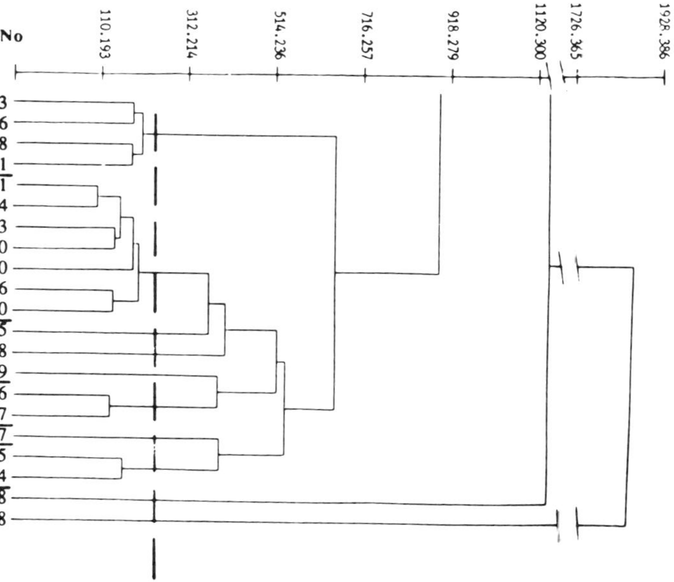

* Antibody in first workshop

Figure 4 The completed dendrogram of the second workshop. (See text for description of the clusters.)

Second Workshop Cluster	Antigen and/or First Workshop Cluster	MAb Name	Donor	Isotype	WS No
		PBS+5%			001
		PBS+5% FCS			032
		S-L10.52	Laurent	?	033
		MOC-143	de Leij	IgM	015
		PBS+5%FCS			051
		PBS+5%FCS			072
	GL6	MBR1	Menard	IgM	040
	Fucosyl GM1	F12.2	Brezicka	IgG3	086
		MLuC2	Menard	IgG2a	042
		MOC-51	de Leij	IgG1	013
		NSEH124	Manderino	IgG2a	038
	Cl 5	LAM8*	Bernal	IgM	002
		SEN2	Stahel	IgG2b	062
		SEN3	Stahel	IgG1	063
		SEN31	Stahel	IgG1	064
		SEN19	Stahel	IgG3	065
	ras p21	NCC-RAS-004	Shimosato	IgG2a	057
		BS152	Ernst	?	023
		MUC54	Johnson	IgM	029
	ICAM-1	P3.58	Johnson	IgM	089
		MUC18	Johnson	IgG2a	030
	Cytokeratin	RCKL05	Broers	IgG1	006
		BS154	Ernst	?	025
		MOC-172	de Leij	IgG1	019
		MLuC4	Menard	IgG1	044
	X-hapten	NCC-LU-279	Shimosato	IgM	055
		43/9F	Pettijohn	IgM	007
		S-L3.5*	Laurent	IgM	035
Cluster w6	Cl w6 Y-hapten	NCC-LU-152*	Shimosato	IgM	047
		MBR8	Menard	IgM	091
		A-80	Manderino	IgM	037
Cluster 8		NCC-LU-35	Shimosato	IgM	092
		NCC-LU-81	Shimosato	IgM	052
		6A3-C8	Chan	IgG	009
		S-L7.3*	Laurent	IgG2a	036
		MOC-153	de Leij	IgM	017

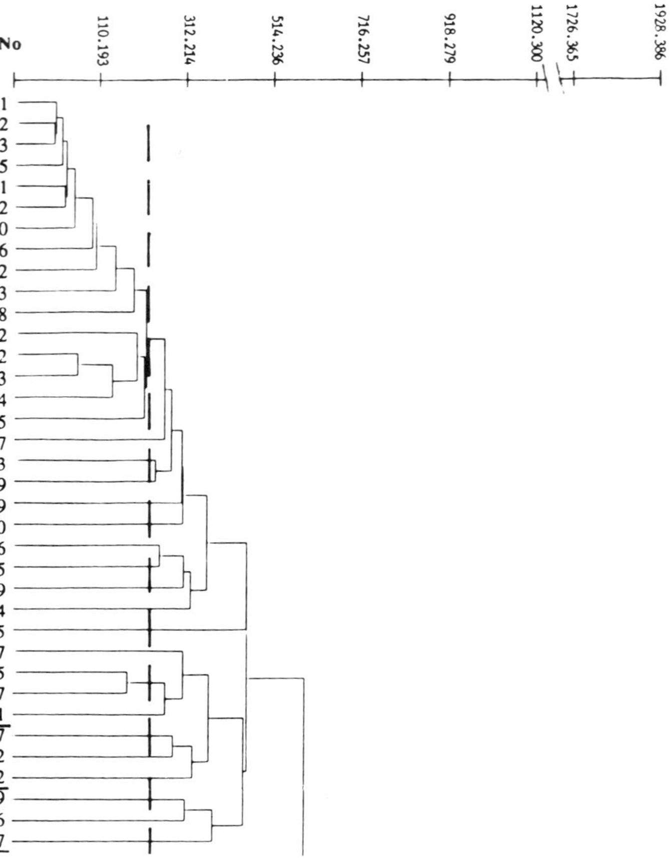

Figure 4 Continued

E. Clusters w7 and w8

The second workshop identified two further clusters. Cluster w7 is an antigen with strong expression on kidney and bronchial epithelium. It is less strongly expressed on SCLC, carcinoid, and neuroblastoma. It may be a high-molecular-weight mucin. The antibodies in this cluster are NCC-ST-439 and NCC-CO-450. Cluster 8 was designated after three antibodies (A80, NCC-LU-35, NCC-LU-81) that had shown association in the cluster analysis were all found to recognize the A trisaccharide.

The workshops have thus started the process of codifying the antigens present on SCLC and other lung cancers, a process that we hope will extend to other cancers and help to prevent duplication of effort. Many antibodies remained unclustered either because they were recognizing different antigens or because there were insufficient data to allow an association to be demonstrated. It is of interest that several of these unclustered antibodies were found to react with sugar molecules in a screening assay. One effect of the workshops has been to encourage groups to define the structure and function of the antigens of the recognizable clusters. The presence of several antibodies will allow epitope mapping.

IV. Neural Cell Adhesion Molecule

The antibodies against cluster 1 antigen (whose structure and function were unknown in 1987) were screened on murine cells infected with the human N-CAM gene and it was shown unambiguously that the cluster 1 group of monoclonal antibodies reacted with the protein N-CAM (Patel et al., 1989a). This suggests that N-CAM is likely to be expressed on SCLC cells and must be quite immunodominant since so many monoclonal antibodies have been generated to this protein. Since there is now a large literature on the structure and function of N-CAM, the aspects that pertain to SCLC are discussed with a view to using N-CAM as a target antigen for antibody therapy. In order to understand N-CAM function it is important to realize that N-CAM is a member of one family of cell adhesion molecules and that cell–cell interactions result in the operation of a number of different cell adhesion molecules. It is clear that the interplay between the relative levels of cell adhesion molecules (CAMs) and substrate adhesion molecules (SAMs) and their appropriate receptors can, in many situations, explain the development of specific cell collectives and, ultimately, tissue form. It is obvious that if we are to understand the molecular basis of specific cell adhesion, we must have available detailed information on the structure and detailed expression of the genes encoding CAMs and SAMs. Until this information is available it is very difficult to interpret the physiological consequences of abnormal patterns of expression in pathologic states such as lung cancer.

As a first step towards this goal we have been studying two different types of CAMs. CAMs can be operationally defined as being Ca^{++} dependent or Ca^{++}

independent, and in the nervous system the major Ca^{++}-dependent CAM is the protein N-Cadherin (Takeichi, 1987), while a major Ca^{++}-independent CAM is the protein N-CAM (Walsh and Dickson, 1989) with which cluster 1 monoclonal antibodies react. The study of these proteins is providing us with a number of rules that appear to be common to different CAM families. The cadherins were originally defined on the basis of antibody perturbation of Ca^{++}-dependent teratocarcinoma cell aggregation. In general there appears to be one cadherin type expressed in each tissue. To date, three members of this gene family have been identified: N-cadherin, which is expressed mainly in nerve and muscle; P-cadherin in placenta; and E-cadherin in epithelial cells (Takeichi, 1987). These proteins appear to be the result of expression of individual genes on different chromosomes and have arisen by gene duplication. The cadherins are homophilic CAMs, meaning that they bind to themselves. The strength of this is such that it allows cells to sort out in model systems. However, although these genes are structurally related, their binding specificities are rigid. Another feature of the cadherins is that there appears to be only a single protein species with no evidence of alternative splicing in the coding regions, although in the case of N-cadherin there are probably three mRNAs. It is likely that the different mRNAs are the result of different polyadenylation events. Glycosylation also does not seem to be particularly important for the function of the cadherins in the same way that it is an important modulatory factor in certain CAMs such as N-CAM. Thus on immunoprecipitation analyses the cadherins are not very polydisperse. The cadherins do, however, appear to interact with elements of the cytoskeleton and a family of proteins called the catenins has been identified as the binding proteins. Deletion of the cytoplasmic tail of the cadherins leads to altered function, which suggests that the cytoskeleton is important for function.

The Ca^{++}-independent CAM called N-CAM is an important CAM in the nervous system and muscle but it shows very different properties to the cadherins. N-CAM was identified originally on the basis of immunologic blockade of an adhesion assay between neural retina cells by Edelman and colleagues (Edelman, 1986). Since then the protein has been extensively studied by a number of groups and the main features of its structure identified. Figure 4 highlights some of the important structural features. In the human genome, N-CAM is present as a single copy at 11q23. The N-CAM gene is large and the coding region is at least 50Kb. There is a single promoter, which is unusual for a nonhousekeeping gene in not containing a TATA box (Barton et al., 1990). The elegant study by Owens et al. (1987) showed that the main protein isoforms could be accounted for by the use of 19 different exons. Since then at least another six exons have been found (Walsh and Dickson, 1989).

Sequence analysis has indicated that N-CAM is a member of the immunoglobulin gene superfamily of recognition molecules. This family of proteins containing members with different functions including adhesion, homing, my-

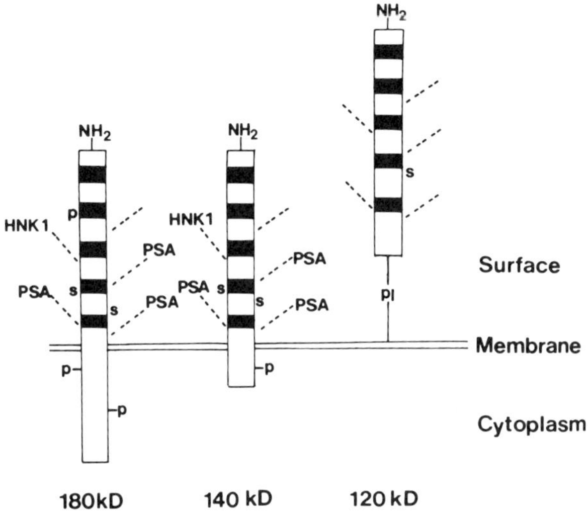

Figure 5 Schematic diagram shows the three main size classes of membrane-associated N-CAM. A fourth form, soluble N-CAM, is not shown since it does not pertain to this review. There are two main types of N-CAM: transmembrane (180 kda and 140 kda) or lipid-tailed (120 kda). Each contains five immunoglobulin domains of the C2 type (shaded blocks). Carbohydrate attachment sites are identified (dashed line), which can carry polysialic acid (PSA) or the HNK1 epitope, depending on the cellular background. Sites of phosphorylation (p) and sulfation (s) are indicated. For simplicity, the sites of novel exon usage are not shown; these can be found in Walsh and Dickson (1989).

elination, and growth factor receptors. N-CAM has five immunoglobulin (Ig) domains of the C2 type and is most closely related to the myelin-associated glycoprotein and the L1 cell adhesion molecule. Each of these Ig domains is made up of 2 exons of about 50 amino acids each; thus the 5 Ig domains are encoded by 10 exons. These are generally invariant between the different protein isoforms and are also the site of the homophilic binding domain. The nature of the binding domain is not known at present, although it is very likely to be found in Ig domain 3. The main region of diversity in N-CAM protein structure is associated with the region involved in membrane attachment. N-CAM can be found associated with the plasma membrane by two mechanisms, first by a classic transmembrane linkage and, second, via covalent attachment to phospholipid via a glycosyl-phosphatidylinositol (GPI) moiety. The transmembrane N-CAMs are of either 180 kilodaltons or 140 kilodaltons and the difference in molecular mass is associated with the usage of a single exon. Another region in the N-CAM gene has been identified that allows the generation of additional protein diversity. This is between exons 12 and 13. Here five new exons have been identified. The first four of these can be found as a single unit in GPI-linked N-CAM in skeletal muscle and here is called the MSD1 region. The first exon, however, appears to be expressed in a subpopulation brain N-CAM isoforms that are both transmembrane and GPI tailed. Since this exon encodes three proline residues, there has been speculation that this region may operate as a hinge region. The fourth exon in this region is responsible for generating secreted N-CAM forms. An unusual splicing mechanism involving the usage of a stop codon in this area called SEC allows the generation of a truncated soluble N-CAM isoform in both muscle and brain. Based on the above patterns of alternative splicing it is now possible to account for over 20 different N-CAM isoforms in muscle and brain cells. This is very different from the situation with N-cadherin, in which there is only one major isoform.

The carbohydrate on N-CAM has also attracted a large amount of study. N-CAM contains mainly N-linked oligosaccharide but, as will be discussed below, there is also evidence of O-linked oligosaccharide in muscle N-CAM. There are probably three main sites of N-linked sugar and these are found attached to sites in the five Ig domains. The oligosaccharides on brain N-CAM are unusual in that they contain an unusual type of sialic acid, an α 2–8 form called polysialic acid. N-CAM is probably the only protein in the nervous system to express this polysialic acid and it can be quite large, often up to 300 residues. The functional consequence of this is to decrease N-CAM homophilic interactions by a steric hindrance mechanism. Since there is extensive variation in polysialic acid content between different brain regions and stages of development, it is highly likely that its expression is involved in regulatory events. In model systems desialylation leads to increase in N-CAM-mediated adhesion. There is great confusion about the sialic acid on N-CAM. Only that sialic acid sensitive to removal by the enzyme endoneuraminidase N, or is reactive with monoclonal antibodies to polysialic acid (generally an antibody that cross-reacts with *Meningococcus* type B capsular polysaccharides), is polysialic acid. The rest of the sialic acid, which can be removed by neuraminidase, is not attached by this specific linkage. The non-α 2–8 linked sialic acid causes N-CAM to move as a broad band on polyacrylamide gels and is neuraminidase sensitive. The polysialic acid is added to N-CAM in a developmentally regulated and tissue-specific manner and is responsible for the so-called embryonic to adult shift in N-CAM mobility on gels (Edelman, 1986). Thus embryonic N-CAM is extensively polysialated while adult N-CAM is not. The only tissue other than brain that can polysialylate N-CAM is kidney, and this has led to the identification of N-CAM-containing polysialic acid in Wilms' tumor (Roth et al., 1988).

The second interesting carbohydrate structure on N-CAM is the HNK1 or L2 epitopes. These are two monoclonal antibodies that react with a sulfoglucuronyl structure, although the exact nature of this is not completely clear at present. The HNK1 reactivity is not specific to N-CAM as other proteins in the nervous system such as the myelin-associated glycoprotein, Po glycoprotein of myelin, and the J1 glycoprotein, also contain this structure. In addition, a similar structure can be found on lymphocytes, since the HNK1 antibody was originally identified as reacting with human killer cells. Whether the carbohydrate is identical in all these situations is not known nor is it very clear if it serves some modulatory role in terms of cell adhesion. It is of interest that not all N-CAM isoforms carry this carbohydrate. Only the transmembrane forms express this structure, while the GPI-tailed forms do not. In addition, it is not found on N-CAM in all tissues; for instance, N-CAM in muscle does not express HNK1 reactivity.

A third interesting carbohydrate structure is the recent identification of O-linked carbohydrate on N-CAM. N-CAM in skeletal muscle has been shown to react with peanut lectin while N-CAM from brain does not (Walsh and Dickson, 1989). With the identification of specific exon usage in skeletal muscle N-CAM, it suggested that these were the site of O-linked carbohydrate attachment. This has indeed been found to be the case and the site has been narrowed down to the first three exons in the muscle-specific domain found in GPI-tailed N-CAM. In terms of structure the O-linked carbohydrate is a sialylated version of the simple disaccharide galactose B1 $\rightarrow$ 3-N-acetylgalactosamine. No function has been ascribed to this modification at present. Thus, in addition to changes in primary amino acid sequence in N-CAM there is also a large amount of diversity in N-CAM carbohydrate. An interesting question is whether there is likely to be any specific modification in N-CAM structural in SCLC. The available evidence, while not complete, would argue that N-CAM is SCLC will be of similar primary amino acid sequence to those forms found in brain.

An extensive analysis by the S1 nuclease technique has not revealed any new exons in addition to those already identified, so it seems unlikely that there will be any novel exons used. There may be a deletion of exons that could lead to altered adhesive function. This possibility has not been addressed in detail but could be done with the polymerase chain reaction using mRNA from SCLC cells of varying metastatic potential. Similar analyses of N-CAM carbohydrate should be carried out.

In order to approach aspects of the function of N-CAM, we have used gene transfer technology to develop cell lines that express individual N-CAM isoforms. Since the only N-CAM in these cell lines is the one that has been introduced, it is possible to use these lines to ask questions about homophilic interactions and whether inclusion or exclusion of certain exons modifies cell adhesion phenomena. We have found that when human N-CAM cDNAs are transfected into 3T3 fibroblast cells, this results in expression of human N-CAM at the cell surface. This N-CAM is also functionally active, since there are changes in the adhesive properties of N-CAM following this procedure (Pizzey et al., 1989). In addition, neurons recognize this N-CAM and can use it to grow over. In some recent studies we found (Doherty et al., 1990) that the major determinant of axonal outgrowth is the level of N-CAM expressed by the 3T3 fibroblasts. In a panel of cells expressing differing amounts of N-CAM, we found that above a specific threshold level, increased amounts of N-CAM led to greatly increased neuronal responsiveness. When the human N-CAM being expressed by the 3T3 fibroblasts is analyzed biochemically, it corresponds in molecular size to the human N-CAM isoform in terms of the core protein size. However, the glycosylation profile is different. While N-CAM expressed by skeletal muscle cells and certain nerve cells are polydisperse because of sialylation effects, the human N-CAM synthesized by the 3T3 fibroblasts migrates on polyacrylamide gels as a very tight band and there is no evidence of extensive polydispersity. There is also no polysialic acid expressed by these cells because, as mentioned earlier, this modification appears to be nervous-system-specific.

These results assist in our interpretation of the SCLC monoclonal antibody workshop data. Since the glycosylation profiles of the transfected cells are relatively simple, we would expect that the majority of the monoclonal antibodies would be reactive with protein determinants. In addition, most of the monoclonal antibodies are species specific and the carbohydrate synthesized by these cells is of murine origin. Antibodies such as HNK1 do not react with the transfected cells. It is also likely that these are multiple epitopes on the N-CAM protein since antibody binding is not cross-blocked by other reagents. Further studies need to be carried out to determine the nature and number of epitopes. One unexpected reactivity was with the monoclonal antibody 3F8 that reacts with ganglioside GD2 (Patel et al., 1989b). GD2 ganglioside has been found expressed in melanoma and neuroblastoma cells. We found that under certain experimental situations we could find reactivity of the GD2-reactive monoclonal antibody 3F8 with human N-CAM. The gene transfer assay is very good at identifying these unexpected cross-reactions of monoclonal antibodies. Whether other GD2 reactive monoclonal antibodies bind N-CAM is not known at present. These studies show the advantages of the cloning and expression of human cell adhesion molecules. The cluster 1 panel of monoclonal antibodies, most of which are human specific, were originally thought to react with a diverse group of surface glycoproteins. The availability of human N-CAM-synthesizing cell lines that reconstitute human N-CAM specific epitopes on a background of murine carbohydrate is an extremely valuable model system. Since cell adhesion phenomena are of crucial importance in determining the metastatic potential of cells, it is likely that CAMs other than N-CAM might be abnormally expressed in SCLC and indeed other monoclonal antibody clusters have neural reactivity. To this end it should be a priority to express CAMs such as N-cadherin and the L1 glycoprotein in 3T3 cells to determine whether other antibody clusters react with these glycoproteins. Finally, it is likely that these panels of transfected cells will be useful test beds for the generation of new monoclonal antibodies of higher affinity that may be of more value for antibody-based therapy.

References

Allan, P. M., Garson, J. A., Harper, E. I., Asser, U., Coakham, H. B., Brownell, B., and Kemshead, J. J. (1983). Biological characterization and clinical application of a monoclonal antibody recognizing an antigen restricted to neuroectodermal tissues. *Int. J. Cancer* **31:**591–598.

Barton, C. H., Gower, H. J., Dwek, R. A., and Rademacher, T. W. (1989). Tissue specific O-linked glycosylation of the neural cell adhesion molecule (N-CAM). *Development* **105:**803–811.

Barton, C. H., Mann, D. A., and Walsh, F. S. (1990). Characterisation of the human N-CAM promoter. *Biochem. J.* (in press).

Bunn, P. A., Linnoila, I., Minna, J. D., Carney, D., and Gazdar, A. F. (1985). Small cell lung cancer, endocrine cells of the fetal bronchus and other neuroendocrine cells express the Leu-7 antigenic determinant present on natural killer cells. *Blood* **65:**764–768.

Cuttita, F., Rosen, S., Bazdar, A. F., and Minna, J. D. (1981). Monoclonal antibodies that demonstrate specificity for several types of human cancer. *Proc. Natl. Acad. Sci.* **78:** 4591–4595.

Doherty, P., Fruns, M., Seaton, P., Dickson, G., Barton, C. H., Sears, T. A., and Walsh, F. S. (1990). A threshold effect of the major isoforms of N-CAM on neurite outgrowth. *Nature* **343:**464–466.

Edelman, G. M. (1986). Cell adhesion molecules in the regulation of animal form and tissue pattern. *Annu. Rev. Cell Biol.* **2:**81–116.

Engel, A. G., Fukuoka, T., Lang, B., Newsom Davis, J., Vincent, A., and Wray, D. (1987). Lambert-Eaton myasthenic syndrome IgG: early morphologic effects and immunolocalization at the motor endplate. *Ann. N.Y. Acad. Sci.* **505:**333–345.

Greenlee, J. E., and Lipton, H. L. (1986). Anticerebellar antibodies in serum and cerebrospinal fluid of a patient with oat cell carcinoma of the lung and paraneoplastic cerebellar degeneration. *Ann. Neurol.* **19:**82–85.

Lambert, E. H., Eaton, L. M., and Rooke, E. D. (1956). Defect of neuromuscular conduction associated with malignant neoplasms. *Am. J. Physiol.* **187:**612–613.

Lehto, V.-P., Stenman, S., Miettingen, M., Dahl, D., and Virtanen, I. (1983). Expression of a neural type of intermediate filament as a distinguishing feature between oat cell carcinoma and other lung cancers. *Am. J. Pathol.* **110:**113–118.

Linnoila, R. I., Mulshine, J. L., Steinberg, S. M., Funa, K., Matthews, M. J., Cotelingam, J. D., and Gazpar, A. F. (1988). Neuroendocrine differentiation in endocrine and non-endocrine lung carcinomas. *Am. J. Clin. Pathol.* **90:**641–652.

Maier, A., Schmidt, U., Waibel, R., Hartung, W., and Stahel, R. A. (1989). Expression of the small cell carcinoma antigens of cluster 5 and cluster 5A in primary lung tumours. *Br. J. Cancer* **59:**692–695.

Okabe, T., Kaizu, T., Fujisawa, M., Watanabe, J., Kojima, K., Yamashita, T., and Takaku, F. (1984). Monoclonal antibodies to surface antigens of small cell carcinoma of the lung. *Cancer Res.* **44:**5273–5378.

Owens, G. S., Edelman, G. M., and Cunningham, B. A. (1987). Organisation of the neural cell adhesion molecule (N-CAM) gene: alternative exon usage as the basis for different membrane associated domains. *Proc. Natl. Acad. Sci. USA* **84:**294–298.

Patel, K., Moore, S. E., Dickson, G., Rossell, R. J., Beverley, P. C. L., Kemshead, J. T., and Walsh, F. S. (1989a). Neural cell adhesion molecule (N-CAM) is the antigen recognised by monoclonal antibodies of similar specificity in small cell lung carcinoma and neuroblastoma. *Int. J. Cancer* **44:**573–578.

Patel, K., Rossell, R. J., Pemberton, L. F., Cheung, N. K., Walsh, F. S., Moore, S. E., Sugimoto, T., and Kemshead, J. T. (1989b). Monoclonal antibody 3F8 recognises the neural cell adhesion molecule (N-CAM) in addition to the ganglioside GD2. *Br. J. Cancer* **60:**861–866.

Pizzey, J. A., Rowett, L. H., Barton, C. H., Dickson, G., and Walsh, F. S. (1989). Intercellular adhesion mediated by human muscle cell adhesion molecule: effects of alternative exon use. *J. Cell Biol.* **109:**3465–3476.

Roberts, A., Perera, S., Lang, B., Vincent, A., and Newsom Davis, J. (1985). Paraneoplastaic myasthenic syndrome IgG inhibits $^{45}Ca^{2+}$ flux in a human small cell carcinoma line. *Nature (Lond.)* **317:**737–739.

Rode, J., Dhillon, A. P., Doran, J. F., Jackson, P., and Thompson, R. J. (1985). PGP 9.5, a new marker for human neuroendocrine tumours. *Histopathology* **9:**147–158.

Roth, J., Zuber, C., Wagner, P., Taajes, D. J., Weisgerber, C., Heitz, P. V., Goridis, C., and Bitter-Suermann, D. (1988). Reexpression of poly (sialic acid) units of the neural cell adhesion molecule in Wilms tumor. *Proc. Natl. Acad. Sci. USA* **85:**2999–3003.

Smith, A., Waibel, R., Wester, G., Martin, A., Zimmerman, A. T., and Stahel, R. A. (1989). Immunolocalisation and imaging of small cell lung cancer xenografts by the IgG2a monoclonal antibody SWA11. *Br. J. Cancer* **59:**174–178.

Souhami, R. L., Beverley, P. C. L., and Bobrow, L. (1988). Proceeding of the first international workshop on small cell lung cancer antigens. *Lung Cancer* **4**.

Strnad, J., Hamilton, A. E., Beavers, L. S., Gamboa, G. C., Apelgren, L. D., Taber, L. D., Sprotsman, J. R., Bumol, T. F., Sharp, J. D., and Gadski, R. A. (1989). Molecular cloning and characterization of a human adenocarcinoma/epithelial cell surface antigen complementary DNA. *Cancer Res.* **49:**314–317.

Takahashi, T., Ueda, R., Song, X., Nishida, K., Shinzato, M., Namikawa, R., Ariyoshi, Y., Ota, K., Nagatsu, T., Imaizumi, M., Abe, T., and Takahashi, T. (1986). Two novel cell surface antigens on small cell lung carcinoma defined by mouse monoclonal antibodies NE-25 and PE-35. *Cancer Res.* **46:**4470–4475.

Takeichi, M. (1987). Cadherins: a molecular family essential for selective cell-cell adhesion and animal morphogenesis. *Trends Genet.* **3:**213–217.

Tapscott, S. J., Bennett, G. S., and Holtzer, H. (1981). Neuronal precursor cells in the chick neural tube express neurofilament proteins. *Nature* **292:**836–838.

Thurkill, C. E., Roth, A. M., and Keltner, J. C. (1987). Cancer associated retinopathy. *Arch. Ophthalmol.* **105:**372–375.

Waibel, R., O'Hara, C., Smith, A., and Stahel, R. A. (1988). Tumor-associated membrane sialoglycoprotein on human small cell lung carcinoma identified by the IgG2a monoclonal antibody SWA20. *Cancer Res.* **48:**4318–4323.

Walsh, F. S., and Dickson, G. (1989). Generation of multiple N-CAM polypeptides from a single gene. *Bioessays* **11:**83–88.

11

Immunohistochemical Analysis of Differentiation Markers for Non-Small-Cell Lung Cancer

JAMES A. RADOSEVICH

Northwestern University
VA Lakeside Medical Center
Chicago, Illinois

STEPHEN G. COMBS†

MacNeal Hospital
Berwyn, Illinois

STEVEN T. ROSEN

Northwestern University Cancer Center
Chicago, Illinois

I. Introduction

The incidence of lung cancer has risen continually over the past decades in the United States. This cancer now accounts for approximately 100,000 deaths annually (Silverberg, 1982). It has been projected that this trend will continue well past the turn of the century, even if all of the implicated environmental factors were removed from our society today. This anticipated rise is in part due to the long and variable latent period of this disease.

The treatment of lung cancer has commanded the attention of many disciplines of medicine and science. Treatment protocols that use surgery, radiation, and/or chemotherapy have all been tested, with at best only moderate success. The average survival remains to be measured in months, for patients presenting with metastatic disease, with few patients living more than several years after diagnosis. This poor prognosis and failure of traditional treatments demand that researchers investigate other treatment modalities and strategies.

---

†Deceased. This chapter is dedicated to his memory.

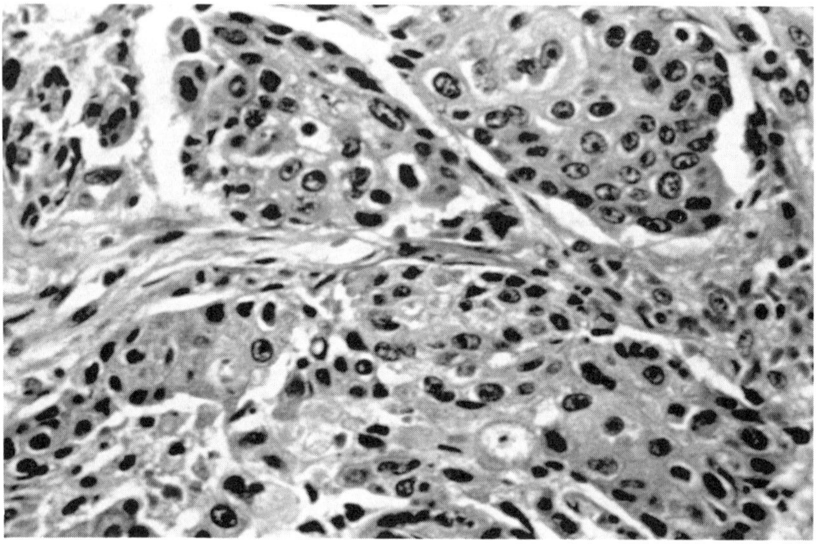

(a)

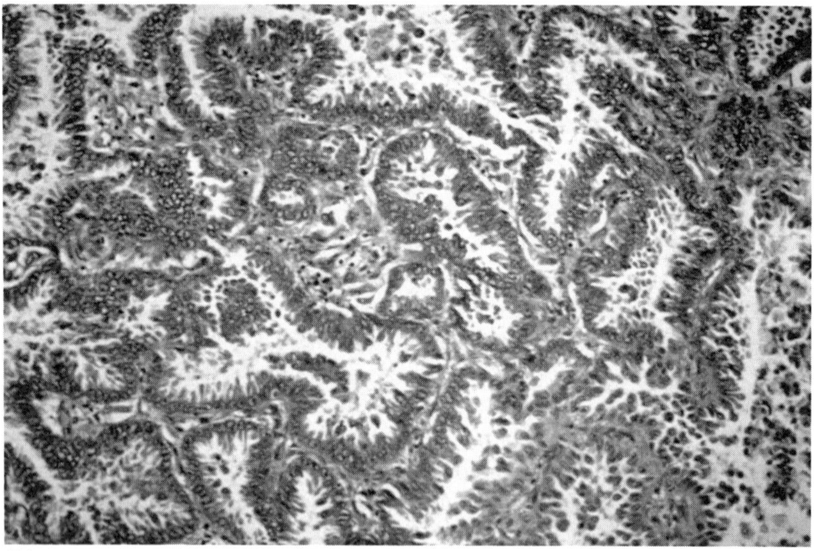

(b)

Figure 1 Primary non-small-cell tumors of the lung. (a) Poorly differentiated squamous cell carcinoma. (b) Adenocarcinoma. (c) Large cell carcinoma. (d) Bronchioloalveolar carcinoma.

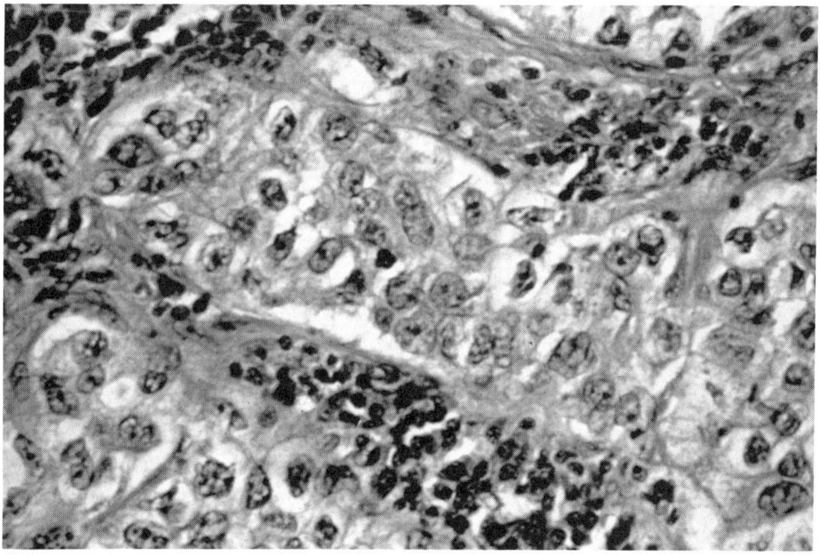

(c)

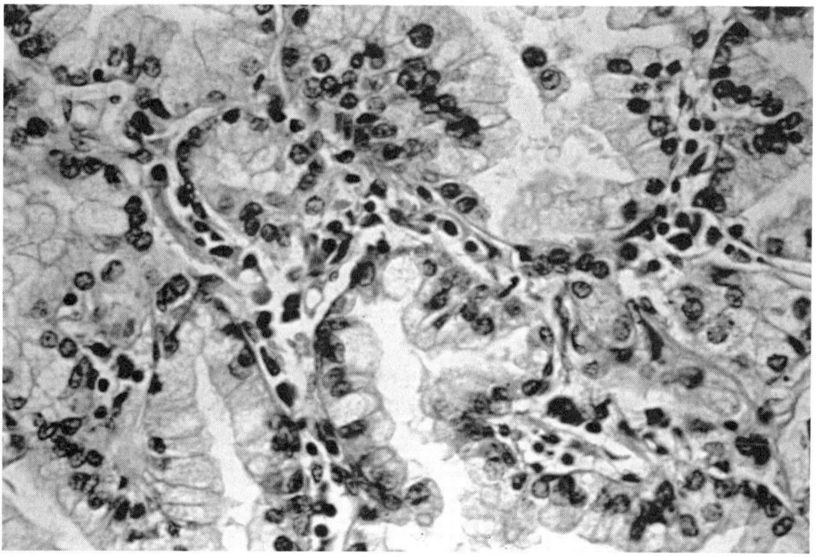

(d)

One of the major obstacles in designing new treatments for pulmonary neoplasms is that these tumors express a great deal of heterogeneity even within the various subtypes. The term "lung cancer" is in itself misleading because it implies a single type of neoplasm that arises in the lungs rather than a group of heterogeneous tumors. In spite of all of these difficulties, classification schemes have been devised using light and electron microscopic criteria (Carter and Eggleton, 1979; Gould et al., 1973; WHO, 1982). This level of evaluation can generally be used to classify these neoplasms into the various subtypes: squamous cell carcinoma (SCC), adenocarcinoma (AC), large cell carcinoma (LCC), bronchioloalveolar carcinoma (BAC), small cell neuroendocrine carcinoma (SCNE), intermediate cell neuroendocrine carcinoma (ICNC), well-differentiated neuroendocrine carcinoma (WDNC), and carcinoid (Carter and Eggleton, 1979; WHO, 1982) (Fig. 1). It is difficult at times, however, to classify these tumors consistently, especially if they lack the salient features of a subtype. The misclassification of these neoplasms has been reported to happen as frequently as 15–20% (Yesner et al., 1965). The LCCs are a prime example of the failure of this type of evaluation, because they are by definition neoplasms that lack the features expressed by tumors in other subgroups. In addition, it is not uncommon for pulmonary neoplasms to express features of more than one morphologic subtype. Another example of how these methods fail is the difficulty in differentiating metastatic adenocarcinoma to the pleura from mesotheliomas. Further evidence that this approach is inadequate lies in the fact that it is unable to predict responsiveness to treatment or prognosis.

The phenotyping of human pulmonary neoplasms, based on their expression of gene products, may allow a more accurate classification of these tumors. Phenotyping would also allow more accurate predictions of treatment sensitivity and prognosis. The classification of tumors that lacked salient features at the light and electron microscopic level could also be consistently classified based on the expression of key gene products. The use of phenotyping data also has the potential to be used to monitor the responsiveness to treatment or the biological evolution of a tumor, that is, the induction of differentiation markers by a biological response modifier. The monitoring of a tumor before and after chemotherapy, for the enhanced expression of the multidrug resistance gene product, is one example of how phenotypic analysis could be useful in assessing the sensitivity of the tumor to additional courses of chemotherapy (Radosevich et al., 1988a).

Many techniques could be used to phenotype pulmonary neoplasms. Two-dimensional polyacrylamide gel electrophoresis, Southern blot analysis, and many other methods have been used to detect differences in human pulmonary tumors or cell lines (Broers et al., 1985; Bunn et al., 1983; Rodenhuis et al., 1987; Branch et al., 1987). Any approach to assessing these tumors at the molecular level on a routine basis must address the limitations of the tissue sample, the need for rapid diagnosis, and the current standard practices used to derive a diagnosis. One approach that overcomes some of the limitations imposed by these techniques is the use of monoclonal antibodies (MCAs) in immunohistochemical analysis.

It is important to note that immunohistochemical analysis is unlikely to be the final and all-encompassing way to analyze these neoplasms. There are several reasons for this. First, a great deal of effort has been expended to produce immunologic reagents that will work in paraffin-embedded tissues, with only moderate success. Second, pulmonary neoplasms may express features that cannot be differentiated by antibodies; chromosomal deletions, gene amplifications or rearrangements, and alteration in enzymatic activity. Third, some antigens may be too labile to serve as useful markers or may be restricted by the immune system so that an antibody cannot be raised against that antigen or epitope. In spite of these and other limitations, MCAs used in immunohistochemical analysis can be useful adjuncts in the molecular dissection of these heterogeneous neoplasms.

II. Monoclonal Antibodies as Probes

With the advent of MCA production by Kohler and Milstein (1975), a new era for the use of immunologic reagents in routine clinical diagnosis began. Polysera from various species have been used, but imposed several limitations. First, polysera are difficult to control in terms of specificity, and vary widely from animal to animal as well as over time within an individual. For this reason, variability is noted from lot to lot of pooled sera. Second, because polysera detect multiple epitopes, it is difficult to be certain that the specific antigen of interest is actually being detected, and not some cross-reactive related antigen.

Monoclonal antibodies offer several features that make them theoretically attractive as probes for tumor markers. First, they recognize only a single epitope and therefore can be highly specific for a given antigen. MCAs can be produced using tissue culture methods that provide large quantities of a uniformly reactive reagent. Since a single hybrid produces a single MCA in relatively high concentration, the MCA can be readily isolated as a pure protein. In addition, a stable hybrid is immortal and serves as a consistent source of a reagent, unlike polysera.

The utility of these reagents can be influenced by many factors. MCAs that detect their antigens in formalin-fixed–paraffin-embedded tissue have the advantageous properties of relatively easy handling requirements, they allow for better assessment of cellular architecture, and permit retrospective studies on routinely processed tissues. Although the antigen profile is greater in frozen tissue, there is considerably more difficulty in both routine handling of these specimens and determination of the tumor's histologic characteristics. Immunoreactive background is also generally higher in frozen tissue sections. The concentration of the MCA and the detection method used can greatly influence the reactivity pattern.

The tumor tissue used to assess the utility of an MCA can influence the results of that evaluation. In general, these tissues are classified using only traditional hematoxylin/eosin-stained tissue sections and by electron microscopic evaluation. This introduces the possibility that the phenotype of a subset of tumors, identified by a MCA, may not correlate with the morphologic appearance of the tissues tested. By carefully controlling these and other parameters to be discussed, it is possible to select MCAs that are useful in the phenotyping of human pulmonary tumors.

III. Methods in Immunohistochemistry

The evaluation of immunohistochemical techniques has led to increasing levels of sensitivity, ease, and reproducibility in the study of the expression of select antigens in tissues. Early methods required the primary antibody to be purified and labeled. This approach was highly variable and laborious. More sophisticated methods employed secondary antibodies that were linked with tracer molecules. Immune complexes (PAP) and other multiple antiantibody systems have been reported (Sternberger et al., 1970). The use of the avidin–biotin complex method (or streptavidin–biotin complex) with a biotinylated secondary MCA has greatly improved the sensitivity, ease, and reproducibility of this approach (Hsu et al., 1981). Commercially available kits that are highly controlled have aided dramatically in this regard.

Although several tracer systems have been used to detect the presence of antigen–antibody complexes in tissues, the ABC method has become the standard. It employs either alkaline phosphatase or horseradish peroxidase enzymatic activity to cause soluble colorless substrates to become a colored, insoluble product. One of the most widely used substrates is diaminobenzidine tetrahydrochloride (DAB), because it results in a deep brown precipitate that has good contrast in hematoxylin counterstained tissue sections. The reaction of DAB can be performed in the presence of $NiCl_2$, which results in the precipitate being black. A green counterstain (light green) is usually used to give the greatest contrast. Caution should be taken when staining lung tissue with this system because anthracotic pigment can be mistaken for a positive reaction. Other substrates have been reported with various counterstains.

When using immunohistochemistry and MCAs as an approach to phenotyping pulmonary neoplasms, one must consider several key controls and conditions. The tissue must be appropriately and uniformly fixed and processed, whether frozen or fixed. Overfixation, embedding temperature, and media can influence immunoreactivity as well as the quality of the reagents used. These parameters must be balanced to ensure that positive tissues exhibit immunoreactivity and have good morphologic and cytologic features. Frozen tissue should be permeabilized with acetone or a mild detergent depending on the antigen to be detected. Both the antibody used and the unique properties of the target antigen dictate the specific conditions to be used during the staining procedure.

Nonspecific binding of the secondary antibodies in the detection system must be totally blocked before application of the primary antibody. This is generally accomplished using nonimmune serum from the same species as the secondary antibody. Caution must be taken to ensure that enzymatic activity is not reintroduced into the tissue. Serum blocking can also introduce interfering activities that affect the avidin–biotin complex formation and the enzymatic activity of the reporting tracer system. Any endogenous enzymatic activity that may result in a false-positive reaction must be inactivated. This inactivation procedure should be titrated to ensure complete blockage without affecting immunoreactivity. Throughout the staining procedure, the tissue and all solutions should have the appropriate pH and salt concentrations so that the antigen–antibody complexes are not dissociated. Substrate solutions need to be tested daily and filtered before use to ensure their activity and to remove insoluble substrate. Wetting agents such as bovine serum albumin or Tween should be used in all solutions to reduce the surface tension of the fluids on the slide. This allows an even coating of the reagents. Any portion of the tissue that does not receive an application of any one of the steps would result in a false-negative reaction for that portion of the tissue. Each lot of wetting agent must be tested to ensure that it does not inhibit the various components from functioning appropriately. Water quality control, especially for contaminating organic compounds, is also critical.

Debate has taken place over the appropriate controls for immunohistochemistry. Generally, a set of daughter slides is stained under the same conditions with no primary MCA and with the substitution of the primary antibody for another irrelevant MCA of the same isotype. The choice of which irrelevant antibody is sometimes difficult. The use of precious tissue samples as controls may be difficult to justify, especially if the MCA reactivity pattern is well known. In some cases, the inhibition of binding by the addition of the isolated epitope to the tissue is used to demonstrate specificity of the antibody. Regardless of the number and type of controls, the primary MCA should be well characterized and the presence of the antigen confirmed by another biochemical method when possible. Without this confirmation, only an inference of specific reactivity in the tissue for any MCA can be made.

IV. Monoclonal Antibodies Reactive with Non-Small-Cell Lung Cancer

Attempts to produce MCAs that react with lung cancer have received much attention. More than 200 MCAs have been reported to react with human lung tumors (Radosevich et al., 1988b). An even larger number of MCAs directed against other tumors has been shown to cross-react with some lung neoplasms. Many of these MCAs have not been extensively studied, nor have their respective antigens been evaluated. Few of the MCAs work in paraffin-embedded tissues and show promise for routine use. The more than 200 MCAs reported not only show the great efforts that have been put forth in this area but also give hope that more durable MCAs may be produced against these epitopes. The demonstration that the resultant immunoreactivity patterns exist confirms the pleomorphic expression of numerous gene products by these tumors and therefore suggests the possible classification of these tumors based on gene expression, rather than strictly on morphologic grounds. No doubt immunohistochemistry will not be the only approach needed to classify this heterogeneous group of neoplasms. Immunohistochemistry does, however, add significant information as an adjunct to light and electron microscopic evaluation.

The remainder of this chapter will be devoted to two MCAs that we have studied in detail and that are representative examples of MCAs with similar binding patterns. The rat MCA 624A12 is one of a panel of MCAs that detects an immunodominant, blood-group-related carbohydrate sequence expressed by many pulmonary and nonpulmonary neoplasms. The aberrant expression of these blood-group-related antigens by tumors is currently under intense study because of their potential clinical relevance. The second MCA, 44-3A6, recognizes a cell surface protein associated with glandular differentiation in adenocarcinomas and normal glandular tissues. The study of these and other antigens detected by MCAs similar to MCA 44-3A6 is directed at understanding the biological roles of these differentiation-related antigens. The possibility of immunophenotyping neoplasms based on the degree of differentiation could have significant clinical importance.

A. MCA 624A12

MCAs were first produced by hybridizing mouse spleen cells to a mouse myeloma cell line (Kohler and Milstein, 1975). It has long been known that different species give different antibody responses to the same antigen. For this reason, rats rather than mice were immunized with lung cancer cell lines in an attempt to elicit unique antibody responses not seen in mice. The rat IgM MCA 624A12 was raised against the classic small cell line NCI-H69 (Rosen et al., 1984a). It has been shown to recognize the ceramide pentasaccharide that contains the lacto-N-fuco-pentose III (LNFP III) sequence of sugars, which is an isomer of the Lewis A blood group antigen.

The initial report of this MCA describes a panel of 21 rat MCAs made against various human small cell lung cancer cell lines (Rosen et al., 1984a). This was found to react with a large number of small cell lung carcinoma cell lines, and with about half of the non small cell lung cancer cell lines tested using a radioimmunoassay. This MCA was found not to react with a variety of human nonpulmonary cell lines. Using this radioimmunoassay, MCA 624A12 was also found to have minimal reactivity with normal lung and liver tissue, but detectable reactivity with normal kidney and with all of the small cell lung cancer necropsy specimens tested. Cross-reactivity was also found with three of four neuroblastoma cell lines tested (Rosen et al., 1984a).

The LNFP III sequence is well preserved in routine formalin-fixed–paraffin-embedded tissues. The radioimmunoassay results were subsequently only partially confirmed using immunohistochemistry on a panel of over 200 primary pulmonary neoplasms (Lee et al., 1987). LNFP III was found to be expressed on adenocarcinomas (49 of 50), bronchioloalveolar carcinomas (10 of 11), and some squamous cell (11 of 38), large cell (11 of 30), and intermediate neuroendocrine carcinomas (7 of 26). Small cell neuroendocrine (0 of 33), well-differentiated neuroendocrine carcinoma (0 of 10), carcinoid (0 of 21), and mesotheliomas (0 of 43) all tested negative. Since MCA 624A12 was raised against the small cell line NCI-H69, the radioimmunoassay and immunohistochemical data seemed inconsistent. Several explanations have been proposed to resolve these findings. The small cell lung cancer cell line has been found to have double to triple the size of a classic small cell carcinoma, and to express neuroendocrine and cytoskeletal markers that are more consistent with the intermediate neuroendocrine carcinomas. An alternative explanation may be that the original tumor phenotype was altered by in vitro culture conditions (Lee et al., 1987).

The monoclonal antibody MCA 624A12 was subsequently studied along with MCA 44-3A6 (to be discussed below) on a panel of malignant pleural mesotheliomas and metastatic pulmonary adenocarcinomas to the pleura (Lee et al., 1986). In all cases, MCA 624A12 was found to be negative for the mesotheliomas, where MCA 44-3A6 showed only rare focal staining that was discernible from adenocarcinomas. Both of these MCAs were found to be immunoreactive on all of the metastatic adenocarcinomas studied. Current studies are using these two MCAs to define further phenotypes expressed by adenocarcinoma, large cell carcinoma, and bronchioloalveolar subtypes.

The expression of LNFP III, as defined by MCA 624A12 immunoreactivity, has been used to map the expression of this epitope through human fetal development using immunohistochemistry (Rosen et al., 1984b). The adult normal organ biodistribution has also been determined (Rosen et al., 1984b). The tissues stained were primarily of epithelial and neuroectodermal origin (Table 1, Fig. 2).

B. MCA 44-3A6

The mouse MCA 44-3A6 is an IgG_1 that was raised against the human lung adenocarcinoma cell line A549. It has been shown to react with 40,000 dalton

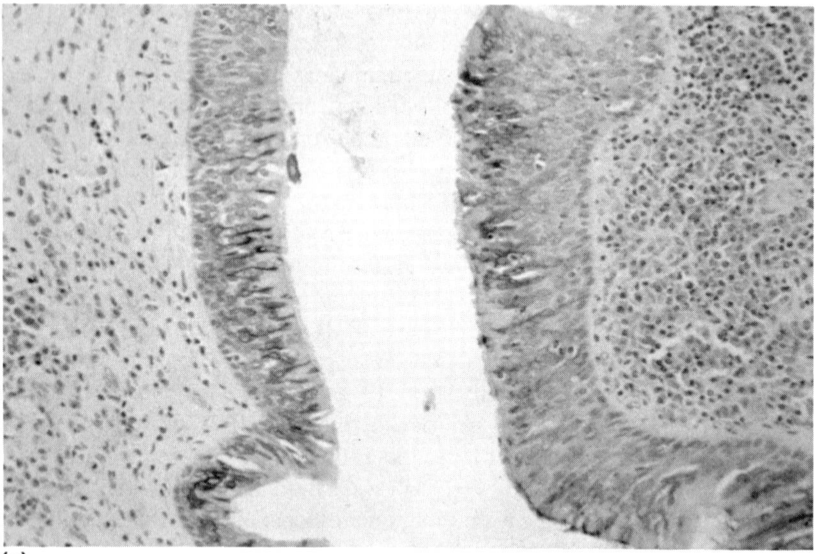

(a)

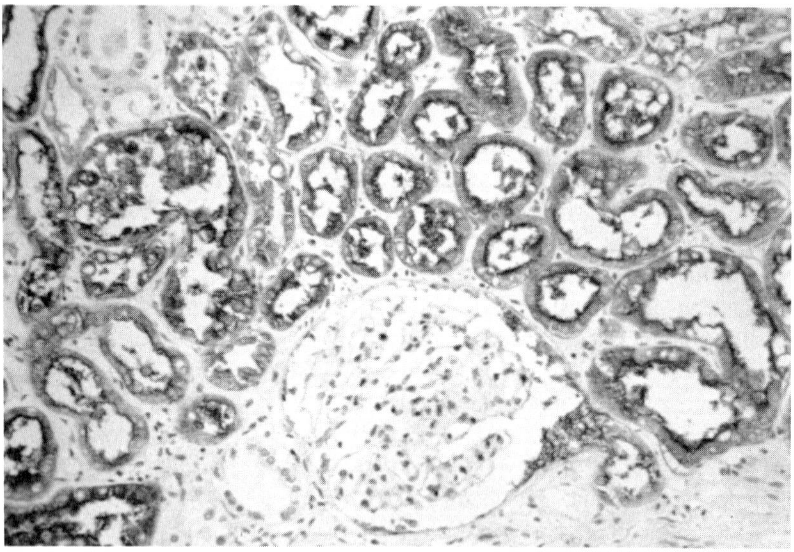

(b)

Figure 2 Normal tissue and tumors show immunohistochemical reactivity with MCA 624A12. (a) Normal adult bronchus. (b) Normal fetal kidney, 22 weeks. (c) Small cell carcinoma of the lung. (d) Wilms tumor.

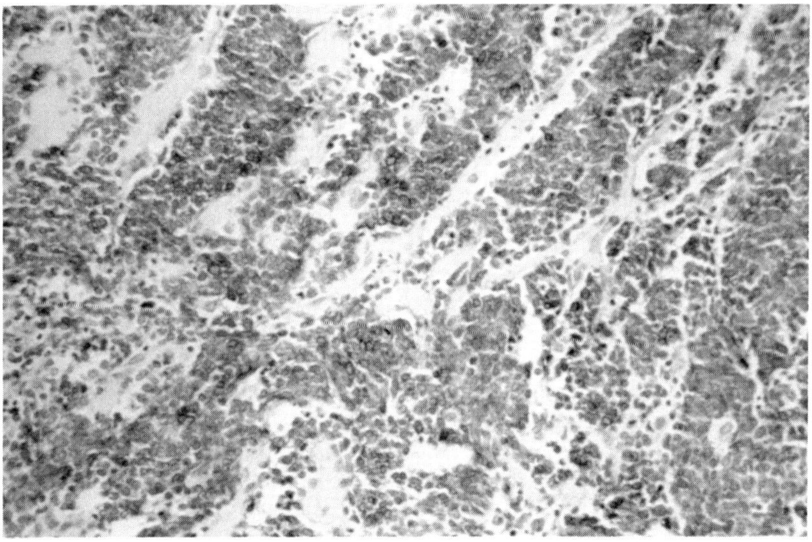

(c)

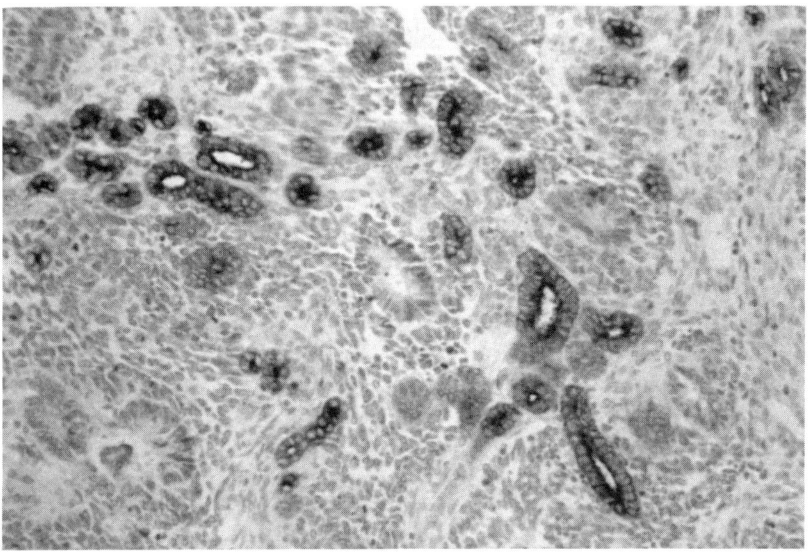

(d)

Table 1 Normal Adult Epithelial Distribution of MCA 624A12

Cells of the anterior pituitary
Bronchial epithelium and mucinous glands
Colonic and jejunal goblet cells
Duodenal goblet cells and Brunner's glands
Exocervical and endocervical cells
Esophageal squamous epithelium
Cells of the gastric crypts
Pancreatic acinar cells
Renal proximal tubular cells
Salivary glands
Skin
Normal adult neuroectodermal distribution of MCA 624A12
Cells of the adrenal medulla
Central nervous system: myelin
Gastric and jejunal argentaffin cells

protein by Western blot analysis (Radosevich et al., 1985). Using live cell radioimmunoassays and fluorescent-activated cell sorter analysis, the antibody has been demonstrated to bind to the cell surface of human adenocarcinoma cell lines (Radosevich et al., 1985). The epitope recognized by MCA 44-3A6 is not affected by treatments that destroy carbohydrate or by the binding of lectins (Radosevich et al., 1988c). Treatments that alter or destroy proteins can affect binding (Radosevich et al., 1985). The behavior of this antigen in purification schemes is consistent with an integral membrane protein (Radosevich et al., 1988c). The antigen is not shed into tissue culture media by positive cell lines and could not be detected in the serum of 80 patients with lung cancer (Radosevich et al., 1985).

The epitope recognized by MCA 44-3A6 is well preserved in routine formalin-fixed, paraffin-embedded tissues (Lee et al., 1985). When the avidin–biotin complex (ABC) method is used to stain tissue sections, the antigen appears to stain the cell surface with weak cytoplasmic staining. This reactive pattern is consistent with a plasma membrane protein antigen. The subcellular localization of this antigen using electron microscopy and immunogold techniques has been completed (Radosevich et al., 1990.)

As a result of the antigen being well preserved in fixed tissues, several studies of human tissues have been reported. In a survey study of over 200 well-characterized human lung carcinomas, MCA 44-3A6 was found to react with all adenocarcinomas, some large cell carcinomas, well-differentiated neuroendocrine carcinomas, and carcinoids, but not with mesotheliomas. Immunoreactivity was not seen with squamous cell carcinomas, bronchioloalveolar carcinomas, or small cell neuroendocrine carcinomas (Lee et al., 1985) (Fig. 3). In an immunocytochemical study of bronchial brushings and their tissue correlates, MCA 44-3A6 was found to react reproducibly in all positive cases (Bannar et al., 1985).

As a result of these findings, a study was undertaken that showed MCA 44-3A6, along with MCA 624A12, to be useful in detecting adenocarcinoma of the lung metastatic to the pleura compared with mesothelioma (Lee et al., 1986). In another study, a panel of large cell carcinomas of the lung were phenotyped immunohistochemically using MCA 44-3A6 and several neuroendocrine markers (Piehl et al., 1988). This study showed that the large cell group could be further subdivided and that MCA 44-3A6 consistently reacted with those neoplasms expressing exocrine features. An additional study was directed at using MCA 44-3A6 to define cytologic subgroups of adenocarcinomas and bronchioloalveolar carcinomas. It was found that adenocarcinomas subclassified as Clara/bronchial surface epithelial cell type and type II alveolar epithelial cell type, that is, adenocarcinoma with no or scanty mucus production, were reactive with MCA 44-3A6 (Radosevich et al., 1990).

The expression of these antigens has also been studied in a wide range of tumors arising outside of the pleural cavity using immunohistochemistry. In one study, more than 200 cases of adenocarcinoma arising in sites other than the lungs were studied (Combs et al., 1988a) (Fig. 4). Immunoreactivity was seen with some but not all of these adenocarcinomas. In another study, a rare case of pleomorphic adenocarcinoma of the pancreas metastatic to the adrenal glands and liver was studied (Combs et al., 1988b). Immunoreactivity was expressed by the tumor, as well as numerous mononuclear and multinucleated tumor giant cells, along with osteoclastlike cells seen in this case. Additional studies are directed at determining the correlation of expression of this antigen with metastases. It is interesting to note that metastatic lesions to the lungs, from tumors arising outside the pleural cavity, express the antigen detected by MCA 44-3A6 at the same frequency as tumors from their respective primary sites (unpublished data). Studies are presently in progress to determine if metastases of pulmonary neoplasms to other organs have altered MCA 44-3A6 antigen expression.

The normal adult and fetal distribution have been investigated using immunohistochemical methods and found to be expressed in a limited number of cell types (unpublished data) (Table 2). This restricted biodistribution, as well as the inability to detect the antigen in the serum of patients with lung cancer, suggest that it may be useful in immunotherapy and immunodiagnosis. Radiolabeled [^{131}I]44-3A6 has been shown to localize in A549 tumors growing as xenografts in male nude mice. The use of MCA 44-3A6 as a cytotoxic agent has been explored. Doxorubicin has been conjugated to MCA 44-3A6 using a five-carbon spacer linker. This conjugated version has proven to be selective and consistently more potent than doxorubicin in vitro (Sinkule et al., 1991).

Future studies are directed at the molecular aspects of this antigen. The purification of this antigen to apparent homogeneity will allow the production of rabbit polysera and amino acid sequencing. (Radosevich et al., 1988c). Recently,

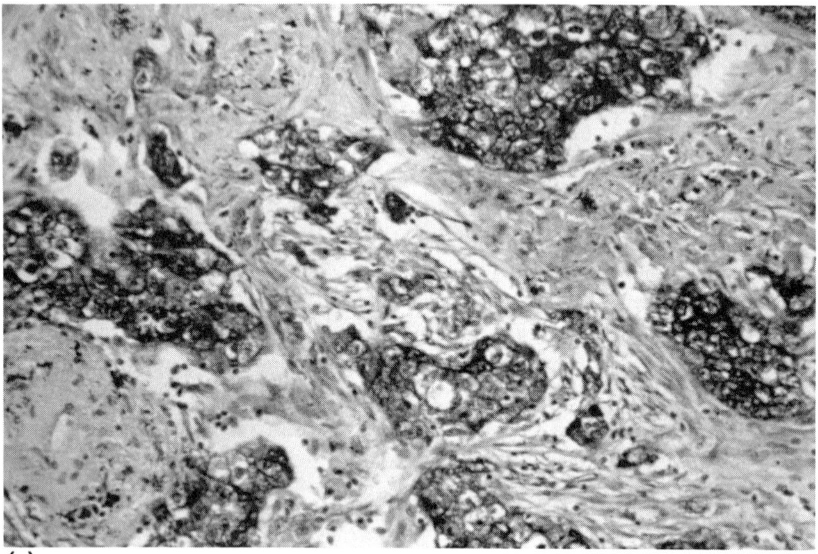

(a)

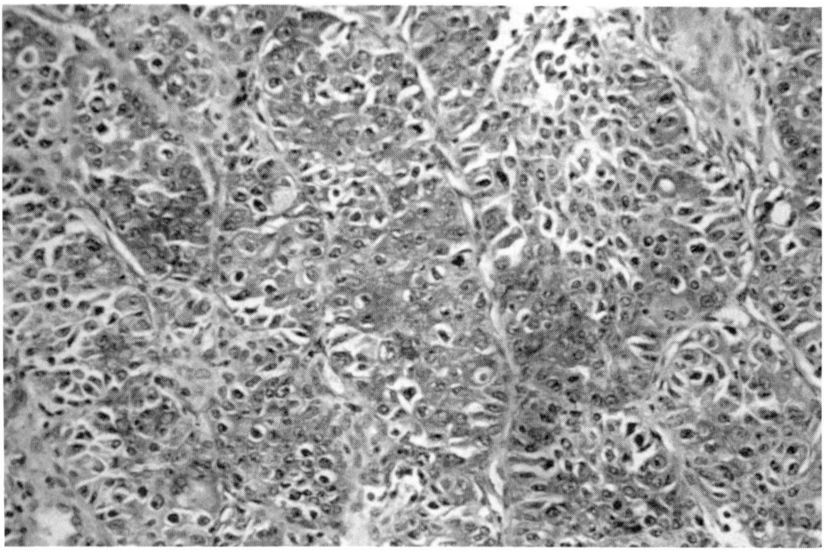

(b)

Figure 3 Immunohistochemical reactivity of primary lung tumors with MCA 44-3A6. (a) Adenocarcinoma. (b) Large cell carcinoma. (c) Adenocarcinoma, sputum cytology. (d) Poorly differentiated squamous cell carcinoma.

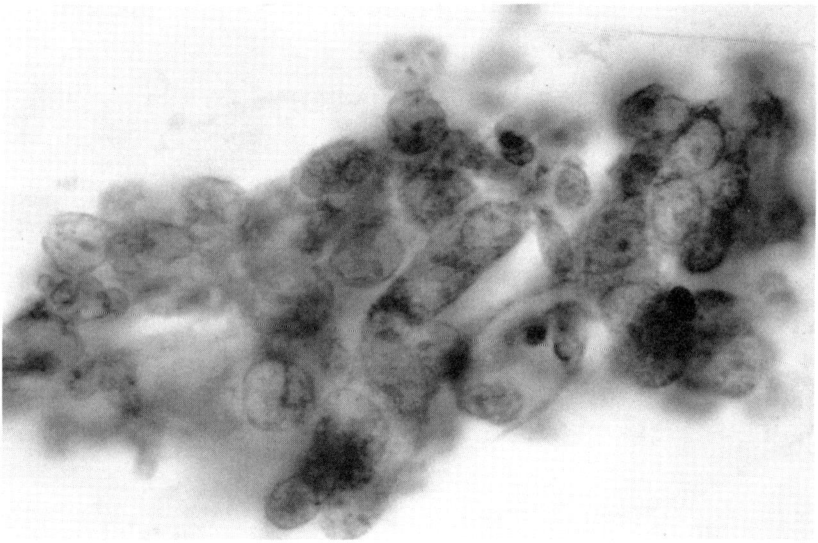

(c)

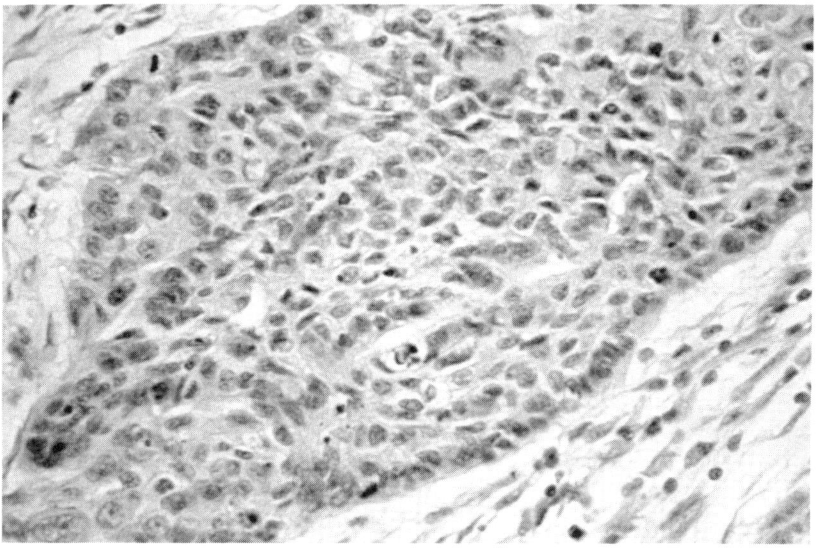

(d)

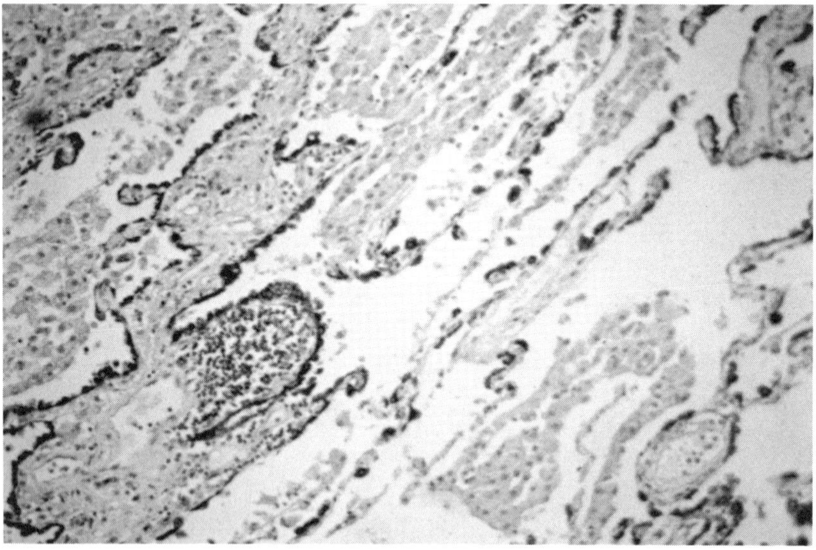

(a)

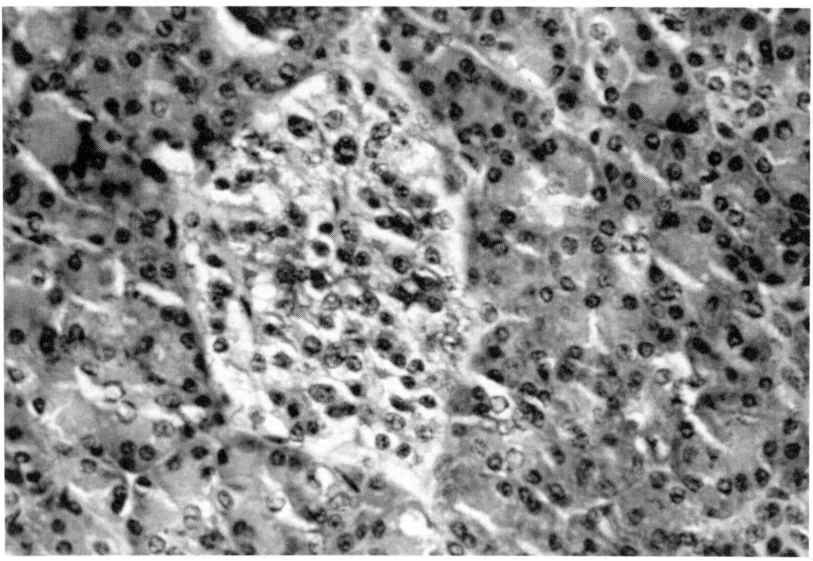

(b)

Figure 4 Immunoreactivity of tumors outside the lung with MCA 44-3A6. (A) Poorly differentiated adenocarcinoma of stomach. (b) Serous cystoadenocarcinoma of ovary. (c) Infiltrating ductal carcinoma of breast. (d) Infiltrating transitional carcinoma of bladder.

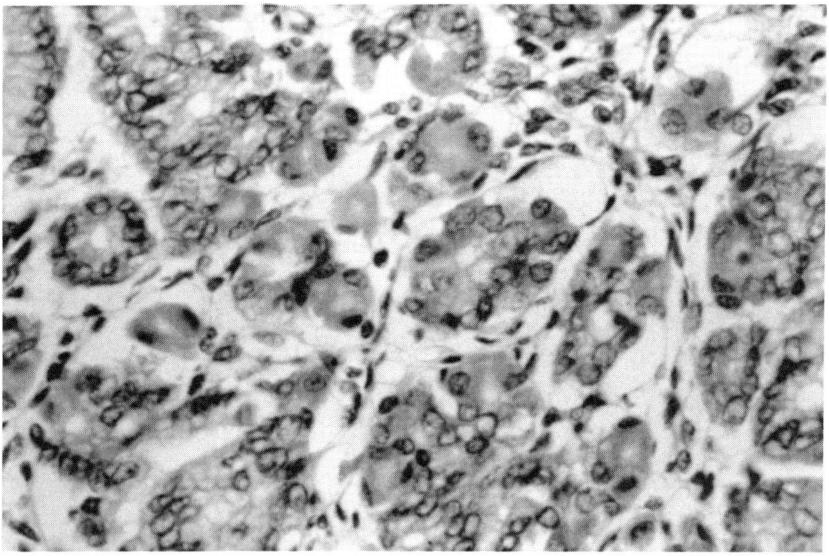

(c)

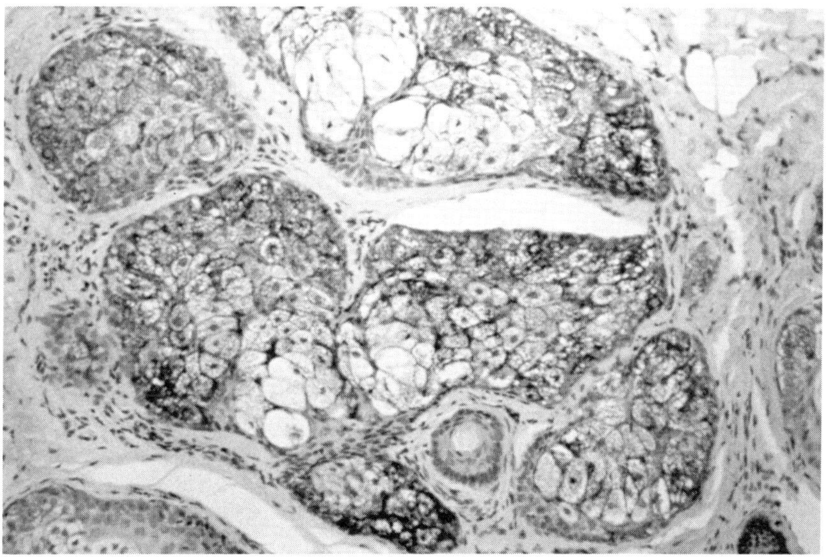

(d)

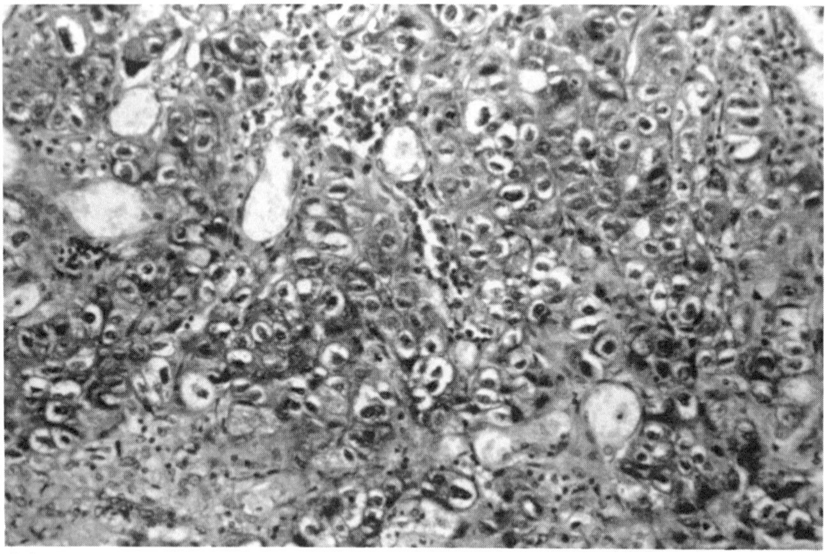

(a)

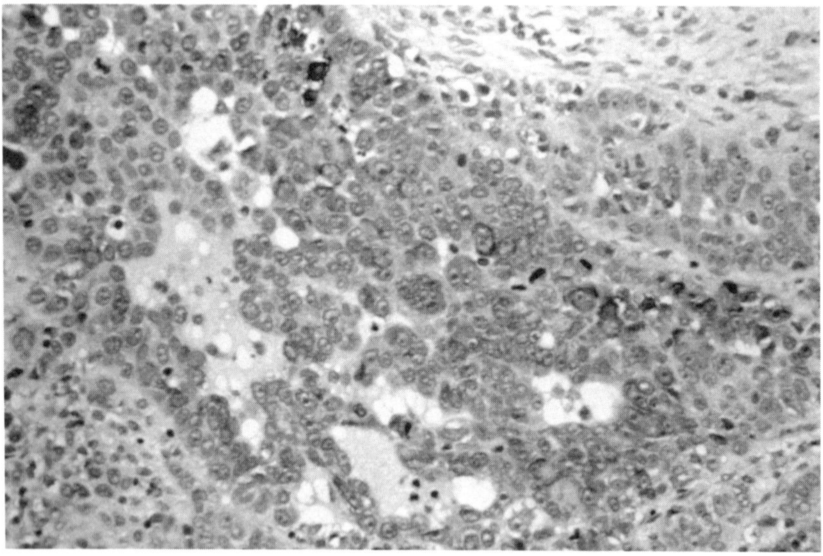

(b)

Figure 5 Normal adult tissue showing immunoreactivity with MCA 44-3A6. (a) Type II pulmonary pneumocytes. (b) Pancreatic islet cells. (c) Parietal cells of stomach. (d) Sebaceous gland.

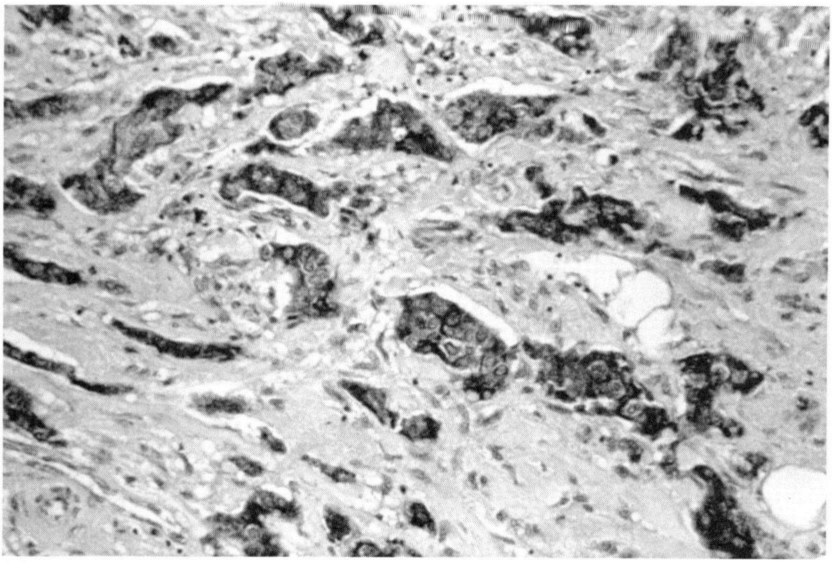

(c)

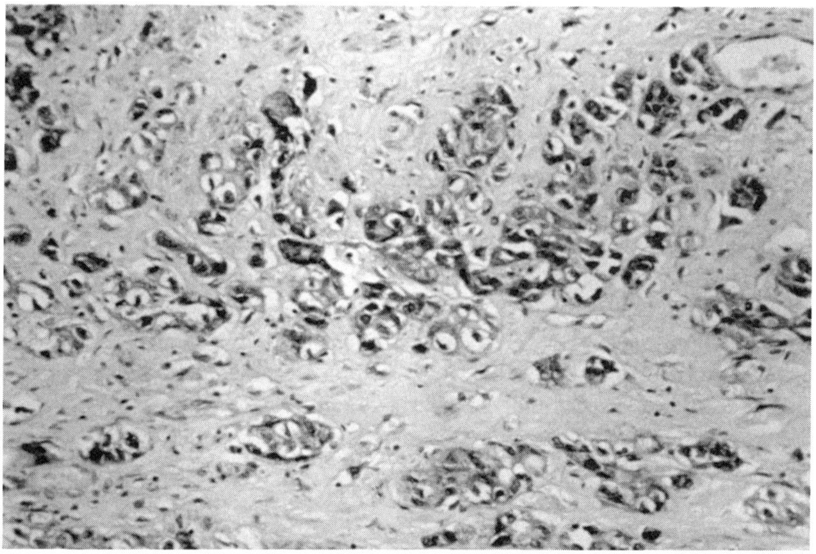

(d)

Table 2 Normal Adult Tissue Distribution of MCA 44-3A6

Pulmonary macrophages and type II pneumocytes
Sebaceous glands of skin
Transitional cells of bladder and renal pelvis
Leydig cells of testes
Colonic enterocytes
Colonic mesenteric ganglion cells
Duodenal Brunner's gland
Pancreatic islet cells
Neuroendocrine cells of the pancreatic ducts and acinar areas
Adrenal cortex
Renal tubular cells
Gastric parietal cells and some chief cells
Rare myoepithelial cells of breast
Rare endothelial cells
Adipocytes

using an A549 cDNA lambda gt11 library, we have been able to screen and isolate a cDNA message encoding the antigen recognized by MCA 44-3A6 (Radosevich, unpublished data).

V. Conclusions

MCAs and immunohistochemistry will continue to be useful tools in the study and diagnosis of human pulmonary carcinomas. As more MCAs become well-characterized reagents, our understanding and ability to apply these reagents to the accurate and consistent classification of these neoplasms will improve. Although the immunophenotyping of these neoplasms is most likely possible, it is important to recall that lung cancer is a very heterogeneous group of neoplasms. Additional techniques and probes will be needed to define tumor characteristics that cannot be measured using MCAs. With the use of multiple levels of analysis, the combined biological potential of an individual neoplasm may be more accurately defined. Understanding the basic biology of these neoplasms and using MCAs with other molecular methods will lead to the design of more meaning clinical trials and potentially effective treatment of this disease.

Acknowledgment

This work was supported by a Veterans Administration Merit Review Grant to J.A.R.

References

Bannar, B. F., Gould, V. E., Radosevich, J. A., Ma, Y., Lee, I., and Rosen, S. T. (1985). Application of monoclonal antibody 44-3A6 in the cytodiagnosis and classification of pulmonary carcinomas. *Diagn. Cytopathol.* **1**:300–307.

Brauch, H., Johnson, B., Hovis, J., Yano, T., Gazdar, A., Pettengill, O. S., Graziano, S., Sorenson, G. D., Poiesz, B. J., Minna, J., Linehan, M., and Zbar, B. (1987). Molecular analysis of the short arm of chromosome 3 in small-cell and non-small-cell carcinoma of the lung. *N. Engl. J. Med.* **317**:1109–1113.

Broers, J. L. V., Carney, D. N., de Ley, L., Vooijs, G. P., and Ramaekers, F. C. S. (1985). Differential expression of intermediate filament proteins distinguishes classic from variant small-cell lung cancer cell lines. *Proc. Natl. Acad. Sci.* USA, **82**:4409–4413.

Bunn, P. A., Jr., Carney, D. N., Gazdar, A. F., Whang-Peng, J., and Matthews, M. J. (1983). Diagnostic and biological implications of flow cytometric DNA content analysis in lung cancer. *Cancer. Res.* **43**:5026–5032.

Carter, D., and Eggleton, J. (1979). Tumors of the lower respiratory tract. In *Atlas of Tumor Pathology*, Fascicle 17. Washington, DC, Armed Forces Institute of Pathology.

Combs, S. G., Radosevich, J. A., Ma, Y., Lee, I., Gould, V. E., Battifora, H., and Rosen, S. T. (1988a). Expression of the antigenic determinant recognized by the monoclonal antibody 44-3A6 on select human adenocarcinomas and normal human tissues. *Tumor Biol.* **9**:116–122.

Combs, S. G., Hidvegi, D. F., Ma, Y., Rosen, S. T., and Radosevich, J. A. (1988b). Pleomorphic carcinoma of the pancreas with osteoclast-like giant cells expressing an epithelial associated antigen detected by monoclonal 44-3A6. *Diagn. Cytopathol.* **4**:316–322.

Gould, V. E., Linnoila, R. L., Memoli, V. A., and Warren, W. H. (1983). Neuroendocrine components of the bronchopulmonary tract: hyperplasias, dysplasias, and neoplasms. *Lab. Invest.* **49**:519–537.

Hsu, S. M., Raine, L., and Fanger, H. (1981). The use of avidin-biotin–peroxidase complex (ABC) in immunoperoxidase techniques: a comparison between ABC and unlabeled antibody (PAP) procedures. *J. Histochem. Cytochem.* **29**:577–581.

Kohler, G., and Milstein, C. (1975). Continuous cultures of fused cells secreting antibody of predefined specificity. *Nature (Lond.)* **256**:495–497.

Lee, I., Radosevich, J. A., Ma, Y., Combs, S. G., Rosen, S. T., and Gould, V. E. (1985). Immunohistochemical analysis of human pulmonary carcinomas using monoclonal antibody 44-3A6. *Cancer Res.* **45**:5813–5817.

Lee, I., Warren, W. H., Gould, V. E., Radosevich, J. A., Ma, Y., and Rosen, S. T. (1987). Immunohistochemical demonstration of lacto-N-fucopentose III in lung carcinomas with monoclonal antibody 624A12. *Pathol. Res. Pract.* **182**:40–47.

Lee, I., Radosevich, J. A., Chejfec, G., Ma, Y., Warren, W. H., Rosen, S. T., and Gould, V. E. (1986). Malignant mesotheliomas—improved differential diagnosis from lung adenocarcinoma using monoclonal antibodies 44-3A6 and 624A123. *Am. J. Pathol.* **123**:497–507.

Piehl, M. R., Gould, V. E., Radosevich, J. A., Ma, Y., Warren, W. H., and Rosen, S. T.

(1988). Immunohistochemical identification of exocrine and neuroendocrine subsets of large cell lung carcinomas. *Pathol. Res. Pract.* **183:**675–682.

Radosevich, J. A., Ma, Y., Lee, I., Salwen, H., Gould, V. E., and Rosen, S. T. (1985). Monoclonal antibody 44-3A6 as a probe for a novel antigen found on human lung carcinomas with glandular differentiation. *Cancer Res.* **35:**5808–5812.

Radosevich, J. A., Robinson, P. G., Rittmann-Grauer, L. A., Wilson, B., Leung, J. P., Ma, Y., Maminta, L., Warren, W., Gould, V. E., and Rosen, S. T. (1988a). Immunohistochemical analysis of pulmonary carcinomas with the monoclonal antibody (MCA) HYB612 directed against a multiple drug resistance related antigen. Abstract, Fifth World Conference on Lung Cancer.

Radosevich, J. A., Lee, I., Gould, V. E., and Rosen, S. T. (1988b). Monoclonal antibody assays for lung cancer. In: *Cancer Diagnosis In Vitro Using Monoclonal Antibodies*. Edited by H. Z. Kupchik. New York, Marcel Dekker.

Radosevich, J. A., Ma, Y., Waibel, R., Maminta, L., Stahel, R. A., and Rosen, S. T. (1988c). Partial purification and characterization of the antigen recognized by the monoclonal antibody (MCA) 44-3A6 from the human adenocarcinoma (AC) cell line A549. Abstract, Fifth World Conference on Lung Cancer.

Radosevich, J. A., Noguchi, M., Rosen, S. T., and Shimosato, Y. (1990). Immunocytochemical analysis of human adenocarcinomas and bronchioloalveolar carcinomas of the lung using the monoclonal antibody 44-3A6. *Tumor Biol.* **11:**181–188.

Radosevich, J. A., Siddiqui, F. S., Rosen, S. T., and W. J. Kabat. (1991). Cell cycle and electron microscopic evaluation of the adenocarcinoma antigen recognized by the monoclonal antibody 44-3A6. *Br. J. Cancer* **63:**86–87.

Rodenhuis, S., van de Wetering, M. L., Mooi, W. J., Evers, S. G., van Zandwijk, N., and Bos, J. L. (1987). Mutational activation of the K-RAS oncogene. *N. Engl. J. Med.* **317:**929–935.

Rosen, S. T., Mulshine, J. L., Cuttitta, F., Fedorko, J., Carney, D. N., Gazdar, A. F., and Minna, J. D. (1984a). Analysis of human small cell lung cancer differentiation antigens using a panel of rat monoclonal antibodies. *Cancer Res.* **44:**2052–2061.

Rosen, S. T., Combs, S., Marder, R., Polovina, M., Minna, J., Mulshine, J., and Radosevich, J. A. (1984b). Immunohistochemical localization of the immunodominant differentiation antigen lacto-N-fucopentose III in normal adult and fetal tissues utilizing monoclonal antibodies. In: *Colloquium: Protides of the Biological Fluids*. Edited by H. Peeters. New York, Pergamon Press, pp. 561–566.

Silverberg, E. (1982). Cancer statistics, 1982. *CA*, 15–31.

Sinkule, J., Rosen, S. T., and Radosevich, J. A. (1991). MCA 44-3A6 douxorubicin (adriamycin) immunoconjugates: comparative in vitro anti-tumor efficacy of different conjugation methods. *Tumor Biol.* **12:**189–248.

Sternberger, L. A., Hardy, P. H., Jr., Cuculis, J. J., and Meyer, H. G. (1970). The unlabeled antibody–enzyme method of immunohistochemistry. Preparation and properties of soluble antigen–antibody complex (horseradish peroxidase–antihorseradish peroxidase) and its use in identification of spirochetes. *J. Histochem. Cytochem.* **18:**315–333.

WHO (1982). Histological typing of lung tumors. *Am. J. Clin. Pathol.* **77:**123–136.

Yesner, R., Gerstl, B., and Auerbach, D. (1965). Application of the World Health Organization classification of lung carcinoma to biopsy material. *Ann. Thorac. Surg.* **1:**33–49.

12

Biomarkers of Small Cell Lung Cancer

DAVID H. JOHNSON and F. ANTHONY GRECO

Vanderbilt University
Nashville, Tennessee

I. Introduction

Considerable progress has been achieved in the management of small cell lung cancer (SCLC) during the past two decades (Morstyn et al., 1984; Johnson and Greco, 1986, 1987). Although it is still somewhat of a rarity, cure can sometimes be realized in patients with tumor confined to the chest (Johnson and Greco, 1986, 1987). Most patients will experience palliation of symptoms during treatment, and prolongation of survival is expected using available chemotherapy programs (Johnson and Greco, 1986). Yet in spite of recent progress, a majority of patients with SCLC eventually die of their disease and few patients survive beyond 5 years (Morstyn et al., 1984; Johnson and Greco, 1986, 1987). There are many reasons for the failure to cure SCLC, the most important of which may be the development of drug resistance by tumor cells (Johnson and Greco, 1986, 1987). Investigators are currently exploring methods of circumventing drug resistance, but these methods will require time for proper development. It is likely that currently available treatments would be more successful if the tumor could be detected earlier in its natural history. That this is true seems evident from the simple fact that patients with limited-stage SCLC enjoy superior survival than those with extensive-stage disease (Johnson and Greco, 1986). Consequently, techniques that would allow clinicians to detect small amounts of tumor are highly desirable. Toward that end, many investigators have searched diligently for a marker or markers that might prove beneficial in the management of SCLC. SCLC is known to be associated with a variety of ectopically produced peptides, many of which have been evaluated as possible tumor markers (Richardson et al., 1978). In addition, during the past 10 years, the extraordinary work of Minna and colleagues has yielded considerable data on the biology of lung cancer in general and SCLC in particular (Minna, 1988; Minna et al., 1984). These investigators have identified several cytoplasmic enzymes that are highly characteristic of SCLC and could potentially serve as useful tumor markers (Minna et al., 1984). In this chapter, we will review recent studies that have evaluated the application of many of these substances as possible markers of SCLC.

II. General Comments

In clinical practice, there is no "ideal" tumor marker. An ideal marker should (McIntire, 1985):

Be produced only by tumor the cells
Reflect the extent of disease present by its concentration in blood and/or urine
Be able to detect microscopic or subclinical disease
Be easy and inexpensive to assay as well as accurate
Be present with sufficient frequency to make its measurement worthwhile

A tumor marker can be used in many ways in the management of disease. For example, a biomarker could be useful for the following purposes:

Initial detection and diagnosis of malignancy
Detection of tumor recurrence
Evaluation of response to therapy
Monitoring disease status during therapy

Currently available biomarkers possess only some of the above properties and yet many are still quite useful in clinical practice [e.g., beta-human chorionic gonadotropin (BHCG) and alpha-fetoprotein (αFP) in testicular cancer and CA-125 in ovarian cancer]. Although it is unlikely that any one particular SCLC-related peptide or enzyme will possess all the above properties, recent data indicate there are some substances of potential value in the management of SCLC.

III. Polypeptides (Adrenocorticotropin, Antidiuretic Hormone, Calcitonin)

The association of pulmonary malignancies with certain hormonal syndromes has been recognized for more than 50 years, but it was not until the early 1960s that the

Table 1 Relationship of Lung Cancer Cell Type to Ectopic Hormone Production

	No. Elevated/total		
Hormone	SCLC (%)	SqCCa (%)	AdenoCa (%)
ACTH	39/190 (36)	0/36 (0)	5/20 (25)
ADH	61/264 (23)	0/18 (0)	4/14 (25)
Calcitonin	115/226 (51)	27/137 (20)	20/60 (33)

SCLC, small cell lung cancer; SqCCa, squamous cell lung cancer; AdenoCa, adenocarcinoma of the lung.
Source: Modified from Bondy (1981).

nature of the association was clearly established (Meador et al., 1962; Bondy, 1981). Subsequently, all lung neoplasms but especially SCLC have been found to be associated with a variety of "ectopically" produced hormones (Table 1). The peptides most extensively evaluated as possible biomarkers for SCLC include adrenocorticotropin (ACTH), vasopressin or antidiuretic hormone (ADH), and calcitonin (Bondy, 1981; Hansen, 1981; Greco et al., 1981). Each of these peptides has been evaluated for its frequency of elevation at diagnosis, its diagnostic value, its relationship to tumor burden, its ability to predict and mirror clinical response and relapse, and for its prognostic value (Tables 1–3). The results of these studies have been extensively reviewed in several recent publications (Hansen, 1981; Greco et al., 1981). Although there was much initial enthusiasm regarding the potential value of these peptides, it would appear that they are inadequate as biomarkers of SCLC (Johnson and Greco, 1986; Hansen et al., 1980) (Tables 2 and 3). All three lack specificity (Table 1) and fail to correlate well with the extent of

Table 2 Pretreatment Peptide Levels; Prediction of Response

Marker		No. Responding/total	Ratio	p Value
ACTH	Normal	30/43	0.70	>0.2
	Elevated	12/18	0.67	
CT	Normal	12/20	0.60	>0.2
	Elevated	30/41	0.73	
SIADH	Absent	30/41	0.73	>0.2
	Present	12/20	0.60	
All 3 normal		6/10	0.60	>0.2
>2 abnormal		16/23	0.73	

Source: Modified from Hansen et al. (1980a).

Table 3 Relationship of Pretreatment Peptide Levels to Survival

Marker		Median survival (days)	p Value	No. alive after >1 yr (%)
ACTH	Normal	325	>0.05	17/44 (39)
	Elevated	298		8/18 (44)
CT	Normal	357	>0.05	9/21 (43)
	Elevated	262		15/40 (38)
SIADH	Absent	360	>0.05	18/41 (44)
	Present	260		6/21 (29)
All normal		363	>0.05	6/11 (55)
>2 abnormal		262		9/24 (38)

Source: Modified from Hansen et al. (1980a).

disease. Changes in serum levels likewise do not adequately reflect changes in disease status and have not proved useful clinically (Hansen, 1981; Greco et al., 1981) (Tables 2 and 3). Even in the case of calcitonin, which appears capable of at least reflecting fairly accurately the development of *recurrent* disease, the increments are modest and usually occur only when progressive disease is clinically evident (Hansen, 1981; Greco et al., 1981; Hansen et al., 1980). Also, false-positive increments in calcitonin may occur when tumor is clinically decreasing in size (Hansen, 1981). Therefore, the routine measurement of these peptides does not appear to be beneficial in the management of SCLC.

One point worth noting, however, is that ectopic ACTH syndrome and "inappropriate" ADH secretion are *primarily* found in patients with SCLC. These clinical syndromes are much less common among the other major histologic types of bronchogenic neoplasms. Thus, the presence of either of these clinical syndromes in a patient with a lung tumor would argue strongly for the diagnosis of SCLC. In this setting, these ectopically produced peptides have limited diagnostic usefulness. However, fewer than 10% of patients with SCLC present with these syndromes.

IV. Carcinoembryonic Antigen

Carcinoembryonic antigen (CEA) has been evaluated as a possible biomarker in a variety of malignancies (Sugarbaker et al., 1976; Lokich et al., 1978; Vincent et al., 1975; Dent et al., 1978). Several investigators have recently explored using CEA determinations in the management of SCLC (McKenzie et al., 1977; Waalkes et al., 1980; Goslin et al., 1981; Woo et al., 1981; Lokich, 1982; Sculier et al., 1985; Laberge et al., 1987; Jaques et al., 1988). Because virtually all patients with SCLC have a history of cigarette smoking, most investigators have required that a CEA level exceed 5–10 ng/ml to be considered "abnormal" (Waalkes et al., 1980; Goslin et al., 1981; Woo et al., 1981; Lokich, 1982; Sculier et al., 1985; Laberge et al., 1987; Jaques et al., 1988). Nevertheless, 35–50% of patients with SCLC have been found to have an elevated pretreatment CEA level (Table 4). Pretreatment CEA levels have correlated reasonably well with the extent of disease (i.e., levels are lowest in patients with limited disease and highest in patients with extensive disease) (Waalkes et al., 1980; Goslin et al., 1981; Lokich, 1982; Sculier et al., 1985; Laberge et al., 1987; Jaques et al., 1988). Not surprisingly, the highest CEA levels (often >50 ng/ml) have been reported in patients with liver metastases (Goslin et al., 1981; Sculier et al., 1985; Jaques et al., 1988). Although it was initially thought that a CEA level ⩾50 ng/ml was virtually diagnostic of liver involvement, several studies have found this not to be the case (Sculier et al., 1985; Laberge et al., 1987; Jaques et al., 1988). Thus, although CEA levels tend to reflect tumor burden, no clear pattern emerges with respect to a particular metastatic site.

Table 4 CEA Elevation at Diagnosis in Small Cell Lung Cancer

Reference	Patient number		Number of patients with abnormal pretherapy CEA	
Waalkes et al. (1980)	Total	42	20	(48%)
	LD	14	3	(21%)
	ED	28	17	(61%)
Aoslin et al. (1981)	Total	85	37	(44%)
	LD	44	6	(13%)
	ED	41	31	(76%)
Lokich (1982)	Total	61	32	(52%)
	LD	29	13	(45%)
	ED	32	19	(59%)
Sailier et al. (1985)	Total	180	61	(34%)
	LD	97	22	(23%)
	ED	83	39	(47%)
Laberge et al. (1987)	Total	147	58	(39%)
	LD	52	9	(17%)
	ED	95	49	(52%)
Jaques et al. (1988)	Total	191	84	(44%)
	LD	62	27	(44%)
	ED	129	57	(44%)
	Totals	706	292	(41%)
	LD	298	80	(27%)
	ED	408	212	(52%)

LD, limited-stage disease; ED, extensive disease.

In general, it has been found that patients with SCLC with raised pretreatment CEA levels are no less likely to obtain an objective response to chemotherapy than patients presenting with normal pretreatment values (Waalkes et al., 1980; Goslin et al., 1981; Woo et al., 1981; Lokich, 1982; Sculier et al., 1985; Laberge et al., 1987; Jaques et al., 1988) (Table 5). However, some investigators have found that *complete* responses are statistically more common among patients with *normal* to *minimally elevated pretreatment* CEA levels (Waalkes et al., 1980; Sculier et al., 1985) (Table 5). For example, Waalkes et al. (1980) noted that among patients with *extensive-stage* disease, *no* complete responses were obtained in those with a pretreatment CEA level >15 ng/ml, whereas 40% with levels <15 ng/ml achieved a complete remission (Waalkes et al., 1980). Likewise, Sculier et al. (1985) reported a substantial difference in the complete response rates based on pretreatment CEA levels. Patients whose pretreatment level exceeded 6 ng/ml achieved complete remission in fewer than 15% of cases, whereas patients with normal values were reported to have experienced a complete response rate of more than 45% ($p = 0.00003$) (Sculier et al., 1985).

Waalkes et al. (1980) reported that pretreatment CEA levels failed to predict survival outcome and that initial stage was more important in this regard. Median survival for patients with raised CEA levels was 12 months compared with 14 months for those with levels <5 ng/ml ($p > 0.3$) (Table 6). Although the higher complete response rate seen in patients with extensive-stage disease with a pretreatment CEA <15 ng/ml translated into an improved median survival compared to patients with CEA >15 ng/ml, this difference was also not statistically significant (12 months vs. 6 months; $p = 0.09$). Similar results have been reported recently by Jaques et al. (1988) when they compared patients with modestly elevated pretherapy CEA levels to those with normal levels. In the latter

Table 5 Association of Pretreatment CEA Level and Response to Treatment

Reference	Response category	Normal (%)		Elevated (%)		p value
Waalkes et al. (1980)	Overall	17/21	(81)	16/20	(80)	>0.5
	Complete	10/21	(48)	6/20	(30)	0.25
Sculier et al. (1985)	Overall	97/112	(87)	42/57	(74)	0.054
	Complete	52/112	(46)	8/57	(14)	<0.00003
Laberge et al. (1987)	Overall	70/89	(79)	35/58	(60)	0.02
	Complete	33/89	(37)	16/58	(28)	0.23
Jaques et al. (1988)	Overall	—		—		—
	Complete	39/109	(36)	22/84	(26)	0.15
Totals	Overall	184/222	(83)	93/135	(67)	
	Complete	134/331	(40)	52/219	(24)	

Table 6 Association of Pretreatment CEA Level with Survival

	Median survival (months)		
Reference	Normal CEA	Elevated CEA	p value
Waalkes et al. (1980)	14.0	12.0	>0.3
Sculier et al. (1985)	12.2	8.8	0.0007
Jaques et al. (1988)	11.6	10.1[a]	
		9.4[b]	<0.05

[a]5–20 ng/ml.
[b]≥20 ng/ml.

study, a survival difference was noted if a higher cutoff level (i.e., >20 ng/ml) was used (Jaques et al., 1988). In contrast, Sculier et al. (1985) reported that patients with a normal pretreatment CEA level enjoyed a statistically superior median survival compared to those with raised levels (12.2 months vs. 8.8 months; $p = 0.0007$) (Sculier et al., 1985) (Table 6). Of interest, this finding proved to be *independent* of pretreatment Eastern Cooperative Oncology Group (ECOG) performance status and stage, which are features generally considered to be most predictive of prognosis in SCLC. Also of note, *no* patient with an elevated pretreatment CEA level experienced a prolonged survival, whereas 11 patients with normal pretherapy values survived more than 2.5 years (Sculier et al., 1985). Jaques et al. (1988) found similar results in comparing patients with pretreatment CEA levels >20 ng/ml with patients with lower CEA levels.

Good to excellent correlation between changes in CEA levels and the clinical course of SCLC has been described by most investigators. Goslin et al. (1981) reported that among patients with raised pretreatment CEA levels, a response was always accompanied by a fall in the CEA level. Likewise, responding patients with abnormal pretreatment CEA levels almost always experienced a rise in the CEA value at relapse (Waalkes et al., 1980; Goslin et al., 1981). Waalkes et al. (1981) found that in nearly 60% of cases, the rise in CEA *preceded* clinical recognition of recurrence by an average of 3 months. Patients with normal pretreatment CEA levels were less likely to experience an increase in plasma CEA with recurrence (Goslin et al., 1981; Laberge et al., 1987). Goslin et al. (1981) noted that of 11 patients whose disease relapsed with *no* change in plasma CEA, 7 (64%) experienced *local* recurrence without developing evidence of extrathoracic metastases before death. In contrast to responding patients, nonresponding patients experienced a progressive rise in plasma CEA levels in most cases (Waalkes et al., 1980; Goslin et al., 1981; Lokich, 1982).

To summarize, plasma CEA levels are elevated (i.e., >5–10 ng/ml) in approximately 40% of untreated patients with SCLC. However, CEA lacks both sensitivity and specificity for SCLC. High pretherapy CEA levels are more common in patients with extensive-stage disease, although levels only roughly correlate with tumor extent. Markedly elevated levels (i.e., >50 ng/ml) are associated with a very poor prognosis perhaps because of the frequent association with hepatic and marrow metastases (Laberge et al., 1987; Jaques et al., 1988). At least some studies suggest that pretreatment CEA levels may be helpful in estimating the probability of achieving a complete remission (Waalkes et al., 1980; Sculier et al., 1985) and prognosis (Sculier et al., 1985; Laberge et al., 1987; Jaques et al., 1988). If the latter data are confirmed, pretreatment CEA levels could be a useful tool for stratifying patients entering randomized treatment trials. Serial CEA determinations tend to mirror the clinical status of patients who present with elevated pretherapy levels (i.e., falling with remission and increasing with recurrence) although this correlation is far from perfect (Goslin et al., 1981; Laberge et al., 1987). Frequently, a rise in plasma CEA will predate clinical recognition of recurrence by several weeks to months, although this finding has not yet been demonstrated to be clinically useful. Patients with apparently local recurrence and normal CEA levels may be candidates for salvage therapy aimed specifically at intrathoracic disease (i.e., radiotherapy and/or surgery) since preliminary data indicate that these patients die primarily without extrathoracic spread (Goslin et al., 1981). In spite of many shortcomings, further study of CEA in the management of SCLC appears warranted.

V. Neuron-Specific Enolase

Enolase is a glycolytic enzyme present in all human cells that catalyzes the conversion of 2-phosphoglycerate to phosphoenol-pyruvate (Marangos et al., 1982a). There are three dimeric isoenzymes consisting of alpha, beta, or gamma subunits. At one time the gamma–gamma isoenzyme was thought to be found exclusively in neurons (hence the name neuron-specific enolase [NSE]) (Marangos et al., 1982a; Schmechel et al., 1978). However, NSE is now known to reside in a variety of endocrine tissues and has been found in many neuroendocrine neoplasms (Tapia et al., 1981; Prinz and Marangos, 1982). Because the cells of endocrine tissues share many common biochemical and cytologic features with neurons and may also share a common embryologic derivation from the neuroectoderm, investigators have explored the potential utility of NSE as a biomarker of SCLC.

Marangos and co-workers (1982b; Parma et al., 1981) were the first investigators to demonstrate abnormal levels of NSE in the supernatants of SCLC cell cultures using a rabbit antisera raised against human NSE. These investigators subsequently reported that approximately 70% of previously untreated patients with SCLC had an elevated serum NSE level compared to healthy adult controls

(Carney et al., 1982). NSE levels were elevated more often in patients with extensive-stage disease and especially in patients with multiple sites of tumor involvement. Among patients with extensive-stage disease, NSE levels tended to correlate well with tumor burden. Virtually all responding patients with an elevated pretreatment NSE level demonstrated a fall in serum NSE level at the time of restaging and all complete responders normalize their serum NSE value. A majority of patients whose disease relapsed demonstrated a rise in NSE with relapse. All four patients in sustained remission at the time of the report had a normal NSE level. It was unfortunate that pretreatment NSE levels did *not* prove predictive of response nor did survival differ in patients with normal or raised NSE levels (Carney et al., 1982).

The aforementioned report was followed by several others that have confirmed and expanded on these initial observations (Jaques et al., 1988; Ariyoshi et al., 1983; Johnson et al., 1984a; Akoun et al., 1985; Esscher et al., 1985; Pahlman et al., 1984; Splinter et al., 1987; Cooper et al., 1985). These studies have demonstrated that 65–85% of patients with SCLC will have raised pretreatment NSE levels and that patients with extensive-stage disease are more likely to present with abnormal pretreatment values (Ariyoshi et al., 1983; Johnson et al., 1984a; Akoun et al., 1985; Esscher et al., 1985; Pahlman et al., 1984; Splinter et al., 1987) (Table 7). Several studies indicate that pretreatment NSE levels correlate well with tumor burden in patients with extensive-stage disease as judged by correlation with number of involved metastatic sites (Ariyoshi et al., 1983; Johnson et al., 1984; Akoun et al., 1985; Esscher et al., 1985).

Serial NSE levels have proved useful in monitoring the clinical course of patients with SCLC since levels tend to decrease with response and rise with relapse (Carney et al., 1982; Ariyoshi et al., 1983; Johnson et al., 1984a; Akoun et al., 1985; Esscher et al., 1985; Splinter et al., 1987). In one study, serial NSE determinations were obtained in 57 patients (Johnson et al., 1984). Forty of the 50

Table 7 Pretreatment NSE Levels in SCLC

Reference	Upper limit of normal (ng/ml)	Limited stage	Extensive stage	Overall %
Carney et al. (1982)	12	15/38 (39%)	49/56 (87%)	68
Ariyoshi et al. (1983)	7.5	—	—	65
Johnson et al. (1984a)	20	23/39 (59%)	45/54 (83%)	73
Akoun et al. (1985)	16	6/16 (38%)	22/27 (81%)	65
Esscher et al. (1985)	12	34/48 (71%)	54/55 (98%)	85
	25	24/48 (50%)	50/55 (91%)	72
Cooper et al. (1985)	13.5	25/38 (66%)	34/39 (87%)	77
Jaques et al. (1988)	12.5	32/53 (60%)	79/113 (70%)	67

(80%) responding patients demonstrated a fall in serum NSE levels toward normal (Fig. 1). Five of 7 (71%) patients with progressive disease had a further increase in NSE levels while 30 of 35 (86%) relapsing patients were found to have increasing NSE levels. In some cases, an increase in NSE occurred several months before the clinical recognition of relapse (Fig. 1) (Johnson et al., 1984a). NSE levels may vary somewhat during remission but several investigators have found that a sustained elevation of NSE levels in an otherwise "disease-free" patient is a harbinger of relapse (Johnson et al., 1984; Splinter et al., 1987; Cooper et al., 1985). In some instances, relapse has occurred in the face of a persistently normal NSE level (including cases that have shown normalization of previously abnormal pretreatment values) suggesting possible heterogeneity of tumor cell NSE content. Indeed, immunoperoxidase studies have confirmed a heterogeneous distribution of staining (Said et al., 1985). However, in some cases in which a raised pretreatment NSE level normalized at response but failed to rise with recurrence, the patient was found to have a non-small-cell lung cancer (NSCLC) rather than SCLC (Splinter et al., 1987). Thus, in a situation in which the pretreatment NSE level was elevated and a patient has clinical evidence of disease recurrence but a *normal* level of NSE, a repeat biopsy should be obtained to confirm the histologic nature of the recurrence (Splinter et al., 1987; Cooper et al., 1985).

In general, most studies have failed to demonstrate convincingly that an elevated pretreatment NSE level per se has prognostic value independent of other

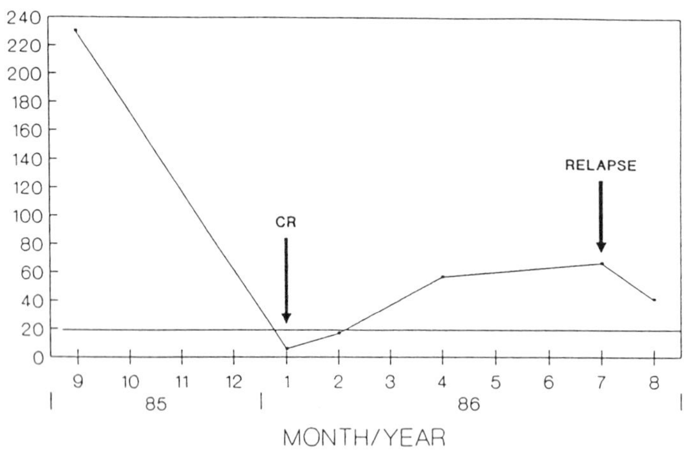

Figure 1 Serial NSE levels in a patient presenting with extensive stage SCLC (liver metastases). Level falls to normal (i.e., <20 ng/ml) at restaging. Chemotherapy is discontinued and NSE level begins to rise. Six months after cessation of treatment the patient experiences a relapse. Note that NSE level rises constantly *prior* to clinical recognition of relapse. NSE level begins to fall with institution of salvage chemotherapy.

known prognostic features (such as stage and performance status). However, this has not been a universal finding; some investigators have shown that a markedly elevated pretreatment level (i.e., >100 ng/ml) is associated with a poor prognosis (Jaques et al., 1988). In the latter study, however, markedly elevated levels were uniformly associated with liver or bone marrow metastases, both of which have poor prognostic implications themselves. Nevertheless, other investigators have shown that patients with pretreatment NSE levels >30 ng/ml have significantly shorter survival times than patients demonstrating normal or less elevated NSE values (Jaques et al., 1988; Akoun et al., 1985). Further studies are needed to clarify this issue.

NSE levels at restaging may have prognostic importance (Johnson et al., 1984; Splinter et al., 1987). For example, Johnson et al. (1984) found that in patients with extensive-stage disease, a normal NSE level at restaging was associated with an improved survival irrespective of the level of response (i.e., partial vs. complete). The duration of response was longer in patients with normal restaging NSE levels than in those achieving a comparable clinical response but with persistently abnormal NSE levels (Johnson et al., 1984).

Akoun et al. (1985) measured serial NSE levels during a 3 day course of induction chemotherapy and found sharp elevations above pretreatment levels in several patients. We have made similar observations (Fig. 2). Because enolase is a cytoplasmic enzyme, this finding was thought to be consistent with tumor cell

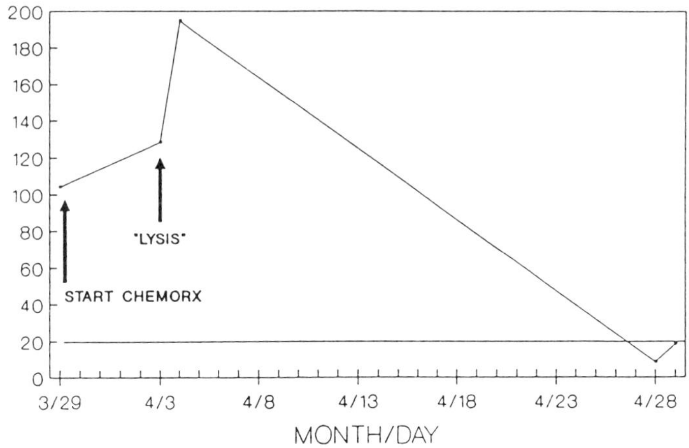

Figure 2 A patient with extensive disease and elevated pretreatment NSE experiences "lysis" during a 3 day course of chemotherapy. Note that the NSE level in serum nearly doubles before falling to within normal range just before cycle 2 of chemotherapy.

lysis and subsequent release of NSE. Such a phenomenon could possibly be used to predict early during the course of treatment whether an objective response will be obtained. For example, of the 13 patients Akoun et al. evaluated for release of NSE during treatment, 7 experienced increases of serum NSE levels to ≥100 ng/ml within 72 hr and all 7 achieved an objective response. On the other hand, only 1 of 6 patients with an acute rise in NSE levels of <100 ng/ml responded objectively. Similar findings have been reported by Cooper et al. (1985) and Ariyoshi et al. (1986).

Although NSE levels are strikingly different in the supernatants of cultured SCLC and NSCLC cell lines (Marangos et al., 1982; Carney et al., 1982; Ariyoshi et al., 1986), NSE can be demonstrated in the cytoplasm of both NSCLC and SCLC by immunoperoxidase staining (Kato et al., 1983; Haimoto et al., 1985). Thus, it is not surprising that serum NSE levels are elevated in some patients with NSCLC (Ariyoshi et al., 1986; Kato et al., 1983; Haimoto et al., 1985). Depending on the reference values used, 10–25% of patients with NSCLC will have an elevated pretreatment NSE level (Ariyoshi et al., 1983; Esscher et al., 1985; Kato et al., 1983) (Table 8). If a high NSE value (≥25 ng/ml) is used as a "cutoff" level, the number of patients with NSCLC with an elevated NSE is small (≤10%) (Esscher et al., 1985), while the number of those with SCLC with abnormal levels remains large (i.e. ≥70%) (Esscher et al., 1985). If patients with nonmalignant lung conditions are tested, a small number will be found to have raised NSE levels (Esscher et al., 1985; Cooper et al., 1985) (Table 9). Of considerable importance is the recent observation that NSE-positive non-small-cell lung cancers may be more responsive to chemotherapy than their NSE-negative counterparts (Ariyoshi et al., 1986; Mulshine et al., 1987). These data are provocative and warrant additional study. A large-scale retrospective study is underway within the ECOG that may help to substantiate these observations.

To summarize, NSE levels are elevated in the serum of a majority of patients with SCLC (i.e., >70%). Pretreatment levels tend to reflect overall tumor burden but are not specific for any particular metastatic site, although marked increases (i.e., >100 ng/ml) may be more common in patients with liver and/or marrow

Table 8 NSE Levels in Non-Small-Cell Lung Cancer

Reference	Upper limit of normal (ng/ml)	Number NSCLC
Ariyoshi et al. (1983)	7.5	6/54 (11%)
Akoun et al. (1985)	16	2/14 (14%)
Esscher et al. (1985)	12	13/51 (25%)
	25	4/51 (8%)
Cooper et al. (1985)	13.5	16/94 (17%)

Table 9 NSE Levels in Conditions Other than SCLC (nl < 13 ng/ml)

Condition	Number	<13 ng/ml	13–25 ng/ml	25–50 ng/ml	>50 ng/ml
Blood donors	33	31 (94%)	2 (6%)		
Non-SCLC	94	78 (83%)	9 (9.5%)	3 (3%)	4 (4%)
Lung metastases	10	8 (80%)	2 (20%)		
Benign lung lesions	11	10 (91%)	1 (9%)		
Pneumonia	20	13 (65%)	6 (30%)	1 (5%)	
Benign GI/liver disease	45	38 (84%)	7 (16%)		
Breast/GI cancer with liver metastases	20	17 (85%)	3 (15%)		
Metastatic prostate cancer	42	31 (74%)	8 (19%)	3 (7%)	
SCLC LD	38	13 (34%)	9 (24%)	11 (29%)	5 (13%)
ED	39	5 (13%)	4 (10%)	12 (31%)	18 (46%)

LD, limited-stage disease; ED, extensive disease.
Source: Modified from Cooper et al. (1985).

metastases. This may simply represent a manifestation of tumor bulk rather than a unique propensity for these metastatic sites to be associated with marked NSE levels. Most studies suggest that response rates and overall survival are not influenced by pretreatment NSE levels, although there are conflicting data. Normalization of previously elevated levels at the time of restaging portends a better survival, at least among patients with extensive-stage disease. Serial NSE levels tend to mirror the clinical course of disease, falling with remission and rising with relapse. An increase in NSE may precede clinical recognition of recurrence by several weeks. Acute elevations of NSE occurring within 72 hr of initiation of chemotherapy appear to be useful in predicting response, but further study is required to confirm this observation. It is unfortunate that NSE lacks specificity and therefore cannot be used as a screening test and, like CEA, is occasionally raised in patients with nonmalignant conditions. Nevertheless, of the many biomarkers studied in patients with SCLC, NSE appears to be a potentially useful clinical tool.

VI. Creatine Kinase BB

Trace amounts of the brain isoenzyme of creatine kinase (CK-BB) can be found in normal serum and may be markedly elevated in patients with a variety of neoplasms including SCLC (Coolen et al., 1979; Zweig et al., 1981). Coolen and colleagues (1979) were the first to report that CK-BB was increased in patients with SCLC. In their study, 12 of 15 (80%) patients with SCLC had an abnormal CK-BB level, although the *total* serum CK levels were usually within normal limits. Although insufficient data were provided, it appears that all patients with SCLC with an abnormal CK-BB level had extensive-stage disease. At least two patients demonstrated a rise in serum CK-BB levels with disease progression.

Other investigators have confirmed and expanded upon Coolen's observations (Jaques et al., 1988; Carney et al., 1984). Zweig et al. (1981) reported that CK-BB levels rarely exceeded 10 ng/ml in healthy adult volunteers. Using this reference point, Carney et al. found that 27 of 105 (26%) previously untreated patients with SCLC had a raised pretreatment level of CK-BB. All but 1 of the 27 patients had extensive-stage disease (limited, 1 of 42; extensive, 26 of 63). a similar or higher frequency of CK-BB elevations has been reported by others (Jaques et al., 1988; Ariyoshi et al., 1986). Carney et al. found no association between an elevated CK-BB level and metastatic disease in any specific site. Jaques et al. (1988), however, noted an association between markedly elevated CK-BB levels (i.e., >30 ng/ml) and the presence of liver and bone marrow metastases. As is true with other putative markers, this could simply represent a manifestation of tumor bulk. For example, Carney et al. did report that as the number of metastatic sites increased, the frequency of elevated CK-BB levels also increased. Among patients with an elevated CK-BB level, those with the higher levels tended to have the greatest number of metastatic sites of disease (Table 10). Survival of patients with a raised pretreatment CK-BB is worse than that of individuals with normal levels (Jaques et al., 1988; Carney et al., 1984). This relationship holds true even when an adjustment is made for the number of metastatic sites present. This observation suggests that both the CK-BB level *and* the number of metastatic sites represent independent variables that correlate with survival (Carney et al., 1984). A surprising finding is that patients with extreme elevations of CK-BB (>30 ng/ml) are also less likely to experience a complete response to chemotherapy (Jaques et al., 1988).

Table 10 Serum CK-BB Levels in SCLC

	No. of patients	Abnormal CK-BB	CK-BB Level (Mean ± SE [ng/ml])
LD	42	1	33.7 ± 0.5
ED			
1 met	31	6	15.5 ± 6.39
2 mets	18	6	43.9 ± 32.06
3 mets	8	6	43.0 ± 12.87
≥4 mets	8	8	82.9 ± 36.57

LD, limited-stage disease; ED, extensive disease; mets, metastases.
Source: Modified from Carney et al. (1984).

Serial CK-BB evaluations have been reported for only a small number of patients. Of 12 patients with extensive disease responding to chemotherapy (5 CR; 7 PR), Carney et al. (1984) reported that 10 demonstrated a normalization or near normalization of the serum CK-BB level at the time of restaging. One nonresponding patient demonstrated a rise in CK-BB level. Among patients experiencing a relapse, previously normalized CK-BB levels were found to have increased in most cases. Four patients remained disease-free at the time of the report and all four had normal CK-BB levels.

These data would seem to indicate that CK-BB isoenzymes may provide some useful prognostic information in patients with SCLC with extensive disease. However, like the other putative markers, CK-BB provides little diagnostic information due to its lack of sensitivity and previously recognized lack of specificity (Zweig et al., 1981; Rubery et al., 1981). Although CK-BB determinations have provided a diagnostic clue to SCLC in certain unique circumstances it cannot be recommended as a routine staging test at this time (Johnson and Greco et al., 1986; Kurtz and Nielson, 1985). CK-BB may be most useful as a parameter for stratifying patients with extensive-stage disease who are entered into investigational studies since it does appear to provide useful prognostic information.

VII. Neurophysins

Neurophysins (HNP) are low-molecular-weight single-chain proteins normally produced by neurons of the hypothalamus (North et al., 1980, 1983). Neurophysins are part of the precursor structure of vasopressin (VP) and oxytocin (OT) and act as carrier molecules for these hormones (North et al., 1983). Their close association with some of the peptides known to be produced ectopically by SCLC has led investigators to evaluate neurophysins as possible markers of SCLC (North et al., 1980, 1983).

In one large study, 64% (96 of 151) of patients had an elevated pretreatment HNP level (i.e., "secretors" of HNP) (North et al., 1983). An additional 13% (19 of 51) had levels two to three times the normal mean (i.e., "possible secretors"). Approximately 50% of secretors produced VP-HNP, 30% produced OT-HNP, and 15% produced both. Neurophysin levels were more commonly elevated in patients with extensive disease (82%) than in those with limited disease (41%). Although this difference may be related solely to tumor burden, North et al. (1983) have suggested that the difference may reflect a *biological* difference (i.e., cells with a proclivity for metastasis may be more likely to produce HNP than are cells less inclined to spread). Evidence for this speculation comes from the observation that neurophysin levels do not necessarily increase serially in relapsing patients. Also, nonsecretors rarely, if ever, develop elevated HNP levels. Indeed, recent data from Johns Hopkins would appear to support the concept of differing clinical behavior

Table 11 Pretreatment Neurophysin Status and Prognosis

	Limited disease		Extensive disease	
HNP secretory status	Response (% complete response)	Median survival (months)	Response (% complete response)	Median survival (months)
Secretor	89% (65%)	9.3	36% (8%)	6.1
Possible secretor	100% (22%)	10.0	50% (50%)	5.8
Nonsecretor	76% (63%)	9.5	44% (11%)	6.5

Source: Modified from North et al. (1983).

based on the presence or absence of various paraneoplastic phenomena (de la Monte et al., 1984).

Although patients with nonsecreting tumors generally maintained normal HNP levels regardless of their clinical status, there appeared to be an excellent correlation between clinical status and HNP levels among the patients with SCLC categorized as secretors (i.e., those with elevated pretreatment levels). As shown with other putative markers, patients achieving a partial or complete response had a concomitant decrease (2–30-fold) in the previously elevated HNP level. Patients failing to respond to therapy typically experienced a progressive rise in plasma HNP level. Among patients enjoying a partial or complete response, relapse was often heralded by a rise in the remission HNP level that *always* preceded clinical recognition of relapse by several weeks (North et al., 1983). In North's study, only one "false-positive" increase in HNP was noted among 103 patients undergoing serial evaluation. Median survival, complete, and overall response rates were not statistically different between secretors, possible secretors, and nonsecretors of HNP (Table 11).

An elevation of neurophysins can be found in patients with NSCLC. However, the HNP levels are usually lower in patients with NSCLC (North et al., 1983). Nevertheless, the measurement of neurophysins does not appear to be a useful discriminatory test for SCLC.

More studies are required to ascertain fully the value of neurophysins in the clinical management of SCLC.

VIII. Chromogranin A

Chromogranin A (CgA) is a high-molecular-weight protein originally isolated from the chromaffin vesicles of the adrenal medulla (Angeletti and Hickey, 1985; O'Connor and Deftos, 1986). The exact function of CgA is not known, although it is released into the blood during sympathoadrenal activation (O'Connor and

Deftos, 1986). For this reason, CgA has been considered to be a potentially useful autonomic probe (O'Connor and Deftos, 1986). The protein is found in a wide variety of neuroendocrine tissues and peptide-producing endocrine neoplasms including pheochromocytomas, medullary thyroid carcinomas, carcinoid tumors, pancreatic islet cell tumors, and several others (O'Connor and Deftos, 1986; Walts et al., 1985). In addition, CgA has recently been described in small cell and non-small-cell tumor lines (Sobol et al., 1986; Deftos et al., 1988; Gazdar and Linnoila, 1988).

Sobol et al (1986) found that pretreatment serum CgA levels were raised (i.e., >175 ng/ml) in more than 50% of patients with limited-stage SCLC and up to 70% of those with extensive-stage disease. Using a radioimmunoassay, these investigators found that serum levels correlated with tumor burden (mean level for limited disease = 234 ± ng/ml vs. 1155 ± 449 ng/ml in extensive disease; p = 0.026). Although an earlier study by these investigators had suggested that CgA levels were rarely elevated in normal individuals or in patients with conditions "in which peptide hormones are not produced" (O'Connor and Deftos, 1986) this later report noted that CgA levels were elevated in patients with a variety of benign processes (Sobel et al., 1986). However, no healthy normal control subject had a value >175 ng/ml (Sobol et al., 1986). Also of interest, four patients with "non-small-cell lung cancers" and raised CgA levels were subsequently found to have mixed tumors (i.e., non-small-cell admixed with small cell elements). Up to one-quarter of the persons with chronic obstructive pulmonary disease had raised CgA and levels were elevated in 28–50% of patients with non-small-cell lung cancer (Sobol et al., 1986).

Although more study is needed to define fully CgA's role in the management of SCLC, some experts believe that CgA is the most useful neuroendocrine marker for differentiating SCLC from non-small-cell lung cancer (Gazdar and Linnoila, 1988). Immunostaining for CgA will yield focal staining in approximately 50% of SCLC tumors while mRNA expression is present in virtually all SCLC tumors and cell lines (Gazdar and Linnoila, 1988). We hope that serum values will prove similarly useful.

IX. Bombesin

Moody and co-workers (1981, 1983) initially described the presence of bombesin, a tetradecapeptide originally isolated from frog skin, in the supernatant of cultured small cell lung cancer cell lines. Although bombesin-like immunoreactivity has been detected in numerous mammalian tissues (including human fetal and neonatal but not adult lung), very low to absent levels have been found in cultured non-small-cell cancer cell lines (Moody et al., 1981). This apparent qualitative difference prompted some investigators to evaluate plasma levels of bombesin as a biomarker in patients with SCLC (Johnson et al., 1984; Pert and Schumacher, 1982; Wood et al., 1982). It is unfortunate that the plasma half-life of bombesin is very brief and it appears that bombesin will not be a useful marker. For example, Johnson et al. (1984b) found plasma bombesin-like activity was raised in only 5% of 31 untreated patients (10 limited-stage; 21 extensive-stage). Pert and Schumacher (1982) found that plasma bombesin levels were raised in six patients with SCLC with limited-stage disease and three with extensive-stage disease. However, raised bombesin levels were also detected in six patients with malignancies other than SCLC. Median bombesin levels were 33 ± 17 and 38 ± 12 pg/200 μl plasma in patients with limited SCLC and non-small cell cancers, respectively. Very high bombesin levels (median = 640 ± 72 pg/μl) were detected only in patients with extensive disease (Pert and Schumacher, 1982). On the other hand, Wood and coworkers (1982) found normal (<10 pmol/L) levels of plasma bombesin in all 31 patients with SCLC they evaluated, 10 of whom had extensive disease.

Thus, based on these preliminary reports, it does not appear that plasma bombesin will be a useful plasma tumor marker. However, bombesin may be a very useful marker for CNS disease (Pederson et al., 1985). Bombesin does, however, appear to be an autocrine factor for SCLC and is potentially exploitable as a therapeutic target (Gazdar and Linnoila, 1988; Cuttitta et al., 1985).

X. Miscellaneous

A variety of additional products have been evaluated as possible biomarkers of SCLC, including neurotensin (Goedert et al., 1984), protein-bound carbohydrates such as mannose and fucose (Waalkes et al., 1983), urinary polyamines including putrescine, spermidine, and spermine (Woo et al., 1983), alpha-1-acid glycoprotein (Ganz et al., 1984), beta-2-microglobulin, (Nissen et al., 1984) as well as more commonly measured serum enzymes such as lactate dehydrogenase (Cohen et al., 1981). In addition to plasma or serum determinations, immunoperoxidase demonstration of some or many of these tumor products have been used as a means of differentiating SCLC from non-small-cell lung cancer with varying degrees of success (Lehto et al., 1983; Walts et al., 1985; Bergh et al., 1985).

Deletion of a portion of the short arm of chromosome 3 (i.e., del 3p (14-23)) has been described in SCLC and may represent yet another method of differentiating SCLC from non-small-cell lung cancers (Whang-Peng et al., 1982). Initially, some investigators were unable to verify the consistent presence of the deletion of the short arm of chromosome 3 (Wurster-Hill et al., 1984). However, more recent studies have employed restriction fragment length polymorphisms to demonstrate that this defect is present in a majority of SCLC specimens (Gazdar et al., 1987; Naylor et al., in press).

SCLC has recently been found to express the Leu-7 antigenic determinant commonly found in natural killer cells and thus may represent yet another method of identifying lung cancer histologic types (Bunn et al., 1985). The emergence of monoclonal antibodies specific for SCLC (described elsewhere in this text) will no doubt improve diagnostic acumen and may lead to the early detection of subclinical amounts of tumor (Bernal et al., 1985; Mulshine et al., 1983).

XI. Conclusions

Small cell lung cancer cells are "biologically active" and are associated with many tumor products. The search for a clinically useful marker remains obviously important. Unfortunately, many of the tumor products reviewed above demonstrate a heterogeneity of expression and therefore it is unlikely that any *one* of these tumor products will be used exclusively as a biomarker of SCLC. However, it is possible that two or more of these substances will be used as a panel of markers to follow the clinical course of individual patients, much like alpha-fetoprotein and beta-HCG are used in the management of germinal neoplasms. However, our results in a small study evaluating three markers (NSE, ADH, and calcitonin) was not particularly promising (Johnson et al., 1984) (Table 12). In fact, NSE proved superior to the panel of markers both in its ability to mirror the clinical status of patients and in its capability of predicting relapse. Similar disappointing results were reported by Aroney et al. Combining NSE, CgA, CK-BB, and CEA may be a better marker composition than those previously employed. The inclusion of CK-BB and CEA determinations may be particularly important since some of the studies cited above indicate that pretreatment CEA and CK-BB levels may provide useful prognostic information.

The evaluation of biomarkers useful in the management of SCLC will undoubtedly continue to be spurred by recent developments in molecular biology. It is anticipated that continued progress in understanding the biology of SCLC will lead to improved methods of tumor detection and therapy.

Table 12 Correlation of NSE, ADH, and Calcitonin (CAL) With Clinical Status of SCLC

Marker	Remission			Relapse		
status	NSE	ADH	CAL	NSE	ADH	CAL
Decrease	15	10	4	0	1	1
Stable	2	8	8	0	9	9
Increase	2	1	4	20	6	9

References

Akoun, G. M., Scarna, H. M., Milleron, B. J., Benichou, M. P., and Herman, D. P. (1985). Serum neuron-specific enolase. A marker for disease extent and response to therapy for small-cell lung cancer. *Chest* **87:**39–43.

Angeletti, R. H., and Hickey, W. H. (1985). A neuroendocrine marker in tissues of the immune system. *Science* **230:**89–90.

Ariyoshi, Y., Kato, K., Ishiguro, Y., Ota, K., Sato, T., and Suchi, T. (1983). Evaluation of serum neuron-specific as a tumor marker for carcinoma of the lung. *Gann* **74:**219–225.

Ariyoshi, Y., Kato, K., Ueda, R., et al. (1986). Biological and clinical implications of neuron-specific enolase and creatinine kinase BB in small cell lung cancer. *Jpn. J. Clin. Oncol.* **16:**213–221.

Bergh, J., Esscher, T., Steinholtz, L., Hilsson, K., and Pahlman, S. (1985). Immunocytochemical demonstration of neuron-specific enolase (NSE) in human lung cancers. *Am. J. Clin. Pathol.* **84:**1–7.

Bernal, S. D., Mabry, M., Stahel, R. A., Griffin, J. D., and Speak, J. A. (1985). Selective cytotoxicity of the SM1 monoclonal antibody towards small cell carcinoma of the lung. *Cancer Res* **45:**1026–1032.

Bondy, P. K. (1981). The pattern of ectopic hormone production in lung cancer. *Yale J. Biol. Med.* **54:**181–185.

Bunn, P. A., Linnoila, I., Minna, J. D., Carney, D., and Gazdar, A. F. (1985). Small cell lung cancer, endocrine cells of the fetal bronchus, and other neuroendocrine cells express the Leu-7 antigenic determinant present on natural killer cells. *Blood* **65:**764–768.

Carney, D. N., Marangos, P. J., Ihde, D. C., et al. (1982). Serum neuron-specific enolase: marker for disease extent and response to therapy of small-cell lung cancer. *Lancet* **1:**583–585.

Carney, D. N., Zweig, M. H., Ihde, D. C., Cohen, M. H., Makuch, R. W., and Gazdar, A. F. (1984). Elevated serum creatine kinase BB levels in patients with small cell lung cancer. *Cancer Res.* **44:**5399–5403.

Cohen, M. H., Makuch, R., Johnston-Early, A., et al. (1981). Laboratory parameters as an alternative to performance status in prognostic stratification of patients with small cell lung cancer. *Cancer Treat. Rep.* **65:**187–195.

Coolen, R. B., Progay, D. A., Nosenchuk, J. S., and Belding, R. (1979). Elevation of brain-type creatine kinase in serum from patients with carcinoma. *Cancer* **44:**1414–1418.

Cooper, E. H., Splinter, T. A. W., Brown, D. A., Muers, M. F., Peake, M. D., and Pearson, S. L. (1985). Evaluation of a radioimmunoassay for neuron specific enolase in small cell lung cancer. *Br. J. Cancer* **52:**333–338.

Cuttitta, F., Carney, D. N., Mulshine, J., et al. (1985). Bombesin-like peptides can function as autocrine growth factors in human small-cell lung cancer. *Nature* **316:**823–826.

Deftos, L. J., Linnoila, R. I., Carney, D. N., et al. (1988). Demonstration of chromogranin A in human neuroendocrine cell lines by immunohistology and immunoassay. *Cancer* **62:**92–97.

Dent, P. B., McCulloch, P. B., Wesley-James, O., et al. (1978). Measurement of carcinoembryonic antigen in patients with bronchogenic carcinoma. *Cancer* **42:**1484–1491.

Esscher, T., Steinholtz, L., Bergh, J., Nou, E., Nilsson, K., and Pahlman, S. (1985).

Neurone specific enolase: a useful diagnostic serum marker for small cell carcinoma of the lung. *Thorax* **40:**85–90.

Ganz, P. A., Baras, M., Ma, P. Y., and Elashoff, R. M. (1984). Monitoring the therapy of lung cancer with α-1-acid glycoprotein. *Cancer Res.* **44:**5415–5421.

Gazdar, A. F., and Linnoila, R. I. (1988). The pathology of lung cancer—changing concepts and newer diagnostic techniques. *Semin. Oncol.* **15:**215–225.

Gazdar, A. F., Mulshine, J. L., Linnoila, R. I., et al. (1987). Deletion of chromosome 3p delineates two groups of human lung cancers expressing neuroendocrine markers. *Proc. Am. Assoc. Cancer Res.* **6:**59.

Goedert, M., Reeve, J. G., Emson, P. C., and Bleehan, N. M. (1984). Neurotensin in human small cell lung carcinoma. *Br. J. Cancer* **50:**179–183.

Goslin, R. H., Skarin, A. T., and Zamchech, N. (1981). Carcinoembryonic antigen: a useful monitor of small cell lung cancer. *JAMA* **246:**2173–2176.

Greco, F. A., Hainsworth, J., Sismani, A., Richardson, R., Hande, K. R., and Oldham, R. K. (1981). Hormone production and paraneoplastic syndromes. In *Small Cell Lung Cancer*. Edited by F. A. Greco, R. K. Oldham, and P. A. Bunn. New York, Grune & Stratton, pp. 117–223.

Haimoto, H., Takahashi, Y., Koshikawa, T., Nagura, H., and Kato, K. (1985). Immunohistochemical localization of α-enolase in normal human tissues other than nervous and neuroendocrine tissues. *Lab. Invest.* **52:**57–63.

Hansen, J., Hammer, M., Hummer, L. (1980b). Diagnostic and therapeutic implications of ectopic hormone production in small cell carcinoma of the lung. *Thorax* **35:**101–106.

Hansen, M. (1981). Clinical implications of ectopic hormone production in small cell carcinoma of the lung. *Dan. Med. Bull.* **23:**221.

Hansen, M., Hammer, M., and Hummer, L. (1980a). ACTH, ADH, and calcitonin as markers of response and relapse in small cell carcinoma of the lung. *Cancer* **46:**2062–2067.

Jaques, G., Bepler, G., Holle, R., et al. (1988). Prognostic value of pretreatment carcinoembryonic antigen, neuron-specific enolase, and creatinine kinase-BB levels in sera of patients with small cell lung cancer. *Cancer* **62:**125–134.

Johnson, D. H., and Greco, F. A. (1986). Small cell carcinoma of the lung. *Crit. Rev. Oncol. Hematol.* **4:**303–336.

Johnson, D. H., and Greco, F. A. (1987). Small cell lung cancer: current prospectives. *Am. J. Med. Sci.* **193:**377–389.

Johnson, D. H., Marangos, P. J., Forbes, J. T., et al. (1984a). Potential utility of serum neuron-specific enolase levels in small cell carcinoma of the lung. *Cancer Res.* **44:** 5409–5414.

Johnson, D. H., Hande, K. R., Marangos, P. J., Forbes, J. T., and Greco, F. A. (1984b). Serum neuron-specific enolase (NSE), a possible biomarker for small cell lung cancer (SCLC). *Proc. Am. Assoc. Cancer Res.* **25:**156.

Kato, K., Ishiguro, Y., and Ariyoshi, Y. (1983). Enolase isoenzymes as disease markers: distribution of three enolase subunits (alpha, beta, and gamma) in various human tissues. *Dis. Markers* **1:**213–220.

Kurtz, K. J., and Nielsen, R. D. (1985). Serum creatine kinase BB isoenzyme as a diagnostic aid in occult small cell lung cancer. *Cancer* **56:**562–566.

Laberge, F., Fritsche, H. A., Umsawasdi, T., et al. (1987). Use of carcinoembryonic antigen in small cell lung cancer. Prognostic value and relation to the clinical course 1. *Cancer* **59:**2047–2052.

Lehto, V. P., Stenman, S., Miettinen, M., Dahl, D., and Vintanen, I. (1983). Expression of a neural type of intermediate filament as a distinguishing feature between oat cell carcinoma and other lung cancers. *Am. J. Pathol.* **110:**113–118.

Lokich, J. J. (1982). Plasma CEA levels in small cell lung cancer: correlation with stage, distribution of metastases, and survival. *Cancer* **50:**2154–2156.

Lokich, J. J., Zamcheck, N., and Lowenstein, M. (1978). Sequential carcinoembryonic antigen levels in the therapy of metastatic breast cancer: a predictor and monitor of response and relapse. *Ann. Intern. Med.* **89:**902–906.

Marangos, P. J., Polak, J. M., and Pearse, A. G. E. (1982a). Neuron-specific enolase: a probe for neurons and neuroendocrine cells. *Trends Neurosci.* **5:**193–196.

Marangos, P. J., Gazdar, A. F., and Carney, D. N. (1982b). Neuron specific enolase in human small cell carcinoma cultures. *Cancer Letts.* **15:**67–71.

McIntire, K. R., (1985). Tumor markers. In *Cancer Principles & Practice of Oncology*. Edited by V. T. DeVita, S. Hellman, and S. A. Rosenberg. Philadelphia, J. B. Lippincott, pp. 375–388.

McKenzie, C. G., Evans, I. M. A., Hillyard, C. J., Carter, H. S., Tan, M. K., and MacIntyre, I. (1977). Biochemical markers in bronchial carcinoma. *Br. J. Cancer* **36:** 700–707.

Meador, C. K., Liddle, G. W., Island, D. P., et al. (1962). Cause of Cushing's syndrome in patients with tumors arising from "nonendocrine" tissue. *J. Clin. Endocrinol.* **22:** 693–703.

Minna, J. D. (1988). Autocrine growth factor production, chromosomal deletions, and oncogene activation in the pathogenesis of lung cancer. *Lung Cancer* **4** (suppl)**:**6–10.

Minna, J. D., Carney, D. N., Cuttitta, F., et al. (1984). Clinical, cellular, and molecular biology of lung cancer. In *Adjuvant Therapy of Cancer IV*. Edited by S. E. Salmon and S. E. Jones. New York, Grune & Stratton, pp. 167–182.

de la Monte, S. M., Hutchins, G. M., and Moore, G. W. (1984). Paraneoplastic syndromes and constitutional symptoms in prediction of metastatic behavior of small cell carcinoma of the lung. *Am. J. Med.* **77:**851–857.

Moody, T. W., Pert, C. B., Gazdar, A. F., Carney, D. N., and Minna, J. D. (1981). High levels of intracellular bombesin characterize human small-cell lung cancer. *Science* **214:**1246–1248.

Moody, T. W., Russell, E. K., O'Donohue, T. L., Linden, C. D., and Gazdar, A. F. (1983). Bombesin-like peptides in small cell lung cancer: biochemical characterization and secretion from a cell line. *Life Sci.* **32:**487–493.

Morstyn, G., Ihde, D. C., Lichter, A. S., et al. (1984). Small cell lung cancer 1973–1983: early progress and recent obstacles. *Int. J. Radiat. Oncol. Biol. Phys.* **10:**515–539.

Mulshine, J. L., Cuttitla, F., Bibro, M., et al. (1983). Monoclonal antibodies that distinguish non-small cell from small cell lung cancer *J. Immunol.* **131:**497–502.

Mulshine, J., Ihde, D., Linnoila, R. I., et al. (1987). Preliminary report of a prospective trial of neuroendocrine marker analysis and in vitro drug sensitivity testing in patients with non-small cell lung cancer. *Proc. Am. Soc. Clin. Oncol.* **6:**181.

Naylor, S. L., Johnson, B. E., Minna, J. D., et al. (199x). Loss of heterozygosity of chromosome 3 short arm markers in small cell lung cancer. *Nature*, in press.

Nissen, M. H., Plesner, T., and Rorth, M. (1984). Modification of β_2-microglobulin in serum from patients with small cell carcinoma of the lung—correlation with the clinical course. *Clin. Chim. Acta* **141:**41–50.

North, W. G., Maurer, L. H., Valtin, H., and O'Donnell, J. F. (1980). Human neurophysins as potential tumor markers for small cell carcinoma of the lung: application of specific radioimmunoassays. *J. Clin. Endocrinol. Metab.* **51:**892–896.

North, W. G., Maurer, L. H., and O'Donnell, J. F. (1983). The neurophysins and small cell lung cancer. In *Biology and Management of Lung Cancer*. Edited by F. A. Greco. Boston, Martinus Nijhoff, pp. 143–169.

O'Connor, D. T., and Deftos, L. H. (1986). Secretion of chromogranin A by peptide-producing endocrine neoplasms. *N. Engl. J. Med.* **314:**1145–1151.

Pahlman, S., Esscher, T., Bergh, J., Steinholtz, L., Hou, E., and Nilsson, K. (1984). Neuron-specific enolase as a marker for neuroblastoma and small-cell carcinoma of the lung. *Tumor Biol.* **5:**119–126.

Parma, A. M., Marangos, P. J., and Goodwin, F. K. (1981). A more sensitive radioimmunoassay for neuron-specific enolase suitable for cerebrospinal fluid determinations. *J. Neurochem.* **36:**1093–1096.

Pederson, A. G., Becker, K., Marangos, P., et al. (1985). Bombesin (BM), creatine kinase BB (CK-BB), calcitonin (C), and neuron-specific enolase (NSE) in the cerebrospinal fluid (CSF) as a marker as CNS metastases and meningeal carcinomatosis (MC) in small cell lung cancer (SCLC). *Proc. Am. Assoc. Cancer Res.* **26:**146.

Pert, C. B., and Schumacher, U. K. (1982). Plasma bombesin concentrations in patients with extensive small cell carcinoma of the lung. *Lancet* **1:**509.

Prinz, R. A., and Marangos, P. J. (1982). Use of neuron-specific enolase as a serum marker for neuroendocrine neoplasms. *Surgery* **92:**887–889.

Richardson, R. L., Greco, F. A., Oldham, R. K., and Liddle, G. W. (1978). Tumor products and potential markers in small cell lung cancer. *Semin. Oncol.* **5:**253–262.

Rubery, E. D., Doran, J. F., and Thompson, R. J. (1981). Brain-type creatine kinase BB as a potential tumour marker—serum levels measured by radioimmunoassay in 1015 patients with histologically confirmed malignancies. *Eur. J. Cancer Clin. Oncol.* **18:** 951–956.

Said, J. W., Vimmadalal, S., Nash, G., et al. (1985). Immunoreactive neuron-specific enolase, bombesin, and chromogranin as markers for neuroendocrine lung tumors. *Hum. Pathol.* **16:**235–240.

Schmechel, D., Marangos, P. J., and Brightman, M. (1978). Neurone-specific enolase is a molecular marker for peripheral and central neuroendocrine cells. *Nature* **276:** 834–836.

Sculier, J. P., Feld, R., Evans, W. K., et al. (1985). Carcinoembryonic antigen: a useful prognostic marker in small-cell lung cancer. *J. Clin. Oncol.* **3:**1349–1354.

Sobel, R. E., O'Connor, D. T., Addison, J., Suchocki, K., Royston, I., and Deftos, L. J. (1986). Elevated serum chromogranin A concentrations in small cell lung carcinoma. *Ann. Intern. Med.* **105:**698–700.

Splinter, T. A. W., Cooper, E. H., Kho, G. S., Osterom, R., and Peake, M. D. (1987).

Neuron-specific enolase as a guide to the treatment of small cell lung cancer. *Eur. J. Cancer Clin. Oncol.* **23:**171–176.

Sugarbaker, P. H., Zamcheck, N., and Moore, F. D. (1976). Assessment of serial carcinoembryonic antigen (CEA) assays in postoperative detection of recurrent colon cancer. *Cancer* **38:**2310–2315.

Tapia, F. J., Polak, J. M., Barbosa, A. J. A., et al. (1981). Neuron-specific enolase is produced by neuroendocrine tumours. *Lancet* **1:**808–811.

Vincent, R. G., Chu, T. M., Fergen, T. B., et al. (1975). Carcinoembryonic antigen in 228 patients with carcinoma of the lung. *Cancer* **36:**2069–2076.

Waalkes, T. P., Abeloff, M. D., Woo, K. B., Ettinger, D. S., Ruddon, R. W., and Aldenderfer, P. (1980). Carcinoembryonic antigen for monitoring patients with small cell carcinoma of the lung during treatment. *Cancer Res.* **40:**4420–4427.

Waalkes, T. P., Abeloff, M. D., Ettinger, D. S., Woo, K. B., Kuo, K. C., and Gehrke, D. W. (1983). Serum protein-bound carbohydrates and small cell carcinoma of the lung. Correlations with extent of disease, tumor burden, survival, and clinical response categories. *Cancer* **52:**131–139.

Walts, A. E., Said, J. W., Shintaku, P., and Lloyd, R. (1985). Chromogranin as a marker of neuroendocrine cells in cytologic material—an immunocytochemical study. *Am. J. Clin. Pathol.* **84:**273–277.

Whang-Peng, J., Kao-Shan, C. S., Lee, E. C., et al. (1982). Specific chromosome defect associated with human small-cell lung cancer: deletion 3p(14–23). *Science* **215:** 181–182.

Woo, K. B., Waalkes, P., Abeloff, M. D., Ettinger, D. S., McNitt, K. L., and Gehrke, C. W. (1981). Multiple biologic markers in the monitoring of treatment for patients with small cell carcinoma of the lung. The use of serial levels of plasma CEA and serum carbohydrates. *Cancer* **48:**1633–1642.

Woo, K. B., Waalkes, T. P., Abeloff, M. D., Lenhard, R. E., Gehrke, C. W., and Kuo, K. C. (1983). Urinary polyamines for evaluating the course of disease for patients with small cell carcinoma of the lung. *Cancer* **52:**1684–1690.

Wood, S. M., Wood, J. R., Ghate, N. A. M., Sorenson, G. D., and Bloom, S. R. (1982). Is bombesin a tumour marker for small-cell carcinoma? *Lancet* **1:**690–691.

Wurster-Hill, D. H., Cannizzaro, L. A., Pettengill, O. S., Sorenson, G. D., Cate, C. C., and Maurer, L. H. (1984). Cytogenetics of small cell carcinoma of the lung. *Cancer Genetics Cytogen.* **13:**303–330.

Zweig, M. H., and Van Steirteghem, A. C. (1981). Assessment by radioimmunoassay of serum creatine kinase BB (CK-BB) as a tumor marker: studies in patients with various cancers and a comparison of CK-BB concentrations to prostate acid phosphatase concentrations. *J. Natl. Cancer Inst.* **66:**859–862.

13

Different Patterns of Expression of Small Cell Lung Cancer (SCLC) Antigens by SCLC "Classic," "Variant," and Carcinoid Phenotypes: Potential Diagnostic and Therapeutic Significance

A. M. C. KOROS and E. C. KLEIN

University of Pittsburgh
Pittsburgh, Pennsylvania

M. J. BUFFO, M. DALBOW, and R. RAIKOW

Allegheny Singer Research Institute
Pittsburgh, Pennsylvania

I. Introduction

A. Lung Cancer is a Public Health Problem

Lung cancer continues to be a serious public health problem, despite an increased understanding of the biology of the tumors. Lung cancer is the leading cause of cancer-related deaths among both men and women in the United States, with approximately 142,000 new cases diagnosed each year and about the same number of deaths (Kadowaki and Ferguson, 1990). Survival rates have not improved in 20 years even though there have been advances in the categorization of lung tumor types.

Lung cancers can be categorized on a clinical basis into two broad groups, small cell lung cancer (SCLC) and non-small-cell lung cancer (NSCLC) (Gazdar, 1989). SCLC comprise about 25% of all lung cancers and are frequently metastatic at diagnosis; they are, however, more responsive to chemotherapy than are the NSCLC. Therefore, the treatment for SCLC has been chiefly chemotherapy, whereas treatment for NSCLC has been primarily surgery and radiation. A small percentage of NSCLC have been identified that share neuroendocrine features with SCLC and may respond to chemotherapy (Gazdar, 1989). Although there have been advances in diagnosis as well as in chemotherapy and radiation therapy concurrent with increased response rates of tumors, patient survival rates are poor. Current strategies are inadequate.

B. Current Treatment Modalities are Inadequate and Not Sufficiently Specific

Chemotherapy is not sufficiently specific for neoplastic cells. Toxicity kills patients either directly or indirectly via suppression of their immune system, which leads to patients' susceptibility to infectious opportunistic agents and subsequent death. There is heterogeneity in tumors, not only in initial lesions but in the evolution of cell types during metastatic progression (Pujol et al., 1989), leading to multidrug resistance. More specific treatments and diagnostic techniques are needed.

C. Future Treatment Strategies Will be "Individualized"

Newer diagnostic methods based on monoclonal antibody (MOAB) panels, immunohistochemistry, flow cytometry, and even molecular probing (Carbone et al., 1991) may ultimately lead to "individualized" patient management. Although there probably are no unique tumor-specific antigens, there is preferential expression of certain antigens by particular tumors; for example, neuroendocrine tumors including SCLC and neuroblastomas (Koros et al., 1988) express CD56 and CD57 antigens defined by MOABS from the 4th Human Leucocyte Differentiation Antigen Workshop (Koros and Hiserodt, 1989). Through the use of such panels of MOABS, individual tumors may be phenotyped very specifically, and in the future appropriate MOABS may be selected for targeted therapy, with either conjugated immunotoxins (Stahel et al., 1990) or radioisotope-targeted therapy (Abrams et al., 1990).

The present study was based on an evaluation of 98 MOABS and controls provided by the Second International Workshop on Small Cell Lung Cancer Antigens (Beverley et al., 1991). Indirect immunofluorescence and flow cytometry were used to determine reactivity of the panel with prototype human continuous cultured lung tumor cell lines as well as normal human peripheral blood lymphocytes.

II. Materials and Methods

Reactivity of MOABS from the workshop (Beverley et al., 1991) was determined on well-characterized prototype cell lines representing SCLC "classic," NCI-H69, SCLC "variant," NCI-N417, and carcinoid, NCI-H727 (Drs. A. F. Gazdar and H. Oie, Bethesda, MD; Carney et al., 1985; Gazdar et al., 1985, 1988; Deftos et al., 1989; Lu et al., 1989). Peripheral blood lymphocytes (PBL) from a normal donor, as well as fresh sea urchin coelomocytes (pooled from six *Eucidaris*) were included as cell controls as described previously (Koros et al., 1987b).

Cultured cells grown in RPMI 1640 medium with 10% heat-inactivated fetal bovine serum without antibiotics were subcultured 24–96 hr before being dispersed mechanically. Cells were washed once with 4°C Hanks' balanced salt solution (HBSS) without Ca^{2+} or Mg^{2+}, containing 0.1% sodium azide and 2% fetal bovine serum (monoclonal wash solution). Approximately 5×10^5 cells were resuspended in 200μl monoclonal wash, and 50μl of the recommended working dilution of workshop antibody was added. Additional control antibodies were anti-HNK1 (prepared from clone HNK1, gift of Dr. A. Tilden) by A. Koros, and anti-NKH1 (N901) (gift of Coulter Immunology). Cells were incubated at 4°C for 1 hr, washed twice in monoclonal wash, resuspended in 200μl monoclonal wash, and stained at 4°C for 1 hr with 50μl of a 1:60 dilution of either fluorescein-conjugated goat $(Fab')_2$ antimouse IgG, IgM, human absorbed fragments (Tago), or a 1:40 dilution of fluorescein-conjugated goat $(Fab')_2$ antirat fragments (Tago). Cells were washed twice in monoclonal wash, resuspended in HBSS without Ca^{2+} or Mg^{2+} containing 1% paraformaldehyde, and analyzed by flow cytometry using a single argon laser (Epics C, Coulter Electronics) and a 200μm diameter biohazard tip. Five thousand cells were analyzed for each antibody. The appropriate working concentration of $(Fab')_2$ fragments was determined by an initial titration using normal PBL as well as cell lines, and a single lot of each fluorescent reagent.

Bit maps were drawn around cell populations falling in regions that were not clumped and free of cell debris. Data were printed as cell frequency vs. log green fluorescence intensity. The autofluorescence of each cell type was used to set the flow cytometer cursors at a baseline. Reactivity of each cell type with the goat $(Fab')_2$ antimouse or antirat IgG, IgM, human absorbed fragments usually was not greater than the autofluorescent controls. If there was any reactivity above autofluorescence, it was recorded as +. Reactivity of each MOAB tested was thereby compared to the baseline control. Intensities of reactivity were scored as −, ±, +, ++, +++. Scores were based not only on percentages of reactive cells but also on the intensity of reactivity. − means no reactivity above baseline with the $(Fab')_2$ control; ± indicates slight reactivity above the $(Fab')_2$ control; + indicates reactivity above baseline $(Fab')_2$ control with respect to either percentages of labeled cells and/or intensity of labeling as determined by peak channel or peak area; ++ indicates reactivity with a peak channel above 100; +++ indicates reactivity with a peak channel above 200.

III. Results

The results of reactivity of the 98 MOABS and controls against the prototype lung cancer cell lines as well as normal PBL and sea urchin coelomocytes are reported

Table 1 MOABS Reacting with Lung Cancer Cell Lines but not Reactive with PBL and Control MOABS

MOABS		CELLS			
			SCLC		
Code	Name	PBL	Classic H69	Variant N417	Carcinoid H727
0	Hanks' BSS	−	−	−	−
5	RNLZ	−	+	+	+
6	RCKL05	−	++	+	+
7	43/9F	−	+	−	++
8[a]	1A9/D4	−	++	++	+++
9	6A3/C8	−	+	+	+
10	10B7	−	++	+	−
11	MOC31	−	++	+	+++
12	MOCCI	−	+++	+	−
37	A80	−	++	+	++
71[a]	5.2	−	+++	++	Not done
93[a]	NCCST421	−	++	+	Not done
A[a,b]	αHNK1	±	++	++	−
B[a,b]	αNKH1	++	+++	++	±

[a]MOABS having reactivity with sea urchin coelomocytes, which may identify evolutionarily conserved antigens.
[b]Control MOABS, not part of the panel.

in detail (Koros et al., 1991). The results of only those MOABS having significant reactivity with either the SCLC "classic" or "variant" or carcinoid prototype cell lines, but no reactivity with PBL, are summarized in Table 1.

Although all of the MOABS in the panel (except number 27, SM1, which was not reactive with any cells) reacted with the SCLC "classic" cell line NCI-H69, most of the MOABS also reacted with PBL. Reactivity of two MOABS, 10 and 12 (10B7 and MOCCI), was greater with the SCLC "classic" NCI-H69 than with the "variant" NCI-N417, and negative with the carcinoid. Of the MOABS tested on those three prototype lines, therefore, 10B7 and MOCCI appear to be the most promising for future toxin or radioisotope targeting of SCLC. Other MOABS may also be useful (Stahel et al., 1990) even though they have some reactivity with PBL; they may still be less toxic than conventional chemotherapeutic agents.

IV. Comments

Although preliminary screening of MOABS with prototype cell lines is useful for identifying potentially useful reagents for clinical application, such MOABS require in vivo testing at several levels beginning with nude mice. Caution is advised regarding reactivity of MOABS with normal tissues as well as tumors (Mechtersheimer et al., 1991). Consequences of interactions between MOABS and cells cannot be predicted; the outcome of the interaction depends on the particular MOAB as well as the entire topography of the cell. The mitogenicity of CD3 MOABS is well known (Transy et al., 1989). The potential toxicity of certain MOABS to normal cells may be no worse than the present status of chemotherapeutic agents, which are cell-cycle-specific and destroy any dividing cells. One example of in vivo testing of a candidate MOAB for future patient use is provided by anti-NKH1 (Koros et al., 1987a). The anti-NKH1 MOAB not conjugated to either an immunotoxin or radioisotope has very limited efficacy in inhibiting the growth of an unusual SCLC line, SHP-77, which has biochemical features of a SCLC "classic" but the histologic features of a SCLC "variant" (Koros et al., 1991). SHP-77 is a SCLC that remains unclassified (Carbone et al., 1991). It is especially useful for emphasizing the plasticity of human tumors that evolve as they metastasize, especially during therapy (Koros, 1991). Results of treatment of nude mice bearing xenografts of SHP-77 were reported in abstract form (Koros et al., 1987a), and are given in detail in Tables 2 and 3 and Figures 1–3.

Table 2 SHP-77 Tumor Volumes (L × W × H) in mm^3 in Individual Mice[a]

Group 1 Treatment	MOAB Anti-NKH1 in RPMI 1640				
Days after tumor cell inoculation	35	40	51	56	59
Mouse 1	60	144	500	1372	1768
	324	336	3800	5280	6750
Mouse 2	245	256	840	2560	3420
	16	18	147	224	360
Mouse 3	147	245	605	1372	1800
Mouse 4	18	32	168	360	660
Mean	810/6	1031/6	6060/6	11168/6	14758
	= 135	= 172	= 1010	= 1861	
Group 2 Treatment	RPMI-1640				
Mouse 1	4	12	120	245	600
	1	6	36	75	210
Mouse 2	45	1575	7150	10800	16896
Mouse 3	128	450	2312	6072	6348
Mouse 4	280	770	2560	5148	5313
	32	210	400	1008	936
Mean	490/6	3023/6	12578/6	23348/6	30303/6
	= 82	= 504	= 2096	= 3891	= 5051

[a]Some mice had two tumors. There is great heterogeneity in tumor sizes.

Table 3 Surface Markers Identified by Flow Cytometry

	Mouse No.	Leu4[a]	Leu7[a]	Leu11[a]	Leu16[a]	T11[b]	MY7[a]	MY9[a]	4B4[b]	2H4[b]	B4[b]	Leu2a[a]	Leu3a[a]	NKH1[b]
SHP-77 xenografts	4	33	18	69	26	28	15	26	44	24	23	0	0	67
from sham-treated	5	31	40	68	38	59	51	32	69	39	36	0	0	69
nude mice	6	52	39	65	39	39	38	41	59	29	15	0	0	75
SHP-77 xenografts	0	0	52	86	52	59	59	71	16	14	8	0	0	not done
from anti-NKH1	1	0	81	84	76	72	67	74	37	28	28	0	0	55
treated	2	0	65	80	68	64	62	66	30	20	30	0	0	23
nude mice	3	0	85	93	93	82	86	81	37	29	28	0	0	37
SHP-77 cultured cells in vitro			76	88							0	0		80

[a]Monoclonal antibodies from Becton Dickinson (Mountain View, CA).
[b]Monoclonal Antibodies from Coulter Immunology (Hialeah, FL).

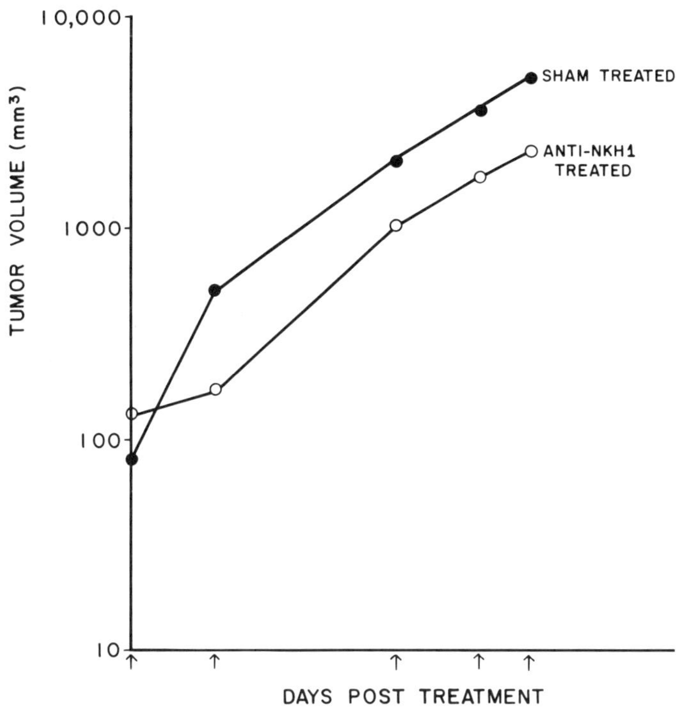

Figure 1 Effect of anti-NKH1 monoclonal antibody on growth of SHP-77 small cell carcinoma in nude mice.

To test the potential therapeutic efficacy of anti-NKH1 (Coulter Immunology), athymic nude mice (Harlan Sprague Dawley) were injected subcutaneously with 3.8×10^6 SHP-77 cells in each of two sites on the abdomen. When visible tumors appeared about 1 month after tumor cell inoculation, mice were classified randomly into two groups. One group was injected intraperitoneally weekly with 0.5 ml containing 0.2 mg of anti-NKH1 murine MOAB in RPMI 1640 cell culture medium. The other group received 0.5 ml of RPMI 1640 alone. Tumors were measured weekly and results are shown in Table 2 and Figure 1. Mice were sacrificed at 54 days after inoculation of SHP-77. Samples of xenografts were fixed in Bouin's fixative and paraffin sections were stained with hematoxylin and eosin. Aliquots of xenografts were dispersed on stainless steel wire mesh and stained with MOABS shown in Table 3 (anti-Leu 4, 3a, 2a, 11, 7, anti-NKH1, and other antileukocyte MOABS). The anti-NKH1-treated group of mice had xenografts of SHP-77 that grew slightly more slowly, were phenotypically different as defined by the MOABS panel (Table 3, Fig. 4), but were histologically indistinguishable in

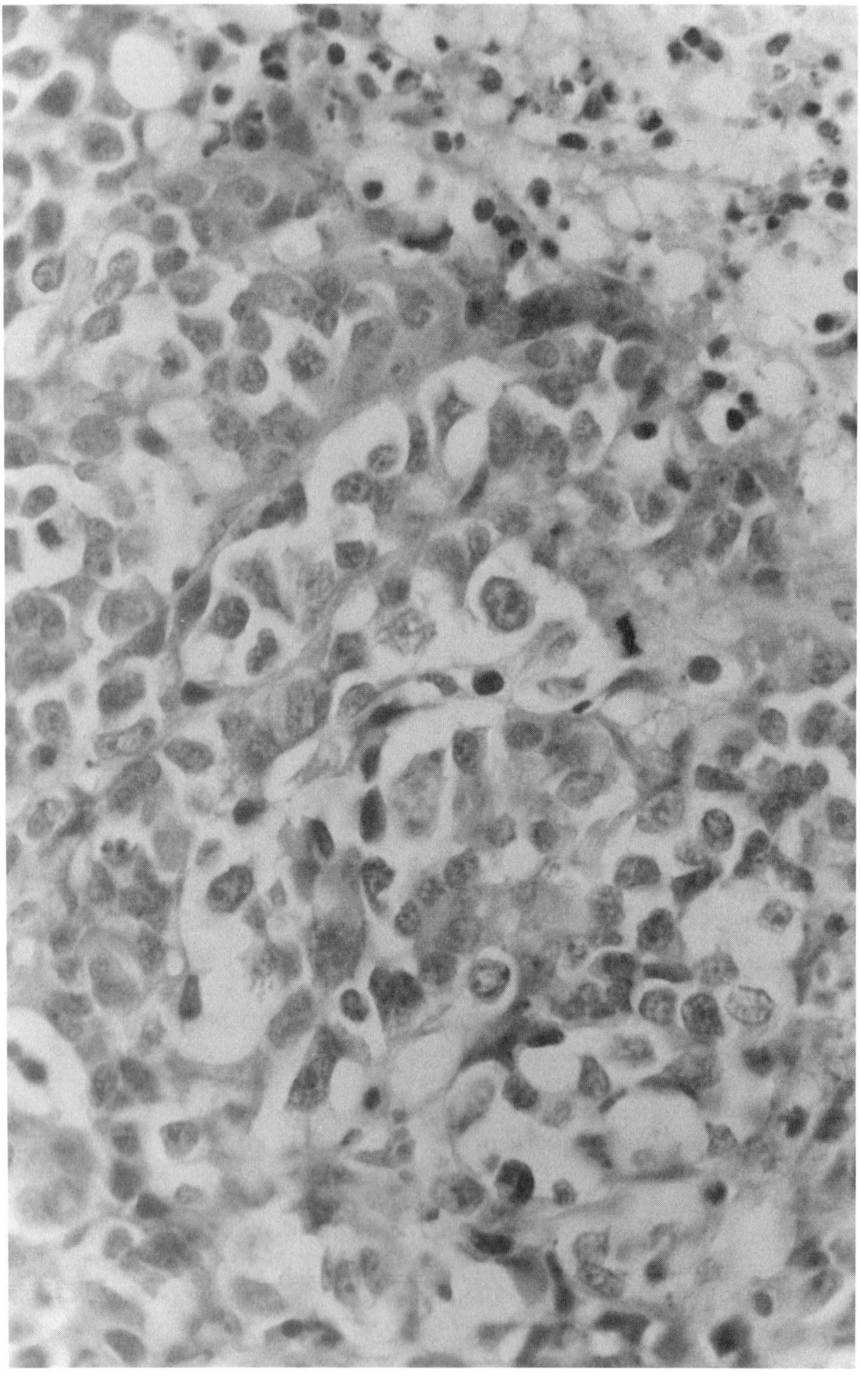

Figure 2 Xenograft from athymic nude mouse inoculated with SHP-77 cells and sham treated with RPMI-1640 tissue culture medium (hematoxylin and eosin, × 1000). Cells are arranged in nests and packets as shown earlier (Koros et al., 1985).

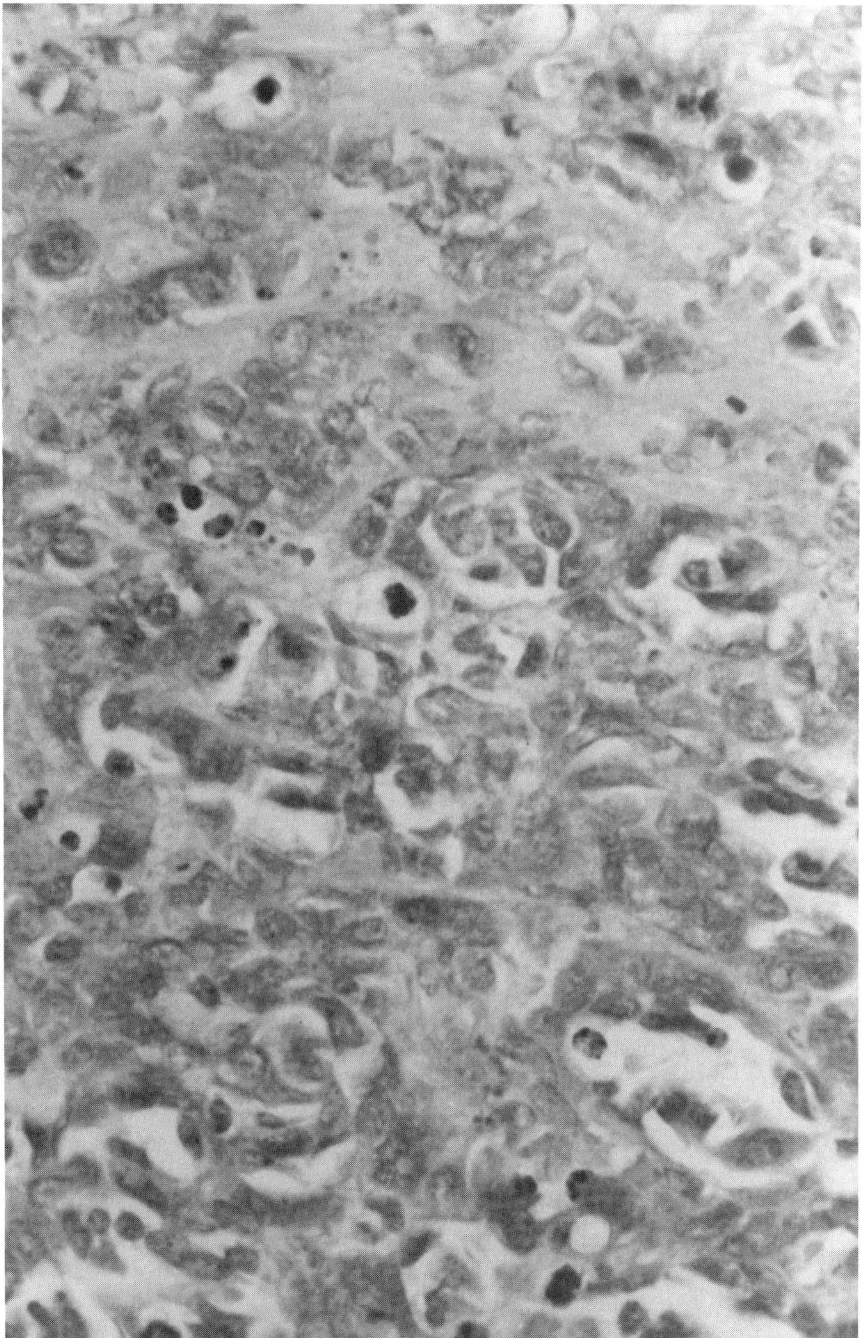

Figure 3 Xenograft from athymic nude mouse inoculated with SHP-77 cells and treated with anti-NKH1 monoclonal antibody. Histopathologic appearance is similar to that shown in Figure 2, with slightly more tissue necrosis (hematoxylin and eosin, × 1000).

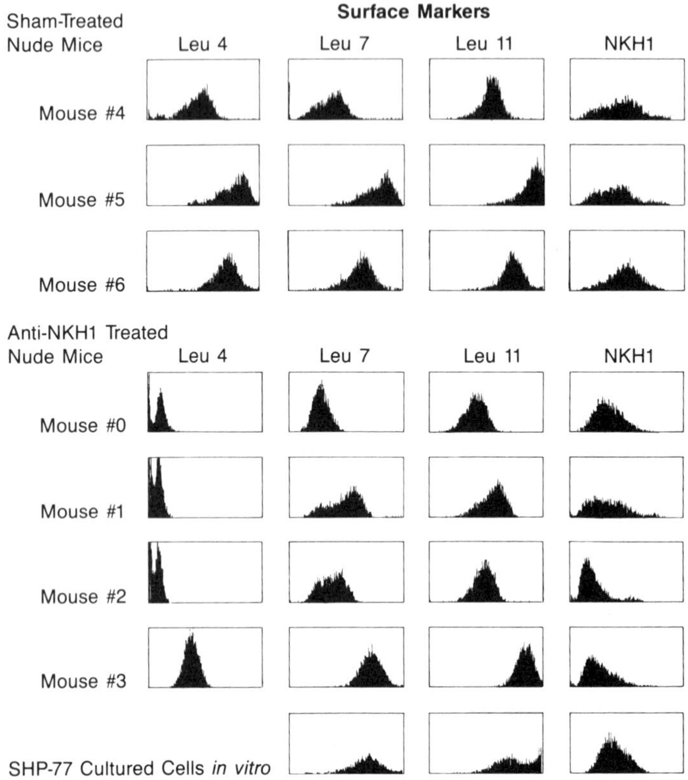

Figure 4 Surface marker expression by SHP-77 xenografts in nude mice treated with anti-NKH1 monoclonal antibody. Ordinate is cell frequency, abcissa is log fluorescence intensity. MOABS are directly conjugated to phycoerythrin except anti-Leu 7, which is conjugated to flurorescein.

Hand E sections compared with controls (Figs. 2, 3). The results show that treatment of mice with anti-NKH1 must be started early after tumor cell inoculation and should be given more frequently than once a week to inhibit tumor growth. More important, however, is that the SHP-77 study emphasizes that future extrapolation to patient treatment requires conjugation of MOABS, because unconjugated MOAB treatment is not completely effective in eliminating tumor cells. There is documented evolution and selection of phenotypically different SHP-77 cell populations in this system and presumably in patient metastases. The utility of phenotyping human tumors with panels of MOABS has limited value (Koros et al., 1988), but more specific treatment requires MOAB targeted therapy (Abrams et al., 1990; Stahel et al., 1990).

Acknowledgments

The support of The Cancer Federation, The Candle Foundation, and Dr. Monto Ho is gratefully acknowledged. We thank Dr. Rinaldo for the use of the Epics C flow cytometer, Drs. Adi Gazdar and Herb Oie for cell lines NCI-H69, NCI-N417, NCI-H727, and Dr. Edwin Fisher for SHP-77. We also thank Coulter Immunology for MOAB anti-NKH1. Preparation of the manuscript by JoEllen Walker is also appreciated.

References

Abrams, P., Salk, D., Fer, M., Fritzberg, A., and Weiden, P. (1990). Specific targeting of lung cancer using monoclonal antibodies. *Lung Cancer* **6:**(5–6), 201.

Beverley, P. C. L., Bobrow, L. G., Gilks, W., and Souhami, R. L. (1991). Second international workshop on small cell lung cancer antigens. *Br. J. Cancer* **63**(Suppl. 15)**:**1–88.

Carbone, D. P., Koros, A. M. C., Linnoila, R. I., Jewett, P., and Gazdar, A. F. (1991). Neural cell adhesion molecule expression and messenger RNA splicing patterns in lung cancer cell lines are correlated with neuroendocrine phenotype and growth morphology. *Cancer Res.* **51:**6142–6149.

Carney, D. N., Gazdar, A. F., Bepler, G., Guccion, J. G., Marangos, P. J., Moody, T. W., Zweig, M. H., and Minna, J. D. (1985). Establishment and identification of small cell lung cancer cell lines having classic and variant features. *Cancer Res.* **45:**2913–2923.

Carney, D. N., and DeLeij, L. (1988). Lung cancer biology. *Semin. Oncol.* **15:**(3), 199–214.

Deftos, L. J., Gazdar, A. F., Ikeda, K., and Broadus, A. E. (1989). The parathyroid hormone-related protein associated with malignancy is secreted by neuroendocrine tumors. *Mol. Endocrinol.* **3:**503–508.

Gazdar, A. F. (1989). Advances in the biology of lung cancer: clinical significance of neuroendocrine differentiation. *Chest* **96**(Suppl.)**:**39S–41S.

Gazdar, A. F., Carney, D. N., Nau, M. M., and Minna, J. D. (1985). Characterization of variant subclasses of cell lines derived from small cell lung cancer having distinctive biochemical, morphological, and growth properties. *Cancer Res.* **45:**2924–2930.

Gazdar, A. F., Helman, L. J., Israel, M. A., Russell, E. K., Linnoila, R. I., Mulshine, J. L., Schuller, H. M., and Park, J. (1988). Expression of neuroendocrine cell markers L-dopa decarboxylase, chromogranin A, and dense core granules in human tumors of endocrine and nonendocrine origin. *Cancer Res.* **48:**4078–4082.

Kadowaki, M. H., and Ferguson, M. K. (1990). The role of chromosome 3 deletions in lung cancer. *Lung Cancer* **6:**165–170.

Koros, A. M. C. (1991). Neuroendocrine antigen expression: practical and theoretical aspects related to lung cancers. In: *Futur Du Cancer Bronchique*. Edited by J.-L. Pujol. Nice, France, Multimed Press, pp. 15–22.

Koros, A. M. C., Atchison, R. W., and Mitchell, D. L. (1991). Small cell lung cancer antigen expression differs on "classic" and variant SCLC and carcinoid cells. *Lung Cancer* **7:**225–234.

Koros, A. M. C., and Hiserodt, J. C. (1989). Monoclonal antibodies directed against human natural killer cells react with human small cell lung-carcinoma cell lines and may have potential therapeutic value. In: *Leucocyte Typing IV*. Edited by W. Knapp et al. Oxford, Oxford University Press, pp. 709–711.

Koros, A. M. C., Klein, E. C., Pan, S., Atchison, R. W., Lakomy, R., Bahnson, A., and Sherer, C. (1985). Stability and utility of the unique human small cell carcinoma line SHP-77. *Cancer Res.* **45:**2725–2731.

Koros, A. M. C., Lange, J. H., Buffo, M. J., Dalbow, M., and Klein, E. (1987a). Anti-NKH1 (N901) monoclonal antibody's effect on oat cell (small cell) lung cancer line SHP-77's growth in nude mice. *Proc. Am. Assoc. Cancer Res.* **28:**42.

Koros, A. M. C., Taylor, M. J., Hiserodt, J. C., Stephens, B., Lakomy, R. J., Dalbow, M., Raikow, R., Lange, J., and Wagner, M. (1987b). Sea urchin coelomocytes, human peripheral blood NK cells and human small cell lung cancer lines may share evolutionarily conserved antigens NKH1 (Leu 7) and N901 (NKH1). *Leukocyte Typing III. Proceedings, Third International Workshop and Conference on Human Leukocyte Differentiation Antigens*. Edited by A. J. Michael. Oxford, Oxford University Press, pp. 866–869.

Koros, A. M. C., Lakomy, R. J., Wagner, M., Lange, J. H., Hiserodt, J. C., and Klein, E. C. (1988). Monoclonal antibodies directed against small cell carcinomas define by flow cytometry phenotypic differences among small cell and non-small cell carcinomas, neuroblastomas, and lymphoblastoid cell lines. *Lung Cancer* **4:**52–54.

Lu, C., Ikeda, K., Deftos, L. J., Gazdar, A. F., Mangin, M., and Broadus, E. D. (1989). Gluocorticoid regulation of parathyroid hormone-related peptide gene transcription in a human neuroendocrine cell line. *Mol. Endocrinol.* **3:**2034–2040.

Mechtersheimer, G., Staudter, M., and Moller, P. (1991). Expression of the natural killer cell-associated antigens CD56 and CD57 in human neural and striated muscle cells and their tumors. *Cancer Res.* **51:**1300–1307.

Pujol, J. L., Simony, J., Laurent, J.-C. Richer, G., Mary, H., Bousquet, J., Godard, P., and Michel, F.-B. (1989). Phenotypic heterogeneity studied by immunohistochemistry and aneuploidy in non-small cell lung cancers. *Cancer Res.* **49:**2797–2802.

Stahel, R. A., Wawrzynczak, E., Collinson, A., Zangemeister, U., Lehmann, H. P., and Waibel, R. (1990). Immunotoxins for small cell lung cancer: results of in vitro investigations. *Lung Cancer* **6:**(5–6)198.

Transy, C., Moingeon, P. E., Marshall, B., Stebbins, C., and Reinherz, E. L. (1989). Most murine anti human CD3 MAB recognize the human CD3 subunit. In: *Leucocyte Typing IV*. Edited by W. Knapp et al. Oxford, Oxford University Press, pp. 293–295.

PART IV

SCREENING, DIAGNOSIS, AND MONITORING OF LUNG CANCER

14

Reversal of Preneoplastic Changes in Upper-Respiratory Epithelium

SCOTT M. LIPPMAN and WAUN K. HONG

The University of Texas M. D. Anderson Cancer Center
Houston, Texas

I. Introduction

Cancer chemoprevention—the inhibition or reversal of carcinogenesis (primarily in the preneoplastic phase) by specific chemical compounds—is an important complement to other cancer-control approaches (Sporn, 1976). This new field brings together basic scientists, epidemiologists, behavioral scientists, nutritionists, statisticians, and clinical investigators interested in carcinogenesis and cancer prevention (Greenwald et al., 1986).

II. Preclinical Studies

In vitro and in vivo model systems are used to screen for new chemopreventive agents (or combinations) and for mechanistic studies. The 7,12-dimethylbenz[a]-anthracene- (DMBA)-induced hamster buccal pouch (oral carcinogenesis) model has greatly influenced clinical trial designs in upper respiratory epithelial cancer chemoprevention. Various retinoids, β-carotene, and vitamin E are active in this system (Lippman and Hong, 1991).

Most of the preclinical work focused on the retinoids (potent regulators of cellular differentiation), which are the best studied and prototypical class of chemopreventive agents (Bollag, 1983; Lippman et al., 1987; Sporn and Roberts, 1984). Recent data suggest that retinoic acid regulates cell growth and differentiation at the level of gene expression by means of nuclear retinoic acid receptors (Blomhoff et al., 1990; Evans, 1988). To date, the genes for three receptors have been cloned and found to be homologous to the steroid/thyroid/vitamin D hormone-receptor family. The homology is most striking in the zinc-finger region (DNA-binding domain). The different nuclear receptors have different binding affinities, chromosomal locations, and tissue distributions. The significance of these patterns is under intense study. There is currently great interest in the possibility that rearrangements in retinoic acid receptor genes may be associated with carcinogenesis. For example, the 15;17 translocation in acute promyelocytic leukemia was recently found to occur within the α-receptor gene (de The et al., 1990). Recent work suggests that the β receptor, which is located at 3p14-24 (the site of a putative tumor-suppressor gene), may play an important role in human lung and head and neck carcinogenesis. Many issues remain unresolved regarding this new area, for example, the role of cytoplasmic receptors (which may function either to shuttle or compete with retinoic acid binding to the nuclear receptors) and the relationship between nuclear retinoic acid receptor message (mRNA) levels and retinoid response.

An important new area of carcinogenesis research is the study of preneoplasia and multistep epithelial transformation. Neoplasias of the upper respiratory epithelium and lung are linked by a process of "field cancerization": the repeated exposure of a region's entire tissue area to carcinogenic insult (e.g., tobacco), which increases the tissue's risk for developing multiple independent preneoplastic and neoplastic foci (Lippman and Hong, 1989). Recent data suggest that epithelial neoplastic transformation arises when specific genetic alterations occur and that primary tumors and second primary tumors may involve both common and distinct genetic changes. Chemoprevention may slow the accumulation of new genetic alterations and/or reregulate the phenotypic changes resulting from genetic events.

III. Pharmacokinetic and Toxicity Studies

Pharmacokinetic studies in chemoprevention trials are critical for monitoring compliance, target-tissue drug levels, and drug interactions (Plezia et al., 1989). The lack of pharmacologic data may have compromised many early trials. This issue is best illustrated with β-carotene: the first pharmacokinetic study was reported in 1988, many years after the initiation of many phase III trials that used this agent at differing and empiric doses and schedules (Dimitrov et al., 1988).

A delicate balance exists between efficacy and toxicity in chemoprevention, informed by the degree of risk. The magnitude of this issue is far greater in chemoprevention than chemotherapy, reflecting the difference between risk and survival, respectively. Although retinoids are the only agents proved to reduce cancer incidence significantly in humans, they have well-described side effects, primarily dose-dependent, reversible mucocutaneous dryness (Lippman et al., 1987). Other promising agents with essentially no toxicity have yet to be proven effective. The major concern with synthetic retinoids is their teratogenic effect.

IV. Clinical Studies

After decades of intense study, uncertainty, cautious optimism, and hope, cancer chemoprevention is now coming of age (Meyskens 1990). Recent positive reports in skin and upper respiratory epithelial cancers established significant site- and drug-specific prevention of invasive cancer in extremely high risk groups (Hong et al., 1990; Kraemer et al., 1988). Chemoprevention trials focus on populations with a spectrum of cancer risk, ranging from the general population to patients with preneoplastic lesions and those at high risk of second primary tumors. Acceptable toxicity will vary with this wide range of cancer risk. Difficult issues of agent(s) selection exist, often based primarily on epidemiologic data. The case for β-carotene is most complex, since even if "carotenoids" have anticarcinogenic activity, it may be impossible to sort out which of the numerous carotenoids are critical. Furthermore, there is no strong scientific basis for the selection of dose and duration of therapy that can be derived from these epidemiologic studies.

A. Tobacco-Related Cancers: Upper Aerodigestive Tract and Lung

The strength of the clinical and biological rationale for developing effective chemopreventive strategies for upper and lower respiratory tract neoplasia is seen in the disproportionate number of phase III trials devoted to these cancers. The clinical importance of developing effective chemoprevention for these epithelial tumors is illustrated by the National Cancer Institute (NCI) SEER data, which indicate that cancers of the head and neck, esophagus, and lung (linked by the tobacco-related field cancerization process) account for one-fifth of all cancers and one-third of all cancer deaths in this country (Boring et al., 1991). These clinical facts, the promising preclinical data, the well-described risk factors, and the biology of the multistep epithelial carcinogenic process support the study of pharmacologic intervention strategies for upper respiratory and lung cancer chemoprevention.

1. Oral Preneoplasia

Leukoplakia is a clinical descriptive term that includes any white patch in the oral cavity that cannot be removed by scraping, reversed by the removal of local irritants, or classified as due to any other specific disease (Silverman, 1988). Leukoplakia is classified as a preneoplastic lesion in part because of its epidemiologic, geographic, and causative similarities to oral cancer and frequent occurrence adjacent to squamous cell carcinoma (median >30%; range, 10–100%). Red (erythroplasia) or speckled sites within lesions are highly associated with dysplastic epithelium. Standard management is close follow-up or surgical excision. Resectability often is limited by lesion extent or location. Furthermore, local therapy does not ameliorate the multifocal carcinogenic process. Effective chemoprevention, therefore, would benefit a significant number of patients with oral premalignancy.

Histologic assessment is critically important since even pure white lesions can be associated with severe dysplasia or even frankly invasive squamous cell carcinoma. Large studies from Silverman and others indicate that hyperplastic lesions are associated with low (<5%) transformation rates, whereas dysplastic lesions (only 10–15% of all leukoplakias) are associated with 10-fold higher rates of transformation (Silverman et al., 1984). These data indicate the variable natural history of this preneoplastic disorder, which is why rigorous histologically documented randomized trials are required to differentiate drug effects from naturally occurring changes. These features further underscore two issues critical to oral chemoprevention trials: first, all clinical "premalignant" lesions must be evaluated histologically; second, to establish drug efficacy, randomized trials must be stratified by histologic characteristics to control for lesions' variable natural histories. In clinical trials, we use the term "oral premalignancy" to refer to the clinical spectrum of lesions defined above, with further classification and stratification based on histologic differences.

The many characteristics of oral preneoplasia—tobacco-related, precursor of squamous cell carcinoma, easily monitored, preclinical models—make it an ideal human in vivo system for the study of chemopreventive and adjuvant agents with potential in other tobacco-related epithelial neoplastic disorders. Oral premalignancy chemoprevention studies already have contributed to the design of a retinoid trial that achieved the suppression of second primary tumors in patients with head and neck cancer.

Upper respiratory cancer chemoprevention programs have focused on retinoids and carotenoids. Stich et al. (1984) studied β-carotene and vitamin A in a series of novel intervention studies in high-risk groups (e.g., betel nut chewers) in India and the Philippines. These investigators were the first to integrate micronuclei frequency (a marker of acute carcinogenic/clastogenic exposure) into chemoprevention trials. Their data indicate that site-specific expression of micronuclei frequency correlates with target-site cancer risk; β-carotene and vitamin A, given alone or in combination, significantly suppress oral micronuclei frequency in high-risk subjects; and canthaxanthin (a synthetic carotenoid with effective electron-scavenging activity, but which is not converted to vitamin A) has no effect on micronuclei frequency. The micronuclei data led to a series of small trials in Asian betel nut chewers testing β-carotene alone or in combination with vitamin A in clinically monitored preneoplastic lesions (Stich et al., 1988). Compared with β-carotene alone, the vitamin A/β-carotene combination produced a twofold higher clinical response and twofold lower rate of new lesion development. During the 6 month β-carotene intervention, the rates of new lesion resolution and of new lesion development were identical (14%) and not significantly different from placebo rates.

To date, the published β-carotene data in oral leukoplakia are limited to five nonrandomized series with mixed results: overall response rates of >70% with 30 mg/day for 3 months contrast with a response rate of <30% with more dose-intensive regimens (90–120 mg/day for 3–6 months) (Wolf et al., 1991). In contrast to the synthetic retinoid trials, no drug-related toxicities occurred in these natural agent trials at the dosages used.

These pilot studies were small, nonrandomized, and their results were not confirmed histologically. Therefore, it is difficult to interpret the limited natural agent results reported thus far. Proving the efficacy of these nontoxic natural agents in a histologically documented, randomized phase III trial in oral premalignancy would have great significance for the control of oral cancer and major implications for the control of other epithelial tobacco-related cancer.

13-*cis*-Retinoic acid is the only agent proved effective in randomized trials of oral preneoplasia as high-dosage induction and as low-dosage maintenance therapy. Several synthetic retinoids at daily dosages of 1 mg/kg/day or greater have produced objective response rates in leukoplakia of 60–90% (Lippman et al., 1987). Hong et al. (1986) reported the only randomized, placebo-controlled retinoid trial in oral leukoplakia, which confirmed the positive results of the earlier, nonrandomized studies. The clinical objective response rate in this high-dosage 13-*cis*-retinoic acid trial (1–2 mg/kg/day) was 67% in the treated group, compared to only 10% in the placebo group ($p = 0.002$). This study was the first to assess all patients histologically before and after therapy. A highly significant finding in this study was the reversal of dysplasia in 54% of the retinoid-treated patients. The two major problems with this short-term study were the notable side effects of 13-*cis*-retinoic acid (mucocutaneous dryness, hypertriglyceridemia) and a relapse rate of over 50% within 2–3 months of discontinuation of therapy.

The high relapse rates noted in essentially all the preclinical and clinical chemoprevention studies led to trials of maintenance therapy following established short-term induction therapy. Hong's randomized 9-month maintenance trial indicated that low-dosage 13-*cis*-retinoic acid (0.5 mg/kg/day) is well tolerated and more effective than β-carotene as monitored by clinical, histologic, and biomarker (micronuclei frequency) data (Wolf et al., 1991).

2. *Adjuvant Retinoid Trial*

Recent results from Hong's randomized, placebo-controlled adjuvant trial of high-dosage 13-*cis*-retinoic acid in head and neck cancer (stage I–IV, M_0) are extremely important. With its rationale primarily in the positive oral preneoplasia data, this adjuvant study of over 100 patients with a median follow up of 3 years detected a highly significant suppression of second primary tumors (Hong et al., 1990). It is instructive that more than 80% of the second primary tumors occurred in the epithelial field at risk (head and neck, esophagus, or lung) and that multiple second primary tumors developed only in the placebo group. The significant retinoid effect on second primary tumor development is even more convincing when the high toxicity-related dropout rate in the treatment arm is considered.

That second primary tumors in head and neck cancer develop at a constant rate of 3–6% per year, that they account for an overall excess mortality of 6–9% per year, and that they are the major cause of death after early-stage presentation are important points of rationale in these studies (Lippman and Hong, 1989). Given the positive data from their high-dosage adjuvant trial and low-dosage oral premalignancy chemoprevention trials, Hong's group has recently designed a multicenter, randomized, placebo-controlled, chemoprevention study of low-dosage 13-*cis*-retinoic acid in more than 1,000 patients with early-stage head and neck cancer rendered disease free by local therapy. Second primary tumor development is the primary study endpoint.

V. Biological Marker Studies

A novel area of study is the role of biological markers both for early detection (screening) and as intermediate endpoints for chemoprevention trials (Lippman et al., 1990). Promising intermediate markers under study in epithelial neoplasia include genomic markers (micronuclei, DNA-adducts, differentially expressed genes); differentiation markers (cytokeratins [K1,K6,K13], involucrin, blood group antigens); growth-regulatory factors (epidermal growth factor receptor, transforming growth factor [TGF]-β; and proliferation markers (polyamines, proliferating cell nuclear antigen, PCNA). Promising early results have already been seen with markers of clastogenic damage and of dysregulated proliferation in studies of high-risk esophageal, colon, head and neck, and lung tissue (Lippman and Hong, 1991). This work is in its infancy, however, and no marker has yet been validated in the context of a chemoprevention trial with the definitive endpoint of invasive cancer. A major direction in the 1990s will be the development and validation of very sensitive biological markers of early and specific events in the multistage process of carcinogenesis; for example, Vogelstein et al. (1988) recently described the dynamic interaction of specific amplification or activation of oncogenes and deletion of suppressor genes in human colon cancer development.

VI. Perspective

Upper respiratory tract and lung epithelial carcinogenesis is an ideal model for the development of chemoprevention strategies given the lack of effective therapy and the shared biological features of cancers in these regions. Upper aerodigestive tract research, both clinical and basic, is becoming a model for research into other epithelial cancers. Current work is focusing on the study of epithelial carcinogenesis and its associated biochemical and molecular alterations and the basic mechanisms of anticarcinogenic activity of chemopreventive agents.

Extensive mechanistic, preclinical, and early clinical data strongly support the chemopreventive efficacy of retinoids and β-carotene in aerodigestive tract epithelial cancers. Preliminary results indicate that it may be possible to reverse the multistep process of tobacco-related carcinogenesis in the respiratory epithelium, halting the progression of premalignant tissue toward often-fatal malignancy and restoring it to normal.

References

Blomhoff, R., Green, M. H., Berg, T., and Norum, K. R. (1990). Transport and storage of vitamin A. *Science* **250:**399–404.

Bollag, W. (1983). Vitamin A and retinoids from nutrition to pharmacotherapy in dermatology and oncology. *Lancet* **1:**860–863.

Boring, C. C., Squires, T. S., and Tong, T. (1991). Cancer statistics, 1991. *CA* **41:**19–36.

de The, H., Chomienne, C., Lanotte, M., Degos, L., and Dejean, A. (1990). The t(15;17) translocation of acute promyelocytic leukemia fuses the retinoic acid receptor α gene to a novel transcribed locus. *Nature* **347:**558–561.

Dimitrov, N. V., Meyer, C., Ullrey, D. E., Ruppenthal, M., Chenoweth W., and Malone, W. (1988). Bioavailability of beta-carotene in humans. *Am. J. Clin. Nutr.* **48:**293–304.

Evans, R. M. (1988). The steroid and thyroid hormone receptor superfamily. *Science* **240:** 889–895.

Greenwald, P., Sondik, E., and Lynch, B. S. (1986). Diet and chemoprevention in NCI research strategy to achieve national cancer control objectives. *Annu. Rev. Public Health* **7:**267–291.

Hong, W. K., Endicott, J., Itri, L. M., Doos, W., Batsakis, J. G., Bell, R., Fofonoff, S., Byers, R., Atkinson, E. N., and Vaughan, C. (1980). 13-*cis*-retinoic acid in the treatment of oral leukoplakia. *N. Engl. J. Med.* **315:**1501–1505.

Hong, W. K., Lippman, S. M., Itri, L. M., Karp, D. D., Lee, J. S., Byers, R. M., Schantz,

S. P., Kramer, A. M., Lotan, R., and Peters, L. J. (1990). Prevention of second primary tumors with isotretinoin in squamous cell carcinoma of the head and neck. *N. Engl. J. Med.* **323:**795–801.

Kraemer, K. H., DiGiovanna, J. J., Moshell, A. N., Tarone, R. E., and Peck, G. L. (1988). Prevention of skin cancer in xeroderma pigmentosum with the use of oral isotretinoin. *N. Engl. J. Med.* **318:**1633–1637.

Lippman, S. M., and Hong, W. K. (1989). Second malignant tumors in head and neck squamous cell carcinoma: the overshadowing threat for patients with early-stage disease (editorial). *Int. J. Radiat. Oncol. Biol. Phys.* **17:**691–694.

Lippman, S. M., and Hong, W. K. (1991). Differentiation therapy for head and neck cancer. In: *Multimodality Therapy for Head and Neck Cancer*. Edited by G. Snow and J. R. Clark. New York, Springer Verlag.

Lippman, S. M., Kessler, J. F., and Meyskens, F. L. Jr. (1987). Retinoids as preventive and therapeutic anticancer agents. *Cancer Treat. Rep.* **71:**391–405, 493–515.

Lippman, S. M., Lee, J. S., Lotan, R., Hittelman, W., Wargovich, M. J., and Hong, W. K. (1990). Biomarkers as intermediate endpoints in chemoprevention trials. *J. Natl. Cancer Inst.* **82:**555–560.

Meyskens, F. L., Jr. (1990). Coming of age—the chemoprevention of cancer. *N. Engl. J. Med.* **323:**825–827.

Plezia, P. M., Alberts, D. S., Peng, Y. M., Xu, M. J., Sayers, S., Davis, T. P., Surwit, E. A., and Meyskens, F. L. (1989). The role of serum and tissue pharmacology studies in the design and interpretation of chemoprevention trials. *Prev. Med.* **18:**680–687.

Silverman, S. (1988). Early diagnosis of oral cancer. *Cancer* **62:**1796–1799.

Silverman, S., Jr., Gorsky, M., and Lozada, F. (1984). Oral leukoplakia and malignant transformation: a follow-up study of 257 patients. *Cancer* **53:**563–568.

Sporn, M. (1976). Approaches to prevention of epithelial cancer during the preneoplastic period. *Cancer Res.* **36:**2699–2702.

Sporn, M. B., and Roberts, A. B. (1984). Role of retinoids in differentiation and carcinogenesis. *J. Natl. Cancer Inst.* **73:**1381–1386.

Stich, H. F., Rosin, M. P., and Vallejera, M. O. (1984). Reduction with vitamin A and beta-carotene administration of proportion of micronucleated buccal mucosal cells in Asian betel nut and tobacco chewers. *Lancet* **1:**1204–1206.

Stich, H. F., Rosin, M. P., Hornby, A. P., Mathew, B., Sankaranarayanan, R., and Nair, M. K. (1988). Remission of oral leukoplakias and micronuclei in tobacco/betel quid chewers treated with beta-carotene and with beta-carotene plus vitamin A. *Int. J. Cancer* **42:**195–199.

Vogelstein, B., Fearon, E. R., Hamilton, S. R., Kern, S. E. Preisinger, A. C., Leppert, M., Nakamura, Y., White, R., Smith, A. M., and Bos, J. L. (1988). Genetic alterations during colorectal-tumor development. *N. Engl. J. Med.* **319:**525–532.

Wolf, G., Lippman, S. M., Laramore, G., and Hong, W. K. (1991). Head and neck cancer. In: *Cancer Medicine*, 3rd ed. Edited by J. F. Holland, E. Frei, R. C. Bast Jr., D. W. Kufe, D. L. Morton, and R. Weichselbaum. Philadelphia, Lea & Febiger.

15

Considerations in Population-Based Screening for the Early Detection of Lung Cancer

JAMES L. MULSHINE

National Cancer Institute
Bethesda, Maryland

MELVYN S. TOCKMAN

The Johns Hopkins School of Hygiene and Public Health
Baltimore, Maryland

I. Lung Cancer Screening: How Do We Get There?

Lung cancer is, at the same time, the most common preventable and most common lethal malignancy in our society (Silverberg et al., 1990). This paradox reflects both the significant addictive quality intrinsic to the habit of smoking cigarettes and the unparalleled profitability of the cigarette industry. Despite intensive, sustained research and application of state-of-the-art treatment, the diagnosis of lung cancer is still associated with a near 90% mortality rate. The net result is a societal tragedy of mind-numbing dimension, as summarized in Table 1 (Sibison, 1990; Council on Scientific Affairs, 1990; National Cancer Institute Annual Cancer Statistics Review, 1988). The simple economic cost of the annual medical care for patients with smoking-related diseases is estimated to be $62 billion in the United States alone. In the current fiscal environment of shrinking health care resources, the magnitude of this problem mandates fresh scrutiny for prevention-

The opinions and assertions herein are the private views of the authors and are not to be construed as official or as reflecting the views of the Department of Health and Human Services.

Table 1 Dimensions of Lung Cancer Problem

1 Billion persons consumed 5 trillion cigarettes in 1986
2.5 Million cigarette-induced deaths annually in the world
United States is world's leading exporter of tobacco
Nearly 150,000 lung cancer deaths projected for 1990 in the United States

based approaches to this disease. The Surgeon General's report (1989) recently outlined a number of proposals to reduce the practice of smoking. Unfortunately, while lung cancer risk declines with time following smoking cessation, lung cancer rates will remain elevated for the remainder of their lives in persons who previously smoked. Therefore, renewed efforts at lung cancer early detection are also required. We recently reviewed the history of early detection approaches in this disease and suggested that certain diagnostic tools were appropriate for evaluation as markers of the development of early lung cancer.

The clinical experience with early detection of two other malignancies, cervical and breast cancer, suggests that in the development of a lung cancer screening program, it is prudent to consider the entire screening process, including steps beyond the development and validation of a useful early detection tool. Given the availability of effective cervical cancer screening tools, why do not all women comply with recommended screening recommendations? As many as 20% of cervical Pap test results are thought to be inaccurate due to technical failure. Why does this failure rate exist? Nevertheless, technical failure alone does not explain the low acceptance of cervical Pap smear screening. In this chapter we will consider issues related to the development of effective early lung cancer detection programs from the published experience with breast and cervical cancer. This discussion includes identifying the components of a screening program and then considering the barriers to screening implementation. Finally, we will review preliminary efforts to develop and validate a sputum immunocytologic approach to lung cancer screening. The goal of this effort is to stimulate thought and ultimately action in developing a more adaptive management strategy to combat the overwhelming clinical problem of lung cancer.

II. Chest-X-Ray-Based Screening

Consideration of radiographic lung cancer screening began in the 1950s with the chest photofluorogram. This type of x-ray technology has since been supplemented by higher-resolution, lower-radiation techniques. Nevertheless, this primitive radiographic technology (in three controlled trials) permitted detection of 60% of the observed lung cancer cases (Tockman et al., 1985, Mulshine et al.,

1989). The remaining 40% of lung cancer cases were found between the 6 month screening intervals during the evaluation of symptomatic individuals. A later (Lilienfeld et al., 1966) study that incorporated state-of-the-art 14 × 17 mm chest x-ray (120 kVP stereo posterior–anterior views; double reading) plus sputum cytology detected 63% of the lung cancer cases with screening. The prevailing sentiment when the National Cancer Institute-sponsored early lung cancer detection trial began was that chest x-ray alone was not sufficiently sensitive as a screening tool. Incorporation of sputum cytology with chest x-ray was considered based on the seminal work of Saccomanno and co-workers (1970, 1974). The combination of the two screening tools was evaluated at the three institutions (Johns Hopkins University, Memorial Sloan Kettering, Mayo Clinic) that conducted the NCI collaborative trial (Berlin et al., 1984; Bailar, 1984a).

The outcome of the randomized NCI-sponsored chest x-ray and sputum cytology study has been extensively discussed in the literature. The use of screening in these trials resulted in an improvement in the detection of cancer at an early stage, increased surgical resectability rate, and reduced postoperative stages of cancer, as well as increased 5 year survival in the screened cohort compared to controls. However, long-term follow up showed that death due to lung cancer was not significantly reduced among the group screened by both cytology and x-ray compared to the control group screened by chest x-ray alone. The basis of this apparently paradoxical outcome was summarized in a thoughtful editorial by Dr. Bailar (1984b) published with the initial reports of the trial. A number of complex issues were identified. The first is the concept of misclassification, in which screening detects lesions such as carcinoma in situ. If an indolent in situ cancer were not to progress to an invasive cancer, the value of screening/detection of such a lesion would not be beneficial.

Another possible explanation of the failure of previous screening programs to reduce lung cancer mortality is the potential influence of a lead-time bias. This possibility arises when detection and treatment of a cancer do not reduce age-specific cancer mortality. An example of lead-time bias might be an apparent stage I, surgically resected lung cancer in which the patient later experiences a solitary, distant metastasis. In that circumstance there may be an increased duration of known disease with early detection but without increased patient survival or delay in the age at death.

A final concern is that indolent cancers, which are associated with a slower progression and prolonged natural history, would be more frequently detected by screening, especially at the initial screening (length-biased sampling). In contrast to a patient with a "benign" lesion misclassified as malignant, a patient with indolent cancer would ultimately die of lung cancer. The apparent benefit associated with length-biased sampling is in reality due to the natural history of the more slowly growing tumors rather than to a uniform benefit of the screening and intervention procedures. With serial screenings the influence of length-biased sampling would be diminished. All three of these factors may have affected the preliminary analysis of the NCI-sponsored early detection trial.

Bailar went on to point out that the NCI-sponsored trial took 15 years to conduct and analyze. During that period the screening technology used was the technology that was available at the beginning of the study and did not reflect any improvements in technology during the study's continuance. The enormous cost of such an effort (which, in the example of the NCI-sponsored trial, was $25 million) imposes constraints. The cost reflects both the large number of subjects required to demonstrate a significant screening-related improvement in survival and the services of many types of professionals. Bailar points out that high-level interaction of biostatisticians, epidemiologists, radiologists, cytopathologists, surgical pathologists, thoracic surgeons, and internists is required for early detection-based clinical trials. Whichever discipline is weakest can become the limiting factor in the success of the study. With even this brief synopsis of Dr. Bailar's editorial, the complex and demanding process of design, execution, and analysis of a trial to validate a screening study is apparent. From the experience with two other validated cancer screening tools, additional limitations in a screening program development and implementation became apparent.

III. Issues in the Historical Development of Cervical and Breast Cancer Screening

More than 20 years ago, Wilson and Junger (1968) provided a basis for determining the essential features of a general population screening program for the World Health Organization. More than 15 years have passed since the 1974 American Thoracic Society Workshop on Screening Programs used these WHO criteria to define the circumstances under which a mass screening program should (or should not) be undertaken (Tockman et al., 1983).

A mass screening program to establish a diagnosis in individuals is not warranted unless there is indisputable scientific evidence that a direct relationship (preferably one to one) exists between the abnormalities to be measured and the definitive disease. The natural history of the disease must also be beneficially modified by therapeutic intervention or by removal of risk factors at the stage of disease identified by screening.

The screening programs for cervical and breast cancer have met these criteria, thereby ensuring the scientific rigor of the programs. Nevertheless, successful application of a valid biomarker to an acceptable program of public mass screening requires the consideration of additional issues.

The relevant issues restricting effective implementation of cervical cancer screening despite the general acceptance of the benefit of this measure are

Table 2 Experience with Papanicolaou Test for Cervical Cancer Screening

Established as clinically beneficial in the 1940s
Screening error rate: approximately 25% under routine conditions
Unresolved issues: optimal specimen acquisition, quality control procedures, interpretation, and subsequent management

summarized in Table 2. Cervical cancer detection with cytologic evaluation was first broadly recognized in the early 1940s. Despite enormous enthusiasm for this approach, the benefit of cervical cytology has never been substantiated in a definitive clinical trial. In a thoughtful review, Dr. Koss (1989) recently outlined the logistical problems associated with obtaining, processing, and interpreting specimens. In contrast to the clinical validation of a suspicious cytologic smear by examination of a histologic specimen, none of these logistical elements of mass cervical cytology screening has been optimized and then formally validated statistically. Many women and surprisingly many physicians seem unaware of these concerns. The issue of cost and the vagaries of establishing guidelines for screening in regard to appropriate study populations and frequency of evaluation are unresolved. These issues have become concerns of national health policy bodies, but the available data are incomplete and static, which impedes making adaptive decisions (Eddy, 1990). These issues are complex, interactive, and dynamic, presenting a daunting analytical challenge.

In contrast to cervical cancer screening, the value of breast cancer screening has been documented in a definitive randomized trial (Shapiro, 1988). In Table 3 issues related to breast cancer screening are considered. Effective population-based screening involves other issues, including the proportion of target populations willing to avail themselves of regular evaluation. Considerably less than half of susceptible women are evaluated with breast or cervical cancer screening at recommended screening intervals. A variety of economic, social, and psychological issues underlying this behavior have been identified (Dodd, 1988; Council on Scientific Affairs, 1989). Steps to overcome barriers to participation emerge as a critical issue. The impact on reduction in overall cancer mortality that may result from early detection programs is greatly diminished when less than 30% of a target population participates in regular screening evaluations.

Table 3 Breast Cancer Screening Experience

Established benefit of mammography in randomized trial
Suboptimal compliance rate (30%) related to cost, fear, and education level
Alternative model: the British National experience

Table 4 British Model of Breast Cancer Control

Comprehensive application to all at-risk populations
Integrated clinical management for the various screening outcomes
Built-in methodologic validation procedures
Continuing review with dynamic process to accommodate feedback

IV. British Breast Cancer Screening Experience

Many of these methodologic concerns have been addressed in a remarkable effort at comprehensive breast cancer screening mounted by the British National Health Service (Table 4). This effort is evolving, but it began with an invitation to all women age 50–64 years to receive a single oblique-view mammogram (Forrest, 1990), every third year. This effort also provided the necessary ancillary medical support personnel and resources to permit appropriate follow-up management. A critical evaluation of the actual level of support required to optimize care was made during this study. A number of quality assurance and other validation tools were developed to refine the process of breast cancer screening. While it is too early to declare the success of these measures, there are a number of hopeful early signs. Most provocative is that this effort uses a technique that may be considered suboptimal for mammographic screening. The power of comprehensive screening application potentially overcomes the deficiencies of a less than perfect biomarker. While this should not be construed as a justification of using less than the optimal screening modality, it does emphasize the importance of optimizing program design and screening implementation.

V. Relevance of Screening Approaches to Lung Cancer

In a (noncurrent) prospective analysis, binding of tumor-associated monoclonal antibodies to dysplastic bronchial epithelial cells shed into the sputum of smokers was associated with a very high predictive accuracy (90%) 2 years before the diagnosis of lung cancer using conventional techniques (including screening by annual chest x-ray and conventional sputum cytology as well as symptomatic clinical presentation) (Tockman et al., 1988). One of the two antibodies used for this analysis was found to bind to the carbohydrate structure, difucosylated Lewis X (Kogashima et al., 1989). This is a member of a class of immunodominant carbohydrate structures that function to provide important differentiation signals in fetal organogenesis (Hakamori, 1986). The work of Fukushi and others suggests the potential for more broadly evaluating the pattern of carbohydrate expression from relevant visceral epithelium to define the stage of malignant progression (or the state of retrodifferentiation) that has occurred in the epithelium of an individual and to relate that phenotype to a defined level of risk for cancer (Fukushi et al., 1989; Mulshine et al., 1990a).

The many basic molecular events that have been described for the early steps of lung carcinogenesis may also find clinical application as signatures of the cellular transformation of the bronchial epithelium and may complement surface antigen phenotyping as indicators of epithelial cell transformation. We have recently reviewed a range of biomarkers that may someday be considered for early detection assays (Mulshine et al., 1990a,b; Gazdar et al., 1990). Immunostaining of sputum cells is currently undergoing extensive evaluation as an early detection technique. As in the case of clinical tests of physiological function, interpretation of the presence of cellular immunomarkers depends upon establishing the source of variation of interest (the signal) compared to all other sources of variation (the noise) (Becklake, 1986). Noise may arise from technical variation in the assay due to biologic variation in the degree of cytologic atypia of the host. Refinements in this approach are being considered to adapt this assay for screening applications. A partial list of these refinements is shown in Table 5. The composition of the list is strongly influenced by the previously discussed experiences with developing cervical and breast cancer screening approaches. Recently developed automated immunostaining instruments help to standardize specimen analysis by eliminating the batch-to-batch staining variation often seen with the manual approach. Adaptation of computer-integrated image analysis systems to quantitate the outcome of immunocytochemical assays will improve the reproducibility of the sputum immunostaining. This process has evolved rapidly with the incorporation of new imaging technologies. Biomarker signal identification depends upon selection of those (spectral, spatial, optical density, and texture) features of the immunoprobe found to correlate, in prospectively collected clinical specimens, with the subsequent development of cancer (Tockman et al., 1991). Neuronal programming or other state-of-the-art computer-analyzed imaging technologies may find practical application in differentiating immunostain-positive bronchial epithelial cells from the multitude of artifacts that can occur in sputum immunocytologic preparations. The integration of new technology will need to be accompanied by rigorous

Table 5 Elements to Refine for a Lung Cancer Screening Approach

Refine antibody panel for immunocytochemistry analysis
Standardize sputum acquisition
Standardize staining procedures
Automate staining interpretation

validation in clinical trials to ensure that computer-assisted, quantitative analyses of specific parameters conform in a predictable way to the ultimate development of lung cancer in a screened population. If standardized, automated procedures can be developed from the complex function of immunostaining analysis, the reproducibility and hence the credibility of the process would be enhanced.

The composite elements of an ideal lung cancer screening assay are summarized in Table 6. The assay(s) that prove to be most predictive of lung cancer risk will likely be predicated upon the fundamental aspect of lung carcinogenesis. Yet it must be appreciated that potentially useful lung cancer biomarkers may merely correlate with, and not necessarily participate in, the disease process. If more than one marker can conform to these specifications, consideration of relative costs become relevant. A disease as common as lung cancer is associated with an enormous population at-risk. However, each year only a small (but increasing) proportion of the population with a high lifetime risk will actually develop lung cancer. To minimize the number of false-positive tests that might be recorded when a large population is screened for a rare disease, a comprehensive early detection approach may include multileveled screening algorithms. Less than totally specific but highly sensitive front-end tests can lead to more specific downstream evaluations. A general discussion of such approaches has been presented previously (Makuch and Muenz, 1987) and this strategy merits further consideration. Screening approaches for lung cancer involve large programmatic as well as personal costs. Misclassifications (both false-positive and false-negative results) may have high psychological as well as medical costs. Thus any cancer biomarkers proposed for screening must undergo rigorous validation to assess their performance against the gold standard of subsequent human lung cancer development. Furthermore, before a program is implemented, the validation must be shown to reflect detection at a stage amenable to successful intervention and mortality reduction. Thoroughness in demonstrating the legitimacy of an early lung cancer detection approach may have a positive impact on the eventual acceptance on the approach by various high-risk target populations. Considerable effort directed at public education will be required to avoid the current levels of resistance to participation experienced with breast and cervical cancer screening. Confidence in participation in cancer screening efforts may grow in the general population as the isolated positive experiences in the first

Table 6 Lung Cancer Screening Goals

Biologically rational test
Algorithm consistent with cost-effective application
Process validated to ensure precision
Comprehensive application to appropriate populations

disease systems mature. The goal of a greater acceptance of preventive medicine approaches must remain a major public education focus, especially for the already proven screening tools.

The availability of effective early diagnostic tools will also affect the manner in which we would treat lung cancer. Very early stages of breast cancer may potentially be controlled by the chronic administration of the antiestrogen agent, tamoxifen (Powles et al., 1989). This is a consequence of the role of estrogen in breast cancer promotion (Pike et al,. 1983). Intervention tools that antagonize fundamental cancer promotion factors may be logical strategies for chemoprevention (Boone et al., 1990). Evidence is mounting to suggest a significant tumor promotion role in lung cancer for gastrin-releasing peptide (GRP). This growth factor has a role in fetal lung development (Sunday et al., 1990), is elevated in the bronchial secretions of smokers (Aguayo et al., 1989), and has an autocrine growth effect in lung cancer cell lines (Mulshine et al., 1990b). Preliminary evaluation of agents to block GRP effects in patients with advanced lung cancer has already begun. If GRP effects can be neutralized without significant host toxicity, this may be an interesting chemoprevention tool. The potential for cross-fertilization in developing treatment and screening strategies for the various epithelial malignancies is considerable and may permit more rapid development of meaningful approaches to the prevention of solid tumor.

The work of the group at M. D. Anderson using 13-*cis*-retinoic acid as a potential intervention agent for upper aerodigestive tract cancer lends support to the credibility of such directions. In a recently reported randomized trial, patients with head and neck cancer treated with curative intent received an additional year of daily oral therapy with either 13-*cis*-retinoic acid or placebo (Hong et al., 1990). This effort was based on the fact that this cigarette-exposed population frequently developed new primary cancers of other sites within the upper aerodigestive tract (including other sites in the head and neck, lungs, or esophagus), and that in vitro, 13-*cis*-retinoic-acid induced benign differentiation of malignantly transformed epithelial cells. In that clinical report, in the group of 51 patients receiving placebo, cancer developed in 12, whereas the equal-sized group receiving 13-*cis*-retinoic-acid included only 2 patients who developed cancer. The trend is in favor of prolongation of survival in the retinoid-treated group. A provocative finding was that the placebo-treated group developed three lung cancers and the 13-*cis*-retinoic-acid-treated group had none. This report is seminal for several reasons, including the demonstration of similar response of adjacent upper aerodigestive organs to common carcinogenic exposures, the value of identifying very early epithelial cancers, and, finally, the significant potential of a biologically rational intervention approach.

In a thoughtful review, Lippman and co-workers (1990) from the M. D. Anderson group suggest that biomarkers, which could be considered for early detection application, might also find application as intermediate endpoints to facilitate the clinical trial process of evaluating new chemointervention agents. Biomarkers that reflect fundamental aspects of tumor induction and evolution may be monitored more readily than some long-term endpoints such as cancer-related survival. The desired result is to shorten the clinical evaluation period of promising intervention tools by incorporating the use of intermediate endpoints. These indicate the success of the intervention tool much more quickly than when one must wait for the traditional clinical trial endpoints (such as cancer-related mortality).

The prospects for developing successful preventive measures for cancer control have never been more promising. Realizing this potential will largely be in the realm of transfer of research techniques from the level of the molecule and cell to the level of the organ (physiology) and the organism (epidemiology). Methodologic precision and attention to detail rival the much more highly visible "molecular biotechnology" in their contribution to the ultimate success of this process.

Acknowledgment

The authors thank Drs. P. Gupta, B. Kramer, D. Ihde, and the late J. Frost for many useful and stimulating discussions on issues related to the contents of the manuscript.

References

Aguayo, S. M., Kane, M., King, Jr., T. E., Schwarz, M. I., Grauer, L., Miller, Y. E. (1989). Increased levels of bombesin-like peptides in the lower respiratory tracts of asymptomatic cigarette for smokers. *J. Clin. Invest.* **84:**1105–1113.

Bailar, J. (1984a). Early lung cancer cooperative study group: early lung cancer detection. Summary and conclusions. *Am. Rev. Respir. Dis.* **130:**565–570.

Bailar, John C., III (1984b). Editorial, Screening for lung cancer—where are we now? *Am. Rev. Resp. Dis.* **130:**541–542.

Becklake, M. R. (1986). Concept of normality applied to measurement of lung function. *Am. J. Med.* **80:**1158–1164.

Berlin, N. I., Buncher, C. R., Fontana, R. S., et al. (1984). The National Institute Cooperative Early Lung Cancer Detection Program. Results of the initial screen (prevalence). Early lung cancer detection: introduction. *Am. Rev. Respir. Dis.* **130:** 545–549.

Boone, C. W., Kelloff, G. J., and Malone, W. E. (1990). Identification of candidate cancer chemopreventive agents and their evaluation in animal models and human clinical trials: a review. *Cancer Res.* **50:**2–9.

Council on Scientific Affairs (1990). The worldwide smoking epidemic tobacco trade, use and control. *J.A.M.A.* **2633**(24):3312–3318.

Dodd, G. D. (1988). Screening for the early detection of breast cancer. *Cancer* **62:**1781–1783.

Eddy, D. M. (1990). Screening for cervical cancer. *Ann. Intern. Med.* **113:**214–216.

Forrest, A. P. (1990). Screening and breast cancer. *Natl. Cancer Inst.* **82**(19):1525–1526.

Fukushi, Y., Ohtani, H., and Orikasa, S. (1989). Expression of lacto series type 2 antigens in human renal cell carcinoma and its clinical significance. *J. Natl. Cancer Inst.* **81:** 352–358.

Gazdar, A. F., Linnoila, I., Kurita, Y., Oie, H. K., Mulshine, J., L., Clark, J. C., and Whitsett, J. A. (1990). Peripheral airway cell differentiation in human lung cancer cell lines. *Cancer Res.* **50:**5481–5487.

Hakomori, S. (1986). Glycosphingolipids. *Sci. Am.* **254:**44–53.

Hong, W. K., Lippman, S. M., Itri, L. M., et al. (1990). Prevention of second primary tumors in squamous cell carcinoma of the head and neck with 13-cis-retinoic acid. *N. Engl. J. Med.* **323:**795–801.

Kogashima, M., Mulshine, J., Linnoila, R. I., et al. (1989). Antibody 624H12, which detects lung cancer at early stages recognizes a sugar sequence in glycosphinogolipid difucosylneolactonorhexaosylceramide. *Arch. Biochem. Biophys.* **275:**309–314.

Koss, L. G. (1989). The Papanicolaou test for cervical cancer detection a triumph and a tragedy. *J.A.M.A.* **261**(5):737–746.

Lilenfeld, A. M., Archer, P. G., Burnett, C. H., et al. (1966). An evaluation of radiographic and cytologic screening for the early detection of lung cancer. A cooperative pilot study of the American Cancer Society and the Veterans Administration. *Cancer Res.* **26:**2083–2121.

Lippman, S. M., Lee, J. S., Lotan, R., et al. (1990). Biomarkers as intermediate end points in chemoprevention trials. *J. Natl. Cancer Inst.* **82:**555–560.

Makuch, R. R., and Muenz, L. R. (1987). Evaluating the adequacy of tumor markers to discriminate among distinct populations. *Semin. Oncol.* **14**(2):89–101.

Mulshine, J. L., Tockman, M. S., and Smart, C. R. (1989). Considerations in the development of lung cancer screening tools. *J. Natl. Cancer Inst.* **18:**900–906.

Mulshine, J. L., Magnani, J. L., and Linnoila, R. I. (1990a). Applications of monoclonal antibodies in treatment of solid tumors. In *Principles of Biotherapy*. Edited by V. DeVita, S. Hellman, and S. Rosenberg. Philadelphia, J. B. Lippincott.

Mulshine, J. L., Treston, A. M., Scott, F. M., Avis, I., Boland, C., Phelps R., Kasprzyk, P. G., Nakanishi, Y., and Cuttitta, F. (1990b). New approaches to the management of lung cancer: rational strategies for early detection and intervention. *Oncol.* **5:**25–32.

National Cancer Institute Annual Cancer Statistics Review: Including Cancer Trends: 1950–1985. (1988). DHHS Publ. No. (NIH) 88–2789. Washington, D.C., Government Printing Office.

NCI Breast Cancer Screening Consortium (1990). Screening mammography: a missed clinical opportunity? *J.A.M.A.* **264**(1):54–58.

Pike, M. C., Krailo, M. D., Henderson, B. E., et al. (1983). "Hormonal" risk factors "breast tissue age" and the age-incidence of breast cancer. *Nature* **303:**767–770.

Powles, T. J., Hardy, J. R., Ashley, S. E., et al. (1989). A pilot trial to evaluate the acute toxicity and feasibility of tamoxifen for prevention of breast cancer. *Br. J. Cancer* **60:** 126–131.

Saccomanno, G., Archer, V. E., Aerbach, O., Saunders, R. P., Brennan, L. M. (1974). Development of carcinoma of the lung as reflected in exfoliated cell. *Cancer* **33:** 256–270.

Shapiro, S. (1988). Determining the efficacy of breast cancer screening. *Cancer* **00:**1873–1880.

Sibison, J. B. (1990). News and comment: King Tobacco under attack. *Cancer* **6:**2875–2882.

Silverberg, E., Boring, C. C., and Squires, T. S. (1990). Cancer statistics. *CA* **40:**9–26.

Sunday, M. E., Hua, J., Dai, H. B., et al. (1990). Bombesin increases fetal lung growth and maturation in utero and in organ culture. *Am. J. Respir. Cell Mol. Biol.*

Surgeon General's Report (1989). Reducing the health consequences of smoking. Superintendent of Documents, Government Printing Office, 1–32.

Tockman, M. S., Becklake, M. R., Clausen, J. L., Cox, P. M., Jr., Fontana, R. S., O'Brien, R. J., Permutt, S., Petty, T. L., Read, C., Reichman, L. B., Stead, W. W. (1983). Screening for adult respiratory disease: the official ATS statement. *Am. Rev. Resp. Dis.* **128:**768–744.

Tockman, M. S., Levin, M. L., Frost, J. K., et al. (1985). Screening and detection of lung cancer. In *Lung Cancer*. Edited by J. Aisner. New York, Churchill Livingstone, pp. 25–48.

Tockman, M. S., Gupta, P. K., Myers, J. D., et al. (1988). Sensitive and specific monoclonal antibody recognition of human lung cancer antigen on preserved sputum cells: a new approach to early lung cancer detection. *J. Clin. Oncol.* **6:**1685–1693.

Tockman, M., Pressman, N., Gill, G., et al. (1991). Quantitation of molecular markers for pre-neoplastic lung cancer. *Proc. Am. Rev. Respir. Dis.*

Wilson, J. M. G., and Junger, F. (1968). Principles and practice of screening for disease. *Public Health Papers 34*. Geneva, WHO, 1968.

16

Recent Advances in the Pathologic Diagnosis of Lung Cancer

Application of Monoclonal Antibodies and Cytofluorometry for Subtyping

YUKIO SHIMOSATO, SETSUO HIROHASHI, MASAYUKI NOGUCHI, YOSHIHIRO MATSUNO, and YOSHIYA TOME

National Cancer Center Research Institute
Tokyo, Japan

I. Introduction

The present World Health Organization (WHO) classification of lung tumors was published in 1981 (World Health Organization, 1981). The increasing amount of knowledge concerning each histologic type of lung cancer that has become available during the last 10 years has made us consider a re-revision of the classification. The Pathology Panel of the International Association for the Study of Lung Cancer proposed new subtyping of small cell carcinoma (SCLC) into "pure" SCLC and SCLC with "large cell components." Because of the similarity in the biological behavior of oat cell type and SCLC of the intermediate cell type, they were put together into the "pure" subtype. Because of some degree of dissimilarity between the pure form and SCLC with large cell components, the latter was separated from intermediate cell type (Hirsch et al., 1988). In this chapter we will first discuss the subtyping of SCLCs.

For adenocarcinoma of the lung, the present WHO classification is based mainly on histologic structure, with no regard for cell type. However, the cell type is known to be important since it determines the growth pattern, and thus the gross features, of the tumor and, probably, sensitivity to therapeutic agents. In Japan, cell typing of adenocarcinoma is performed, but typing is, of course, difficult or almost impossible in poorly differentiated adenocarcinoma, which represents an obstacle to its worldwide diffusion. However, while working on differentiation antigens in each cell type of lung adenocarcinoma, we found a very useful differentiation antigen common to each cell type of adenocarcinoma, that is, surfactant apoprotein, which we discuss here.

Factors associated with proliferating activity, or degree of malignancy other than histology and cytology, are also discussed because they are important aids to physicians and surgeons in deciding on the most appropriate therapeutic approach. Representative parameters are nuclear DNA content, incidence of cells in DNA synthesis (S-phase), and antigen associated with proliferative activity of tumor cells.

II. Subtyping of Small Cell Lung Cancer

It is easy to define verbally "SCLC with large cell components," but the degree of diagnostic agreement does not appear to be high in actual practice. It may be partially due to the quality of histologic sections and interpretation of degenerating tumor cells and artifact. Therefore, methods of subtyping other than histology are desired. Immunohistochemistry is one.

In 1987, the Workshop on SCLC Antigens held in London partially characterized "cluster 1 SCLC antigen," against which several monoclonal antibodies had been produced in different laboratories (Okabe et al., 1984; de Leij et al., 1985; Takahashi et al., 1986; Hirohashi et al., 1988). We produced three monoclonal antibodies, NCC-LU-243, -244, and -246, that reacted with cluster 1 SCLC antigen (145 kD cell membrane antigen) but with different epitopes (Hirano et al., 1989). All of these antibodies reacted immunohistochemically, with the cell membrane of almost every SCLC cell in every case, on frozen sections or AMeX sections (cold acetone fixed, methylbenzoate cleared, and paraffin-embedded sections) (Sato et al., 1986). However, the antigen was labile in formalin solution, and only NCC-LU-243 was found to be reactive with SCLC cells that were formalin-fixed for a short period of time (overnight). Later, we noted that addition of 2% zinc sulfate to formalin solution preserved the antigenicity relatively well (Tome et al., 1990).

With proper fixation, either using AMeX or zinc–formalin-fixed paraffin-embedded sections, almost every cell of all pure SCLC specimens, either oat cell or intermediate cell type, reacted with the antibody. However, SCLC with large-cell components reacted focally (Fig. 1). This finding indicates that some tumor cells of SCLC with large-cell components might have lost the cluster 1 SCLC antigen or that the antigenicity was reduced to the immunohistochemically undetectable level. The cluster 1 SCLC antigen was preserved very well in ethyl-alcohol-fixed cytologic smears. Pure SCLC cells were also positively stained but

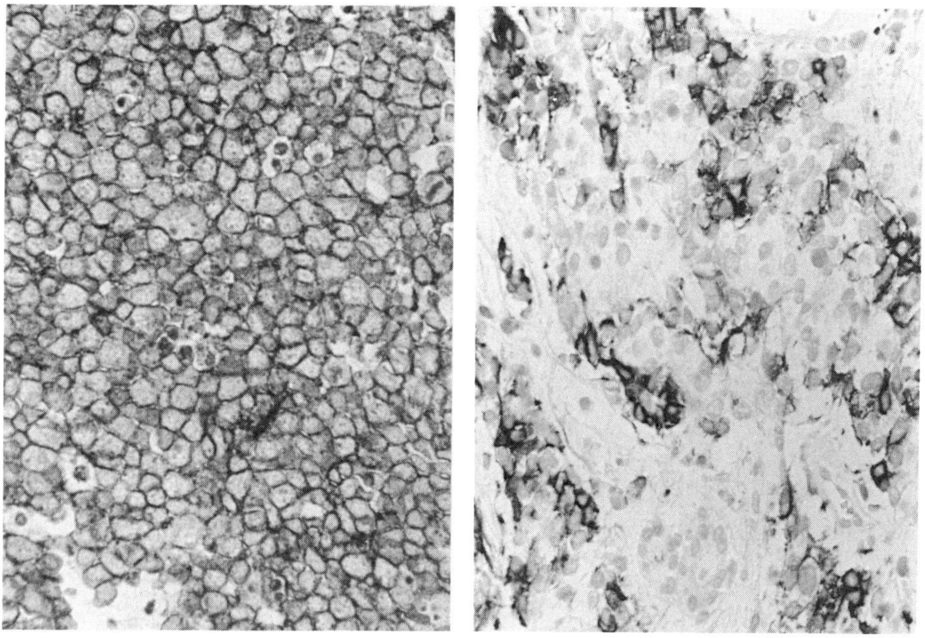

A B

Figure 1 Immunostaining of histologic section for cluster 1 small cell lung cancer antigen (NCAM) with NCC-LU-243. A. "Pure" small cell carcinoma shows positive reaction in the cell membrane of all tumor cells. B. Small cell/large cell carcinoma, however, is only focally stained.

some cells of the small-cell/large-cell type were unstained (Fig. 2). Differences in staining patterns may be useful for differentiating pure SCLC from SCLC with large-cell components, provided that sections are properly fixed. Although we described good preservation of antigenicity for at least 1 week in zinc–formalin (Tome et al., 1990), results were much better with a short fixation time (i.e., 1 or 2 days).

Positive reaction with NCC-LU-243, although focal, was occasionally noted in non-SCLCs, 7 in 26 large-cell carcinoma, 5 in 36 adenocarcinomas, and 7 in 20 squamous cell carcinomas, when zinc-formalin fixed large sections were examined. Among these, only one large cell carcinoma was found to contain a few neurosecretory granules among four tumors examined by an electron microscope.

Two of five adenocarcinomas with positive immunostaining were tubular type with rosettelike structures and fine cytoplasmic granularity, suggesting neuroendocrine carcinoma, although no secretory granules were found (Fig. 3). One was well-differentiated papillary adenocarcinoma, in which chromogranin-

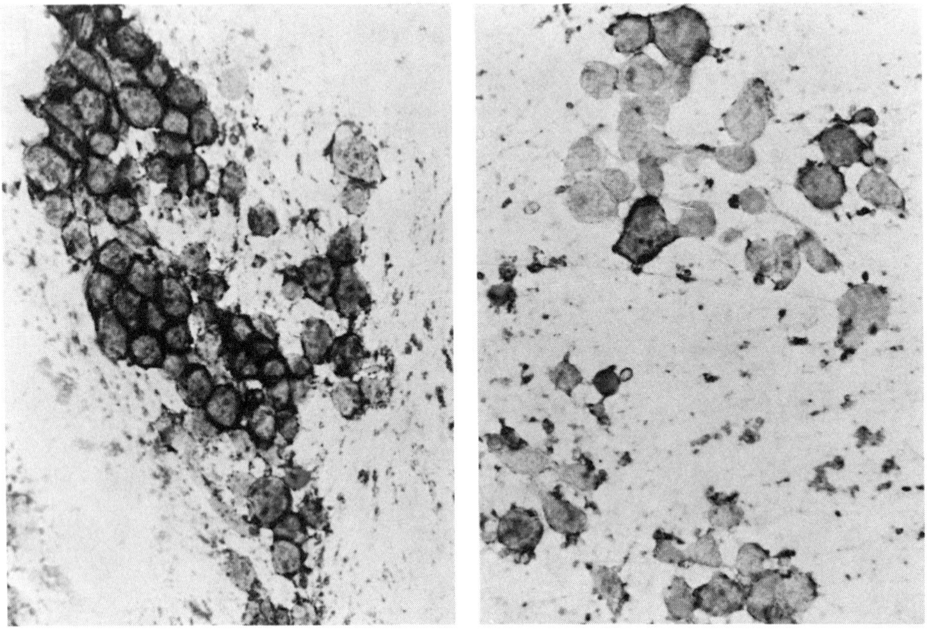

A B

Figure 2 Immunostaining of cytologic imprints for cluster 1 small cell lung cancer antigen (NCAM) with NCC-LU-243. A. Every tumor cell of "pure" small cell carcinoma reveals positive reaction in the cell membrane. B. Small cell/large cell carcinoma shows positive reaction in some but negative in others.

A-positive cells were scattered in cells with positive cluster 1 SCLC antigen. The remaining two cases were poorly differentiated.

Very recently these antibodies, which reacted with cluster 1 SCLC antigen, were found to react with neural cell adhesion molecule (NCAM) (Patel et al., 1989). However, immunohistochemical reactivity between our NCC-LU-243, -244, and -246 and MoAb 735, which was said to be reactive with the polysialyl acid portion of NCAM (Kibbelaar et al., 1989), was somewhat different. On the other hand, one of the antibodies recognizing cluster 1 SCLC antigen was found to react with fetal lung epithelium (Fukayama et al., 1990). From these findings it is too early to conclude that non-SCLCs reactive with antibodies against cluster 1 SCLC antigen contain NCAM and thus possess neural or neuroendocrine properties. Those non-SCLCs may merely show oncofetal changes rather than neural characteristics. It is necessary to confirm expression of NCAM by Northern blot analysis. From our experience, however, MoAb 735 can also be used for routine diagnosis because the carbohydrate epitope is more stable in formalin solution,

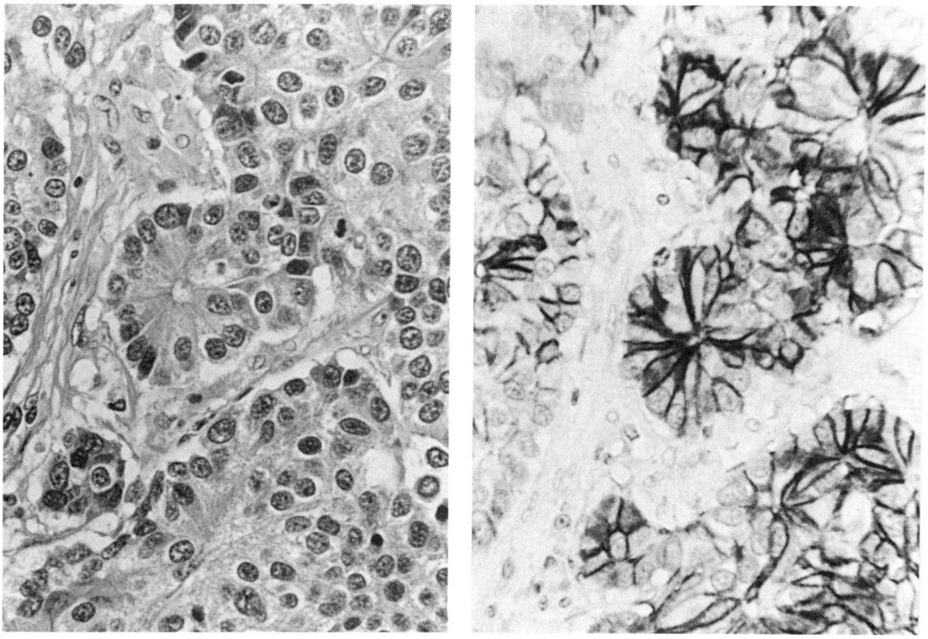

A B

Figure 3 Adenocarcinoma with some neuroendocrine features. A. Histologic section shows rosette-like structures and individual cells have finely granular cytoplasm. B. Although focal, tumor cells are strongly positive for cluster 1 small cell lung cancer antigen (immunostaining with NCC-LU-243). This tumor was stained negative with monoclonal antibody 735, which reacts with sugar chain of NCAM. It was also negative for chromagranin A.

although the number of cells reactive with the antibody is less than that stained with NCC-LU-243. Non-small-cell neuroendocrine carcinoma (Gazdar et al., 1988) should be re-examined in terms of NCAM.

III. Subtyping of Adenocarcinoma

Adenocarcinoma has been subtyped by histologic structure in the WHO classification as mentioned previously. However, many pathologists recognize that there were several cell types even within a single histologic subtype of papillary adenocarcinoma, among which Clara cell type, type II alveolar epithelial cell type (type II pneumocyte type), and mucin-producing (goblet) cell type were already recognized as entities (Montes et al., 1977; Torikata and Ishiwata, 1977; Kimula, 1978; Morningstar and Hassan, 1979; Shimosato et al., 1982). To these three subtypes we added "bronchial surface epithelial cell type" and "bronchial gland cell type" (Kodama et al., 1982, 1984; Shimosato and Kodama, 1986). The latter is not a papillary but tubular adenocarcinoma. Most well-to-moderately differentiated adenocarcinomas can be classified into the above five cell types, but unanimity of diagnosis based on cell type decreases significantly among pathologists when the tumor is less differentiated. This necessitates a search for marker substances for each cell type. Among marker substances identified so far, lactoferrin is a good marker for bronchial gland cell type adenocarcinoma, and lysozyme for goblet cell type, although some cases did not show positive reaction (Shimosato, 1983).

Surfactant apoproteins are differentiation antigens of type II pneumocytes, the antibody against which clearly recognizes not only type II pneumocytes in nonneoplastic lung but also individual cells of type II pneumocyte type (Singh et al., 1981; Kuroki et al., 1986) and Clara cell type adenocarcinomas (Fig. 4) (Mizutani et al., 1988).

By using monoclonal antibody against surfactant apoproteins, PE-10, about one-half of adenocarcinomas of the lung irrespective of the degree of differentiation were immunostained, while no small cell, large cell, squamous cell carcinomas of the lung or adenocarcinomas of other organs metastatic to the lung were stained (Mizutani et al., 1988). Further study disclosed that all cell types, except for goblet cell type adenocarcinoma (bronchioloalveolar carcinoma with abundant mucin production) were found to be reactive. Bronchial gland cell type adenocarcinoma arising in cartilage-bearing bronchi was also immunoreactive, more so in cells producing little or no mucin (Noguchi et al., unpublished data). This finding indicates that differentiation antigen specific for type II pneumocytes may be expressed in cells of pulmonary adenocarcinoma of other than type II pneumocyte type. The absence of reaction in goblet cell type adenocarcinoma may be due to filling of cytoplasm with mucin. We also examined the immunoreactivity of this antibody with various adenocarcinomas. As seen in Table 1, no gastric, pancreatic, bile duct, or breast carcinomas reacted, but 3 of 22 thyroid cancers reacted. However, there were few positive cells and much of the reaction product was present in colloid and free cell borders of tumor cells. Difference in staining patterns from that of pulmonary adenocarcinoma suggests that PE-10 may have recognized antigen in neoplastic thyroid tissue different from surfactant apoproteins. In fact, Western blotting of the thyroid cancer tissue with positive immunostaining with PE-10 did not reveal surfactant apoproteins (Matsuno et al., unpublished data).

This antibody is also useful for the identification of mesothelioma, which was nonreactive, from peripheral adenocarcinoma with involvement of the pleural cavity. In such instances, combination of immunostaining with antibodies against Lewis a and Tn is helpful in the diagnosis of mesothelioma because they are frequently positive in pulmonary adenocarcinoma and very rarely so in mesothe-

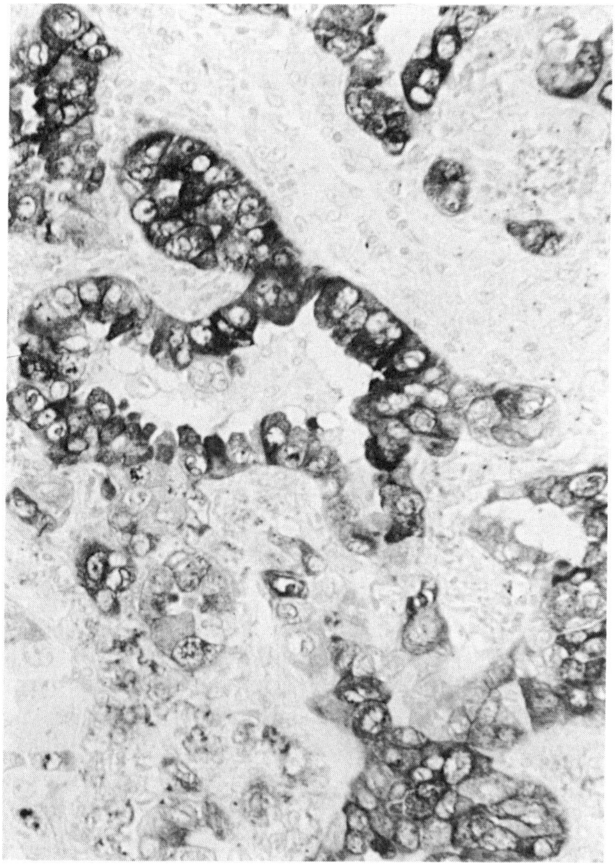

Figure 4 Immunostaining of papillary adenocarcinoma of Clara cell type with PE-10, a monoclonal antibody for surfactant apoproteins. Cytoplasm of majority of tumor cells is stained positively. Nuclear inclusions are also reactive.

lioma (Noguchi et al., 1989). From the above findings, adenocarcinoma of unknown primary can be suspected to be of lung origin, if surfactant apoproteins are found.

IV. Factors Associated with Degree of Malignancy

Many factors affecting the prognosis of patients with cancers are associated with degree of malignancy of the tumor. Of course, the TNM factors are most important. However, one-third of patients with pulmonary adenocarcinoma in

Table 1 Surfactant Apoprotein-Positive Lung Cancer and Adenocarcinoma of Other Organs

	No. of cases positive/ no. cases examined	%
Lung cancer		
Adenocarcinoma	36/75	48
Well-differentiated	19/41	46
Moderately differentiated	11/24	46
Poorly differentiated	6/10	60
Squamous cell carcinoma	0/5	0
Large cell carcinoma	0/8	0
Small cell carcinoma	0/1	0
Metastases from other organs	0/23	0
Gastric cancer	0/40	0
Pancreatic cancer	0/39	0
Biliary tract cancer	0/27	0
Breast cancer	0/20	0
Thyroid cancer	3/22	14

stage Ia (T1N0M0) died of recurrence within 5 years after undergoing "curative" resection. This indicates the need to identify factors affecting prognosis other than TNM. Accordingly, we found that nuclear atypia and the mitotic index were very important prognostically or associated with degree of malignancy (Takise et al., 1988). Nuclear atypia expressed by nuclear area or standard deviation of nuclear area was found to be associated with nuclear DNA content (NDC) ($p < 0.01$ and $p < 0.05$, respectively) (Asamura et al., 1989a) and mitotic index with frequency of S-phase cells or proliferating cells.

A. Cytofluorometry of Nuclear DNA Content

NDC of tumor cells was measured by cytofluorometry, and occurrence of aneuploidy and histogram patterns was checked. Flow cytometry is another method to evaluate DNA content but pathologists tend to prefer the former. First, we analyzed the mean nuclear DNA content (MNDC) of tumor cells in imprint smears of 72 surgically resected adenocarcinomas of the lung (Asamura et al., 1989a). The MNDC of poorly differentiated adenocarcinoma was significantly larger than that of well-differentiated adenocarcinoma both in stages I + II and III + IV ($p < 0.001$ each), and the MNDC of stages III + IV was significantly larger than that of I + II in poorly differentiated adenocarcinoma ($p < 0.01$). There was a tendency for histogram patterns III + IV, in which more aneuploid cells were present than in I + II, to be more common and for the incidence of the aneuploid stem cell line to be higher in less differentiated and more advanced adenocarcinomas, although differences were not statistically significant.

Subsequently, 46 cases of adenocarcinoma of the lung in stage I (pT1-2N0M0) were studied in terms of NDC (Asamura et al., 1989b). They consisted of 23 cases each with and without tumor recurrence within 5 years postoperatively. The NDC was compared, in which the tumor size and the degree of histologic differentiation were completely matched. The NDC was larger in the recurrent group than in the nonrecurrent group in terms of MNDC, and the DNA histogram pattern was more abnormal with more frequent occurrence of an aneuploid stem cell line, of which the difference in MNDC was statistically significant ($p < 0.05$). The differences were more significant in well-differentiated ($p < 0.01$) and T1 ($p < 0.05$) subgroups than in moderately to poorly differentiated and T2 subgroups, respectively. The results indicated that the NDC was a good predictor of prognosis in stage I adenocarcinoma of the lung. Its prognostic importance increases in more differentiated and smaller tumors, compared to less differentiated and larger tumors.

Subsequently, we compared the MNDC of 60 primary tumors and 20 cases each of regional lymph node metastases, and brain and liver metastases. In the lymph node metastasis group, tumor tissues were obtained surgically as in the brain metastasis group, in which primary tumors were removed first and brain metastases later. The liver metastases were obtained at autopsy with corresponding primary tumors. The average MNDCs of hematogenous brain and liver metastases were significantly larger than that of primary tumors ($p < 0.01$ and $p < 0.01$, respectively). From these findings, together with analysis of histogram patterns, we concluded that a minor subclone with significantly larger MNDC in the primary tumor was the source of metastasis, or a more abnormal subclone with larger MNDC developed after metastatic tumors were established (Nomori et al., 1991).

B. Analysis of Proliferative Activity

As to the proliferative activity of tumor cells, we first studied 52 resected adenocarcinomas of the lung by an immunoperoxidase procedure after bromodeoxyuridine labeling (Yoshida et al., 1989). The labeling index (LI) was highest in SCLC (4 cases with average LI of 19.0%), followed by squamous cell carcinoma (10 cases with average LI of 11.9%), which were analyzed as controls for adenocarcinoma. The LI of adenocarcinoma ranged from 0.1 to 19.2% (average, 3.6%), with two-thirds of the cases showing LI values of 3.0% or less. Metastatic tumors in the brain from pulmonary adenocarcinoma showed an LI of more than 5.0%, although in these cases labeling was carried out in vivo (Cho et al., 1988). These findings may indicate that hematogenous metastasis rarely develops in pulmonary adenocarcinoma with an LI of 3.0% or less. Concerning the cell type of adenocarcinoma, the LI was low in goblet cell type and type II pneumocyte type, whereas the values for the bronchial surface epithelial cell type varied widely (average, 5.2%) and those for the Clara cell type were intermediate (average, 1.8%). Comparison of LI with known prognostic factors, such as TNM factors, histologic differentiation, degree of nuclear atypia, and others, showed a significant correlation. Thus, BrdU LI was suggested to be a useful new prognostic factor for pulmonary adenocarcinoma.

Another approach to assess the proliferative activity of tumors is to use monoclonal antibodies for DNA polymerase alpha, proliferation-associated nuclear antigen (Ki-67), proliferating cell nuclear antigen (PCNA, CYCLIN), and others. In relation to such studies, there is a disadvantage in the inactivation of antigens by formalin fixation. However, very recently a monoconal antibody TOB 7 against PCNA has become available, which can be used to some extent for formalin-fixed paraffin-embedded tissue sections. Matsuno et al. (1990) analyzed the proliferative activity of nodules in lesions of the liver with the antibody and showed correlation between the number of cells with positive staining and the degree of nuclear atypia. A preliminary study on pulmonary adenocarcinoma possibly arising in adenoma (or atypical adenomatous hyperplasia) shows frequent positively stained tumor cell nuclei in the adenocarcinoma focus and almost no positive staining in the adenoma area (Matsuno, et al., unpublished data) (Fig. 5).

From the findings described above, adenocarcinoma of the lung should better be classified by degree of nuclear atypia (mild, moderate, and severe), more preferably by nuclear DNA content (MNDC, occurrence of aneuploidy, and histogram pattern), and by degree of proliferative activity (frequency of S-phase cells, ≦3%; >3%, ≦6%; >6%) or percentage of PCNA-positive cells. By doing so, patients with adenocarcinoma in stage I with aneuploid stem cell line and S-phase cells of larger than 3% could become candidates for postoperative therapy to prevent recurrence.

C. Abnormal Genes

Other factors associated with degree of malignancy of tumors are amplification or overexpression of oncogenes and deletion or inactivation of antioncogenes. In neuroblastoma, amplification of N-*myc* gene (Tsuda, et al., 1988) and in breast cancer amplification and overexpression of *c-erb*B-2 gene (Tsuda et al., 1989, 1990) were associated with poorer prognosis of patients. In lung cancer, abnormality in *myc* family oncogenes appears to be associated with higher malignancy of tumors, although this has not been completely verified yet. Evidence suggesting a relationship between gene abnormality and increase in degree of malignancy includes that in vitro SCLC cell lines with shorter doubling time often showed amplification of *c-myc*, and in one strain overexpression of L-*myc* (Terassaki et al., unpublished data); in adenocarcinoma, none of 18 primary tumors showed

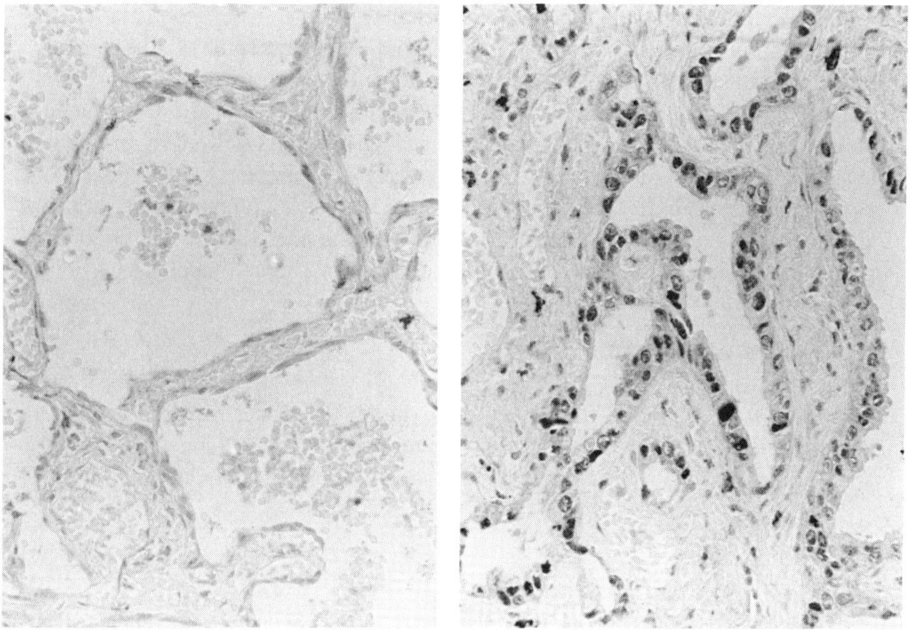

A B

Figure 5 Immunostaining of adenocarcinoma in adenoma (or atypical adenomatous hyperplasia) for proliferating cell nuclear antigen. A. There is almost no nuclear staining in areas with features of adenoma. B. Many nuclei are positively stained in areas with features of well-differentiated adenocarcinoma.

amplification of c-*myc* but 9 of 17 brain metastases did show amplification (Nakajima et al., unpublished data); and in lung cancer in general, tumors without *myc* gene abnormality rarely showed tumor-take in nude mice, but tumors with abnormal *myc* gene often showed tumor take (Gemma et al., 1988). Deletion of chromosome 16 was associated with a higher grade of cell atypia, and thus poorer prognosis of patients with hepatocellular carcinoma (Tsuda et al., 1990b), but so far no such association has been found in lung cancer.

V. Conclusions

This chapter has described the usefulness of monoclonal antibodies against cluster 1 SCLC antigen (NCAM) in histologic subtyping of SCLC, particularly NCC-LU-243, which can be applied to zinc–formalin-fixed paraffin-embedded tissue sections. Differences between "pure" SCLC and SCLC with large-cell components at the immunohistochemical level were emphasized.

In adenocarcinoma, surfactant apoprotein was found to be a good marker for differentiating pulmonary adenocarcinoma from adenocarcinoma of other organs. In addition to subtyping of lung adenocarcinoma by histology and cytology, it is suggested that mean nuclear DNA content of tumor cells, occurrence of aneuploidy, and abnormal histogram pattern as well as proliferative activity of tumors are important factors associated with the degree of malignancy or prognosis of patients. Data on these factors should be added to routine diagnosis of surgical specimens for better management of patients. In the near future, data on oncogenes and antioncogenes may also become useful in clinical oncology.

Acknowledgments

This work was supported in part by grants-in-aid for cancer research and for a comprehensive 10-year strategy for cancer research from the Ministry of Health and Welfare and from the Ministry of Education, Science and Culture, Japan.

References

Asamura, H., Nakajima, T., Mukai, K., Noguchi, M., and Shimosato, Y. (1989a). DNA cytofluorometric and nuclear morphometric analyses of lung adenocarcinoma. *Cancer* **64:**1657–1664.

Asamura, H., Nakajima, T., Mukai, K., and Shimosato, Y. (1989b). Nuclear DNA content by cytofluorometry of stage I adenocarcinoma of the lung in relation to postoperative recurrence. *Chest* **96:**312–318.

Cho, K. G., Hoshino, T., Pitts, L. H., Nomura, K., and Shimosato, Y. (1988). Proliferative potential of brain metastases. *Cancer* **62:**512–515.

de Leij, L., Poppema, S., Klein, N. J., ter Haar, A., Schwander, E., Ebbens, F., Postmus, P. E., and The, T. H. (1985). Neuroendocrine differentiation antigen on human lung carcinoma and Kulchitski cells. *Cancer Res.* **45:**2192–2200.

Fukayama, M., Funata, N., Hayashi, Y., Maeda, Y., Koike, M., Watanabe, J., and Okabe, T. (1990). Brain associated small-cell lung cancer antigen (BASCA) is expressed in developing lung: an immunohistochemical and immunoelectron microscopic study. *J. Histochem. Cytochem.* **38:**51–57.

Gazdar, A. F., Helman, L. J., Israel, M. A., Russell, E. K., Linnoila, R. I., Mulshine, J. L., Schuller, H. M., and Park, J.-G. (1988). Expression of neuroendocrine cell markers L-dopa decarboxylase, chromagranin A, and dense core granules in human tumors of endocrine and nonendocrine origin. *Cancer Res.* **48:**4078–4982.

Gemma, A., Nakajima, T., Shiraishi, M., Noguchi, M., Gotoh, M., Sekiya, T., Niitani, H., and Shimosato, Y. (1988). *myc* family gene abnormality in lung cancers and its relation to xenotransplantability. *Cancer Res.* **48:**6025–6028.

Hirano, T., Hirohashi, S., Kunii, T., Noguchi, M., Shimosato, Y., and Hayata, Y. (1989). Quantitative distribution of cluster I small cell lung cancer antigen in cancerous and non-cancerous tissues, cultured cells and sera. *Jpn. J. Cancer Res.* **80:**348–355.

Hirohashi, S., Kunii, T., Hirano, T., and Shimosato, Y. (1988). 145 kDa cell membrane antigen on SCLCs as a common target for several monoclonal antibodies raised against SCLCs. *Lung Cancer* **4:**103–104.

Hirsch, F. R., Matthews, M. J., Aisner, S., Campobasso, O., Elema, J. D., Gazdar, A. F., MacKay, B., Nasiell, M., Shimosato, Y., Steele, R. H., Yesner, R., and Zettergren, L. (1988). Histopathological classification of small cell lung cancer. Changing concepts and terminology. *Cancer* **62:**973–977.

Kibbelaar, R. E., Moolenaar, C. E. C., Michalides, A. J. A. M., Bitter-Suermann, D., Addis, B. J., and Mooi, W. J. (1989). Expression of the embryonic neural cell adhesion molecule N-CAM in lung carcinoma. Diagnostic usefulness of monoclonal antibody 735 for the distinction between small cell lung cancer and non-small cell lung cancer. *J. Pathol.* **159:**23–28.

Kimula, Y. (1978). A histochemical and ultrastructural study of adenocarcinoma of the lung. *Am. J. Surg. Pathol.* **2:**253–264.

Kodama, T., Shimosato, Y., and Kameya, T. (1982). Histology and ultrastructure of bronchogenic and bronchial gland adenocarcinomas (including adenoid cystic and mucoepidermoid carcinomas) in relation to histogenesis. In *Morphogenesis of Lung Cancer*. Edited by Y. Shiomosato, M. R. Melamed, and P. Nettesheim. Boca Raton, FL, CRC Press, pp. 147–166.

Kodama, T., Shimosato,Y., Koide, T., Watanabe, S., and Yoneyama, T. (1984). Endobronchial polypoid adenocarcinoma of the lung. Histological and ultrastructural studies of five cases. *Am. J. Surg. Pathol.* **8:**845–854.

Kuroki, Y., Dempo, K., and Akino, T. (1986). Immunohistochemical study of human pulmonary surfactant apoproteins with monoclonal antibody. Pathologic application for hyaline membrane disease. *Am. J. Pathol.* **124:**25–33.

Matsuno, Y., Hirohashi, S., Furuya, S., Sakamoto, M., Mukai, K., and Shimosato, Y. (1990). Heterogeneity of proliferative activity in nodule-in-nodule lesions of small hepatocellular carcinoma. *Jpn. J. Cancer Res.* **81:**1137–1140.

Mizutani, Y., Nakajima, T., Morinaga, S., Gotoh, M., Shimosato, Y., Akino, T., and Suzuki, A. (1988). Immunohistochemical localization of pulmonary surfactant apoproteins in various lung tumors. Special reference to nonmucus producing lung adenocarcinomas. *Cancer* **61:**532–537.

Montes, M., Binette, J. P., Adler, R. H., and Guarino, R. (1977). Clara cell adenocarcinoma. Light and electron microscopic studies. *Am. J. Surg. Pathol.* **1:**245–253.

Morningstar, W. A., and Hassan, M. O. (1979). Bronchioloalveolar carcinoma with nodal metastases. An ultrastructural study. *Am. J. Surg. Pathol.* **3:**273–278.

Noguchi, M., Nakajima, T., Hirohashi, S., Akiba, T., and Shimosato, Y. (1989). Immunohistochemical distinction of malignant mesothelioma from pulmonary adenocarcinoma with anti-surfactant apoprotein, anti-Lewis a, and anti-Tn antibodies. *Hum. Pathol.* **20:**53–57.

Nomori, H., Nakajima, T., Noguchi, M., Iga, R., and Shimosato, Y. (1991). Cytofluorometric analysis of metastases from lung adenocarcinoma with special reference to the difference between hematogenous and lymphatic metastases. *Cancer* **67:** 2941–2947.

Okabe, T., Kaizu, T., Fujisawa, M., Watanabe, J., Kojima, K., Yamashita, T., and Takaku,

F. (1984). Monoclonal antibodies to surface antigens of small cell carcinoma of the lung. *Cancer Res.* **44:**5273–5278.

Patel, K., Moore, S. E., Dickson, G., Rossell, R. J., Beverley, P. C., Kemshead, J. T., and Walsh, F. S. (1989). Neural cell adhesion molecule (NCAM) is the antigen recognized by monoclonal antibodies of similar specificity in small-cell lung carcinoma and neuroblastoma. *Int. J. Cancer* **44:**573–578.

Sato, Y., Mukai, K., Watanabe, S., Gotoh, M., and Shimosato, Y. (1986). The AMeX method. A simplified technique of tissue processing and paraffin embedding with improved preservation of antigens for immunostaining. *Am. J. Pathol.* **125:**431–435.

Shimosato, Y. (1983). Lung cancer: histogenesis, differentiation, and prognostic factors. *Trans. Soc. Pathol. Jpn.* **72:**29–57.

Shimosato, Y., Kodama, T., and Kameya, T. (1982). Morphogenesis of peripheral type adenocarcinoma of the lung. In *Morphogenesis of Lung Cancer*, vol. 1. Edited by Y. Shimosato, M. R. Melamed, and P. Nettesheim. Boca Raton, FL, CRC Press, pp. 65–89.

Shimosato, Y., and Kodama, T. (1986). Adenocarcinoma: clinical significance of subtyping and other morphologic factors. In *Clinical and Experimental Pathology of Lung Cancer*. Edited by J. G. McVie, W. Bakker, S. Wagenaar, and D. Carney. Dordrecht/Boston/Lancaster, Martinus Nijhoff, pp. 19–33.

Singh, G., Katyal, S. L., and Torikata, C. (1981). Carcinoma of type II pneumocytes. Immunodiagnosis of a subtype of bronchiolo-alveolar carcinomas. *Am. J. Pathol.* **102:**195–208.

Takahashi, T., Ueda, R., Song, X., Nishida, K., Shinzato, K., Namikawa, R., Ariyoshi, Y., Ota, K., Kato, K., Nagatsu, T., Imaizumi, M., Abe, T., and Takahashi, T. (1986). Two novel surface antigens on small cell lung carcinoma defined by mouse monoclonal antibodies NE-25 and PE-35. *Cancer Res.* **46:**4770–4775.

Takise, A., Kodama, T., Shimosato, Y., Watanabe, S., and Suemasu, K. (1988). Histopathologic prognostic factors in adenocarcinomas of the peripheral lung less than 2 cm in diameter. *Cancer* **61:**2083–2088.

Tome, Y., Hirohashi, S., Noguchi, M., and Shimosato, Y. (1990). Preservation of cluster I small cell lung cancer antigen in zinc-formalin fixative and its application to immunological diagnosis. *Histopathology* **16:**469–474.

Torikata, C., and Ishiwata, R. (1977). Intranuclear tubular structures observed in the cells of an alveolar cell carcinoma of the lung. *Cancer* **40:**1194–2101.

Tsuda, H., Shimosato, Y., Upton, M. P., Yokota, J., Terada, M., Ohira, M., Sugimura, T., and Hirohashi, S. (1988). Retrospective study on amplification of N-*myc* and c-*myc* genes in pediatric solid tumors and its association with prognosis and tumor differentiation. *Lab. Invest.* **59:**321–327.

Tsuda, H., Hirohashi, S., Shimosato, Y., Hirota, T., Tsugane, S., Yamamoto, H., Miyajima, N., Toyoshima, K., Yamamoto, T., Yokota, J., Yoshida, T., Sakamoto, H., Harada, M., and Sugimura, T. (1989). Correlation between long-term survival in breast cancer patients and amplification of two putative oncogene-coamplification units: *hst*-1/*int*-2 and *c-erb*B-2/*ear*-1. *Cancer Res.* **49:**3104–3108.

Tsuda, H., Hirohashi, S., Shimosato, Y., Tanaka, Y., Hirota, T., Tsugane, S., Shiraishi, M., Toyoshima, K., Yamamoto, T., Terada, M., and Sugimura, T. (1990a). Immunohistochemical study on overexpression of *c-erb*B-2 protein in human breast cancer: its correlation with gene amplification and long-term survival of patients. *Jpn. J. Cancer Res.* **81:**327–332.

Tsuda, H., Zhang, W., Shimosato, Y., Yokota, J., Terada, M., Sugimura, T., Miyamura, T., and Hirohashi, S. (1990b). Allele loss on chromosome 16 associated with progression of human hepatocellular carcinoma. *Proc. Natl. Acad. Sci. USA* **87:**6791–6794.

World Health Organization (1981). *Histological Typing of Lung Tumours*, 2nd ed. Geneva, World Health Organization, pp. 19–32.

Yoshida, K., Morinaga, S., Shimosato, Y., and Hayata, Y. (1989). A cell kinetic study of pulmonary adenocarcinoma by an immunoperoxidase procedure after bromodeoxyuridine labeling. *Cancer* **64:**2284–2291.

PART V

NON-SMALL-CELL LUNG CANCER: SCIENTIFIC RATIONALE FOR COMBINED TREATMENT APPROACHES

17

Neoadjuvant Therapy for Stage III Non-Small-Cell Lung Cancer: A Review

JACOB D. BITRAN, EVERETT E. VOKES, PHILIP C. HOFFMAN, WILLIAM GRADISHAR, CHRIS ENGLISH, and HARVEY M. GOLOMB

University of Chicago
Chicago, Illinois

I. Standard Therapy for Stage III Non-Small-Cell Lung Cancer

Patients with stage III non-small-cell lung cancer (NSCLC) have a dismal prognosis. The median survival for patients with unresectable NSCLC is less than 12 months and the 2 year survival rate is less than 20% (Johnson, 1988; Perez et al., 1982; Eagan et al., 1977). Patients with regionally advanced NSCLC undergoing resection have a similar poor prognosis that is not altered by the use of postoperative radiotherapy (Johnson, 1988; Perez et al., 1982; Eagan et al., 1977). In both groups, local and distant disease recurrence is frequently observed and reflects the inability of currently available therapeutic approaches to eradicate local bulky disease and to control systemic micrometastatic disease.

A new staging classification for lung cancer has recently been adopted (Mountain, 1988) that allows for patients with regionally advanced (stage III) NSCLC to be classified into two categories. Patients with stage IIIA disease have T_1, T_2, or T_3, primary lesions with only ipsilateral mediastinal involvement, which are considered resectable. These patients can, therefore, be treated with curative intent. Patients with stage IIIB NSCLC have regionally advanced disease including T_4 primaries or contralateral mediastinal lymph nodes or contralateral supraclavicular lymph nodes. T_4 primaries include extensive involvement of the mediastinum, invasion of the heart or great vessels, or invasion of the trachea and esophagus. Despite apparent regional confinement of the NSCLC, patients with such regionally advanced disease cannot undergo complete resection of their primaries and are frequently treated with radiation alone, administered with a palliative intent.

Although the overall cure rates for patients with stage III NSCLC are poor, the prognosis for patients with stage IIIB disease remains particularly dismal. Only an occasional patient achieves long-term disease-free status (Mountain, 1988).

The new staging classification can serve to facilitate clinical research and a better understanding of the treatment outcome of a given patient cohort. However, it has only recently been adopted, and most published literature still refers to "resectable" or "unresectable" stage III disease, without applying the new staging criteria.

II. Experimental Treatment Approaches

If surgery and/or radiotherapy defines the standard of care for patients with stage III NSCLC, the results of this therapy are less than optimal. Therefore, there is a need for continued investigational trials. For the last decade, these approaches have focused on the integration of chemotherapy in the overall treatment plan. Several options for doing so are available (see Table 1).

Both adjuvant chemotherapy and concomitant chemoradiotherapy are theoretically attractive concepts. Induction or neoadjuvant chemotherapy is a concept that has been under clinical investigation in patients with several types of solid tumors. It is particularly attractive for those with NSCLC, and a substantial amount of clinical information has been generated over the last decade regarding its use in this disease.

Table 1 Combined Modality Therapy: Theoretical Considerations

Local therapy → adjuvant chemotherapy (stage III A)
Neoadjuvant chemotherapy → local therapy
Neoadjuvant chemotherapy → local therapy → adjuvant chemotherapy
Concomitant chemotherapy (± surgery)
Neoadjuvant chemotherapy → concomitant chemoradiotherapy → (± surgery) adjuvant chemotherapy

Source: Modified from Vokes, 1990.

III. Principles of Neoadjuvant Chemotherapy

The term *neoadjuvant chemotherapy* implies the initial administration of chemotherapy for the treatment of regionally advanced solid tumors (Frei, 1988). This is then followed by local therapy, usually consisting of surgery and/or radiotherapy. Following a defined number of chemotherapy cycles, the response of the disease is evaluated. The response assessment provides a direct measurement of the activity of the chemotherapy regimen in a given malignancy. Local therapy with "curative intent" is not altered from that administered without prior chemotherapy (i.e., the extent of surgical resection, the radiotherapy dose, or portals). It is clear that this approach mandates a multispecialty team composed of a medical oncologist, a radiation oncologist, a chest surgeon, and nursing and social service support.

The rationale for using chemotherapy before surgery and radiotherapy has been reviewed previously (Steel and Lamberton, 1968; Shabel, 1976; Van Putten, 1986). The rationales include improved delivery of the cytotoxic agent to the tumor cell before destruction of the local vasculature by surgery and/or radiation; it can also be postulated based on the Goldie and Coldman (1979) hypothesis that the use of chemotherapy earlier in the natural history of the disease will result in higher efficacy due to the prevalence of fewer drug-resistant cells; initial chemotherapy can decrease the tumor size, allowing the subsequent radiotherapy to be administered to less bulky local disease, which might result in a better outcome; surgical margins might be less likely involved with tumor. All these factors might contribute to improved locoregional tumor controls, therefore, chemotherapy might succeed at eradicating microscopic distant metastases if given early in the course of the disease. Such micrometastases are presumed to be present in a high percentage of patients with regionally advanced NSCLC and, thus, represent a frequent cause of treatment failure. The use of neoadjuvant chemotherapy might also result in less morbid local therapy and spare the sacrifice of an organ (McNeil et al., 1981). This goal is less obviously applicable to NSCLC than it is to bladder or head and neck cancer.

These theoretical advantages for neoadjuvant chemotherapy must be considered against a number of potential theoretic disadvantages (Table 2). These include

Table 2 Theoretical Disadvantages of Neoadjuvant Chemotherapy

Toxicity
Long overall treatment duration
Possible increased incidence of distant metastases
Possible loss of option for curative surgery in nonresponders
Selection of radioresistant cells by chemotherapy

Source: Modified from Vokes, 1990.

the toxicity associated with various chemotherapy regimens and the length of time required for its administration and increased expense. There is the concern that preoperative chemotherapy might not be able to eradicate distant micrometastases and might increase the incidence of distant metastases (Van Putten et al., 1975). Patients whose disease fails to improve with chemotherapy lose the option of surgical treatment.

Neoadjuvant chemotherapy has been investigated in patients with several solid tumors, including sarcomas (Rosen et al., 1982) and head and neck cancer (Vokes et al., 1989a; Ervin et al., 1987; Rooney et al., 1985). The principles that guide its use include the need to use the most active available combination of drugs available for a given neoplasm to maximize its therapeutic potential. In diseases for which few such drugs are available, the investigation of new drugs can be performed cautiously on patients with an otherwise very poor prognosis, provided that patients whose disease improves with neoadjuvant therapy receive standard therapy with surgery and/or radiotherapy.

Time intervals in a protocol must also be defined. These include the duration of chemotherapy cycles: the maximum time interval that can be allowed between the different treatment modalities. There can be little benefit from neoadjuvant chemotherapy, even in the responding patient, if the time interval between chemotherapy and local therapy is long enough to allow for regrowth of tumor cells. The need for a rapid sequencing of treatment modalities may at times run counter to sentiments by chest surgeons, who may prefer to operate on patients who have "completely recovered" from combination chemotherapy. Similar thoughts apply to the scheduling of postoperative chest radiotherapy.

The clinical experience with neoadjuvant chemotherapy to date indicates that higher overall response rates can be achieved in patients with regionally advanced tumors compared to those patients with recurrent or metastatic disease. In some patients even histologically complete remissions can be achieved. In patients with head and neck cancer, those who achieve a complete response to neoadjuvant chemotherapy have a very good overall prognosis (Vokes et al., 1989a; Ervin et al., 1987; Rooney et al., 1985) and the subsequent administration of standard therapy is not compromised by the initial use of chemotherapy.

IV. Clinical Experience

NSCLC was not among the first tumors for which neoadjuvant chemotherapy was investigated. One reason for this is that until recently no combination of drugs had ever convincingly been shown to influence the natural history of the disease in patients with metastatic NSCLC. Only in the last few years have cisplatin-based combination chemotherapy regimens resulted in a modest improvement in survival (Rapp et al., 1988; Cormier et al., 1982; Woods et al., 1985; Ganz et al., 1989).

Based on the experience in other diseases, this modest activity in the stage IV setting might translate into more substantial activity in the stage III setting. Neoadjuvant chemotherapy could be helpful in identifying new drugs or combinations of drugs that are active. The use of neoadjuvant chemotherapy in NSCLC is well justified by the pattern of relapse of stage III disease that is systemic.

In the next section we review some of the clinical studies that specifically address the investigation of neoadjuvant chemotherapy in NSCLC and have been fully published.

An early trial of neoadjuvant chemotherapy in NSCLC was conducted at our own institution, the University of Chicago, between 1983 and 1985. We treated 27 patients with regionally advanced NSCLC using two cycles of neoadjuvant etoposide, vindesine, and cisplatin (Vokes et al., 1989b). Most of these patients were inoperable and would now be classified as having stage IIIB disease. Four patients were unevaluable for response to chemotherapy. Of 23 evaluable patients, 13 had a partial response and 10 had stable disease or disease progression. The overall response rate was therefore 48%. Five patients received no subsequent local therapy due to early disease progression. Local therapy consisted of either surgery followed by radiotherapy in only 4 patients or radiotherapy alone in 14 unresectable patients. At completion of local therapy, seven patients were considered free of disease including all four who had undergone surgery. The median time to disease progression for the 13 patients who had a partial response to neoadjuvant chemotherapy was 8 months. The median survival for all 27 patients registered on study was 8 months (range, 3 days–53+ months), and one patient is currently alive at 60+ months of follow-up. Chemotherapy's toxic effects included moderate degree of myelosuppression, nausea and vomiting, and, in selected patients, ototoxicity, neurotoxicity, and a wasting syndrome. One patient died of intracerebral hemorrhage while thrombocytopenic from chemotherapy during cycle 1. Although this study has an encouraging response rate with acceptable toxicity, the median survival achieved is no better than that achieved with standard therapy. We have subsequently abandoned further investigation of this regimen.

Two trials conducted at the Dana-Farber Cancer Institute included patients with marginally resectable and with unresectable disease (Van Putten et al., 1975; Skarin et al., 1989). Forty-one patients had stage IIIA disease and received two cycles of neoadjuvant cyclophosphamide, doxorubicin, and cisplatin (CAP) followed by radiotherapy (3000 CGy preoperatively) and resection (Skarin et al., 1989). Postoperative therapy included additional radiation and CAP chemotherapy in some patients. The response rate after two cycles of CAP (minimal and partial responses) was 53%. The response rate to all preoperative therapy was 72% (complete response [CR]-rate 2.5%); an improvement in response between CAP chemotherapy and subsequent radiotherapy was noted in 14 patients. Subsequently 37 patients (90%) underwent thoracotomy and all gross disease was successfully removed in 36 patients.

At a median follow-up of 32 months for all 41 patients entered on study, 22 of the 37 resected patients (61%) developed disease recurrence. This involved both the chest and distant sites in nine patients, the chest only in four, and distant sites only in nine patients. The central nervous system (CNS) was involved as a site of relapse in three resected patients. The use of prophylactic cranial radiation was not mandated by the trial. The CNS relapse occurred in only 1 of 7 patients receiving prophylactic cranial irradiation, compared to 7 of 27 patients not receiving prophylactic cranial irradiation. The median survival for all patients was 32 months and the 1 year survival rate was 75%. Fourteen patients (34%) are alive, with survival times ranging from 38 to 71 months. Three relapses were noted after 20 months from diagnosis. This study, therefore, demonstrated a high response rate in these resectable patients, and, in addition, suggests that improved survival figures can also be achieved.

Fram et al. (1985) reported on the same CAP regimen administrated to 30 patients with unresectable disease for 2 cycles before radiotherapy (55–57 Gy) followed by additional chemotherapy for those patients with documented response to initial chemotherapy. A response rate of 47% to CAP was documented (13 patients with partial response, 1 with complete response). Following radiotherapy, 66% of the patients had objective disease regression (7 complete, 12 partial responses). Of 13 patients with partial response to CAP chemotherapy, 5 achieved complete response with subsequent radiotherapy. In contrast, of 12 patients with no response to neoadjuvant chemotherapy, 5 had a partial response to radiotherapy. The median survival for all patients was only 9 months. Locoregional recurrence was observed less frequently in patients having partial or complete response after radiotherapy (5 of 19) than in those patients who had less than a partial response (8 of 10).

When comparing these two studies from Dana Farber Cancer Center, it is of interest that high response rates were achieved in both resectable and unresectable patients. A possible improvement in survival, on the other hand, is suggested only for resectable patients but not for unresectable patients.

Eagan et al. (1987) reported on 39 patients with regionally advanced inoperable NSCLC treated with 2 cycles of cyclophosphamide, doxorubicin, and cisplatin. Although 20 patients (51%) had an initial response to chemotherapy, the median survival for all patients was only 11 months. For 19 patients who underwent subsequent thoracotomy (all 19 had responded to neoadjuvant chemotherapy), the median survival was 15 months and the 2 year survival rate was 10%. These patients who underwent thoracotomy were noted to have a low local recurrence rate; however, a high distant failure rate was observed, presumably due to inability of the chemotherapy used in this study to eradicate distant micrometastases.

Cox et al. (1986) reported on a trial by the Radiation Therapy Oncology Group (RTOG). Thirty evaluable patients with inoperable NSCLC received 2 cycles of neoadjuvant cisplatin and etoposide followed by radiotherapy (50–60

Gy. Two patients achieved a clinical CR and 4 a partial response (PR) to chemotherapy alone. Fifty three percent of patients developed recurrence within the radiation treatment field and 43% developed distant metastases. The 1 and 2 year survival rates were 47% and 20%, respectively. These survival data were similar to those of prior RTOG studies using radiotherapy alone and, therefore, again were not suggestive of a significant impact of this regimen on survival. On the other hand, the number of patients studied was small. In addition, the dosage of cisplatin was low and may have been suboptimal for achieving responses.

A frequently used regimen in patients with NSCLC is the combination of cisplatin, mitomycin C, and a vinca alkaloid (vindesine or vinblastine) (MVP) (Kris et al., 1986; Martini et al., 1988; Pisters et al., 1990). This combination was initially developed by Gralla and his co-workers at Memorial–Sloan Kettering Cancer Center and has also been investigated at other institutions (Kris et al., 1986; Martini et al., 1988; Pisters et al., 1990; Spain, 1988). Although not clearly superior to similar regimens when studied in patients with stage IV disease (Ruckdeschel et al., 1986), it is composed of single agents all known to be active in NSCLC (Joss et al., 1984). The experimental use of this regimen in the neoadjuvant setting, therefore, is well justified.

Pisters and colleagues (1990) recently reported the results achieved in a study underway involving 58 patients with stage IIIA NSCLC. These patients were treated with three cycles of MVP chemotherapy followed by surgery and two additional cycles of chemotherapy. Mediastinal radiotherapy was administered to patients with evidence of residual disease at the time of thoracotomy. Of 58 patients evaluated for response to MVP, 7 (12%) had a clinical complete response (4 of these with no residual disease at surgery) and 37 (63%) a partial response (5 of these with pathologic complete response), for an overall response rate of 76%. Forty-two patients subsequently underwent thoracotomy with complete removal of tumor in 33 (57% of total study population). At a follow-up time ranging from 4 months to 4 years, the median survival is 20 months.

This study clearly demonstrates the feasibility of performing surgery following MVP chemotherapy and, in the opinion of the investigator, also suggests an increased resectability rate compared to historic control (Kris et al., 1985). The survival data in this study also appear favorable and justify the further testing of MVP in randomized clinical trials. In view of these positive survival data it is important to stress that this study, like that by Skarin et al. (1989), focused on patients with resectable disease.

Spain (1988) investigated a variant of the MVP regimen using mitomycin C, cisplatin, and continuous infusion vinblastine. Thirty-one patients with mostly unresectable NSCLC were included in this study. The specific treatment design initially included initial or concomitant radiotherapy, while later in the course of the study patients received 3 to 4 cycles of MVP followed by surgery (5 patients) and/or radiotherapy of 50–66 Gy.

Response to MVP was assessed in 22 patients. Five (23%) achieved a complete response and 11 (50%) a partial response for an overall response rate of 73%. All patients undergoing surgery were found to have residual disease in the pathologic specimen. Two of 5 patients undergoing resection remain alive and disease-free at 49 and 62 months of follow-up. The median survival for 26 patients receiving radiotherapy is 19 months, with 6 patients alive and free of disease at 127–77 months of follow-up. These encouraging survival data contrast positively with a historic control group of patients treated with radiotherapy alone at the same institution. An important side effect of MVP chemotherapy is its potential for lung injury; in this trial the administration of dexamethasone seemed to prevent this.

Nittamo-Korhonen et al. (1989) compared cisplatin plus vindesine to cisplatin plus etoposide, each administered for three cycles before radiotherapy. Overall response rates were 66% and 50%, respectively. However, median survival times of 241 days and 409 days were not thought to be different from figures achieved with standard therapy alone.

Additional studies have been published by Takita et al. (1986), who administered nonstandardized neoadjuvant chemotherapy to 29 patients with inoperable NSCLC and by Osoba et al. (1986). In the latter study, two cycles of bleomycin, etoposide, and cisplatin were followed by split-course radiotherapy. The objective response rate to chemotherapy was 60%. At early follow-up the median survival time had not been reached in these unresectable patients.

In summary, these pilot trials clearly demonstrate the feasibility of administering neoadjuvant chemotherapy to patients with stage III NSCLC. Response rates in most of these trials reach or exceed 50%, indicating increased activity of chemotherapy in NSCLC when used earlier in the natural history of the disease, as has been shown in other diseases. In addition, histologic confirmation of complete response can occasionally be achieved.

Most of the studies reviewed here have included patients with unresectable disease, who would nowadays frequently be classified with stage IIIB. For these patient cohorts the survival data reported are frequently disappointing, suggesting that the high response rates to neoadjuvant chemotherapy do not necessarily translate into improved survival. On the other hand, when patients with stage IIIA disease were treated and surgery was included in the overall treatment plan, the survival data were more encouraging (Cormier et al., 1982; Skarin et al., 1989).

Although most chemotherapy regimens have included cisplatin, it is not clear which combination of drugs and which schedule are superior. Clinical research therefore clearly needs to continue to focus on the development of innovative drug combinations and the evaluation of new drugs in NSCLC in an attempt to increase further overall and complete response rates to neoadjuvant chemotherapy. At the same time, randomized studies are needed to establish unequivocally whether the addition of neoadjuvant chemotherapy to standard therapy improves survival for stage IIIA and/or stage IIIB NSCLC compared to standard therapy alone.

Results from one such randomized study conducted by the Cancer and Leukemia Group B have recently been reported (Dillman et al., 1990). One hundred and eighty patients with unresectable NSCLC were randomized to receive radiotherapy alone or two cycles of cisplatin and vinblastine followed by radiotherapy. One hundred and fifty-five eligible patients were analyzed for response. Of 77 patients receiving radiotherapy alone, 43% responded, including 16% with a complete response. Of 78 patients receiving neoadjuvant chemotherapy, 55% responded to both treatment modalities, including 19% with complete response. With a median follow-up of 19 months, the median survival was 13.8 months for patients receiving combined modality therapy and 9.7 months for patients receiving radiotherapy alone. The pattern of relapse was identical in both study arms, showing a predominance of local recurrence or of combined local and distant recurrence, while few patients experienced distant disease progression alone.

These data are highly encouraging: for the first time they conclusively demonstrate a (small) survival advantage through combined modality therapy in stage III NSCLC. This advantage is achieved despite using only a moderately active combination chemotherapy regimen (complete response rate after two cycles 4%, overall response rate 36%). It is also of interest, that the study population in this trial, although classified as having "unresectable" disease according to the study eligibility criteria, would nowadays be predominantly staged as having stage IIIA disease. The survival advantage demonstrated in this study therefore confirms the suggested benefit in some of the pilot studies investigating neoadjuvant chemotherapy in patients with stage IIIA disease.

Despite these positive results, this CALGB trial does not represent an endpoint in itself. A median survival of 13.8 months is still very unsatisfying. Rather than define a new standard therapy, this CALGB trial therefore merely leads the way to continuing the investigation of sequential combined modality therapy with the goal of further improving the survival rate and eventually defining curative approaches for regionally advanced NSCLC.

References

Cormier, Y., Bergeron, D., LaForge, J., et al. (1982). Benefits of polychemotherapy in advanced non-small cell bronchogenic carcinoma. *Cancer* **50:**845–849.

Cox, J. D., Samson, M. K., Herskovic, A. M., et al. (1986). Cisplatin and etoposide before definitive radiation therapy for inoperable squamous carcinoma, adenocarcinoma, and large cell carcinoma of the lung: a phase I-II study of the Radiation Therapy Oncology Group. *Cancer Treat. Rep.* **70:**1219–1220.

Dillman, R. O., Seagren, S. L., Propert, K., et al. (1990). A randomized trial of induction chemotherapy plus high-dose radiation versus radiation alone in Stage III non-small cell lung cancer. *N. Eng. J. Med.* **323:**940–945.

Eagan, R. T., Ingle, J. N., Frytak, S., et al. (1977). Platinum-based poly-chemotherapy versus diaphydrogalactitol in advanced non-small cell lung cancer. *Cancer Treat. Rep.* **61:**1339–1345.

Eagan, R. T., Ruud, C., Lee, R. E., et al. (1987). Pilot study of induction therapy with cyclophosphamide, doxorubicin, and cisplatin and chest irradiation prior to thoracotomy in initially inoperable stage III M_0 non-small cell lung cancer. *Cancer Treat. Rep.* **71:**895–900.

Ervin, T. J., Clark, J. R., Weichselbaum, R. R., et al. (1987). An analysis of induction and adjuvant chemotherapy in the multidisciplinary treatment of squamous-cell carcinoma of the head and neck. *J. Clin. Oncol.* **5:**10–20.

Fram, R., Skarin, A., Balikian, J., et al. (1985). Combination chemotherapy followed by radiation therapy in patients with regional stage III unresectable non-small cell lung cancer. *Cancer Treat. Rep.* **69:**587–590.

Frei, E. III (1988) What's in a name—neoadjuvant. *J. Natl. Cancer Inst.* **80:**1088–1089.

Ganz, P. A., Figlin, R. A., Haskel, C. M., et al. (1989). Supportive care versus supportive care and combination chemotherapy to metastatic non-small cell lung cancer. Does chemotherapy make a difference? *Cancer* **63:**1271–1278.

Goldie, J. H., and Coldman, A. J. (1979). A mathematical model for relating the drug sensitivity of tumors to their spontaneous mutation rate. *Cancer Treat. Rep.* **63:**1727–1733.

Johnson, M. R. (1988). Selecting patients with lung cancer for surgical therapy. *Semin. Oncol.* **15:**246–254.

Joss, R. A., et al. (1984). New agents in non-small cell lung cancer. *Cancer Treat. Rev.* **11:** 205–236.

Kris, M. G., Gralla, R. J., Kalman, L. A., et al. (1985). Randomized trial comparing vindesine plus cisplatin with vinblastine plus cisplatin in patients with non-small cell lung cancer with analysis of methods of response assessment. *Cancer Treat. Rep* **69:** 387–395.

Kris, M. G., Gralla, R. J., Wertheim, M. S., et al. (1986). Trial of the combination of mitomycin, vindesine, and cisplatin and patients with advanced non-small cell lung cancer. *Cancer Treat. Rep.* **70:**1091–1096.

Martini, N., Kris, M. G., Gralla, R. T., et al. (1988). The effects of preoperative chemotherapy in the resectability of non-small cell lung carcinoma with mediastinal lymph-node metastases (N_2 M_0). *Ann. Thorac. Surg.* **45:**370–379.

McNeil, B. J., Weichselbaum, R. R., and Pauker, S. (1981). Speech and survival: tradeoff between quality and quantity of life in laryngeal cancer. *N. Eng. J. Med.* **305:** 982–987.

Mountain, C. F. (1988). Prognostic implications of the international staging system for lung cancer. *Semin. Oncol.* **15:**236–245.

Niitamo-Korhonen, S., Holsti, L. R., et al. (1989). A comparison of Cis-platinum–vindesine and cisplatinum–etoposide combined with radiotherapy for previously untreated localized inoperable non-small cell lung cancer. *Eur. J. Cancer Clin. Oncol.* **7:**1039–1043.

Osoba, D., Rusthoven, J. J., Evans, H. K., et al. (1986). Combined chemotherapy and radiation therapy for non-small cell lung cancer. *Semin. Oncol.* **13** (Suppl. 3): 121–124.

Perez, C. A., Stanley, K., and Grundy, G. (1982). Impact of irradiation technique and tumor extent in tumor control and survival of patients with unresectable non-oat cell carcinoma of the lung. *Cancer* **50:**1091–1099.

Pisters, K. M. W., Kris, M. G., Gralla, R. J., and Martini, N. (1990). Paraoperative chemotherapy in non-small cell lung cancer. An analysis of a trial in patients with clinically Stage III A apparent mediastinal lymph node involvement. In *Adjuvant Therapy of Cancer*. Edited by S. E. Salmon. Philadelphia, W. B. Saunders, pp. 125–132.

Rooney, M., Kish, J., Jacobs, J., et al. (1985). Improved complete response rate and survival in advanced head and neck cancer after three course induction therapy with 120-hour 5-FU infusion and cisplatin. *Cancer* **55:**1123–1128.

Rapp, E., Pater, J. L., Willan, A., et al. (1988). Chemotherapy can prolong survival in patients with advanced non-small cell lung cancer. Report of a Canadian multicenter randomized trial *J. Clin. Oncol.* **6:**641–663.

Rosen, G., Caparros, B., Huvos, A. G., et al. (1982). Preoperative chemotherapy for osteogenic sarcoma: selection of postoperative adjuvant chemotherapy based on the response of the primary tumor to preoperative chemotherapy. *Cancer* **49:**1221–1230.

Ruckdeschel, J. C., Finkelstein, D. M., Ettinger, D. S., et al. (1986). A randomized trial of the four most active regimens for metastatic non-small cell lung cancer. *J. Clin. Oncol.* **4:**14–22.

Shabel, F. M., Jr. (1976). Concepts for treatment of micrometastases developed in murine systems. *Am. J. Roentgenol.* **126:**500–511.

Skarin, A., Jochelson, M., Sheldon, T., et al. (1989). Neoadjuvant chemotherapy in marginally resectable Stage III M_0 non-small cell lung cancer: long-term follow-up in 41 patients. *J. Surg. Oncol.* **40:**266–274.

Spain, R. C. (1988). Neoadjuvant mitomycin C., cisplatin, and infusion vinblastine in locally and regionally advanced non-small cell lung cancer: problems and progress from the perspective of long-term follow-up. *Semin. Oncol.* **15:**6–15.

Steel, G. G., and Lamberton, L. F. (1968). Cell population kinetics and chemotherapy. *Natl. Cancer Inst. Monogr.* **30:**29–50.

Takita, H., Regal, A. M., Antkowiak, J. G., et al. (1986). Chemotherapy followed by lung resection in inoperable non-small cell lung carcinoma due to locally far-advanced disease. *Cancer* **57:**630–635.

Van Putten, L. M. (1986). Experimental preoperative chemotherapy. In *Recent Results in Cancer Research, Preoperative (Neoadjuvant) Chemotherapy*. Edited by J. Ragaz, P. R. Bank, and J. H. Goldie. New York, Springer-Verlag, pp. 36–40.

Van Putten, L. M., Kram, L. K. J., Van Dierendonck, H. H. C., et al. (1975). Enhancement by drugs of metastatic lung nodule formation after intravenous tumor cell injection. *Int. J. Cancer* **15:**588–595.

Vokes, E. E., Moran, W. J., Mick, R., et al. (1989a). Neoadjuvant and adjuvant methotrexate, cisplatin and fluorouracil in multinodal therapy of head and neck cancer. *J. Clin. Oncol.* **7:**838–845.

Vokes, E. E., Bitran, J. D., Hoffman, P. C., et al. (1989b). Neoadjuvant vindesine, etoposide, and cisplatin for locally advanced non-small cell lung cancer. Final report of a phase II study. *Chest* **96:**110–113.

Woods, R. L., Kui, J. A., Page, J., et al. (1985). Non-small cell cancer: a randomized comparison of chemotherapy with no chemotherapy. *Proc. Am. Soc. Clin. Oncol.* **4:**177 (abstr.).

18

Rapidly Alternating Radiotherapy and High-Dose Cisplatin in Stage III Non-Small-Cell Lung Cancer

EDITH A. PEREZ and DAVID R. GANDARA

University of California, Davis
VA Medical Center
Martinez, California
and
Northern California Oncology Group
Belmont, California

FRANK H. VALONE and THEODORE PHILLIPS

University of California
San Francisco, California
and
Northern California Oncology Group
Belmont, California

ALBERT B. DEISSEROTH

The University of Texas M. D. Anderson Cancer Center
Houston, Texas

MACK ROACH, III

University of California
San Francisco, California

DAVID K. AHN

Northern California Oncology Group
Belmont, California

I. Introduction

Locally advanced non-small-cell lung cancer (NSCLC) accounts for approximately one-third of all bronchogenic cancers, or approximately 50,000 cases per year in the United States. Radiotherapy has been widely used in the treatment of locally advanced disease with little impact on long-term survival (Perez et al., 1987). Traditional radiotherapy yields median survival times of only 9–12 months and 5-year survival rates of 10–15% (Arriagada et al., 1990; Choi and Couchette, 1981; Cox et al., 1991; Perez et al., 1982; Salazar et al., 1986) in spite of its well documented palliative benefit. Substaging of locally advanced NSCLC is described in the current American Joint Committee on Cancer (AJCC) system, based on the extent of the primary tumor and nodal disease and is designated as stages III_A and III_B (Mountain, 1986). Patients with stage III_B are generally reported to have a worse prognosis with a median survival of less than 8 months and a 5-year survival rate of only 3–5%. By comparison, patients with stage III_A disease have median survival times of approximately 12 months and 5-year survival rates of 13–15% (Talton et al., 1990), although there is some controversy about this point (Curran and Stafford, 1990).

In view of the poor survival with radiation therapy alone for patients with unresectable NSCLC, a number of trials adding chemotherapy to radiotherapy have been performed. Although results have varied, some studies have shown survival benefit when combined modality treatment is used (Dillman et al., 1990; Mattson et al., 1988; Mira et al., 1990). The goals of combined modality therapy are both to improve local control and eradicate distant metastases. Methods of combining these modalities include sequential use of chemotherapy followed by radiotherapy, concurrent use, or alternation of these modalities.

In some experimental models, alternating radiotherapy and chemotherapy enhances tumor cell kill compared to either modality alone or sequential use of both modalities (Goldie et al., 1988). Alternation also reduces host toxicity and normal tissue reaction compared to concurrent use (Looney et al., 1984). In addition, mathematical models of tumor resistance predict that alternation of radiotherapy and chemotherapy will decrease the emergence of both drug resistant and radiation resistant tumor cells (Looney, 1988). The chemotherapeutic agent cisplatin is of particular interest when used in this setting in NSCLC, in view of its documented activity in the treatment of metastatic disease (Gandara et al., 1989) and its radiosensitizing potential (Dewit, 1986).

In view of these data, we designed this study to determine the feasibility of combining radiotherapy with a day 1 and 8 high-dosage cisplatin regimen in patients with locally unresectable NSCLC. The following report updates our preliminary findings (Gandara et al., 1991) with more patients and a longer follow-up time.

II. Materials and Methods

A. Patients

Twenty-nine patients gave written informed consent and were registered in this cooperative group study between February 1986 and June 1989. All patients had histologically or cytologically confirmed unresectable NSCLC (stage III_A or III_B). Prior surgical resection, radiotherapy, chemotherapy, or biological response modifier therapy was not allowed. Karnofsky performance status (KPS) >60%, age <70 years, and adequate hematologic, renal, and hepatic function were required. All patients underwent pretreatment staging with bronchoscopy, chest and upper abdominal computed tomographic (CT) scan, as well as bone and brain CT scans. All patients had measurable disease.

Table 1 Patient Characteristics at Study Entry

Characteristic		Number
Total patients		29
Age in years	Mean	59
	Range	(40–70)
Sex	Male	27
	Female	2
Karnofsky performance status	70–80	13
	90–100	16
Histologic subtype:	Squamous	14
	Adenocarcinoma	8
	Large cell	3
	Unspecified	3
	Mixed	1
Stage of disease	IIIA	6
	IIIB	23

Patients' characteristics at study entry are shown in Table 1. The mean age for all patients was 59 years, with a range from 40 to 70 years. There were 27 (93%) male and 2 (7%) female patients. Median KPS was 90% with a range between 70 and 100%. Seventeen (59%) of the patients had squamous cell cancer. Six (22%) of patients had stage IIIA, and the majority (23 or 78%) had stage III_B disease. Seventy-five percent of patients had weight loss of more than 5%.

B. Therapy

The treatment plan schema is shown in Table 2. This consisted of radiation therapy to a total of 60 Gy given in three courses over 10 weeks and high-dosage cisplatin chemotherapy on alternating weeks. Radiotherapy was given as three 10-day courses of 200 cGy/fraction/day, starting on weeks 1 and 2 of therapy, course two on weeks 5 and 6, and course three on weeks 9 and 10. The first and third radiotherapy courses included a large field encompassing the entire target volume, hila, and mediastinal structures, using anteroposterior/posteroanterior ports. One centimeter margins were subsequently modified to 0.5 cm during courses 1 and 3 because of concern of enhanced radiation (RT) pneumonitis. The treatment volume during the second RT course consisted of a smaller boost to gross disease only, including the primary lung lesion, ipsilateral hilum, mediastinal lymph nodes, and supraclavicular nodes if involved, with shielding of the spinal cord. Oblique and lateral ports were used. High-dosage cisplatin was given at a dosage of 100 mg/m^2 in 250 ml 3% saline as a 3 h infusion, on weeks 3 and 4, 7 and 8, 11 and 12, and a consolidation on weeks 15 and 16.

Table 2 Schema for NCOG P2N-85-1, Alternating Radiotherapy and High-Dosage Cisplatin in NSCLC

Week	1	2	3	4	5	6	7	8	9	10	11	12	13	14	15	16	17	18	19	20	21	22
Radiotherapy	XL	XL			XB	XB			XL	XL												
Chemotherapy			C	C			C	C			C	C			C	C						
Staging	X																					
Restage																						X

XL, large field 200 cGy daily for 10 days = 2000 cGy to gross tumor and prophylactic areas; XB, boost field 200 cGy daily for 10 days = 2000 cGy to gross disease only, avoiding esophagus and spinal cord; C, 100 mg/m^2 cisplatin in 250ml of 3% saline IV over 3 h.

During chemotherapy, patients received pretherapy and posttherapy saline hydration of at least 3 L and were aggressively treated with parenteral and oral antiemetics before, during, and for 3–5 days after cisplatin administration.

The program was designed to deliver radiotherapy courses without delay whenever possible. Dose reduction of cisplatin was not allowed. Patients received drug therapy if the creatinine clearance was ≥50 ml/min, WBC ≥3500/mm^3, and platelet count ≥125,000/mm^3. If these criteria were not met, day 1 chemotherapy was deleted from that course of therapy. Before each day 8 drug treatment, only a serum creatinine measurement was required. Day 8 cisplatin was given if the change in serum creatinine was ≤0.5 mg/100 ml and the serum creatinine level was ≤1.5 mg/100 ml. For any changes above that, a creatinine clearance level was obtained, with requirements for treatment as for day 1. If treatment criteria were not met, day 8 cisplatin was deleted from that course.

Standard Northern California Oncology Group (NCOG) criteria were used to assess response and toxicity, as previously described (Gandara et al., 1989).

Statistical analysis was plotted by the method of Kaplan and Meier (1958).

III. Results

A. Response and Survival

Twenty-eight patients were eligible for response and survival analysis. One patient was ineligible due to the presence of metastatic disease. As shown in Table 3, a complete response was achieved in 6 patients (21%) and a partial response ≥50% by bidimensional measurements in 14 patients (50%). The overall response rate was 71% (20/28). Partial response of <50% occurred in 5 patients.

Table 3 Detailed Overall Response

	Number of patients (N = 29)
Complete response	6
Partial response >50%	14
Partial response <50%	5
No response/progression	3
Ineligible	1
Overall response rate (n = 28)	
Complete response rate (CR/Eligible)	6/28 (21%)
Partial response (PR >50%/Eligible)	14/28 (50%)
Overall objective response rate (CR + PR >50%/Eligible)	20/28 (71%)

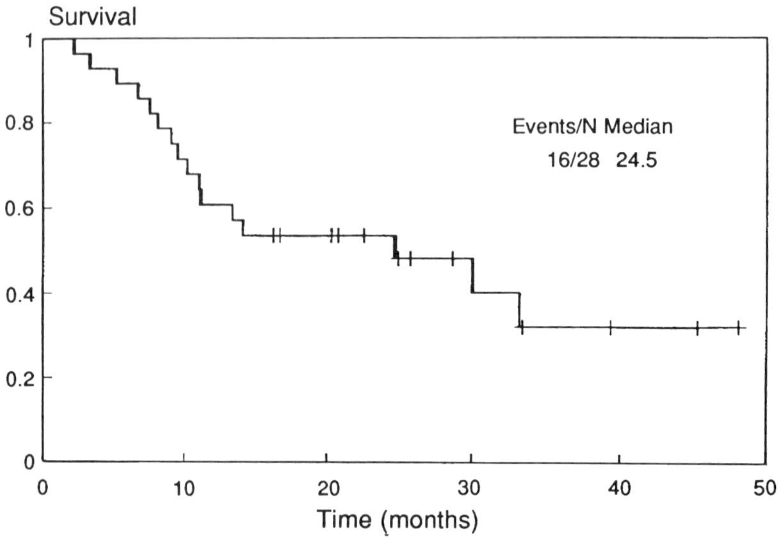

Figure 1 Actuarial survival distribution for all eligible patients.

Median survival time by Kaplan and Meier plot was 24.5 months with a range of 2–48+ months, as shown in Figure 1. The median survival time for 22 patients with stage III_B disease was 11.2 months. One- and 2-year overall survival rates are 62% (17/28) and 32% (9/28), respectively.

All patients in this report have been evaluated for a minimum of 1 year or until death. Twelve of 28 patients remain alive, 9 without evidence of progression. Sixteen patients have died, 13 of progressive cancer, and 3 of other causes. Sites of failure are chest only (21%), chest plus distant (7%), and distant only (25%). Three patients developed brain metastases.

B. Toxicity

The toxicity of this regimen was significant but manageable. There were no treatment-related deaths. As described in Table 4, mild to moderate radiation-related and/or chemotherapy-related toxicity occurred in most patients. Demonstrating feasibility, 25 of 28 patients completed the planned radiotherapy program and a median dosage of 500 mg/m^2 (or 2.5 cycles) of cisplatin was delivered. Four patients had delays in radiotherapy courses as specified by hematologic criteria for continued treatment.

Severe myelosuppression (white blood cell count $<1000/mm^3$) occurred in two patients. Four patients had nadir platelet counts between 25,000 and 49,000/mm^3. No patients showed a platelet count $<25,000/mm^3$. A maximum serum creatinine level between 1.5 and 3.0 mg/100 ml was observed in 10 patients, but in

Table 4 Hematologic and Nonhematologic Toxic Reactions

Toxic Reactions	Grade	Total (n = 29)	Percent
WBC Count ($1000/mm^3$)			
3.0 –4.4	1	3	10
2.0–2.9	2	10	34
1.0–1.9	3	10	34
<1.0	4	2	7
Platelet Count ($1000/mm^3$)			
90–129	1	5	17
50–89	2	4	14
25–49	3	4	0
<25	4	0	0
Serum creatinine level (mg/100 ml)			
1.5–3.0	1	10	34
3.1–5.0	2	0	0
5.0–10.0	3	0	0
<10.0	4	0	0
Peripheral Neuropathy	1	9	31
	2	2	7
	3	1	3
	4	0	0
Ototoxicity	1	2	7
	2	2	7
	3	2	7
	4	0	0
Radiation Pneumonitis	1	3	10
	2	2	7
	3	1	3
	4	0	0
Radiation Esophagitis	1	7	24
	2	1	3
	3	0	0
	4	0	0

only 4 was this >2 mg/100 ml. Peripheral neuropathy occurred in 41% of patients. Grade 3 neuropathy (gait disturbance) was observed in only 1 patient.

Radiation pneumonitis occurred in 6 patients (21%) and was clinically severe in one patient. Mild esophagitis occurred in 8 patients (28%). Radiation pericarditis occurred in one patient 8 months after radiation therapy, and resolved with corticosteroid therapy and serial pericardiocentesis. The patient remains alive without evidence of disease 51 months after initiating protocol therapy.

IV. Discussion

We conclude that rapid alternation of radiotherapy and high-dosage cisplatin is feasible, that toxicity is manageable, and that survival data in this small pilot study are encouraging. Twenty-five of 28 patients completed the planned radiation therapy program. The median number of cycles of cisplatin administered was 2.5. In addition, our data suggest that alternating radiotherapy and high-dosage cisplatin may have a positive impact on survival in patients with locally advanced NSCLC. The 1-year survival rate was 61% and the 2-year survival rate was 32%. The median survival time for all patients was 24.5 months and 11.2 months for patients with stage III_B disease.

One interesting aspect of this study has been the time to maximal response, which has been prolonged in some patients. Responses have continued to evolve on chest x-ray and CT scans for 1 year or more after completion of therapy. Several patients have stable abnormalities on CT scan over many months or even years, suggesting that these prolonged partial responses represent only residual disease.

Approaches to combining radiotherapy and chemotherapy in NSCLC include sequential, concurrent, and integrated alternating therapy. Although a large number of pilot studies of combined modality therapy have reported encouraging results, few randomized phase III trials have been performed (Mattson et al., 1988; Mira et al., 1990; Pisch et al., 1990; Schaake-Konig et al., 1986; Van Haskamp et al., 1987). The current interest in sequential induction chemotherapy followed by radiotherapy is based primarily on the positive results of a single study, that of the CALGB (Dillman et al., 1990) and confirmation is required. In theory, alternating radiotherapy and cisplatin-based chemotherapy offers advantages over the sequential approach by the early use of both modalities and enhanced radiosensitizing effects of cisplatin, while avoiding the excess toxicity of concurrent combined modality therapy.

Our observations of encouraging response and survival data, as well as acceptable toxicity in a subset of patients with a historically defined poor prognosis, confirm the feasibility of the integrated alternating approach. Issues to be addressed in future studies are the optimal dosage schedule of radiotherapy and cisplatin and the importance of the actual sequence of alternation of these modalities.

References

Arriagada, R., LeChevalier, T., Quoix, E., Ruffie, P., Tarayre, M., Douillard, J. Y., and Martin, M. (1990). Chemotherapy effect on locally advanced non-small cell lung carcinoma: a randomized study of 363 patients. *Proc. ASTRO* **19**(1):195 (#137).

Choi, N. C., and Couchette, J. A. (1981). Improved survival of patients with unresectable non small cell bronchogenic carcinoma by an innovative high-dose en-bloc radiotherapeutic approach. *Cancer* **48:**101–109.

Cox, J. D., Azarnia, N., Byhardt, R. W., Shink, H., Emami, B., and Pajak, T. (1991). A randomized phase I/II trial of hyperfractionated radiation therapy with total doses of 60.0 Gy to 79.2 Gy: possible survival benefit with ⩾ 69.6 Gy in favorable patients with radiation therapy oncology group stage III non-small cell lung carcinoma: report of Radiation Therapy Group 83–11. *J. Clin. Oncol.* **8:**1543–1551.

Curran, W. J., and Stafford, P. M. (1990). Lack of apparent difference in outcome between clinically staged III_A and III_B non-small cell lung cancer treated with radiation therapy. *J. Clin. Oncol.* **8:**409–415.

Dewit, L. (1986). Combined treatment of radiation and cisdiamminedichloroplatinum (II): a review of experimental and clinical data. *Int. J. Radiat. Oncol. Biol. Phys.* **13:**403–426.

Dillman, R. O., Seagren, S. L., Propert, K. J., Guerra, J., Eaton, W. L., Perry, M. C., Carey, R. W., Frei, E. F., and Green, M. R. (1990). A randomized trial of induction chemotherapy plus high-dose radiation versus radiation alone in Stage III non-small cell lung cancer. *N. Engl. J. Med.* **323:**940–945.

Gandara, D. R., Wold, H., Perez, E. A., Deisseroth, A. B., Doroshow, J., Meyers, F., McWhirter, K., Hannigan, J., and DeGregorio, M. W. (1989). Cisplatin dose intensity in non-small cell lung cancer: phase II results of a day 1 and 8 high-dose regimen. *J. Natl. Cancer Inst.* **81:**790–794.

Gandara, D. R., Valone, F. H., Perez, E. A., Deisseroth, A. B., Roach, M., Ahn, D. K., and Phillips, T. (1991). Rapidly alternating radiotherapy and high-dose cisplatin chemotherapy in stage III_B non-small cell lung cancer: results of a Phase I-II study. *Int. J. Radiat. Oncol. Biol. Phys.* **20:**1047–1052.

Goldie, J. H., Coldman, A. J., Ng, V., Hopkins, H. A., and Looney, W. (1988). Mathematical and computer-based model of alternating chemotherapy and radiation therapy in experimental neoplasms. *Antibiot. Chemother.* **41:**11–20.

Kaplan, E. L., and Meier, P. (1958). Non-parametric estimation from incomplete observations. *J. Am. Stat. Assoc.* **53:**457–481.

Looney, W. B. (1988). Special lecture: alternating chemotherapy and radiotherapy. *NCI Monog.* **6:**85–94.

Looney, W. B., Hopkins, H. A., and Carter, W. H. (1984). Solid tumor models for the assessment of different treatment modalities: XXII. The alternate utilization of radiotherapy and chemotherapy. *Cancer* **54:**416–425.

Mattson, K., Holsti, L. R., Holsti, P., Jakobsson, M., Kajnti, M., Liioppo, K., Mantual, M., Nitamo-Korhonem, S. (1988). Inoperable non-small cell lung cancer: radiation with or without chemotherapy. *Eur. J. Cancer Clin. Oncol.* **24:**477–482.

Mira, J. G., Miller, T. P., and Crowley, J. J. (1990). Chest irradiation (RT) versus chest RT + chemotherapy: prophylactic brain RT in localized non-small cell lung cancer: a Southwest Oncology Group randomized study. *Proc. ASTRO* **19**(1):145 (#9).

Mountain, C. F. (1986). A new international staging system for lung cancer. *Chest* **89:**225–233 (suppl).

Perez, C. A., Stanley, K., Grundy, G., Hanson, W., Rubin, P., Kramer, S., Brady, L. W., Marks, J., Perez-Tomayo, R., Brown, G. S., Concannon, J. P., and Rotman, M. (1982). Impact of irradiation technique and tumor extent in tumor control and survival of patients with unresectable non-oat cell carcinoma of the lung: report by the RTOG. *Cancer* **50:**1091–1099.

Perez, C. A., Pajack, T. F., Rubin, P., Simpson, J., Mohiuddin, M., Brady, L., Perez-Tomayo, R., and Rotman, M. (1987). Long term observations of the patterns of failure in patients with unresectable non-oat cell carcinoma of the lung treated with definite radiotherapy: report by the Radiation Therapy Oncology Group. *Cancer* **59:**1874–1881.

Pisch, J., Malamud, S., Beattie, E., and Vikram, B. (1990). Cisplatin based chemotherapy with accelerated, b.i.d. radiation therapy for advanced non-small cell lung cancer (NSCLC). Abstract, *International Conference on Lung Cancer.*

Salazar, O. M., Slawson, R. G., Poussin-Rosillo, H. P., Amin, P. P., Sewchand, W., and Strohl, R. (1986). A prospective randomized trial comparing once a week versus daily radiation therapy for locally advanced, non-metastatic lung cancer, a preliminary report. *Int. J. Radiat. Oncol. Biol. Phys.* **12:**770–787.

Schaake-Konig, C., Barelink, H., Adema, B. H., Schuster-Uitterhoeve, I., and Van Zandwijk, N. (1986). Radiotherapy and cis-diammedichloroplatinum (II) as combined treatment modality for inoperable non-small cell lung cancer: a dose finding study. *Int. J. Radiat. Oncol. Biol. Phys.* **12:**379–383.

Talton, B. M., Constable, W. C., and Kersh, C. R. (1990). Curative radiotherapy in non-small cell carcinoma of the lung. *Int. J. Radiat. Oncol. Biol. Phys.* **19:**15–21.

Van Haskamp, G., Boven, E., Vermorkin, J. B., Van Deutekom, H., Stam, J., Njo, K. H., Karim, A. B. M. F., Tierih, A. H., Golding, R. P., and Pinedo, H. M. (1987). Phase II trial of combined radiotherapy and daily low dose cisplatin for inoperable, locally advanced non-small cell lung cancer. *Int. J. Radiat. Oncol. Biol. Phys.* **13:**1735–1738.

19

Neoadjuvant Chemotherapy and Radiotherapy in Stage IIIA Non-Small-Cell Carcinoma of the Lung: A Cancer and Leukemia Group B Study

G. STRAUSS

Brigham and Women's Hospital/Harvard Medical School
and Harvard Community Health Plan
Boston, Massachusetts

M. GOUTSOU and K. PROPERT

Harvard School of Public Health
Boston, Massachusetts

C. MODEAS

Frontier Science and Technology Research Foundation, Inc.
Amherst, New York

D. SHERMAN

St. Joseph's Hospital
Milwaukee, Wisconsin

D. MATHISEN, R. CAREY, and N. CHOI

Massachusetts General Hospital
Boston, Massachusetts

V. REGE

Rhode Island Hospital
Providence, Rhode Island

M. GREEN

University of California Medical Center
San Diego, California

I. Introduction

Approximately one-third of patients with non-small-cell lung cancer (NSCLC) present with regionally advanced (stage III) disease. This is subdivided by the new International Staging System (Mountain, 1986) into stage IIIA disease, which is marginally resectable, and stage IIB disease, which is categorically unresectable.

The optimal treatment for stage IIIA disease is undefined. The conventional therapy most frequently used for such patients is radiation alone. While radiation is effective in the short-term palliation of such patients, long-term survival with this approach is achieved in fewer than 10% of patients and median survival times are generally less than 1 year (Perez et al., 1982).

Surgery, which is thought to represent the most effective modality in patients with NSCLC is usually not offered to patients with stage IIIA disease. While many of these patients have disease that is technically resectable at outset or can be rendered resectable by preoperative treatment, it has not been clearly shown that this approach translates into improvements in survival.

The present study is the first attempt by the Cancer and Leukemia Group B (CALGB) to use combined modality therapy in selected patients with stage IIIA disease, utilizing a combination of initial chemotherapy and radiation, followed by surgery. The study was designed as a phase II trial to evaluate the overall feasibility, efficacy, and toxicity of this approach in a multi-institutional setting.

II. Materials and Methods

Patients were required to have histologically confirmed NSCLC and stage IIIA disease as defined by the International Staging System (a T3 primary lesion and/or N2 disease). They were required to have either measurable or evaluable disease. They had to be of performance status 0–1 and have normal hemotologic, renal, and hepatic function.

Surgical staging was carried out on two occasions during the course of the protocol. Initial surgical staging was done before protocol treatment was started; surgical restaging was done after initial chemotherapy and radiotherapy were completed before the patient was considered for surgical resection.

Initial surgical staging consisted of posteroanterior (PA) and lateral chest x-ray, computed tomographic (CT) scan of the chest and upper abdomen, and bone scan. Bronchoscopy with biopsies and brushings was performed to determine the exact extent of involvement of the tracheobronchial tree. Mediastinoscopy was performed in 38 of 41 patients before they entered the study.

Surgical restaging included the following procedures: PA and lateral chest x-ray, CT scan of chest and upper abdomen, and bronchoscopy with biopsy and brushings. Repeat mediastinoscopy was not performed.

Patients were treated initially with concurrent chemotherapy and radiation. The chemotherapy consisted of 5-fluorouracil, vinblastine, and cisplatin (FVP). Two cycles were administered in a neoadjuvant fashion beginning on days 1 and 29. Radiation therapy (3000 cGy) was initiated concurrently with chemotherapy on day 1. Patients were then restaged, and those whose disease was judged to be resectable underwent thoracotomy (approximately day 57). Patients then received an additional 3000 cGy of radiation with one additional cycle of FVP given concurrently.

The 5-fluorouracil (5-FU) was given at a dosage of 30 mg/kg/day by 72 hr continuous infusion beginning on day 1 of each cycle. The cisplatin was given at a dosage of 100 mg/m^2 over 30 min, also on day 1. Vinblastine was given at a dosage of 3 mg/m^2/day as an intravenous bolus on days 1 and 3 of each cycle.

Radiation was initially delivered to a large field utilizing equally weighted anterior–posterior parallel opposed fields with megavoltage cobalt 60 or 4–10 MEV. The first field included the primary lesion, the ipsilateral pulmonary hilum, mediastinum, and ipsilateral supraclavicular fossa, with a 1.5 cm margin around the primary lesion. The subcarinal region was routinely treated with a 4 cm margin below the carina. A total of 3000 cGy in 15 fractions over 3 weeks was given concurrently with the first cycle of chemotherapy.

The boost volume included the original (pretherapy) radiologically defined primary tumor volume (minimum 1 cm margin) as well as involved hilar or mediastinal nodes.

Surgical resection was performed on approximately day 57 of the protocol. Patients were considered for surgery if their disease was thought to be technically resectable. Radiographic response to the initial chemotherapy and radiation was not required for consideration for surgery.

Surgery was performed to remove the entire known tumor volume while preserving as much functional lung as possible. It encompassed the tumor extent found at the time of surgery rather than the possibly larger volume present at the time of initial surgical staging.

Responses were graded according to standard response criteria. The categories of response recorded were complete response (CR), partial response (PR), regression, stable disease, and progression. Partial response was used only when there was measurable disease, while regression was applied to evaluable disease only.

Responses were determined on two occasions during the course of the protocol. The first determination was made following the initial chemotherapy and radiation at the time of surgical restaging. The response status was reassessed after all protocol treatment was completed. If patients underwent complete resection and thus were rendered completely disease-free, then they were judged to be in complete remission (CR).

III. Results

The study was open to patient accrual from May 1986 to February 1988. Forty-one eligible patients were enrolled in the study. As of November 1, 1990, the median follow-up of surviving patients was 46 months, with a range from 37 to 52 months.

The patient population consisted of 32 men and 9 women. Their median age was 58 years, with a range of 34–72 years.

There was a similar number of each of the three major histologic subtypes. Thirteen patients had squamous cell carcinoma, 14 had adenocarcinoma, 13 had large cell carcinoma, and 1 patient had mixed adenosquamous histologic findings.

Analysis of the tumor/node/metastases (TNM) subsets making up stage IIIA disease indicates that the most common grouping was T2N2; 68% of the patients' disease was classifiable in this category. Eighty percent of the patients had N2 disease (1 T1N2, 28 T2N2, and 4 T3N2), while 29% had T3 primary lesions (5 T3N0, 3 T3N1, and 4 T3N2).

Overall, 33 of the 41 patients were judged to have N2 disease (ipsilateral mediastinal adenopathy). Of these, 8 were so assigned because of positive findings on mediastinoscopy, while 18 had positive findings on mediastinoscopy as well as meeting CT scan (and/or chest x-ray) criteria. In addition, seven were judged to have N2 disease because of gross involvement of mediastinal structures on CT and/or chest x-ray, despite negative mediastinoscopic findings in 5 and no mediastinoscopy performed in two. Accordingly, 25 of 33 patients (76%) who had N2 disease had gross radiographic evidence of N2 disease, while 8 (24%) had only microscopic evidence of such involvement.

The response to initial chemotherapy and radiation was determined by restaging studies just prior to surgery. No patient achieved a complete response. Fifty-four percent achieved a partial response while 5% had a regression of evaluable disease. Accordingly, 59% achieved a clear antitumor effect. Thirty-nine percent had stable disease. One patient (2%), who developed liver metastases, progressed during the period of neoadjuvant therapy.

Of the 41 patients, 31 (76%) eventually underwent thoracotomy. Twenty-five patients were resected. Accordingly, the resectability rate was 81% of those operated on and 61% of all patients. The surgical procedures that were performed included pneumonectomy in 10, pneumonectomy and chest wall resection in 1, lobectomy in 10, and lobectomy and chest wall resection in 4.

Ten patients (24%) did not undergo surgery; this was due to severe toxicity in two patients and early failure in two others (one in the liver and the other in the brain). In the other six patients in whom thoracotomy was not attempted, this decision was made by each attending surgeon. Two were rejected specifically because they had stable disease. The other four did achieve response, but the attending surgeon, nevertheless, thought that a successful resection could not be accomplished. It is clear in retrospect that despite protocol guidelines, surgical "judgment" varied significantly among the cooperating surgeons.

The response to neoadjuvant chemotherapy and radiation in relation to the results of surgery is shown in Table 1. While numbers are small, there are no major differences between the "no surgery," "unresectable," and "resectable" groups with respect to the response rates to initial therapy, thus indicating that response to neoadjuvant therapy did not predict the surgical outcome.

Pathologic findings were analyzed on surgical specimens from the 31 patients who underwent thoracotomy. Among the 25 patients who underwent resection, viable tumor was present in 21 resection specimens, including 11 in which both the lung and nodes contained tumor and 10 in which the lung was

Table 1 Results of Initial Chemotherapy/Radiation Compared to Results of Surgery

	No surgery (n = 10)	Unresectable (n = 6)	Resectable (n = 25)
Partial response	3 (30%)	3 (50%)	16 (64%)
Regression	1 (10%)	1 (17%)	0
Stable	5 (50%)	2 (33%)	9 (36%)
Progression	1 (10%)	0	0

positive but the regional nodes were negative. In the remaining four specimens, only necrotic tumor was found.

In the 6 unresectable patients, all of whom underwent extensive biopsies, three specimens contained viable tumor, while the other three contained only necrotic tumor.

Accordingly, 7 of 31 patients (23%) who underwent surgery did not have viable tumor in the specimen. In the 4 completely resected patients who can be considered pathologic complete responders, 3 patients had a partial response to the chemotherapy and radiation, but 1 patient in this group had stable disease. Three of these 4 pathologic complete responders have remained disease-free for 39, 43, and 50 months, while the fourth died without evidence of recurrent cancer at 16 months.

Among the three unresectable patients with no viable tumor, all had either a partial response or regression documented by prethoracotomy assessment. It should be further noted that two of these three resectable patients went on to achieve a complete response to their postoperative therapy as determined by subsequent CT scan and chest x-ray, and both have remained disease-free with current follow-up times of 46 months and 53 months, respectively.

Table 2 indicates the comparative response rates achieved following neoadjuvant therapy and following all protocol treatment (indicated as "best response" achieved). On the left are the responses to neoadjuvant chemotherapy and radiation: there were no complete responses and an overall response and regression rate of 59%. In contrast, following the completion of all protocol treatment, 65% of patients were judged to have achieved a complete response. The 27 patients in this category includes the 25 who underwent complete surgical resection, as well as two unresectable patients judged to have attained complete remission with their postoperative chemotherapy/radiation. Overall, 82% of patients were judged to have achieved a complete response, partial response, or regression as their best response following all protocol treatment, while 15% had stable disease, and 2% had progressive disease.

Table 2 Comparative Clinical Response Status at Different Steps of Protocol

	Chemotherapy/Radiation		Best Response	
	Number	Percentage	Number	Percentage
Complete response	0	0	27	65
Partial response	22	54	6	15
Regression	2	5	1	2
Stable disease	16	39	6	15
Progression	1	2	1	2

Treatment-related morbidity and mortality were major problems for many patients on this protocol. The most common serious toxicity encountered during the chemotherapy/radiation was leukopenia: 68% of patients experienced severe or life-threatening decreases in their white cell count. Severe thrombocytopenia was seen in 22%, while severe anemia was seen in 20%. Virtually all patients experienced some degree of nausea and vomiting. Renal toxicity was a problem for only one patient who developed severe renal failure shortly after his first cycle of chemotherapy; his creatinine level maximized at 14 mg/100 ml 17 days after treatment was initiated.

In 6 patients (15%) treatment may have contributed to their deaths. These included 2 patients who died from sepsis in the setting of chemotherapy-related neutropenia. A third patient died of pneumonia after recovering from leukopenia, but was still considered to have died from chemotherapy-induced toxicity.

Three other patients' deaths were considered to be perioperative. The first patient developed a massive pulmonary hemorrhage 2 h postoperatively. The second died of surgical complications 8 days postoperatively. The third patient had a stenosis at the anastomotic site and experienced a fatal out-of-hospital respiratory arrest 8 weeks postoperatively.

At present, 11 patients (27%) are disease-free, with a median follow-up of 46 months. This includes 10 patients who have been continuously disease-free, and one who had a solitary recurrence in a supraclavicular node that was resected and irradiated and who has been disease-free for 42 months following recurrence.

Thirty patients (73%) have died. Twenty (49%) have died of progressive disease. Three (7%) experienced chemotherapy-related toxic deaths and 3 (7%) perioperative deaths. One patient developed chronic respiratory insufficiency following pneumonectomy that required a long-term tracheostomy and died after 16 months without known metastatic disease. One died of a second primary cancer of the colon. In addition, 2 (5%) out-of-hospital sudden deaths were thought likely to represent cardiac or thromboembolic events.

The Kaplan-Meier survival curve of the entire group is shown in Figure 1.

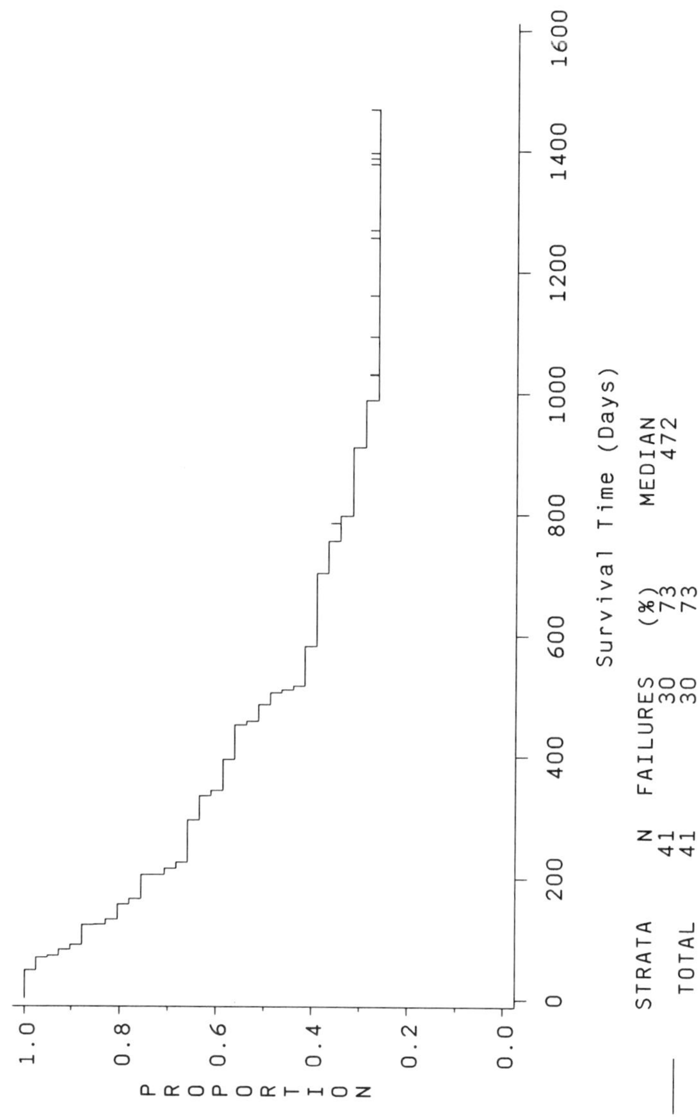

Figure 1 Kaplan-Meier survival curve.

The one-year survival was 58%, the median survival was 15.7 months, and 27% remain alive.

Of the 20 patients who have died of progressive disease, the median survival was 14 months, with a range of 4–29 months. As already indicated, among the 11 patients who remain free of disease, the median follow-up is currently 46 months with a range of follow-up of 37 to 52 months. These data suggest that a cohort of patients will enjoy prolonged disease-free survival and possibly cure. Longer follow-up on this group of patients will be necessary to verify this hypothesis.

IV. Discussion

This trial was intended as a phase II study to determine the effectiveness and tolerability of an aggressive combined approach utilizing all three modalities in patients with stage IIIA NSCLC. A basic aim of the study was to determine the feasibility of the overall approach within the cooperative group setting.

A relatively high response rate of 59% was achieved from the neoadjuvant chemotherapy and radiation, although complete responses were not observed. Sixty-one percent of the patients underwent successful tumor resection. If one also factors in the therapeutic effects of the postoperative treatment, 65% of patients were ultimately rendered completely disease-free, and 82% of patients attained at least a partial remission. A majority of the patients entered in this study had very advanced disease, as indicated, for example, by the fact that 61% of the patients had gross mediastinal involvement at presentation. The advanced nature of the patients' disease underscores the importance of the highly encouraging therapeutic effects observed.

It was of interest that the radiographic response achieved with the initial chemotherapy and radiation was not reliably predictive for subsequent resectability or for the pathologic response observed. As previously noted, radiographic response was not required by the protocol for surgical resection to be attempted. More than one-third of the 25 patients who underwent resection had demonstrated no radiographic response to initial treatment, while, conversely, 4 of the 6 patients who could not undergo resection had, in fact, responded to treatment. It was also of significant interest that one of the four patients whose resection specimen revealed no viable tumor (pathologic complete responder) was judged to be a nonresponder based on preoperative radiographic criteria.

While the protocol treatment was reasonably tolerated and safely delivered to the majority of patients treated, very substantial toxicity was observed, much of which was perhaps predictable from the intensive nature of the therapies used. The fact that there were six deaths attributable to the therapy (three from chemotherapy and three from surgery) underscores the hazards of this aggressive approach and the need for careful patient selection. It also underscores the need to set as a clear goal for future phase II trials a reduction in treatment-related morbidity and mortality.

The median survival of 15.7 months is somewhat longer than is usually reported for patients with regionally advanced NSCLC. This apparently improved survival may be explainable by patient selection factors rather than improved efficacy of the treatment utilized. Our data indicate that currently 27% (11 patients) remain free of disease with a median and minimum follow-up of 46 months and 39 months, respectively. In contrast, the median and maximum survival of those who have died of progressive disease was 14 and 29 months, respectively. These data suggest that most or all of 27 percent of patients who continue to have no evidence of recurrence have, in fact, been cured of their disease.

This is one of several phase II trials performed in recent years that confirm the feasibility of a multimodality approach in patients with regionally advanced NSCLC (Ihde, 1988). Several other studies have also indicated that median survival is better than is usually achieved with radiation alone, and that a sizable minority of patients achieve prolonged disease-free survival (Skarin et al., 1989; Strauss et al., 1987; Taylor et al., 1987; Gralla, 1988). The major question at this point is whether a treatment approach such as is utilized in this trial is responsible for the better outcome observed in the group of patients treated, or whether patient selection factors account for the apparent difference. Phase II trials such as this do not address this question. Furthermore, even if the therapeutic strategy used in this trial is responsible for the improved results compared to that of radiation alone, it does not addresss the question of whether equivalent results could be achieved with the combination of two modalities, rather than combining all three treatment modalities.

Questions about the real efficacy of this treatment approach can only be answered through randomized phase III trials. Such a trial could assume many potential designs. Some would argue that such a trial should simply compare radiation therapy alone to a treatment arm combining chemotherapy, radiation, and surgery such as was used here. Such a design, however, would not allow us to evaluate the contribution of each treatment modality.

To evaluate better the role of each treatment modality, a strategy comparing "triple modality" therapy as was used here with a control arm utilizing two treatment modalities would be preferable. Since the most highly "experimental" modality in the treatment of NSCLC is chemotherapy, perhaps the most interesting study would evaluate the role of chemotherapy in the context of combined modality treatment. Such a study might compare preoperative radiation followed by surgery to a treatment arm utilizing neoadjuvant chemotherapy followed by surgery and radiation.

Phase II studies such as this only address issues of feasibility but cannot adequately address questions of efficacy. Only through the mechanism of the randomized phase III trial can fundamental questions about optimal therapy be answered.

References

Gralla, R. J. (1988). Preoperative and adjuvant chemotherapy in non-small cell lung cancer. *Semin. Oncol.* **15:**8–12 (suppl. 7).

Ihde, D. C. (1988). Neoadjuvant chemotherapy for non-small cell lung cancer: current North American experience. *Semin. Oncol.* **15:**3–7 (suppl. 7).

Mountain, C. F. (1986). A new international staging system for lung cancer. *Chest* **89:**225S–233S.

Perez, C. A., Stanley, K., and Grundy, G. (1982). Impact of irradiation technique and tumor extent in tumor control and survival of patients with unresectable non-oat cell carcinoma of the lung: report by the Radiation Therapy Oncology Group. *Cancer* **50:** 1091–1099.

Skarin, A., Jochelson, M., Sheldon, T., et al. (1989). Neoadjuvant chemotherapy in marginally resectable stage III MO non-small cell lung cancer: long-term follow-up in 41 patients. *J. Surg. Oncol.* **40:**266–274.

Strauss, G., Sherman, D., Schwartz, J., et al. (1987). Combined modality therapy for regionally advanced stage III non-small cell carcinoma of the lung employing neoadjuvant chemotherapy, radiotherapy, and surgery (abstract). *Proceedings of the Fifth International Conference on the Adjuvant Therapy of Cancer* **5:**81.

Taylor, S. G., Trybula, M., Bonomi, P., et al. Simultaneous cisplatin fluorouracil infusion and radiation followed by surgical resection in regionally localized stage III, non-small cell lung cancer. *Ann. Thorac. Surg.* **43:**87–91.

20

A Pilot Study of Radiation Therapy with or without Concomitant Cisplatinum and Etoposide as Adjuvant Therapy in Non-Small-Cell Lung Cancer

DANIEL D. KARP, BENEDICT D. T. DALY, JAMES T. DIEHL, DAVID WAZER, RICHARD HEIDBREDER, MARK S. BANKOFF, and BARRY FANBURG

Tufts University/New England Medical Center
Boston, Massachusetts

ROSS ABRAMS

Johns Hopkins Oncology Center
Baltimore, Maryland

NANCY A. DIMARTINO

Boston VA Medical Center
Boston, Massachusetts

NICHOLAS J. ROBERT

Fairfax Hospital
Falls Church, Virginia

TIMOTHY O'CONNOR

Newton-Wellesley Hospital
Newton, Massachusetts

BERNARD WILLETT and L. JACK FALING

Boston VA Medical Center and Tufts University School of Medicine
Boston, Massachusetts

I. Introduction

Despite recent improvements in staging and preoperative diagnosis (Mountain, 1986), most patients with non-small-cell lung cancer (NSCLC) have advanced disease at the time of initial treatment and only 30% of patients are candidates for a curative resection. Patients with completely resected pathologic stage I disease have a tumor-free survival that ranges from 60 to 70%. For patients with locally or regionally advanced non-small-cell lung cancer, radiation therapy is the standard treatment, but survival rates remain poor (Holmes, 1989).

It has recently been shown that even in patients with unresectable stage III

NSCLC a short course of cisplatin and vinblastine prior to radiation significantly improves median survival (by about 4 months) and doubles the number of long-term survivors, as compared with radiation therapy alone (Dillman et al., 1990). Rates of survival in the chemotherapy-treated group were 55% after 1 year, 26% after 2 years, and 23% after 3 years, compared with 40, 13, and 11% in the radiation-only-treated group, respectively. Since this combined strategy appears to produce a modest but definite improvement in unresectable lung cancer, the use of combined treatment in patients eligible for resection might have the ability to produce survival benefit. However, since three-quarters of the patients reported by Dillman and colleagues still died of their disease within 3 years, further improvements in systemic and local therapy are clearly needed.

In recent years, there has been increasing evidence that the use of *concomitant* chemotherapy and radiotherapy is feasible in the treatment of non-small-cell lung cancer. The Mayo Clinic group reported a clinical trial in patients with unresectable regionally advanced disease (Eagan et al., 1979). Patients received either cyclophosphamide, doxorubicin, and cisplatinum (CAP) or cyclophosphamide, doxorubicin, and dacarbazine (CAD). The first two cycles were administered simultaneously with radiotherapy. Time to progression was slightly better in the CAP-treated group (303 days vs. 271 days) but the lack of a radiation-only control group does not allow for any further conclusions. A series of papers from the University of Chicago has reported the use of infusional 5-fluorouracil (5-FU) and cisplatinum and radiation therapy on an alternate-week schedule (Byfield et al., 1983). Later, etoposide was added to this regimen (Bonomi et al., 1986). These studies also showed the feasibility of using such strategies before definitive surgery.

There are several theoretical reasons why a simultaneous approach would be advantageous. First, in a situation where local recurrence and systemic metastases are both such formidable problems, there is the early delivery of each treatment modality–each with its independent activity. In the postoperative setting, each treatment can be initiated within 6 weeks of surgery. This eliminates the concern that chemotherapy administered before radiation might produce an unwelcome delay that could compromise local control or even produce resistance of the tumor cell to radiation. On the other hand, one of the arguments in favor of induction or "neoadjuvant" chemotherapy is that initial radiation may alter tumor blood flow or other host factors that decrease patient tolerance or sensitivity to chemotherapy (Clark et al., 1987). This neutralizes the debate over which treatment sequence might be more advantageous (Ervin et al., 1981). Second, the toxicity profiles of the two modalities are sufficiently different to allow high doses of each in order not to compromise the effects of either. The toxicity of radiation is for the most part limited to localized inflammation in the mediastinum, esophagus, and lung. The dosage-limiting side effects of chemotherapy often involve the bone marrow and other organs such as the kidneys and liver. Finally, cisplatinum and radiation have synergistic cytotoxicity. Cisplatinum forms DNA, RNA, and protein crosslinks that occur within a single strand (intrastrand) as well as across (interstrand) double-stranded forms. Cisplatinum can generate free radicals that will enhance radiation and can inhibit repair of the damage caused by radiation.

Enhanced survival with concomitant chemoradiotherapy has been shown for patients treated in randomized studies for anal, pancreatic, colorectal, small cell lung, head and neck, and cervical cancer. This is presumed to work by improving local and systemic control due to a decrease in radioresistance as well as the elimination of sites of early metastases (Vokes and Weichselbaum, 1990).

II. Objective and Rationale

We are reporting the preliminary results of a randomized prospective pilot study using conventional radiation therapy with or without concomitant cisplatinum and etoposide as classic adjuvant treatment in patients who have undergone resection as well as initial therapy for those with marginally resectable disease. The goals were to assess the feasibility and toxicity of the combined regimen and to evaluate its ability to improve local control and quality of life by compressing the duration of treatment. The choice of cisplatinum and etoposide was based on several factors. As mentioned above, cisplatinum is a well-known and extensively studied radiation sensitizer (Douple and Richmond, 1979) whose toxicity profile and delivery were well managed, even when the dosage was much higher (Hesketh et al., 1990). The combination of cisplatinum and etoposide has clear synergistic effects against a variety of human tumors and can produce a response rate of 30–40% in patients with non-small-cell cancer (Klastersky, 1986). The Eastern Cooperative Oncology Group (ECOG) carried out a large prospective study in patients with advanced metastatic non-small-cell cancer who were randomized to receive one of four treatment combinations. In that trial, patients randomized to the cisplatinum and etoposide arm had a modest but increased survival over patients treated with the other drug regimens (Ruckdeschel et al., 1986).

III. Patients and Methods

Thirty-four patients (20 men, 14 women) participated in this study. All had histologically proven non-small-cell cancer. Their median age was 60 (range, 33–69). With one exception (1 patient with stage IIIB), all patients had stage II or IIIA disease. All patients had an ECOG performance status of 0 or 1 and had experienced no weight loss.

Staging evaluation included bronchoscopy, bone scan, and computed tomographic (CT) scan of the chest, upper abdomen, and brain. Invasive staging of mediastinal lymph nodes was performed as indicated by the CT scan (Daly et al.,

1987). Patients were discussed at a weekly multidisciplinary lung cancer conference and judged suitable for aggressive therapy. Standard clinical criteria for immediate operability and resectability were used (Daly et al., 1987). Patients who were judged to have marginally resectable disease were randomized to receive radiation or chemoradiation before possible surgery.

Surgery was performed by one of two senior surgeons (BDTD, JTD). All patients who underwent resection had complete mediastinal lymph node dissection performed as part of their surgery. Chemotherapy consisted of cisplatinum 60 mg/m^2 on day 1 and etoposide 100 mg/m^2 on days 1, 2, and 3 repeated at 21–28 day intervals, based on recovery of white blood count to a minimum of 4,000/mm^3 and platelet count of 100,000/mm^3. Patients with marginally resectable disease received two cycles of chemotherapy preoperatively and a maximum of four cycles postoperatively. Patients with initially resectable tumors received four cycles of chemotherapy postoperatively. Radiation therapy was begun on day 1 or 2. Treatment consisted of thirty-three 180 cGy fractions (total dose, 5940 cGy) for patients receiving radiation only or 30 fractions (5400 cGy total) for those undergoing concomitant chemoradiation. Treatment volumes were tightly defined. The contralateral hilum was not treated in its entirety. Supraclavicular regions were treated only if involved by identified tumor masses. Doses to critical normal structures were strictly limited. Treatment was withheld if white blood cell counts were lower than 2000/mm^3 or platelet levels were below 50,000/mm^3.

Patients' characteristics are listed in Tables 1 and 2. Despite the small numbers, the two groups were well matched for age, histologic type, and stage of tumor.

IV. Results

The toxicity of chemotherapy was acceptable; early discontinuation of treatment was required in 4 patients due to an anaphylactoid reaction, patient refusal, *Candida* esophagitis, and cardiac arrhythmia. Temporary discontinuation was necessary for fungal sinusitis in a diabetic patient who later completed therapy.

Esophagitis was graded from 0 to 4 using standard criteria analogous to World Health Organization criteria for stomatitis and other gastrointestinal toxicity. Scoring was judged independently by a senior radiation oncologist (DW) who was not primarily involved in the initial treatment. The incidence and severity of esophagitis were increased in the combined treatment group, as shown in Table 3.

Radiation pneumonitis requiring steroid treatment occurred in two patients, one from each group. Neutropenia was managed with prophylactic ciprofloxicin in selected patients at the discretion of the oncologist caring for the patient. There were no deaths.

A. Survival

Standard survival curves were constructed using Kaplan–Meier analysis. Groups were analyzed using Pearson Chi square and Mantel–Cox statistics. The median survival for all patients is 23 months. Eighteen remain alive at 4+–35+ months (Fig. 1). Sixteen have died. Given the small size of the study, it is hazardous to draw conclusions regarding survival. However, in those patients with initially resectable tumors undergoing complete resection, followed by either chemoradiation or radiation alone (Fig. 2), 10 of 11 receiving cisplatinum and etoposide (CE) plus radiation remain alive (median, 19+ months), compared with 3 of 7 (11+ months) who received only adjuvant radiation ($p = 0.014$). One patient randomized to receive CE plus radiation was lost to follow-up and is not included in the analysis.

B. Cause of Death

One patient with known brain metastases was lost to follow-up at 9 months and is presumed dead. Causes of death among patients include brain metastases (four), cardiovascular causes with no evidence of disease (three), predominantly local recurrence (two), unknown causes (two), and second primary cancers (two). One patient died from complications of bone metastases and one terminally ill patient with extensive locoregional recurrence committed suicide.

V. Discussion

This adjuvant prospective randomized study was designed to explore the feasibility of delivering concomitant chemoradiation using moderate-dosage cisplatin on day 1 plus etoposide on days 1, 2, and 3 in 21–28 day cycles with a goal of 4 cycles of treatment. Esophagitis was a manageable but major source of toxicity in the patients receiving combined therapy. No fatal toxicity occurred. Radiation pneumonitis occurred in 2 patients (1 received radiation only). Only 4 of the 15 patients with marginally resectable stage IIIA NSCLC were ultimately rendered candidates for surgery. All four underwent definitive resection without undue surgical complications.

Overall, local control was satisfactory, with only three instances in which local recurrence predominated as the major source of morbidity and/or death. No correlation was noted in this small series between local control and use of combined modality therapy.

Caution is required in drawing any conclusions regarding survival given the small size of this group (Piantadosi, 1990). The main conclusion to be drawn from this study is that a combined modality approach is feasible and does not appear to have an adverse impact on survival. In fact, survival in the combined surgery plus

Table 1 Patients' Characteristics and Outcome

Patient	Age	Stage	T	N	M	Treatment	Timing	Radiation esophagitis	Survival (mos.)	Histologic type	Comments
CT	56	IIIA	2	2	0	Chemo/rad	Unresect	2	4+	NSC/NOS	Withdrew from therapy
SP	66	IIIA	2	2	0	Chemo/rad	Unresect	0	11+	NSC/NOS	Persistent disease
PO	54	IIIA	2	2	0	Chemo/rad	Unresect	2	28	Lge cell	Brain mets
JH	69	IIIA	3	0	0	Chemo/rad	Pre-op	2	23+	Squamous	Alive, NED
WC	6	IIIB	4	0	0	Chemo/rad	Unresect	4	3	Lge cell	Brain mets
HO	50	II	2	1	0	Chemo/rad	Post-op	2	19+	Squamous	
WM	69	II	2	1	0	Chemo/rad	Post-op	0	14	Adeno	Anaphylactoid rxn cycle 3
NH	47	II	2	1	0	Chemo/rad	Post-op	2	23+	Adeno	
HW	65	IIIA	3	2	0	Chemo/rad	Post-op	3	17+	Adeno	Candida esophagitis
JW	58	IIIA	1	2	0	Chemo/rad	Post-op	0	15+	Adeno	NED
EC	61	IIIA	2	2	0	Chemo/rad	Post-op	1	35+	Adeno	
LT	58	IIIA	1	2	0	Chemo/rad	Post-op	3	34+	Adeno	NED; *Aspergillus* sinusitis
RO	33	IIIA	3	0	0	Chemo/rad	Post-op	3	32+	Lge cell	NED
JB	51	IIIA	2	2	0	Chemo/rad	Post-op	0	4+	Adenosq	NED
MF	67	IIIA	2	2	0	Chemo/rad	Post-op	0	0+	Adenosq	Too early
HL	63	IIIA	3	1	0	Chemo/rad	Post-op	2	16+	Adeno	NED
BT	58	IIIA	2	2	0	Chemo/rad	Post-op	2	22+	Squamous	NED; coexistent systemic lupus

RP	52	IIIA	3	0	0	Radiation	Pre-op	0	14	Squamous	Suicide; recurrent disease
PS	45	IIIA	3	X	0	Radiation	Unresect	2	4	Squamous	Local–regional recurrence
AH	66	IIIA	3	X	0	Radiation	Unresect	0	10	Adeno	
DD	60	IIIA	3	X	0	Radiation	Unresect	2	2	Squamous	Local disease
GP	53	IIIA	3	0	0	Radiation	Unresect	0	9	Lge cell	Brain mets; lost
OC	63	IIIA	2	X	0	Radiation	Unresect	0	27	Lge cell	Developed 2nd H&N cancer
CE	55	IIIA	1	2	0	Radiation	Pre-op	0	6	Adeno	
JR	59	IIIA	X	2	0	Radiation	Pre-op	2	16+	Lge cell	Adrenal metastasis
DB	64	IIIA	3	0	0	Radiation	Unresect	0	10	Adeno	Bone mets
RG	63	IIIA	3	0	0	Radiation	Unresect	0	4	Squamous	Brain mets
NT	67	II	1	1	0	Radiation	Post-op	2	11+	Adeno	Alive, NED
RD	66	II	2	1	0	Radiation	Post-op	0	22	Squamous	2nd primary lung CA
GB	47	IIIA	1	2	0	Radiation	Post-op	1	10+	Adeno	Working, NED
WW	63	IIIA	1	2	0	Radiation	Post-op	0	11	Lge cell	Died NED; myocardial infarction
JA	66	IIIA	2	2	0	Radiation	Post-op	0	7	Adeno	Radiation pneumonitis
RW	55	IIIA	3	0	0	Radiation	Post-op	0	4	Adenosq	Brain mets
RC	64	IIIA	1	2	0	Radiation	Post-op	0	25+	Adeno	Alive, NED

CHEMO/RAD, concomitant chemotherapy and radiation; PRE-OP, treatment prior to definitive resection; UNRESECT, lesion not resectable following initial therapy; POST-OP, postsurgical adjuvant treatment, +, patients remaining alive, NED, no evidence of disease.

Table 2 Patients' Characteristics

	Concomitant chemoradiation	Radiation
Number	17	17
Median age	58	59
Histologic type		
Adenocarcinoma/Large cell	12	12
Squamous	3	5
NSC/NOS	2	0
Stage		
II	3	2
IIIA	13	15
IIIB	1	0

chemotherapy/radiation group appears superior to that of patients receiving radiation alone following surgery.

Concomitant cisplatinum, etoposide, and radiation therapy is feasible as adjuvant treatment in non-small-cell lung cancer. The Eastern Cooperative Group will soon initiate a large-scale multicenter trial in patients with resected stage II and III non-small-cell lung cancer using a similar treatment program. This trial is designed to determine whether cisplatinum, etoposide, and concurrent radiation can produce survival benefit on a national level. It is expected that approximately 420 eligible patients will need to be accrued over 3.5 years, with a required follow-up period of 18 months to complete this trial.

Table 3 Incidence of Esophagitis According to Treatment Regimen(s)

	Treatment	
Grade of esophagitis	Chemotherapy/ radiation	Radiation alone
2	7	4
3	3	0
4	1	0

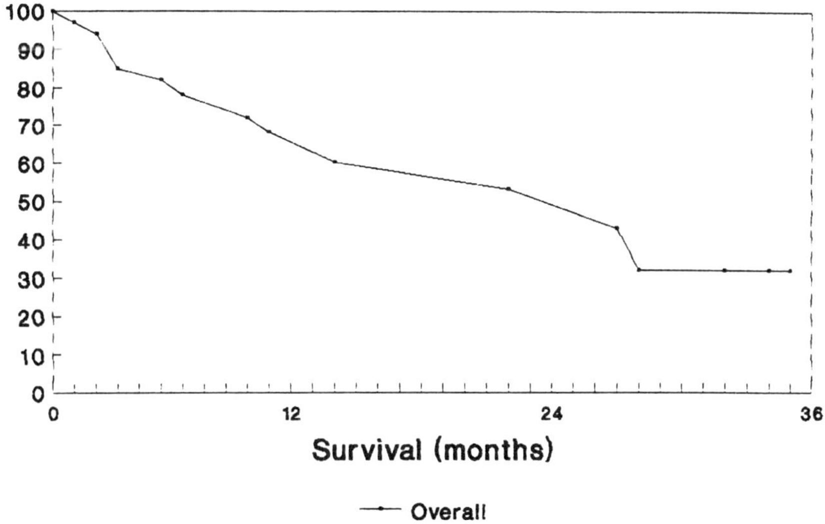

Figure 1 Overall survival.

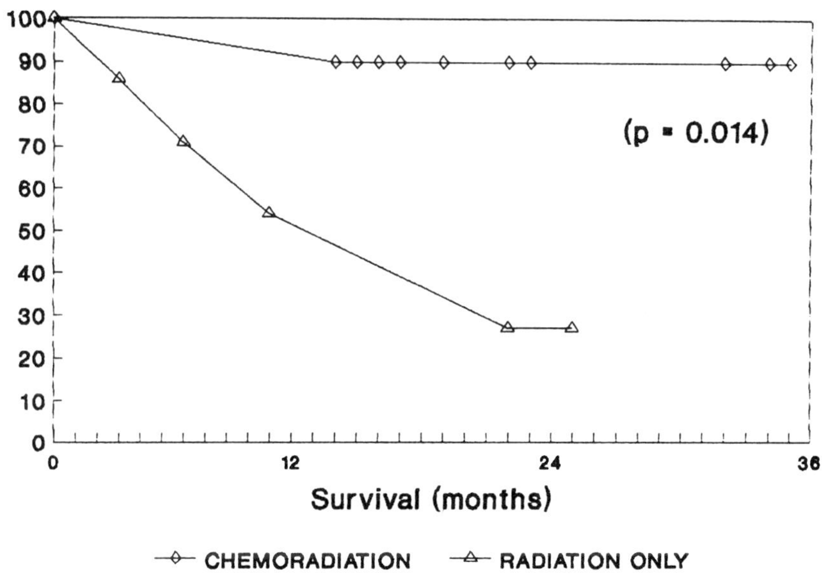

Figure 2 Survival of patients undergoing surgery followed by chemoradiation versus radiation only.

References

Bonomi, P., Rowland, K., Taylor, S. G., IV, et al. (1986). Phase II trial of etoposide, cisplatin, continuous infusion 5-fluorouracil, and simultaneous split-course radiation therapy in stage III non-small cell bronchogenic carcinoma. *Semin. Oncol.* **13:**115–120 (suppl. 3).

Byfield, J. E., Stanton, W., Sharp, T. R., et al. (1983). Phase I–II study of 120-hour infused 5-FU and split-course radiation therapy in localized non-small-cell lung cancer. *Cancer Treat. Rep.* **67:**933–936.

Clark, J. R., Fallon, B. G., and Frei, E. F. III (1987). Induction chemotherapy as initial and treatment for advanced head and neck cancer: a model for the multidisciplinary treatment of solid tumors. In *Important Advances in Oncology*. Edited by V. DeVita, S. Hellman, and S. A. Rosenberg. Philadelphia, J. B. Lippincott, pp. 175–196.

Daly, B. D. T. Jr., Faling, L. J., Bite, G., Gale, M. E., Bankoff, M. S., Jung-Legg, Y., Cooper, A. G., and Snider, G. L. (1987). Mediastinal lymph node evaluation by computed tomography in lung cancer. An analysis of 345 patients grouped by TNM staging, tumor size, and tumor location. *J. Thorac. Cardiovasc. Surg.* **94**(5): 664–672.

Dillman, R. O., Seagren, S. L., Propert, K. J., Guerra, J., Eaton, W. L., Perry, M. C., Carey, R. W., Frei, E. F., and Green, M. R. (1990). Randomized trial of induction chemotherapy plus high-dose radiation versus radiation alone in stage III non-small-cell lung cancer. *N. Engl. J. Med.* **323**(14)**:**940–945.

Douple, E. B., and Richmond, R. C. (1979). A review of platinum complex biochemistry suggests a rationale for combined platinum-radiotherapy. *Int. J. Radiat. Oncol. Biol. Phys.* **5:**1335–1339.

Eagan, R. T., Lee, R. E., Frytak, S., et al. (1979). Randomized trial of thoracic irradiation plus combination chemotherapy for unresectable adenocarcinoma and large cell carcinoma of the lung. *Int. J. Radiat. Oncol. Biol. Phys.* **5:**1401–1405.

Ervin, T. J., Karp, D. D., Weichselbaum, R. R., et al. (1981). The role of chemotherapy in the multidisciplinary approach to advanced head and neck cancer: potentials and problems. *Ann. Otol. Rhinol. Laryngol.* **90:**506–511.

Hesketh, P., Tansan, S., Hesketh, A., Karp, D., et al. (1990). Very high dose cisplatin and etoposide and mitomycin in advanced non-small-cell lung cancer. *Proc. Am. Soc. Clin. Oncol.* **9:**248.

Holmes, E. C. (1989). Surgical adjuvant therapy of non-small-cell lung cancer. *Cancer Treat. Res.* **45:**245–258.

Klastersky, J. (1986). Therapy with cisplatin and etoposide for non-small cell lung cancer. *Semin. Oncol.* **13**(3)**:**(suppl. 3), 104–114.

Mountain, C. F. (1986). A new international staging system for lung cancer. *Chest.* **89:** 2255–2335.

Piantadosi, S. (1990), Hazards of small clinical trials. *J. Clin. Oncol.* **8**(1)**:**1–3.

Ruckdeschel, J. C., Finkelstein, D., Ettinger, D. S., et al. (1986). A randomized trial of the four most active regimens for metastatic non-small-cell lung cancer. *J. Clin. Oncol.* **4:**14–22.

Vokes, E. E., and Weichselbaum, R. R. (1990). Concomitant chemoradiotherapy: rationale and clinical experience in patients with solid tumors. *J. Clin. Oncol.* **8**(5)**:**911–934.

PART VI

NON-SMALL-CELL LUNG CANCER: NEW THERAPEUTIC AGENTS

21

Edatrexate: An Antifolate with Activity in Non-Small-Cell Lung Cancer

Results of Trials at Memorial–Sloan Kettering Cancer Center

STEFAN C. GRANT and MARK G. KRIS

Memorial–Sloan Kettering Cancer Center
New York, New York

I. Introduction

Edatrexate (also known as 10-ethyl-10-deazaaminopterin or 10EdAM) is an antifolate antimetabolite developed jointly at the Sloan Kettering Institute and SRI International. In clinical trials antitumor activity has been demonstrated in patients with advanced non-small-cell lung cancer, cancer of the head and neck, breast cancer, and non-Hodgkin's lymphoma. We review the preclinical data and results of the trials in patients with non-small-cell lung cancer undertaken at Memorial–Sloan Kettering Cancer Center (MSKCC).

II. Structural Design and Biochemical Properties

A. Mechanisms of Action

Antifolates prevent the synthesis of reduced folates by inhibiting the enzyme dihydrofolate reductase. This causes an accumulation of inactive folates resulting in a cessation first of thymidylate, and then of purine nucleotide accumulation. Because the depletion of intracellular reduced folates is only partial, the exact mechanism by which antifolates exert their toxicity is uncertain. Exposure of cells to antifolates generates a number of toxic polyglutamate derivatives of the parent compound. These polyglutamate forms have direct inhibitory effects on thymidylate synthetase as well as on the enzymes of de novo purine synthesis. In mouse and human systems mediated membrane transport has an important influence on the cytotoxic action of antifolates (Sirotnak, 1982). There is also evidence in animal tumor models (Chello et al., 1977) that suggests that differences between the ability of normal proliferative cells and tumor cells to transport these compounds, as well as differences in polyglutamylation account, to a large extent, for the selectivity of the observed antitumor activity of this class of drug (Sirotnak and DeGraw, 1984; Rumberger et al., 1984).

B. Development and Therapeutic Advantage of Edatrexate

Differences in specificity for substituents at three sites of the folate molecule (the 5-position, the 10-position, and the γ-carboxyl group) account for differences in accumulation of various folate analogs between normal proliferating cells and tumor cells (Sirotnak, 1980). Edatrexate is one of a number of compounds developed by substitutions at the N^{10} position of 4 aminofolate, and differs from methotrexate by the presence of an alkyl group at the N^{10} position. The structural

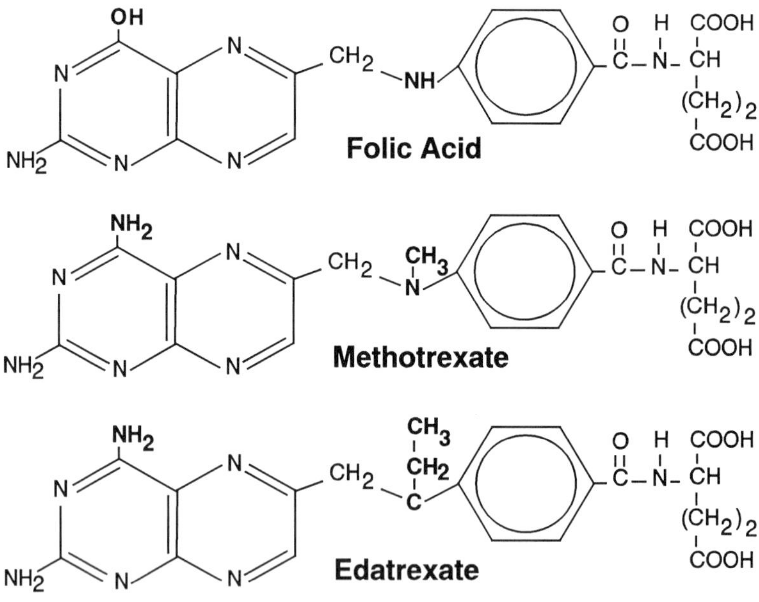

Figure 1 Chemical structures of folic acid, methotrexate, and edatrexate. Structural differences are shown in bold type.

differences between these two antifolates and folic acid are shown in Figure 1. This substitution has little effect on the inhibition of dihydrofolate reductase (Sirotnak and DeGraw, 1984). The increased selectivity of edatrexate compared to other antifolates appears to be due to an increased differential in membrane transport between normal tissues and tumor cells, as well as an increase in the polyglutamylation and intracellular accumulation as cytotoxic polyglutamates in tumor cells (Sirotnak et al., 1984; Rumberger et al., 1984). The transport of edatrexate into tumor cells is 3–12-fold greater than that of methotrexate and once inside the tumor cells the polyglutamylation is 2–3 times greater. In contrast, the transportation into and formation of polyglutamate forms within normal proliferating cells are lower than that of methotrexate. The plasma pharmacokinetics are similar to methotrexate.

III. Antitumor Activity in Preclinical Studies

Antitumor activity superior to other antifolates has been demonstrated against a number of tumors. In studies by Sirotnak et al. (1984) activity superior to methotrexate was demonstrated. In a series of in vivo experiments $BD2F_1$ mice were transplanted with 10^6 mouse tumor cells, either subcutaneously or intraperitoneally. The animals were then treated with methotrexate or edatrexate. In methotrexate-sensitive tumor cell lines the antitumor activity of edatrexate was much greater and even in methotrexate-resistant lines edatrexate had substantial antitumor activity. In other studies (Schmid et al., 1985) with Swiss nude mice, human xenografts were transplanted 2 days before treatment with the LD_{10} dose of these analogs. Antitumor activity was substantially higher for edatrexate and, in the case of those animals transplanted with the MX-1 breast carcinoma, tumor-free animals were identified after one cycle of therapy. Only in mice receiving edatrexate were complete regressions and prolonged survival seen. The tumors used and the effects of therapy are shown in Table 1.

IV. Clinical Studies of Edatrexate

A. Phase I Trials

1. Study Design

Two phase I trials were undertaken treating 62 patients (Kris et al., 1988). Initially 35 patients were treated weekly for 3 weeks followed by a 2 week "rest period." Edatrexate was administered at dosage levels of 5, 10, 20, 30, 40, 55, 70, 85, 100, and 120 mg/m^2 intravenously; 27 patients were also treated at a weekly dosage of 80 or 100 mg/m^2 without a planned "rest period."

Table 1 In Vivo Activity of Edatrexate Against Mouse Tumors and Human Xenografts

			Average reduction in tumor burden[a]	
Tumor	Species	Type	Methotrexate	Edatrexate
L1210	Mouse	Lymphoid leukemia	+	++++
S180	Mouse	Ascites sarcoma	±	++++
E0771	Mouse	Breast adenocarcinoma	−	++
T241	Mouse	Fibrosarcoma	−	++
MX1	Human	Breast carcinoma	−	+++
LX1	Human	Lung carcinoma	−	++
CX1	Human	Colon carcinoma	−	+

[a]Degree of reduction: −, 0%; ±, 0–25%; ++, 50–75%; +++, 75–90%; ++++, 100%

Source: Adapted from Schmid et al., 1985.

2. *Results*

The most common and dose-limiting toxic reaction was mucositis, which increased in frequency and severity with increasing dosage levels. In the majority of patients with mucositis it was self-limited and lasted 3–7 days. The median leukocyte nadir was within the normal range. Fifteen percent of all patients' courses were complicated by 2+ or greater leukopenia, 30% occurring in patients on the weekly schedule. In addition 2+ or greater thrombocytopenia occurred in 15% of patient courses. At a dosage of 80mg/m^2/week (the dosage eventually selected for phase II study), 72% of patients had either no or grade 1 myelosuppression. At this dosage level 29% of patients had grade 3 or 4 mucositis. Significant myelosuppression was not observed in the absence of mucositis of comparable severity.

Other toxic effects observed were mild and included elevated levels of serum glutamic oxaloacetic transaminase (SGOT) (without evidence of jaundice or a hepatitis-like illness), fatigue (30% of courses), and nausea/vomiting (18% of courses). These effects were seen at all dosage levels and their incidence and severity did not correlate with dosage levels. A macular rash on the trunk and extremities was noted in 12 patients (19%) and occurred more commonly in those patients receiving edatrexate on the weekly schedule. Mild transient elevations in partial thromboplastin times or prothrombin times were noted occasionally and four patients developed mild alopecia.

Objective antitumor responses were observed. Partial remissions lasting 6 to 73+ months were seen in patients with non-small-cell lung cancer. One partial response lasting 15 months was observed in a previously treated patient with breast cancer.

B. Phase II Trial

1. *Study Design and Patient Characteristics*

After completion of the phase I studies, a phase II trial was undertaken in patients with stage III or IV non-small-cell lung cancer (Shum et al., 1988). In this study 20 patients who had not previously received chemotherapy were treated. Patient pretreatment characteristics are shown in Table 2. Fourteen had stage IV disease, five had stage IIIB, and one had stage IIIA disease. All had a Karnofsky performance status (KPS) of at least 50% (median KPS 70%), 60% had an elevated serum lactate dehydrogenase level, and 7 patients had a pretreatment weight loss ≥ 6%. All patients were evaluable for toxicity, 19 for response. Edatrexate was

Table 2 Pretreatment Patient Characteristics in Phase II Trial of Edatrexate in Non-Small-Cell Lung Cancer

Number of patients	
Entered	20
Adequate for response	19
Adequate for toxicity	20
Stage of disease (%)	
IIIA	5
IIIB	25
IV	70
Karnofsky performance status (%)	
80–90%	45
60–70%	35
50%	20
Men:women ratio (%)	45:55
Pretreatment weight loss ≥ 6% (%)	35
Elevated serum lactate/dehydrogenase (%)	60
Bone metastases (%)	25
Median age (range)	61 (56–78)
Histologic subtype (%)	
Adenocarcinoma	50
Epidermoid carcinoma	35
Large cell carcinoma	15

Source: Adapted from Shum et al., 1988.

administered intravenously at a dosage of 80 mg/m^2 weekly for 5 weeks. Dosages were increased or attenuated based on the absence or presence of toxic effects; the median dosage administered weekly was 60mg/m^2.

2. Response Data

A major response rate of 32% (95% confidence interval for predicted response rate 15–55%) was observed. Four partial responses were seen in patients with measurable disease and two patients with evaluable disease had improvement in their indicator lesions. The median response duration was 15.4 months (range, 5.5–41 months). The median survival duration in this group of 20 patients with advanced disease was 10.8 months, with a 1 year survival rate of 45%.

3. Adverse Effects

In this group of previously untreated patients the toxic reactions seen were qualitatively similar but generally milder than those seen in the phase I trials. Hematologic toxicity was infrequent, with only two patients (10%) experiencing leukocyte nadirs below the normal range and only three patients (15%) having platelet nadirs <100,000/μl. Although 25% of patients experienced grade 3+ or 4+ mucositis, only one patient required hospitalization. Other side effects seen were mild and consisted of fatigue, nausea, vomiting, a macular rash, elevated SGOT levels, diarrhea, and mild alopecia.

V. Edatrexate in Combination with Other Agents

A. Preclinical Studies

A synergistic effect had been demonstrated in preclinical studies when edatrexate was combined with other chemotherapeutic agents.

In one study edatrexate was compared to methotrexate, in combination with 5-fluorouracil, cyclophosphamide, cisplatin, or melphalan (Schmid et al., 1987). These agents were tested in $BD2F_1$ mice against three tumor models: E0771 mammary adenocarcinoma and T241 fibrosarcoma metastatic to lung, and L1210 leukemia. The endpoint of the study was the measurement of survival duration. In all three tumor models, edatrexate in combination with cyclophosphamide was the most active combination. The therapeutic activity was far greater than that obtained with each agent given alone and a substantial number of long-term survivors were seen. Edatrexate was also highly active with melphalan and with cisplatin against the E0771 tumors and with cisplatin against the L1210 leukemia. Most striking was the fact that when the agents were given in various combinations, only in those groups of mice receiving a combination of an alkylating

Table 3 Antitumor Effects of Edatrexate Combinations Against Mammary Adenocarcinoma E0771

LD_{10} dose	Agent	Median survival time (days)	Increase in lifespan (%)	45-Day survivors/ total treated
1	Methotrexate	14 ± 2.8	17	0/14
1	Edatrexate	24 ± 3.5	100	0/13
1	Cisplatin	22 ± 3.4	83	0/14
1	Cyclophosphamide	21.5 ± 2	87	0/14
0.5	Methotrexate + cisplatin	19.5 ± 3	63	0/14
0.5	Edatrexate + cisplatin	30	150	4/14
0.5	Methotrexate + cyclophosphamide	25 ± 4.2	108	0/14
0.5	Edatrexate + cyclophosphamide	>45	>275	9/14

Therapy began 6 days after transplantation of 10^6 tumor cells intravenously.
Source: Adapted from Schmid et al., 1987.

agent plus edatrexate were long-term survivors (beyond 45 days) seen (see Table 3).

In subsequent experiments by the same group (Sirotnak et al., 1989), the activity of edatrexate, methotrexate, and cisplatin alone and in combination was studied against an established mouse ovarian cancer tumor model. After 10^6 cells of a mouse ovarian teratoma were transplanted as ascites into C3HeB/Fe mice and the tumor was established, either edatrexate or cisplatin was administered, either intraperitoneally or subcutaneously. When given intraperitoneally at the LD_{10} dose, both edatrexate and cisplatin were highly effective. Methotrexate was minimally active when given by this route. When cisplatin was administered in combination with either edatrexate or methotrexate, all at half the LD_{10} dose, the former combination was substantially more effective than the latter, as assessed by the increased lifespan of treated animals compared to controls (percentage increase in lifespan = 160% vs. 60%, $p < 0.001$). In addition, tumor-free long-term survivors were seen only with the edatrexate plus cisplatin combination.

B. Phase II Trial of Edatrexate with Mitomycin and Vinblastine

1. Study Design Rationale

This trial was based on the phase II trial of edatrexate in non-small-cell lung cancer along with the demonstration, in preclinical studies, of enhanced activity when edatrexate was administered with other antitumor agents. The trial was designed to establish a dosage of edatrexate when used in combination with mitomycin and vinblastine (Kris et al., 1990). These latter two agents were each selected because of their demonstrated activity in phase II trials, their differing mechanisms of action from each other and edatrexate, and the absence of overlapping toxicities. Dosages and schedules were based on the single-agent phase II data for edatrexate and results of earlier combination studies for mitomycin and vinblastine. The ability to administer the regimen entirely in an outpatient setting was a particular advantage of this combination.

2. Treatment Schedule

Edatrexate was given at dosages of 40, 50, 60, 70, and 80 mg/m^2 weekly for 5 weeks, and then every 2 weeks. At the 50 and 80 mg/m^2 dosages additional levels with a 50% dosage reduction on day 8 were incorporated. Vinblastine was given on the same schedule as edatrexate at a dosage of 4 mg/m^2 on day 1, 2 mg/m^2 on day 8, and then 4.5 mg/m^2. Mitomycin was given at a dosage of 8 mg/m^2 on days 1, 29, and 71.

3. Eligibility Criteria and Patient Characteristics

Requirements for entry into the study included no prior chemotherapy, pathologically confirmed stage III or IV disease, a Karnofsky performance status of at least 60%, normal renal and hepatic function, a normal peripheral blood count, and measurable or evaluable indicator lesions that had not been irradiated. A total of 99 patients with stage III (35% stage IIIB, 7% stage IIIA) or stage IV (58%) non-small-cell lung cancer were entered and all were evaluable for both response and toxicity. Patient characteristics are shown in Table 4. They included a performance status of 80 or 90% in 60% and 34% of patients had a weight loss $\geq$ 6% in the six months before entry into the study. Two-thirds of the patients were men, and 36% of patients had elevated serum lactate dehydrogenase (LDH) levels. The median age was 58 years (range, 29–82) and 63% of patients had adenocarcinoma, 21% epidermoid, and 16% large cell carcinoma.

4. Results

A major objective response of 58% (95% confidence interval 47–67%) was observed. Similar response rates were seen at all dosage levels of edatrexate. Three percent of patients had a complete response and 55% of patients had a partial response or improvement. The median response duration was 9.5 months, the median survival was 13.6 months, and the 1 year survival rate was 54%, with a median follow up of 13.3 months (range, 3–23 months). During the course of this study 82% of patients improved or maintained their performance status and two-thirds gained weight. Fifty-three percent of patients were not hospitalized for any reason while on the study. In order to assess objectively changes in the symptoms of cough, dyspnea, pain, and hemoptysis during the course of the study, a

Table 4 Pretreatment Patient Characteristics in Trial of Edatrexate in Combination with Mitomycin and Vinblastine

Number of patients	
Entered	99
Adequate for response	99
Adequate for toxicity	99
Stage of disease (%)	
IIIA	7
IIIB	35
IV	58
Karnofsky performance status (%)	
80–90%	60
60–70%	40
Men:women ratio (%)	68:32
Pretreatment weight loss $\geqslant$ 6% (%)	32
Elevated serum lactate/dehydrogenase (%)	36
Bone metastases (%)	21
Median age (range)	58 (29–82)
Histologic subtype (%)	
Adenocarcinoma	63
Epidermoid carcinoma	21
Large cell carcinoma	16

Source: Kris et al., 1990.

previously established 100 mm linear visual analog scale was utilized. There was a significant improvement in symptoms for all patients during the study. Those patients who had a major response had a statistically greater improvement in these four symptoms compared to nonresponders.

5. *Adverse Reactions*

The toxic reactions seen in this study were similar to those seen in the single-agent phase II trials and were generally mild to moderate. Overall grade 3 or 4 leukopenia and stomatitis occurred in 32% and 13% of patients, respectively. When the 80 mg/m^2 edatrexate dosage level with or without a 50% dose attenuation on day 8 was compared, the value of the dose attenuation in reducing side effects was apparent. Grade 2 or greater mucositis was reduced from 52% to 36%. Similar effects were seen with myelosuppression. The incidence of grade 2 of greater leukopenia fell from 63% to 41% and grade 2 or greater thrombocytopenia fell from 18% to 0%. There were no treatment-related deaths in this study (0% observed rate, 95% confidence interval 0–4%).

6. Summary of Findings

This trial showed the combination of edatrexate, mitomycin, and vinblastine (EMV) to be an active regimen in patients with non-small-cell lung cancer. Treatment with this regimen led to prolonged survival and improvement in patients' performance status and symptoms. It was shown that the full phase II dosage of edatrexate could be given in combination with mitomycin and vinblastine. The recommended dosage and schedule of edatrexate (80 mg/m^2 on day 1, 40 mg/m^2 on day 8, 80 mg/m^2 on days 15, 22, and 29, then every 2 weeks) for phase III study was established. The optimal EMV regimen is currently being evaluated in a randomized multicenter phase III trial involving 30 centers across North America, in which it is being compared to the combination of mitomycin and vinblastine alone. The study began in December, 1989, and patient accrual was completed in 1991.

VI. Conclusions

Edatrexate has shown antitumor activity against advanced non-small-cell lung cancer in phase I and II studies undertaken at Memorial–Sloan Kettering Cancer Center. The combination of edatrexate with mitomycin and vinblastine has been demonstrated to be both active and well tolerated. During the course of our phase II study, patients showed improvement in their symptoms and the observed survival data are encouraging. Adverse effects are tolerable. The major and dose-limiting toxicity is mucositis. It is generally self-limiting when edatrexate is given at the dosages studied. Other side effects have been mild and include myelosuppression, nausea, vomiting, and skin rashes.

The therapeutic advantage of this compound appears to be related to its relative exclusion and rapid elimination from normal proliferating tissues and its concentration within tumor cells. The increased formation of polyglutamate forms within tumor cells appears to be, at least in part, related to this effect. There is preclinical evidence that the antitumor activity of edatrexate can be enhanced by increased dosages followed by leucovorin "rescue," altered dosing schedules, and other combination chemotherapy regimens. Edatrexate is currently being studied in a multicenter randomized phase III trial in patients with non-small-cell lung cancer comparing edatrexate, mitomycin, and vinblastine to mitomycin and vinblastine alone.

References

Chello, P. L., Sirotnak, F. M., Dorick, D. M., and Donsbach, R. C. (1977). Therapeutic relevance of differences in the structural specificity of the transport systems for folate analogs in L1210 tumor cells and in isolated murine intestinal epithelial cells. *Cancer Res.* **37**(12):4297–4303.

Kris, M. G., Kinahan, J. J., Gralla, R. J., Fanucchi, M. P., Wertheim, M. S., O'Connell, J. P., Marks, L. D., Williams, L., Farag, F., Young, C. W., and Sirotnak, F. M. (1988). Phase I trial and clinical pharmacological evaluation of 10-ethyl-10-deazaaminopterin in adult patients with advanced cancer. *Cancer Res.* **48:**5573–5579.

Kris, M. G., Gralla, R. J., Potanovich, L. M., Marks, L. D., and Heelan, R. T. (1990). Assessment of pretreatment symptoms and improvement after edam + mitomycin + vinblastine (EMV) in patients (pts) with inoperable non-small cell lung cancer (NSCLC) (abstr.). *Proc. Am. Soc. Clin. Oncol.* **9:**883.

Rumberger, B. G., Barrueco, J. R., and Sirotnak, F. M. (1990). Differing specificities for 4-aminofolate analogs of folylpolyglutamyl synthetase from tumors and proliferating intestinal epithelium of the mouse with significance for selective antitumor action. *Cancer Res.* **50:**4639–4643.

Sirotnak, F. M., DeGraw, J. I., Moccio, D. M., Samuels, L. L., and Goutas, L. J. (1984). New folate analogs of the 10-deaza-aminopterin series. Basis for structural design and biochemical and pharmacologic properties. *Cancer Chemother. Pharmacol.* **12:** 18–25.

Schmid, F. A., Sirotnak, F. M., Otter, G. M., and DeGraw, J. I. (1985). New folate analogs of the 10-deazaaminopterin series: markedly increased antitumor activity of the 10-ethyl analog compared to the parent compound and methotrexate against some human tumor xenografts in nude mice. *Cancer Treat. Rep.* **69:**551–553.

Schmid, F. A., Sirotnak, F. M., Otter, G. M., and DeGraw, J. I. (1987). Combination chemotherapy with a new folate analog: activity of 10-ethyl-10-deaza-aminopterin compared to methotrexate with 5-fluorouracil and alkylating agents against advanced metastatic disease in murine tumor models. *Cancer Treat. Rep.* **71:**727–732.

Shum, K. Y., Kris, M. G., Gralla, R. J., Burke, T., Marks, L. D., Heelan, R. T. (1988). Phase II study of 10-ethyl-10-deaza-aminopterin in patients with stage III and IV non-small cell lung cancer. *J. Clin. Oncol.* **6:**446–450.

Sirotnak, F. M. (1980). Correlates of folate analog transport, pharmacokinetic and selective antitumor action. *Pharmacol. Ther.* **8:**71–103.

Sirotnak, F. M., Chello, P. L., DeGraw, J. I., Piper, J. R., and Montgomery, J. A. (1982). Membrane transport and the molecular basis for selective antitumor action of folate analogs. In: *Molecular Actions and Targets for Cancer Chemotherapeutic Agents.* Edited by A. Sartorelli. New York, Academic Press, p. 349.

Sirotnak, F. M., and DeGraw, J. I. (1984). Selective antitumor action of folate analogs. In: *Folate Antagonists as Therapeutic Agents*, vol 2. Edited by F. M. Sirotnak. New York, Academic Press, pp. 43–91.

Sirotnak, F. M., Schmid, F. A., and DeGraw, J. I. (1989). Intracavitary therapy of murine ovarian cancer with *cis*-diamminedichloroplatinum (II) and 10-ethyl-10-deaza-aminopterin incorporating systemic leucovorin protection. *Cancer Res.* **49:**2890–2893.

22

Chronic Oral Etoposide in the Treatment of Lung Cancer

JOHN D. HAINSWORTH, DAVID H. JOHNSON, and F. ANTHONY GRECO

Vanderbilt University
Nashville, Tennessee

Etoposide is a semisynthetic podophyllotoxin derivative with a wide spectrum of antineoplastic activity. In addition to widespread use in the treatment of germ cell tumors and hematologic malignancies, etoposide has become a standard part of most treatment regimens for small cell lung cancer (Evans et al., 1985; Porter et al., 1985). Although much less active against non-small-cell lung cancer, etoposide shows some single-agent activity, and has been widely used in combination with cisplatin (Klastersky et al., 1986; Hainsworth et al., 1989a).

Since its development as an antineoplastic agent, etoposide has shown evidence of schedule dependency. Until recently, however, this schedule dependency has not been studied clinically. The recent availability of etoposide in an oral preparation has allowed its administration in a chronic, low-dosage schedule. In this chapter, the rationale for this schedule of administration is reviewed, and results of phase II studies in small cell and non-small-cell lung cancer are presented.

I. Rationale for a Chronic Dosing Schedule

A. Mechanism of Action

Although originally assumed to act as an antimicrotubule agent like the parent compound podophyllotoxin, it soon was evident that etoposide inhibited cells in the G_2 phase of the cell cycle rather than during mitosis (Greider et al., 1974). In addition, the detection of both single-strand and double-strand DNA breaks after exposure to low concentrations of etoposide indicated that DNA damage was the primary mechanism of cytotoxicity (Wozniak and Koss, 1983; Kalwinsky et al., 1983). Therefore, even before the exact mechanism of action was known, it was appreciated that etoposide had a unique mechanism of action, being a phase-specific agent with primary activity against DNA itself.

Etoposide is now known to produce DNA damage by interaction with topoisomerase II. This enzyme catalyzes DNA topoform interconversions by introducing a transient enzyme-bridged break in one of the two crossing DNA segments. This intermediate DNA–enzyme complex has been isolated, and presumably represents the reaction intermediate of the breaking–rejoining mechanism (Liu et al., 1983). Etoposide stabilizes the DNA–topoisomerase II complex, resulting in the inability of the DNA strands to rejoin and producing double-strand breaks (Chen et al., 1984). Topoisomerase II is most active during the G_2 phase of the cell cycle, thus accounting for the cycle-specific activity of etoposide (Sullivan et al., 1986).

Recent data indicate that the interaction of etoposide with topoisomerase II is reversible following withdrawal of etoposide. Reversal of the DNA–topoisomerase II–etoposide interaction could theoretically allow subsequent DNA repair and thereby lessen cytotoxicity. Therefore, both the cell-cycle-specific mechanism of action and the reversibility of the etoposide–topoisomerase II interaction suggest that prolonged exposure to etoposide would enhance its antineoplastic efficacy.

B. Preclinical Studies

The schedule dependency of etoposide in the treatment of murine L1210 leukemia was demonstrated by Dombernowsky and Nissen in 1973. In this animal model, a variety of treatment schedules were investigated, including a 1-day only schedule, a daily schedule for 5 days, and intermittent dosing schedules with dosing intervals ranging from 2–10 days. The daily dosing schedule and the intermittent schedules with dosing intervals of 2–5 days were both superior to the single dosing schedule. Efficacy decreased when the dosing interval was prolonged beyond 5 days. Intermittent dosing every fifth day produced a median survival of 60 days and a cure rate of 50–63%. In contrast, only 13% of mice were cured with a single dose, and 21% were cured with a 5-day divided-dose schedule.

In a second part of this study, the same total dose was administered either as a single daily dose, or as a divided dose given every 3 hr over a 24-hr period. The divided-dose schedule produced a 50% cure rate, compared to only a 13% cure rate for the single-dose schedule (Dombernowsky and Nissen, 1973). Because of these results, early clinical trials with etoposide used daily dosing for 3–5 days, or intermittent dosing in a day 1,3,5 schedule.

C. Clinical Data

Although early retrospective studies in patients with small cell lung cancer suggested etoposide schedule dependency (Cavalli et al., 1978), definitive evidence has become available only recently. In a prospective study, Slevin et al. (1989a) randomized patients with extensive stage small cell lung cancer to receive single-agent etoposide, administered either as a 24-hr continuous infusion or in daily divided doses for 5 days. All patients received the same total etoposide dose (500 mg/m^2 every 3 weeks). Response rates in this randomized study differed markedly: 89% of patients who received the 5-day etoposide schedule responded, compared to only 10% of those who received the 24-hr infusion ($p < 0.001$). Pharmacokinetic studies showed that the total exposure to etoposide was almost identical with these two regimens. However, patients receiving the 5-day divided-dose schedule maintained serum levels of etoposide > 1μg/ml for approximately twice as long. Therefore, the time of exposure to etoposide appears more important in determining cytotoxicity than do the peak serum concentrations achieved.

In a subsequent study, Slevin and co-workers (1989b; Clark et al., 1989) further extended the schedule of etoposide administration, and compared a 5-day with an 8-day regimen. Again, all patients had extensive stage small cell lung cancer, and all received a total etoposide dose of 500 mg/m^2. No statistically significant efficacy differences were seen between the two groups, although the 8-day-treated group had a slightly better response rate (80% versus 72%), remission duration (5.6 versus 4.7 months), and survival (9.1 versus 7.0 months). However, the 8-day schedule produced less myelosuppression; median leukocyte nadir during the first course was 1500/μl with 8-day administration vs. 800/μl for the 5-day-treated group ($p < 0.05$). In this study, the etoposide schedules produced serum levels > 1 μg/ml for similar time durations.

In summary, considerable evidence now exists to support the schedule dependency of etoposide in the treatment of extensive-stage small cell lung cancer. Pharmacokinetic data suggest that the maintenance of etoposide exposure for long periods, even at low levels, is an important determinant of drug activity. The minimum serum level of etoposide necessary to achieve tumoricidal activity has not been defined.

D. Phase I Study with a 21-Day Oral Etoposide Regimen

Based on increasing evidence supporting the schedule dependency of etoposide, we evaluated further prolongation of etoposide administration. We arbitrarily chose a 21-day oral schedule, and performed a phase I study to determine the maximum tolerated dose using this schedule (Hainsworth et al., 1989b). Eighteen patients with advanced, treatment-refractory malignancies were treated. The etoposide dosage was 25 mg/m^2/day; subsequent patients received 50 mg/m^2/day and 80 mg/m^2/day.

In these pretreated patients, the maximum tolerated dosage of etoposide was 50 mg/m^2/day. As expected, myelosuppression was the dose-limiting toxicity, with leukocyte nadirs occurring between days 22 and 29, and repeat courses possible beginning on day 36. Severe leukopenia ($<$1000/μl) occurred in 4 of 20 courses, and resulted in 1 infection-related fatality. Two patients required platelet transfusions. Total alopecia occurred in all patients receiving etoposide 50 mg/m^2/day; other toxicity, including gastrointestinal effects, was mild and easily tolerated.

Five partial responses were observed in this phase I study (soft tissue sarcoma, 2; breast cancer, 1; ovarian cancer, 1; non-Hodgkin's lymphoma, 1). Four of these patients had tumor types in which other schedules of etoposide have not shown a high level of activity.

Based on these results, we and others have investigated chronic, low-dose, oral etoposide in the treatment of a variety of malignancies. We have used 50 mg/m^2 for 21 days, since this was the maximum tolerated dosage determined by our phase I study. The remainder of this chapter summarizes results to date in the treatment of lung cancer.

II. Small Cell Lung Cancer

A. Single-Agent Oral Etoposide

Between July 1988 and January 1990, we treated 22 patients with relapsed or refractory small cell lung cancer with oral etoposide (Johnson et al., 1990). Eligibility criteria for this trial are outlined in Table 1. Etoposide was administered orally in the form of soft gelatin capsules for 21 consecutive days at a dosage of 50 mg/m^2/day. Since etoposide is available only in 50 mg capsules, it was necessary to make some approximations in the calculated daily dose. For example, if a patient was calculated to receive 85 mg/day, etoposide was given 100 mg, 100 mg, and 50 mg on 3 consecutive days, and the schedule was repeated for 21 days (i.e., average daily dose of 83.3 mg).

During treatment, weekly blood counts were obtained, and etoposide was discontinued if the leukocyte count fell below 2000/μl or platelet levels fell below 75,000/μl. Therapy was reinitiated when leukocyte counts rose to $>$3000/μl, usually on day 28 or day 35. Patients who had leukocyte nadirs $<$2000/μl or who

Table 1 Phase II Oral Etoposide Trial in Patients with Relapsed or Refractory Small Cell Lung Cancer: Eligibility Criteria

Histologic diagnosis of small cell lung cancer
Prior treatment with at least one combination chemotherapy regimen
ECOG performance status 0, 1, or 2
Leukocytes >3000/μl, platelets >100,000/μl
Serum bilirubin <2 mg/dl (unless due to liver metastases)
Life expectancy ≥12 weeks
No previous therapy for at least 3 weeks
Informed consent

required discontinuation of etoposide prior to day 21 had a dosage reduction to 75% on subsequent cycles. Tumor response was assessed after two courses of treatment; responding patients received a maximum of four courses.

Patient characteristics are detailed in Table 2. Clinical features were typical of a population with small cell lung cancer. Eighteen of 22 patients had received prior intravenous etoposide as part of a combination regimen.

Objective responses were achieved in 10 patients (46%; 95% confidence interval [CI], 27–65%). Two patients had complete response. Median response duration was 4 months (range, 1.5–9.5 months). Two of four patients with no previous etoposide exposure responded, compared to 8 of 18 who had received previous intravenous etoposide. Response rate was better in patients who had been off therapy for >90 days (64% versus 13%).

Previous trials using standard intravenous schedules of etoposide in second-line therapy of small cell lung cancer yielded response rates of 10% or less (Issell et al., 1985; Antman et al., 1984). The high response rate to chronic oral etoposide in these previously treated patients therefore suggests that the schedule of adminis-

Table 2 Phase II Small Cell Lung Cancer Study: Patient Characteristics (n = 22)

Median age, yrs (range)	62 (46–82)
Male:female ratio	15:7
Median number previous combination chemotherapy regimens (range)	1 (1–3)
Previous intravenous etoposide	18 (82%)
Response to previous therapy	
CR	6
PR	12
No response	4
Median interval since most recent treatment, months (range)	4.5 (1–29)

CR, complete response; PR, partial response.

tration is an important factor. In addition, most of the patients who received chronic oral etoposide had received previous intravenous etoposide; patients in previously reported second-line studies were previously untreated with etoposide. Unfortunately, the short response duration in most patients indicates that chronic oral etoposide as a second-line treatment will not make a major impact in the treatment of small cell lung cancer. It remains to be seen whether the incorporation of this "more active" agent into first-line combination regimens will improve treatment results.

Preliminary results using single-agent chronic daily etoposide as initial therapy for small cell lung cancer are also recently available. Clark et al. (1990) reported initial results of therapy in 20 patients with small cell lung cancer who were considered too elderly or otherwise unfit to receive combination chemotherapy. Median age of these patients was 70 years, and median Karnofsky performance status was 60%. Fifteen of 20 patients had extensive-stage disease. All patients received oral etoposide 50 mg twice daily for 14 consecutive days, followed by 1 week without therapy. Responding patients received a maximum of six courses.

Seventeen of 20 patients (85%; 95% CI, 62%–97%) responded to therapy, with two complete responses. After a short median follow-up, remission durations ranged from 2+ to 8+ months. Median nadir leukocyte count was 2900/μl, and occurred on day 15. No thrombocytopenia was encountered. Gastrointestinal toxicity was mild; all patients experienced total alopecia.

This single-agent regimen, which is active and easily tolerated, provides a useful therapeutic alternative for patients with small cell lung cancer who are elderly or who have poor performance status. These patients are difficult to treat with standard combination regimens due to their prohibitive toxicity. Many refuse treatment when informed of potential side effects, and others cannot complete therapy due to declining clinical status. While it is doubtful that the response duration with single-agent oral etoposide will prove to be equivalent to combination regimens, it will probably prove superior to other available choices in selected elderly or unfit patients.

B. Chronic Oral Etoposide in Combination Regimens

Experience with the use of our 21–day schedule of oral etoposide in combination regimens remains limited. We are currently conducting a phase II study using high-dose cisplatin and oral etoposide (Table 3). Full dosages of both agents are combined in this regimen; the primary aim of the study is to evaluate toxicity in previously untreated patients.

Preliminary results indicate that this combination regimen is feasible and well tolerated by most patients. Twenty-two patients have now been treated; all were previously untreated and had extensive-stage small cell lung cancer. Fifteen

Table 3 Combination Regimens Being Evaluated for Initial Therapy

Small cell lung cancer
Cisplatin 100 mg/m^2 iv day 1
Etoposide 50 mg/m^2 orally days 1–21
Repeat every 4–5 weeks
Non-small-cell lung cancer
Carboplatin 300–400 mg/m^2 iv day 1
Etoposide 50 mg/m^2 orally days 1–21
Repeat every 4–5 weeks

patients were male; median age was 56 years (range, 44–74 years). Eighteen of 22 patients responded (82%; 95% CI, 62–93%), with 2 complete and 18 partial responses. Myelosuppression was moderate and was usually easily managed, although some patients required early discontinuation of oral etoposide. Severe leukopenia (<1000/μl) occurred in only 3 of 75 courses (4%), and severe thrombocytopenia (<50,000/μl) occurred in 14 of 75 courses (19%). Additional toxicity included alopecia (100%), nausea/vomiting (29%), and nephrotoxicity (4%).

Results from this phase II trial indicate that oral etoposide 50 mg/m^2 for 21 days can be safely combined with full-dose cisplatin in previously untreated patients with extensive-stage small cell lung cancer. As expected, this regimen produced a high response rate, but its efficacy compared to standard cisplatin/etoposide regimens remains unknown.

III. Non-Small-Cell Lung Cancer

A. Single-Agent Oral Etoposide

Two phase II studies have now been completed evaluating chronic oral etoposide in patients with previously untreated non-small-cell lung cancer. Results of these studies are conflicting.

Saxman et al. (1990) reported a cooperative trial by the Hoosier Oncology Group, in which 45 patients received oral etoposide 50 mg/m^2 daily for 21 consecutive days. Cycles were repeated every 28 days, with courses delayed if the day 28 leukocyte count was <2500/μl. Among the first 30 evaluable patients, only 2 partial responses were observed (7% response rate). Eight additional patients had stable disease after a median of four treatment courses. Toxicity was tolerable, with only six episodes of severe neutropenia, and mild gastrointestinal toxicity.

We achieved somewhat better results in a recently completed phase II study. Twenty-five patients who had locally unresectable or metastatic non-small-cell lung cancer and were previously untreated with systemic therapy received oral etoposide 50 mg/m^2 daily for 21 consecutive days. Courses were repeated at 28 day intervals, or when the leukocyte count was >3000/μl. Five of 25 patients (20%; 95% CI, 9–39%) had partial responses, with a median response duration of 4 months. Myelosuppression was less severe than we observed in the previously treated patients in our small cell lung cancer study. Median leukocyte nadir during course 1 was 3200/μl; leukocyte nadirs of <1000/μl occurred in only 4 of 69 courses (6%). Anemia was cumulative with repeat courses. Other than alopecia in all patients, extramedullary toxicity was unusual.

Chronic oral etoposide therefore appears to have some activity in the treatment of patients with advanced non-small-cell lung cancer, but the objective response rate is probably 20% or less. The schedule of administration may improve the level of activity, but probably not enough to make a major clinical difference in this relatively resistant tumor type.

B. Combination Regimens Containing Chronic Etoposide

We are currently investigating a combination of carboplatin and chronic oral etoposide in the treatment of advanced non-small-cell lung cancer. Carboplatin was chosen in an attempt to design an outpatient regimen with limited toxicity. Because of the anticipated addition of the carboplatin to overall myelosuppression, we chose a moderate carboplatin starting dosage of 300 mg/m^2, in addition to etoposide 50 mg/m^2/day for 21 days. We subsequently escalated the carboplatin dosage to 350 mg/m^2, and are currently evaluating a dosage of 400 mg/m^2.

Preliminary results form this phase II trial indicate that this regimen is feasible and well tolerated using carboplatin dosages of 300 mg/m^2 or 350 mg/m^2 in addition to oral etoposide. Thirty-seven patients have now been treated, and 30 are evaluable for response. Twenty-nine patients were male, median age was 58 years (range, 40–70 years), and the majority of patients had Eastern Cooperative Oncology Group (ECOG) performance status of 1. Twenty-seven patients had metastatic lung cancer while 10 had locally advanced (stage IIIB) disease. Eight of 30 patients (27%; 95% CI, 14–44%) had partial responses; there were no complete responses. Median duration of response has not been reached at 5 months. Myelosuppression was moderate, and was not different with the two carboplatin dosage levels: median leukocyte nadir was 2900/μl and median platelet nadir was 172,000/μl.

From these preliminary results, it appears that carboplatin combined with oral etoposide produces a response rate similar to those reported for other cisplatin-based treatment regimens for non-small-cell lung cancer. This regimen has the advantage of being well tolerated in the outpatient setting. However, it is doubtful that the incorporation of chronic oral etoposide into regimens for patients with non-small-cell lung cancer will markedly improve treatment results.

C. Summary and Conclusions

The schedule dependency of etoposide has been suspected since the initial preclinical and clinical development of this drug, and recent clinical trials have substantiated the importance of schedule. Most data now support the concept that the activity of etoposide depends more on the time of exposure to a threshold serum level, rather than to the peak level achieved. As might be expected, the toxicity profile of etoposide can also be changed by administering the drug by different schedules. Neither the "optimal" time of exposure nor the minimum serum drug level required for activity has been defined.

In patients with small cell lung cancer, phase II data suggest that a 21 day etoposide schedule is more active than the standard 3–5 day intravenous schedules. Similar increased activity has also been suggested in patients with lymphoma and testicular cancer, tumor types that are also highly sensitive to etoposide (Hainsworth et al., 1990; Miller et al., 1989). The impact of chronic etoposide schedules in the treatment of small cell lung cancer, particularly with respect to its incorporation in combination regimens, awaits further definition. For elderly patients, single-agent oral etoposide provides an active and easily tolerated alternative to combination chemotherapy.

The role of chronic etoposide in the treatment of non-small-cell lung cancer is even less clear. The level of activity against non-small-cell lung cancer is relatively low, but may be comparable to other "active" agents. Based on results to date, it seems unlikely that changes in the etoposide schedule will cause markedly increased activity in non-small-cell lung cancer, or in any tumor that is relatively resistant to etoposide given by standard schedule.

Many unanswered questions remain. What is the minimum serum level of etoposide that is tumoricidal in sensitive malignancies? Is there a level that is tumoricidal but nonmyelosuppressive? If so, can this dosage be given for periods longer than 21 days, and will this further enhance efficacy? What is the best way to incorporate chronic etoposide into combination regimens? Answers to these questions will be needed before the place of chronic etoposide in the treatment of cancer can be determined.

References

Antman, K., Pomfret, E., Karp, G., Skarin, A., and Canellos, G. (1984). Phase II trial of etoposide in previously treated small cell carcinoma of the lung. *Cancer Treat. Rep.* **68:**1413–1414.

Cavalli, F., Sonntag, R. W., Jungi, F., Senn, H. J., and Brunner, K. W. (1978). VP-16-213 monotherapy for remission induction of small cell lung cancer. A randomized trial using three dosage schedules. *Cancer Treat. Rep.* **62:**473–475.

Chen, G. L., Yang, L., Rowe, T. C., Halligan, B. D., Tewey, K. M., and Liu, L. F. (1984).

Non intercalative antitumor drugs interfere with the breakage–reunion reaction of mammalian DNA topoisomerase II. *J. Biol. Chem.* **259:**13560–13566.

Clark, P. I., Joel, S. P., and Slevin, M. L. (1989). A pharmacokinetic hypothesis for the clinical efficacy of etoposide in small cell lung cancer. *Proc. Am. Soc. Clin. Oncol.* **8:**66 (abstr).

Clark, P. I., Cottier, B., Joel, S. P., Thompson, P. I., and Slevin, M. L. (1990). Prolonged administration of single-agent oral etoposide in patients with untreated small cell lung cancer (SCLC). *Proc. Am. Soc. Clin. Oncol.* **9:**226.

Dombernowsky, P., and Nissen, N. I. (1973). Schedule dependency of the antileukemic activity of the podophyllotoxin-derivative VP 16-213 (NSC-141540) in L1210 leukemia. *Acta Pathol. Microbiol. Scand.* [A], **81:**715–724.

Evans, W. K., Shepherd, F. A., Feld, R., Osoba, D., Dang, P., and Deboer, G. (1985). VP-16 and cisplatin as first-line therapy of small-cell lung cancer. *J. Clin. Oncol.* **3:**1471–1477.

Greider, A., Maurer, R., and Stahelin, H. (1974). Effect of an epipodophyllotoxin derivative (VP 16-213) on macromolecular synthesis and mitosis in mastocytoma cells in vitro. *Cancer Res.* **34:**1788–1793.

Hainsworth, J. D., Johnson, D. H., Hande, K. R., and Greco, F. A. (1989a). Chemotherapy of advanced non-small cell lung cancer: a randomized trial of three cisplatin-based chemotherapy regimens. *Am. J. Clin. Oncol.* **12:**345–349.

Hainsworth, J. D., Johnson, D. H., Frazier, S. R., and Greco, F. A. (1989b). Chronic daily administration of oral etoposide—a phase I trial. *J. Clin. Oncol.* **7:**396–401.

Hainsworth, J. D., Johnson, D. H., and Greco, F. A. (1990). Chronic daily administration of oral etoposide in refractory lymphoma—a phase II trial. *Eur. J. Cancer* **26:**818–821.

Issell, B. F., Einhorn, L. H., Comis, R. L., et al. (1985). Multicenter phase II trial of etoposide in refractory small cell lung cancer. *Cancer Treat. Rep.* **69:**127–128.

Johnson, D. H., Greco, F. A., Strupp, J., Hande, K. R., and Hainsworth, J. D. (1990). Prolonged administration of oral etoposide in patients with relapsed or refractory small-cell lung cancer: a phase II trial. *J. Clin. Oncol.* **8:**1613–1617.

Kalwinsky, D. K., Look, A. T., Ducore, J., and Fridland, A. (1983). Effects of the epipodophyllotoxin VP-16-213 on cell cycle traverse, DNA synthesis, and DNA strand size in cultures of human leukemic fibroblasts. *Cancer Res.* **43:**1592–1597.

Klastersky, J., Sculier, J. P., Ravez, P., et al. (1986). A randomized study comparing a high and standard dose of cisplatin in combination with etoposide in the treatment of advanced non-small cell lung cancer. *J. Clin. Oncol.* **4:**1780–1786.

Liu, L. F., Rowe, T. C., Yang, L., Tewey, K. M., and Chen, G. L. (1983). Cleavage of DNA by mammalian DNA topoisomerase II. *J. Biol. Chem.* **258:**15365–15370.

Miller, J. C., Loehrer, P. J., Williams, S. D., and Einhorn, L. H. (1989). Phase II study of daily oral VP-16 in refractory germ cell tumors. *Proc. Am. Soc. Clin. Oncol.* **8:**145 (abstr).

Porter, L. L., Johnson, D. H., Hainsworth, J. D., Hande, K. R., Greco, F. A. (1985). Cisplatinum and VP-16 combination chemotherapy for refractory small cell carcinoma of the lung. *Cancer Treat. Rep.* **69:**479–481.

Saxman, S., Logie, K., Stephens, D., Workman, F., Scullin, D., Loehrer, P. J. (1990). Phase

II trial of daily oral etoposide in patients with surgically unresectable non-small cell lung cancer. *Proc. Am. Soc. Clin. Oncol.* **9:**238. (abstr).

Slevin, M. L., Clark, P. I., Joel, S. P., Malik, S., Osborne, R. J., Gregory, W. M., Lowe, D. G., Reznak, R. H., and Wrigley, P. F. M. (1989a). A randomized trial to evaluate the effect of schedule on the activity of etoposide in small-cell lung cancer. *J. Clin. Oncol.* **7:**1333–1340.

Slevin, M. L., Clark, P. I., Joel, J. P., Thompson, P., Talbot, D., Price, C., and Wrigley, P. F. M. (1989b). A randomized trial to examine the effect of more extended scheduling of etoposide administration in small cell lung cancer. *Proc. Am. Soc. Clin. Oncol.* **8:**236 (abstr).

Sullivan, D. M., Glisson, B. S., Hodges, P. K., Smallwood-Kentro, S., Ross, W. E. (1986). Proliferation dependence of topoisomerase II mediated drug action. *Biochemistry* **25:**2248–2256.

Wozniak, A. J., and Ross, W. E. (1983). DNA damage as a basis for 4-dimethyl epipodophyllotoxin-9 (4, 6-0-ethylidene-B-D-glucopyranoside) (etoposide) cytotoxicity. *Cancer Res.* **43:**120–124.

23

Oral Ifosfamide in Advanced Non-Small-Cell Lung Cancer: Results of a Phase I/II Study

C. MANEGOLD, H. BISCHOFF, J. R. FISCHER, A. SCHMÄHL, and P. DRINGS

Chest Hospital
Heidelberg, Germany

M. PEUKERT

Asta Medical AG
Frankfurt, Germany

I. Introduction

Non-small-cell lung cancer (NSCLC) is one of the most common malignant diseases in the world, appearing throughout both developed and underdeveloped countries. For limited stages of the disease, surgery and radiotherapy are the leading treatment options (Cox et al., 1983; Mountain, 1983; Johnson, 1988; Wannenmacher et al., 1990). Chemotherapy is reserved solely for patients with advanced stages of NSCLC, but up until now it has only brought marginal benefits (Aisner et al., 1983; Hoffman et al., 1983).

The search for an effective systemic chemotherapy regimen continues, not only because the majority of patients present initially with advanced inoperable disease, but also because the survival of operable patients originally presenting with limited disease remains poor, with only 25% alive after 5 years. In these latter cases, local tumor relapses or distant metastases frequently occur, despite the fact that these patients were primarily treated by surgery with curative intent (Vogt-Moykopf et al., 1988; Martini et al., 1988; Drings, 1987).

Ifosfamide is considered to be one of the most effective cytotoxic agents in the treatment of NSCLC (Drings, 1989; Johnson, 1990; Worrall, 1982). It has been shown that when ifosfamide is administered parenterally as a single agent, a remission rate of approximately 20% can be achieved. Similar results have been cited in a variety of studies involving large numbers of patients receiving various fractionated and single-dose treatment schedules (Thatcher et al., 1986; Constanzi et al., 1982; Souhami, 1985; Nohile et al., 1984). Combination chemotherapy using ifosfamide with cisplatin and mitomycin C or etoposide has also demonstrated a relatively high response rate in various clinical phase II studies, including complete remissions in about 10% of the cases (Drings et al., 1986; Shepherd et al., 1990; Ardizzoni et al., 1987; Cullen et al., 1988). However, toxicity in such intensive combination chemotherapy regimens continues to be a major clinical problem. An attempt to reduce treatment toxicity must be one of the main considerations in clinical trials.

The oxazaphosphorines tend to differ greatly in their physiochemical, pharmacologic, toxicologic, and therapeutic properties. Antitumor activity is greater for ifosfamide than for cyclophosphamide in several experimental tumor systems, some of which are primarily resistant to cyclophosphamide (Goldin, 1982). The metabolization profile of cyclophosphamide also differs greatly from that shown by ifosfamide (Colvin, 1982).

As a result, ifosfamide's therapeutic index has largely been determined by the schedules used for its medical application. Investigations by Klein et al. (1984) gave evidence that daily fractionated administration or continuous infusion of ifosfamide is less toxic and more effective in animals and humans than a single bolus injection.

Wagner and Drings (1986) as well as Cerny et al. (1986) were able to demonstrate that the bioavailability of oral ifosfamide is comparable to the intravenous form (i.e., close to 100%). Blood level curves (Fig. 1) demonstrated rapid absorption kinetics for oral ifosfamide. With the exception of the first hour,

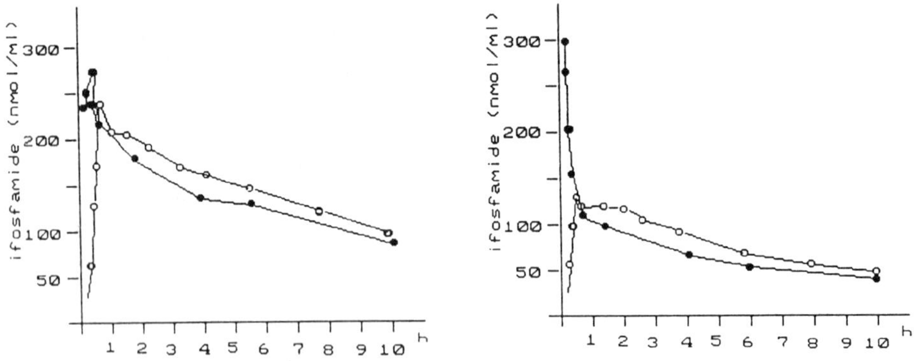

Figure 1 Mean blood concentration of ifosfamide after intravenous injection (●—●) and oral administration (○—○). Left, 2 g/m² (n = 6); right, 1 g/m² (n = 12).

Table 1 Pharmacokinetic Parameters and Bioavailability of Ifosfamide

Ifosfamide	$t_{1/2}$ (h)	$AUC^{0-\infty}$ (μmol/h/ml^{-1})	$\frac{AUC_{oral}}{AUC_{i.v.}}$
1 g/m^2, i.v.	5.89 ± 2.6	1.28 ± 0.86	1.049 ± 0.27
n = 22, oral	5.76 ± 2.1	1.32 ± 0.46	0.67 − 1.55
2 g/m^2, i.v.	5.71 ± 2.8	2.24 ± 0.85	0.59 ± 0.42
n = 6, oral	5.33 ± 1.8	2.14 ± 0.81	0.42 − 1.43

$t_{1/2}$, terminal elimination half-life; AUC, area under the blood concentration curve.

during the absorption phase the mean blood level curves of oral and intravenously administered ifosfamide were identical. There were also no significant differences between the terminal half-life times reached by the oral and intravenous forms of ifosfamide (Table 1), which in both cases ranged from 5 to 6 h. Since the pharmacokinetic figures for oral ifosfamide do not differ from those noted for its intravenous equivalent, it would appear to be advantageous to replace the intravenous administration of ifosfamide with equal doses of the more easily administered oral version, especially when fractionated dose schedules are required.

To establish the maximum tolerated dose of oral ifosfamide and to determine its tumor response effectiveness, we decided to initiate a dose escalation study, believing that ifosfamide in its oral form would most likely be better accepted by patients.

II. Materials and Methods

A. Participation Criteria

Entry criteria included histologically confirmed, advanced NSCLC; an Eastern Cooperative Oncology Group (ECOG) performance status of 0–2; life expectancy of at least 3 months; patients' age of 75 years or less; measurable or evaluable disease; and informed, written consent to participation. Reasons for exclusion from the study were previous chemotherapy; severe accompanying diseases; elevation of alkaline phosphatase or bilirubin levels more than 1.5 times higher than the normal range; a transaminase level more than 4 times above normal; a serum-creatinine level greater than 1.6 mg/100 ml; persistent bone marrow insufficiency; a history of noncompliance; severe cerebral sclerosis; brain metastasis; hypercalcemia; a history of alcohol abuse; pregnancy or lactation; and any second malignancy, except for in situ carcinoma of the cervix or adequately treated basal cell carcinoma of the skin.

B. Treatment

Oral ifosfamide was given in four different treatment schedules (Table 2): 1, 1000 mg for 5 consecutive days; 2, 750 mg for 14 consecutive days; 3, 1000 mg for 14 consecutive days; and 4, 1250 mg for 14 consecutive days. Cycles were repeated every 4 weeks. Mesna was given orally with each single dose of oral ifosfamide (300–500 mg from drinking ampules).

C. Evaluation

1. *Response*

Responses were evaluated according to the International Union Against Cancer (UICC) criteria. A complete response (CR) was defined as the disappearance of all measurable lesions for at least 2 months. A partial remission (PR) was defined as a reduction in tumor size of more than 50% and the absence of new lesions for at least 2 months. Effusions and bone lesions were not regarded as being objectively measurable. No change (NC) was defined as either stabilization of disease or a reduction in tumor parameters of less than 50% without progression of other lesions for at least 3 months. Progression of disease (PD) was defined as an increase of more than 25% in any of the metastatic lesions based on the maximal response observed. Duration of response was calculated from the start of treatment until disease progression. A minimum of two treatment cycles was required to be considered for response evaluation.

2. *Toxicity*

Toxicity (except for neurotoxic reactions) was evaluated according to World Health Organization criteria. For central nervous system (CNS) toxicity the clinical grading system proposed by Meanwell and colleagues (1986) was used. For each patient, the highest grade of toxicity that occurred is cited.

Table 2 Treatment Plans

Group	Schedule	Dose per cycle
1	1000 mg/day × 5	5,000 mg (3.0 g/m^2)
2	750 mg/day × 14	10,500 mg (6.0 g/m^2)
3	1000 mg/day × 14	14,000 mg (7.5 g/m^2)
4	1250 mg/day × 14	17,500 mg (10 g/m^2)

Table 3 Patient Population

	Group			
	1	2	3	4
No.	15	19	23	7
Gender				
Male	14	14	20	6
Female	1	5	3	1
Age (years)				
Median	54	60	61	60
Range	47–67	47–69	51–73	55–65
ECOG performance status				
Grade 0	4	—	2	—
Grade 1	5	15	7	4
Grade 2	6	4	14	3
Histologic type				
Adenocarcinoma	9	14	16	3
Epidermoid carcinoma	4	5	5	2
Large cell carcinoma	2	—	1	2
Mixed adenocarcinoma	—	—	1	—

D. Patient Population

A total of 64 patients were included in the study (Table 3). Most of the patients were male. The median age was 60 years (range, 47–73). The performance status (ECOG) was grade 0 in 6 patients, grade 1 in 31, and grade 2 in 27 patients. Most of the patients had either adenocarcinoma (n = 42) or a squamous cell carcinoma (n = 16).

III. Results

A. Evaluability

Treatment according to schedule 1 was given to 15 patients, schedule 2 to 19 patients, schedule 3 to 23 patients, and schedule 4 to 7 patients. Fifty-nine of the 64 patients included in the study were evaluable for response and/or toxicity (Table 4). Reasons for exclusion from evaluation were protocol violations (n = 3) or tumor-related early death (n = 2).

Table 4 Patients' Evaluability (n = 64)

	Group			
	1	2	3	4
Evaluable for response and toxicity	12	14	16	2
Evaluable for toxicity only	2	4	5	4
Not evaluable	1	1	2	1

B. Toxicity

A total of 308 treatment cycles was administered with no evidence of severe neurotoxicity (grade 3 or 4). Sixteen patients developed grade 1 or 2 CNS toxicity before the 14-day 1000 mg/day schedule was exceeded: 13% on schedule 1, 44% on schedule 2, and 35% on schedule 3 (Table 5). However, in 4 of the 5 patients (80%) on schedule 4, CNS toxicity appeared within the first two treatment cycles. None of the patients showed myelosuppression, gastrointestinal toxicity, nausea or vomiting, or alopecia exceeding WHO grade 2. Urotoxicity was not a clinical problem.

C. Response

Forty-four of the 64 patients included in this study received two or more cycles of therapy and were thus eligible for evaluation of tumor response (Table 6): 12 patients in treatment group 1, 14 patients in treatment group 2, 16 patients in treatment group 3, and 2 patients in treatment group 4. Three patients in group 1 showed no change after documented tumor progression, while 3 patients on

Table 5 Treatment-Related Toxicity (Maximal WHO Grade of Symptom per Patient, %)

Grade	0				1				2			
Group	1	2	3	4	1	2	3	4	1	2	3	4
Alopecia	87	69	30	43	13	31	35	43	0	0	35	14
Leukopenia	92	90	76	80	8	0	0	0	0	10	24	20
Thrombocytopenia	100	100	95	100	0	0	0	0	0	0	5	0
Anemia	77	68	62	80	23	16	14	20	0	16	24	0
Nausea/vomiting	53	42	39	100	13	14	17	0	34	46	44	0
Urotoxicity	100	100	95	100	0	5	0	0	0	0	0	0
Encephalopathy[a]	87	56	55	20	0	12	0	20	13	32	35	60

[a]Grading according to Meanwell et al. (1986).

Table 6 Tumor Response Efficacy[a]

	Group			
	1 (n = 12)	2 (n = 14)	3 (n = 16)	4 (n = 2)
CR	—	—	—	—
PR	—	3 (21%)	4 (25%)	—
NC	3	8	10	1
PD	9	3	2	1

[a]Following second treatment cycle.
CR, complete response; PR, partial response; NC, no change; PD, progression of disease.

schedule 2 had a partial remission and 8 showed no change. On schedule 3, 4 patients obtained a partial remission and 10 patients showed no change. The median duration of response was 6 months (range, 4–16) for patients on treatment schedule 1, 7 months (range, 4–20) on schedule 2, and 6 months (range, 3–12) on schedule 3.

IV. Discussion

Ifosfamide has long been recognized as one of the most effective substances in oncology (Bramwell et al., 1987; Drings, 1989; Einhorn and Loehrer, 1986; Hunter and Harrison, 1982; Thatcher et al., 1987; Wheeler et al., 1986; Williams, 1984). The intravenous form of ifosfamide has also proven effective in the treatment of NSCLC, both in single-agent and combination chemotherapy. The purpose of our study was to clarify the effectiveness and to evaluate the toxicity of oral ifosfamide.

One of the most serious drawbacks noted in previous studies using ifosfamide is one of the most common problems of cancer chemotherapy: treatment-related toxicity. The toxicity most often associated with ifosfamide's use was hemorrhagic cystitis (Spechter et al., 1965). Studies have shown that this cystitis most likely stems from acrolein, one of the metabolites of ifosfamide. Acrolein is an α,β-unsaturated aldehyde, which is a bladder mucosa irritant (Brock et al., 1979). It has been found, however, that the sulfhydryl compound mesna combines with 4-hydroxyisophosphamide and acrolein in the efferent urinary tract, and is thus able to prevent hemorrhagic cystitis (Brock et al., 1982; Scheef et al., 1979; Burkert, 1983).

The effectiveness of mesna's uroprotective properties in its oral form (drinking ampules) could be substantiated in this study. No urotoxicity exceeding

WHO grade 1 was observed in the 59 patients evaluable for toxicity in our phase I/II trial, which encompassed a total of 308 treatment cycles. Urotoxicity was therefore not a significant clinical problem.

Instead, neurotoxic reactions have proven to be the major limiting toxicity factor in ifosfamide therapy. CNS toxicity has been reported to develop clinically in 5–10% of the patients treated with ifosfamide (Scheulen et al., 1983; Klein et al., 1983; Meanwell et al., 1986). Moreover, electroencephalographic abnormalities, with or without clinical CNS toxicity, developed in an additional 56% of the patients treated with 36 h continuous ifosfamide infusions (Meanwell et al., 1986).

CNS toxicity in ifosfamide therapy is still not completely understood. Among its metabolites, chloracetaldehyde is considered to be the principal source of such neurotoxic reactions (Goren et al., 1986). Other short-lived metabolites that may contribute to this toxicity include acrolein and chlorethanol, with its dimer aldehydes. The development of CNS toxicity also is related to the form of ifosfamide administration selected. Such toxicity appears most frequently with oral application, whereas it is rarely to be found when administered by continuous infusion over 3–5 days (Cerny and Küpfer, 1989). Furthermore, it could be shown that a history of impaired renal function and low serum albumin concentrations, which may also be reflected in neoplasia-associated catabolic states or hepatocellular insufficiency, predisposes to ifosfamide-induced encephalopathy (Meanwell et al., 1986).

In our study using the oral form of ifosfamide in different daily fractionated dose schedules, CNS toxicity was not a serious clinical problem until the 14-day 1000 mg/day schedule was exceeded. At this point about 15% of the patients developed clinically recognizable, mild neurotoxic reactions ranging from grade 1 to grade 2. However, it was discovered retrospectively that most of these patients had either a history of chronic alcoholism or previous CNS involvement that was not known at study entry.

The number of patients in our study affected by CNS toxicity was actually lower than expected, which we attribute to our strict adherence to the acceptance criteria delineated in our protocol. We did not include patients with limited renal function and low serum albumin concentrations. We also rejected patients with concomitant diseases that could affect or impair CNS function: chronic alcoholism, hypercalcemia, brain metastasis, severe cerebral sclerosis, or a history of drug abuse. The use of certain drugs that might interfere with CNS function (i.e., narcotic analgesics, tranquilizers, and dopamine antagonists) was allowed when clinically indicated, but these were to be used with caution. The fact that an increase in the daily ifosfamide dosage to 1250 mg led to a significant increase in neurotoxic reactions would suggest that there is a definite relationship between dosage and toxicity. This is not surprising and has been noted in previous studies.

Nonetheless, the daily oral dosage reportedly administered by Cerny and Küpfer (1989) is significantly higher (1500 mg/m^2) than that used in our study.

It can be stated that the fractionated oral ifosfamide therapy utilized in our study was well tolerated by the patients and that the oral treatment schedule proved to have a more positive objective toxicity spectrum than the intravenous schedules. None of our patients showed myelosuppression or nausea and vomiting exceeding WHO grade 2. Moreover, a factor of perhaps even greater significance for the general tolerance of this therapy was that alopecia exceeding WHO grade 2 was not observed; hair loss was therefore not a problem. despite the fact that CNS toxicity was mild in patients receiving our oral ifosfamide therapy regimens, it is suggested that the daily dosage of 1000 mg in a 14-day fractionated dose treatment schedule not be exceeded.

The tumor response efficacy of oral ifosfamide in patients with NSCLC is comparable to the rate achieved in various phase II studies using ifosfamide intravenously. A remission rate of about 20% was reached, but only partial responses were seen. The median duration of response was approximately 7 months. To obtain these results, our study indicated that daily oral ifosfamide dosages should not be less than 750 mg within a fractionated 14-day treatment schedule. The high rate of disease stabilization after documented progression is a phenomenon recently observed in other phase II studies of NSCLC (Khanavkar et al., 1989). The weight that should be given to the rubric "no change" in the context of treatment efficacy has yet to be clarified. It is very clear, however, that the clinical value of disease stabilization after documented progression can and should not be dismissed, especially within the scope of palliative treatment, when the main goal is to achieve a relatively long-lasting, symptom-free interval with an acceptably high quality of life.

We conclude from our study that ifosfamide can easily be tolerated utilizing fractionated doses in a 14-day treatment regimen. The CNS toxicity encountered could be categorized as mild and was generally temporary. Although CNS toxicity remains the main concern with oral ifosfamide therapy, it can be significantly reduced when high-risk patients (i.e., those with inadequate renal or hepatic function, a history of alcohol and/or drug abuse, hypercalcemia, advanced cerebral sclerosis, or CNS metastases) are excluded from therapy.

Urotoxicity was rarely seen, which would indicate that when mesna is administered orally concurrently with oral ifosfamide, its protective qualities are sufficiently effective. Myelotoxicity, a well-known problem in cyclophosphamide treatment, and one that is moderate in intravenous ifosfamide use, was not a clinical problem with oral ifosfamide. Because oral ifosfamide produces little myelotoxicity, it would appear to be a better choice as a partner in combination chemotherapy than other alkylating agents, and would be especially suitable for combining with myelotoxic agents.

The encouraging results obtained in this phase I/II trial of oral ifosfamide concerning both response effectiveness and degree of toxicity in patients with NSCLC must be confirmed in further trials. We remain hopeful, however, that our positive findings will be substantiated by randomized trials comparing oral ifosfamide with its intravenous equivalent, at which time more conclusive results can be drawn.

References

Aisner, J., Alberto, P., Bitran, J., Conus, R., Daniels, J., Hausen, M. W., and Smyth, J. (1983). Role of chemotherapy in small cell lung cancer: a consensus report of the International Association for the Study of Lung Cancer Workshop. *Cancer Treat. Rep.* **67**:37–43.

Ardizzoni, A., Fusco, V., and Guilisano, M. (1987). Etoposide, ifosfamide and cisplatin in the treatment of advanced non small cell lung cancer. *Cancer Treat. Rep.* **71**:1311–1312.

Bramwell, V. H. C. Mouridsen, H. T., Santoro, A., Blackledge, G., Somers, R., Verwey, J., Dombernowsky, P., Onsrud, M., Thomas, D., Sylvester, Oosterom, A., van (1987). Cyclophosphamide versus ifosfamide: final report of a randomized phase II trial in adult soft tissue sarcoma. *Eur. J. Cancer Clin. Oncol.* **23**:311.

Brock, N., Stekar, J., and Pohl, J. (1979). Acrolein, the causative factor of urotoxic side effects of cyclophosphamide, ifosfamide and sulfosfamide. *Arzneimittelforsch.* **29**: 659–661.

Brock, N., Pohl, J., Stekar, J., and Scheef, W. (1982). Studies on the urotoxicity of oxazaphosphorine cytostatics and its prevention—3. Profile of action of sodium 2-mercaptoethane sulfonate (mesna). *Eur. J. Cancer Clin. Oncol.* **18**:1377–1387.

Burkert, H. (1983). Clinical overview of mesna. *Cancer Treat. Rev.* **10**:175–181.

Cerny, T., Marginson, J., Thatcher, N., and Wilkinson, P. M. (1986). Bioavailability and tolerance of oral ifosfamide in patients with bronchial carcinoma. *Br. J. Cancer* **54**:197.

Cerny, T., and Küpfer, A. (1989). Anmerkungen zum pharmakologischen Profil von Ifosfamid/Mesna. *Schweiz Krebs Bull.* **4**:7–9.

Colvin, M. (1982). The comparative pharmacology of cyclophosphamide and ifosfamide. *Semin. Oncol.* **9**(4)(suppl 1):2–7.

Constanzi, J. J., Morgan, L. R., and Kokanson, J. (1982). Ifosfamide in the treatment of extensive non-oat cell carcinoma of the lung. *Semin. Oncol.* **9**(4)(suppl 1):61–65.

Cox, I. D., Byhardt, R. W., and Kornaki, R. (1983). The role of radiotherapy in squamous, large cell and adenocarcinoma of the lung. *Semin. Oncol.* **10**(suppl 4):81–94.

Cullen, M. H., Joshi, R., Chetiyawardana, A. D., and Woodroffe, C. M. (1988). Mitomycin, ifosfamide and cisplatin in non small cell lung cancer: treatment good enough to compare. *Br. J. Cancer* **58**:359–361.

Drings, P. (1987). European experience with ifosfamide in non small cell lung cancer. *Semin. Oncol.* **16**(1)(suppl 3):22–30.

Drings, P. (1989). Ifosfamide in the treatment of bronchial carcinoma. *Contrib. Oncol.* **26:** 294–318.

Drings, P., Abel, U., Blzebruck, H., Stiefel, P., Kleckow, M., and Manke, H. G. (1986). Experience with ifosfamide combinations (etoposide or DDP) in non small cell lung cancer. *Cancer Chemother. Pharmacol.* **18**(suppl 2)**:**34–39.

Einhorn, L. H., and Loehrer, P. J. (1986). Ifosfamide chemotherapy for pancreatic cancer. *Cancer Chemother. Pharmacol.* **18**(suppl 2)**:**51.

Goldin, A. (1982). Ifosfamide in experimental tumor systems. *Semin. Oncol.* **9**(4)(suppl 1)**:** 14–23.

Goren, M. R., Wright, R. K., Pratt, C. B., and Pell, F. E. (1986). Dechlorethylation of ifosfamide and neurotoxicity. *Lancet* **2:**1219–1220.

Hoffman, P. C., Bitan, I. D., and Golomb, H. M. (1983). Chemotherapy of metastatic non small cell bronchogenic carcinoma. *Semin. Oncol.* **10**(suppl 4)**:**111–122.

Hunter, H. L., and Harrison, E. F. (1982). The anticancer spectrum of ifosfamide. *Semin. Oncol.* **4**(suppl 1)**:**96.

Johnson, D. H., (1990). Overview of ifosfamide in small cell and non small cell lung cancer. *Semin. Oncol.* **17**(2)(suppl 4)**:**22–30.

Johnson, M. R. (1988). Selecting patients with lung cancer for surgical treatment. *Semin. Oncol.* **15**(3)**:**246–254.

Khanavkar, B., Gatzemeier, U. F., Meyer-Schwickerath, E., Lorenz, J., Schreml, W., Brugger, R., Schick, H. D., von Pawel, J., Nordstrom, R., and Drings, P. (1989). Treatment of non-small-cell-lung-cancer with the alkyllysophospholipid edelfosine. Intermediate data analysis. *Contrib. Oncol.* **37:**224–235.

Klein, H. O., Dias Wickramanayake, P., Coerper, C. I., Christian, E., Pohl, J.N., and Brock, N. (1983). High dose ifosfamide and mesna as continuous infusion over five days—a phase I/II trial. *Cancer Treat. Rev.* **10**(10)**:**167–173.

Klein, H. O., Wickramanayake, P. D., Christian, E., and Coerper, C. (1984). Therapeutic effects of single-push or fractionated injections or continuous infusion of oxazaphosphorines (cyclophosphamide, ifosfamide, Asta 2 7557). *Cancer* **54:**1193–1203.

Martini, N., Bains, M. S., Kaiser, I. R., Bert, M. E., and Pomerantz, A. H. (1988). Surgical treatment of non small cell carcinoma of the lung. The Memorial Sloan Kettering experience. In: *Lung Tumors.* Edited by B. Hoogstraten, F. J., Adis, H. H. Hansen, N. Martini, and S. G. Spiro. pp. 111–119.

Meanwell, C. A., Blake, E. B., Kelly, K. A., Honigsberger, L., and Blackledge, G. (1986). Prediction of ifosfamide/mesna associated encephalopathy. *Eur. J. Cancer Clin. Oncol.* **22**(7)**:**815–819.

Mountain, C. F. (1983). Therapy of stage I and II non small cell lung cancer. *Semin. Oncol.* **10**(suppl 4)**:**71–80.

Nohile, M. T., Rosso, R., Brema, F., et al. (1984). Phase II-study of ifosfamide combined with mesna uroprotection in advanced non small cell carcinoma and other solid tumors. *Tumori* **70:**433–437.

Scheef, W., Klein, H. O., Burkert, H., Gunther, U., Hoefer-Janker, H., Mitrenga, D., Schnitker, J., and Voigtmann, R. (1979). Controlled clinical studies with an antidote against the urotoxicity of oxazaphosphorines: preliminary results. *Cancer Treat. Rep.* **63:**501–505.

Scheulen, M. E., Niederle, N., Bremer, K., Schutte, J., and Seeber, S. (1983). Efficacy of ifosfamide in refractory malignant diseases and uroprotection by mesna: results of a clinical phase II study with 151 patients. *Cancer Treat. Rev.* **10**(A)**:**93–101.

Shepherd, A. F., Goss, E. P., Latreille, J., Steward, D., Logan, D., Evans, W. K., Maroun, J., and Warner, E. (1990). A phase II study of ifosfamide, cisplatin, etoposide in patients with advanced non small cell lung cancer: a preliminary report. *Semin. Oncol.* **17**(2)(suppl 4)**:**19–23.

Souhami, R. (1985). Chemotherapy in non small cell bronchial carcinoma. *Thorax* **40:** 641–645.

Thatcher, N., Anderson, H., Smith, D. B., Harrison, E. F., Hawke, J. E., Hunter, H. L., Constanzi, J. J., Morgan, L. R., Plotkin, D., and Tucker, W. G. (1986). Ifosfamide by bolus: a treatment for advanced non small cell lung cancer. *Chemother. Pharmacol.* **18**(suppl)**:**30–33.

Thatcher, N., Cerny, T., Stout, R., Anderson, H., Barber, P. V., Wolstenholme, R. I., Barnes, P., and Deiraniya, A. (1987). Ifosfamide, etoposide, and thoracic irradiation therapy in 163 patients with unresectable small cell lung cancer. *Cancer* **60:**2382.

Vogt-Moykopf, I., Drings, P., Blzebruck, H., Probst, G., and Merkle, N. (1986). Das Bronchialkarzinom. *Z. Herz Thorax Gefsschir.* **2:**62–70.

Wagner, T., and Drings, P. (1986). Pharmacokinetics and bioavailability of oral ifosfamide. *Arzneim.* **26:**878–880.

Wannenmacher, M., Kimming, B., and Vogel, D. (1990). Strahlentherapie des Bronchialkarzinoms. *Chirung* **61:**565–570.

Wheeler, B. J., Loehrer, P. J., Williams, S. D., and Einhorn, L. H. (1986). Ifosfamide in refractory male germ cell. *J. Clin. Oncol.* **4:**28.

Williams, M. (1984). Ifosfamide in the treatment of advanced breast cancer. In: *Proceedings: Ifosfamide in Solid Tumors*. Croydon, U.K., Boehringer Ingelheim, p. 32.

Worrall, P. M. (1982). Single-dose ifosfamide: efficacy studies in non small cell lung cancer. *Semin. Oncol.* **9**(4)(suppl 1)**:**56–60.

24

Controversies in the Management of Non-Small-Cell Lung Cancer with Radiotherapy

ANDREW T. TURRISI, III

University of Michigan Medical Center
Ann Arbor, Michigan

I. Rationale for Combined-Modality Therapy

Modern concepts of the development of lung cancer are causing us to rethink our ideas about carcinogenesis. Instead of a simple isolated event leading to cancer, the process of oncogenesis may be multifactorial. In addition to the association of tobacco excess in the development of lung cancers, recent evidence from epidemiologic sources and the laboratory is showing lung cancer to be a genetic disease.

Tumors may be composed of heterogeneous populations of cells. Some cells may have intrinsic or acquired resistance since resistance to therapy, either chemotherapy or radiotherapy, may lead to persistence of tumor and ultimately the death of the patient. An interesting model of resistance can be drawn from small cell lung cancer. The prototype model of resistance to radiotherapy has been hypoxic cells. Based on difference in oxygen tension in tumors, biologists planned experiments with cells treated in oxygen, air, and hypoxic conditions. Hypoxic cells were relatively radioresistant. Subsequent to this, other models have been developed. Investigators used radiobiological techniques to test radiation responses in cell lines developed from human small cell lung cancers (Carney et al., 1983). These cell lines were developed both from primary tumors and from metastatic sites. They maintain their morphologic phenotype, but were also characterized by a variety of different parameters. The admixture of small cell lung cancer with large cell, now known as variant histology, has remarkably different radiobiological characteristics compared to small cell lung cancer of the classic types. The variant histology has a radiobiological shoulder. This shoulder region indicates early resistance; that is, one has to achieve a threshold dose accumulation before starting exponential cell kill. The variant histology has been associated with the c-myc oncogene (Little et al., 1983). Using normal rat embryo cell lines, McKenna and colleagues (1990) transfected the myc oncogene into this cell line. This created a broader shoulder than that in the wild-type cells. However, the slope of the exponential cell kill was not remarkably altered. When H-ras was transfected into the c-myc positive cells, resistance increased, manifest by alteration in the slope of the survival curve. These pieces of the puzzle suggest that molecular events, as well as oxygen tension, influence radiation resistance.

II. Radiotherapy for Lung Cancer

For years, radiation therapy has been used to treat patients with unresectable non-small-cell lung cancer. One year survival ranges between 8 and 12 months and 2-year survival ranges between 10 and 20%. The 5-year survival in all of these studies and in other studies is less than 10% (Katz and Alberts, 1983). The undisclosed selection criteria may be important. The radiotherapy technical variables may also exert influence. Some of these variables are course, dosage (both total and individual daily fraction), total time of therapy, and volume. In one fractionation technique, hyperfractionation, the dosage is less than or equal to 140 cGy per fraction. The interval between treatments ranges from 4 to 8 h to allow for intertreatment repair of radiation-induced damage. An alternative technique is to use dosages greater than or equal to 140 rad per fraction, twice a day, with 4–8 h between fractions, for 2–3 fractions per day. This strategy is referred to as *accelerated fractionation*, which gives two or more doses of radiation therapy a day. This twice a day strategy has a double purpose. First, for tumors without shoulders, this allows for exponential killing of the tumor, but it applies a lower dose of radiation to normal tissues. Second, tumors with rapid proliferative rates may be radiated initially during a period of relative radioresistance. After the interfraction interval, the cells cycle through to a more sensitive phase of the cell cycles.

Table 1 lists the variables by which we can compare and contrast most radiotherapy trials. For full discussion of survival, an excellent review of older trials is provided by Katz and colleagues (1983). In most trials, the median survival for patients with non-small-cell lung cancer ranges between 9 and 13 months. The 1-year survival is between 30 and 50%, 2-year survival about 10–15%, and the 5-year survival between 3 and 10%. Our understanding of radiation therapy and its

Table 1 Variables of Radiotherapy Trials

Volume
Margin of normal tissue for build-up and motion
Regional lymphatics
Dose
Total
Individual daily
Fractionation
Standard: 2 Gy ± 10%
Hyperfractionation: large individual daily dose, shorter course, shorter total dose
Hyperfractionation: doses between 100 and 140 cGy, 4–8 hr between doses, total time approximately constant
Accelerated fractionation: doses of 140–200 cGy, 4–8 hr between doses, total time foreshortened
Course
Split with planned breaks of 2–4 weeks
Continuous course with no interruptions (? weekends)

responses in normal tissue has expanded over the last few years. Since the early days of radiotherapy, it has been shown that multiple doses are better at controlling dividing tissues than larger, single doses. To achieve the identical effect (isoeffect), a multiple fraction scheme needs to provide a larger total dose than a single fraction dose. Because this repair occurs between fractions, this is commonly known as the repair of sublethal damage or "split-dose repair." Linear-quadratic formulations are now used to describe acute and late effects (Fowler, 1989). The alpha exponent describes the population of cells (either tumor or normal cells) destroyed by single-hit kinetics with no ability to repair. The quadratic portion causes the beta effect, which describes the amount of damage capable of being repaired. This expression acknowledges that most tumors and normal tissues are heterogeneous: composed of individual cells with different radiation sensitivities. Tissues with the predominance of alpha responding cells produce predominantly acute effects. Most tumors with a rapidly dividing population fall into this category. However, many normal tissues, such as hair follicles, oral and esophageal mucosa, and renewing stem cells of the hematopoietic system mainly have an alpha component. Radiotherapy trials or schedules limited by acute effects, for instance, those with split does or that have unlimited amounts of breaks due to the observed acute clinical effects, commonly allow for the regeneration of tumor cells and repopulation of cells that resisted the initial therapy. Tissues that have predominating beta effects may manifest very little acute responding difficulties, but may be limited by debilitating late effects. One of the pioneers of fractionation,

Regaud, aptly demonstrated this (Regaud and Nogier, 1911). When radiating rams' testes, a large single fraction caused scrotal necrosis at a delayed time point; the acute responding germinal cells, however, were not totally eliminated by this single large fraction. In human beings, the lethal late effects for single-dose 10 Gy total body irradiation are pronounced in the lungs, a late responding tissue, but that large single fraction may incompletely eliminate the rapidly proliferating tissues composing the tumor or normal bone marrow cells. Radiotherapists and radiobiologists for decades have described these by parallel sigmoid curves, which assume sharp and narrow ranges for the rapidly responding tissues. At the higher end of the dose scale, small increases in dosage may result in an increase in tumor control, but increasing the dosage causes a more pronounced increase in the complication rate. The variables expressed in Table 1 affect both tumor control and late normal tissue damage.

The RTOG study 73-01 compared four dosage levels of radiotherapy (Perez et al., 1980). The dose of 40 Gy was administered by two different fraction schedules. One was a split-course technique using 4 Gy fractions with 2 separate courses of 20 Gy, and then a fall off for 2–3 weeks. Another method of delivering 40 Gy was to use 2 Gy fractions continuously for 4 weeks. The other 2 arms use 50 and 60 Gy, respectively, both employing continuous techniques for 5 and 6 weeks, respectively. Many reports on this study have been published. Analysis has indicated that the larger dosages in smaller dosage per fraction provide more local control, more complete responses, and better survival at the 2- and 3-year endpoints, but identical survival at the 5-year endpoint. When one isolates the complete responders, of whom there are more in the higher-dosage, more protracted regimens, their survival rate is nearly 20% at 5 years. Although these data have been used to establish 60 Gy in 6 weeks as the standard regimen in the United States, this standard is not universal throughout the world. In the United States, the use of expanded field radiotherapy, covering the regional lymph nodes, including contralateral lymph nodes and supraclavicular lymph nodes, is commonplace. There are virtually no data indicating that this larger-volume technique produces better survival. The definition of local control is also somewhat arbitrary. In the RTOG study described above, the split-course and the lower dosage per fraction studies both produce local failures in the range of 55%. In the study using the 60 Gy dose, the RTOG reported local failure at a rate of only 40%. It is often difficult to score local control and local failure in cooperative trials because the sites of failure are generally more global, such as "lung," which includes contralateral lung perhaps better categorized as distant disease, even in the ipsilateral lung, which may reflect more bloodborne metastasis than a regional extension of disease. In a recent study of early stage lung cancer from the University of Pennsylvania, investigators found that tumor size was important in long-term local control but that even in tumors that are 3 cm or less and in which a dose of 60 Gy is used, the local control rate is only 50% (Sandler et al., 1990). A reasonable figure for local control with a dose of 60 Gy is 50%. Moreover, 60 Gy, with its ability to produce local control of only 50%, can hardly be expected to improve survival in a disease likely to have distant dissemination in all cell types. Distant dissemination cause death in the majority of cases.

The Mountain staging system was instituted in this country in 1986. Studies before that rarely classified patients into the IIIA and IIIB categories. The new staging system provided a rational basis for the increasing use of surgery for patients formerly treated with nonsurgical methods. This staging system has been adopted by the International Union Against Cancer (UICC) and the American Joint Commission for Cancer Staging. One of the most important features includes the acknowledgment that the T3 category included a vast range of tumor presentations. This system now separates out some of the more ominous ones. Tumors with direct invasion into critical structures that cannot be resected are now labeled T4 (i.e., invasion of a vertebral body or of any major mediastinal structure: esophagus, aorta, heart, or trachea). Nodal stations are now precisely mapped, and this system's generalized use has been put into action by the Lung Cancer Study Group (LCSG) (Weisenburger and Gail, 1986). This group has used a disciplined approach to dissecting the mediastinum and reported results of treatment interventions based on this careful assessment and pathologic staging of mediastinal and hilar lymph nodes. It is important to understand that surgical results are principally reported using pathologic assessment of lymph nodes whereas most, if not all, radiotherapy reports have been based on the clinical assessment of lymph nodes. Radiographic assessment of mediastinal lymph nodes is fraught with hazard; there are no adopted criteria that clearly and unequivocally identify positive or negative lymph nodes (Libshitz, 1990).

III. Postoperative Radiotherapy

Radiotherapy traditionally was applied to postoperative patients with positive lymph nodes or positive margins. Retrospective data supported the use of postoperative radiotherapy. However, these studies compared patients selected to receive postoperative radiotherapy with those who refused it, were denied it, or were too sick to receive it. The radiotherapy-treated groups commonly experienced superior survival irrespective of histologic type or nodal station. In randomized studies of patients with negative nodes, there was an excess mortality rate in patients treated with radiotherapy (Van Houtte et al., 1980). Recently, the LCSG reported a rigorous, uniform assessment of nodes in patients with squamous tumors in stage II and stage III (Weisenburger and Gail, 1986). The patients were randomized to receive postoperative 50 Gy radiotherapy or observation. There was a statistically significant improvement in local control among the treated patients. Only 1 patient failed in the chest, whereas more than 20 patients on the observation arm failed in the chest. In this study with roughly 80 patients on each arm, local control did not improve long-term survival. Despite the squamous histologic type required for entry, the majority of the patients died of distant disease. The 5-year survival, with positive lymph nodes completely dissected, ranged between 30 and 40%. Although some investigators were disappointed with radiotherapy's failure to improve survival, it is logical that a local form of therapy can improve local control but cannot improve survival in patients with occult distant metastatic disease. This study shows that patients with positive lymph nodes have a high frequency of occult distant metastatic disease that elude detection by the available clinical means. Even squamous tumors, once thought to be exclusively local problems, have a propensity for distant metastasis when their local disease is controlled. In the LCSG study it is not clear from the postoperative observations how patients who fail in the chest respond to radiotherapy. Undoubtedly, virtually none are long-term survivors or experience cure. Although some have taken this study to indicate that postoperative radiotherapy is not useful, it is quite clear that it reduces the frequency of local failure. Without data showing that salvage is possible for all failures, we continue to recommend postoperative radiotherapy whenever positive nodes are found. In a companion LCSG study of patients with residual nodes or adenocarcinoma with any node found to be positive, patients were randomized to receive chest radiotherapy as the control group or chest radiotherapy plus CAP (cyclophosphamide, Adriamycin [doxorubicin], platinum) chemotherapy. The overall survival for the squamous and adenocarcinoma groups was not influenced by the addition of the chemotherapy, but there was a modest prolongation of median survival and disease-free survival when chemotherapy was added. Investigators indicate that this is a "biological effect" of the chemotherapy (Lad et al., 1988).

IV. Preoperative Radiotherapy

In the preoperative radiotherapy reports of Bromley and Szur (1955) and of Bloedorn (1961), as well as the autopsy report by Rissanen et al. (1968), radiotherapy produces a pathologic response in patients brought to the operating room or autopsy suite in 30–50% of instances. In randomized prospective trials, this technique produced no benefit in survival (Shields, 1972; Warram, 1975).

V. Superior Sulcus Tumors

Preoperative therapy continues to be used, as in superior pulmonary sulcus tumors. A number of series have used preoperative radiotherapy (Table 2). Fewer studies are reporting the results of radiotherapy alone and these are also included in Table 3. Although the raw numbers appear to show better results, there is a

Table 2 Superior Pulmonary Sulcus Tumors: Preoperative Series

Institution	Patients	Dose	2 or 3 year survival (%)	5 year survival (%)
Baylor (Paulson et al., 1975, 1979)	107	30	34	32
Memorial (Hilaris et al., 1987)	82	20–40	~50	25
UCLA (Anderson et al., 1986)	55	30–45	—	34
Wilford Hall (Stanford et al., 1980)	53	—	$N_0$50% N_+15%	50
Florida (Devine et al., 1986)	40	30–50	20	10
Michigan (Kirsh et al., 1973)	35	50–60	—	0
Emory (Miller et al., 1978)	26	20–40	54	31
Mass. Gen. Hosp. (Wright et al., 1988)	21	30–45	55	27
Maryland (Attar et al., 1979)	19	55–60	23	—

selection bias for patients receiving surgery. In order to be included in these trials patients must be medically fit and have lesions that surgeons think they can excise. The radiotherapy-treated groups include all patients irrespective of their underlying medical conditions. Many practitioners advocate mediastinoscopy in patients with superior pulmonary sulcus, since patients with nodal or bony disease have poorer survival. Patients with affected lymph nodes, major bone invasion, phrenic nerve paralysis, or superior vena cava syndrome are commonly excluded from surgical consideration but are included in the radiotherapy group. Because of these selection biases, it is difficult to draw firm conclusions from these retrospective studies. Most believe that this tumor is too rare to permit national, multi-institutional trials comparing preoperative radiotherapy plus surgery with radiotherapy alone. Many physicians and some patients have biases against trials in which one arm involves surgery and the other does not.

Table 3 Superior Pulmonary Sulcus Tumors: Radiotherapy Alone

Institution	Patients	Dose	2 or 3 year survival (%)	5 year survival (%)
Michigan (Kirsh et al., 1973)	48	50–60	28	21
Med. Coll. Wisc. (Komacki et al., 1981)	36	40–64	32	28
Rochester (VanHoutte et al., 1984)	31	20–70	—	18
Florida (Devine et al., 1986)	7	61–70	29	29

VI. Intraoperative Techniques for Radiotherapy

Intraoperative radiotherapy sources (either "hot" or afterloaded) have not been commonly used. One institution, Memorial–Sloan Kettering, has used this technique extensively; however, they have never done so in a controlled fashion. The use of interstitial radiotherapy sources has the potential to add higher doses to the tumor without exceeding the tolerance of surrounding normal tissues. This could be done with the permanent implantation of iodine 125 seeds or by leaving catheters in place and afterloading them with strands of radioactive iridium 192 so that they can be removed. The Memorial Group reports a low complication rate and local control rates of roughly 50% when margins are positive and 90% when margins are negative. The further use and relative benefits of this technique, as well as intraoperative therapy of any kind, need further study (Hilaris and Martini, 1988).

VII. Chemotherapy Strategies

The use of chemotherapy and radiotherapy is now referred to as "neoadjuvant" or "protoadjuvant" chemotherapy. Up-front use of this method is appealing because the blood supplies of the tumors are uncompromised before use of local forms of therapy. The early use of chemotherapy also allows for ready access of the drugs to the primary tumor. This may render them less capable of metastasizing and, potentially, sensitize them to the effect of radiotherapy, which is to reduce the size of tumors. A noteworthy trial has recently been published (Dillman et al., 1990).

In this study, two doses of platinum were given on days 1 and 29, and 5 weekly doses of Velban prior to the use of 60 Gy radiotherapy. This was compared to a group of patients randomized to receive 60 Gy of radiotherapy. The neoadjuvant group survived a median of 13.8 months compared to a median of 9.7 months for the radiotherapy-alone group. The 2 year survival was roughly 26% in the neoadjuvant group and 13% in the radiotherapy-alone group. A report from the RTOG used multiple, twice-a-day fractions of 1.2 Gy, and escalated the dose to 69.6 Gy and then higher. The 69.6 Gy dose is highlighted because the higher doses had slightly higher complication rates. The median and 2 year survival rates were similar to the neoadjuvant arm of Dillman's CALGB study (Cox et al., 1990). As a consequence, the RTOG and Eastern Cooperative Oncology Group have joined together in a confirmatory trial comparing radiotherapy in 60 Gy in 6 weeks with 69.6 Gy using the hyperfractionated technique in comparison with the two cycles of platinum prior to 60 Gy radiotherapy.

Besides the up-front use of chemotherapeutic agents, the concurrent use of chemotherapy allows it to sensitize tumors. Schaake-Koning and co-workers (1990) reported a recent example from the EORTC. This trial used a split-course technique of 55 Gy in 8 weeks (30 Gy in ten 3 Gy fractions for the first 2 weeks, 4 weeks off, and then 25 Gy in 2 weeks in ten 2.5 Gy fractions). This schedule was compared to identical radiotherapy with weekly platinum (30 mg/m^2) as experimental arm 1 and daily platinum (6 mg/m^2) during the course of the radiotherapy as experimental arm 2. This report shows trends favoring the weekly and daily administration in causing response, reducing time to progression, and improving local control.

VIII. New Ideas Using Radiotherapy

Perhaps the most innovative use of radiotherapy comes from Mount Vernon Hospital in the United Kingdom, where Saunders and colleagues have reported using 1.5 Gy fractions every 8 hr for 12 consecutive days: total dose was 54 Gy in 12 days. This enables a large does of radiotherapy to be administered in a brief time. This eliminates the population of cells that proliferates during the course of radiotherapy. These active, evolving cells may make up for the clones evolving to resistance or to metastasis. A final report is not yet available but 60% 1 year survival rates are reported, with excellent local control. This accelerated method of radiotherapy gives a very intense course of treatment in a very short period of time.

The concept of three-dimensional treatment planning techniques may allow us to provide larger doses of radiotherapy without increasing their toxicity. They allow for more accurate targeting of tumor, but may require compromises in volumes or fields. These techniques allow separation of the "tumor control" and "complication curves" by increasing tumor doses but minimizing the normal tissue exposure. Inclusion of regional nodes has become commonplace. Since the irradiation of regional lymphatics *has not* improved long-term survival, it is not clear why this must be a part of radiotherapeutic management of non-small-cell lung cancer. In early stage lung cancer, some trials from Europe disregard prophylactic irradiation of lymph nodes. The survival reported is at least as good as those studies in the United States, in which mediastinal irradiation was routine (Noordijk et al., 1988). Exclusive sites of failure in regional lymph nodes are probably very uncommon. As in patients with breast cancer, nodal spread is likely to predict a higher frequency of systemic disease.

IX. Prophylactic Cranial Irradiation

The subject of prophylactic cranial irradiation is usually found in discussions of small cell lung cancer. However, in a review of Veterans Administration patients, it was found that those with adenocarcinoma and large cell carcinoma had brain relapse in approximately 50% of instances. In one report, this rate exceeded that found for small cell lung cancer (Cox and Yesner, 1979). Many have found isolated late brain relapses; these sometimes have been rather difficult to control. Unlike the treatment of small cell lung cancer, no generally accepted standard combination chemotherapeutic regimen produces a high frequency of complete responses. With neoadjuvant approaches used prior to surgery, some data now being collected show a 20–30% complete response rate when evaluated pathologically. Nevertheless, the frequency of isolated central nervous system failure is not common. Certainly fewer than 10% of patients have the central nervous system as the exclusive site of metastasis.

In the early 1980s, a series of reports identified major clinical and radiographic findings in patients subjected to prophylactic cranial irradiation. Many have suggested that long-term survival was infrequent and uniformly compromised by the use of the prophylactic cranial irradiation and the high frequency of adverse reactions. Even in patients with small cell lung cancer, the use of prophylactic cranial irradiation remains extraordinarily controversial. In non-small-cell cancer, some investigators began to incorporate brain irradiation along with systemic therapy (Umsawasdi et al., 1982; Skarin et al., 1989). The use of prophylactic cranial irradiation did seem to reduce the overt central nervous system failure. A recent SWOG trial randomized prophylactic cranial irradiation in patients on non-small-cell lung cancer studies. This trial is showing a slight detriment in survival in patients randomized to receive brain radiotherapy, but, again, a slight but definite reduction in the central nervous system failure pattern (Mira et al., 1990).

There are a number of continuing controversies in the radiotherapy of lung cancer: the different techniques; the volumes, doses, and courses of treatment to be applied for localized disease; and how best to integrate radiotherapy with chemotherapeutic strategies. Whether surgery for stage IIIA disease will provide superior results or not is yet to be proven; however, in an era with a new staging system and new imaging modalities, how things look may not be how things are. We must be very cautious in interpreting retrospective results and must carefully design prospective randomized trials. Lung cancer kills patients due to systemic disease. This is a firmly established fact and provides the rationale for the use of systemic therapy in this disease. However, we must be very careful in assessing the relative benefits and toxicities that systemic therapy provide for patients, and learn to integrate local and systemic modalities of therapy.

References

Anderson, T. M., May, P. M., and Holmes, E. C. (1986). Factors affecting survival in superior sulcus tumors. *J. Clin. Oncol.* **4:**1598–1603.

Attar, S., Miller, J. E., Satterfeld, J., Ho, C. K., Slawson, R. G., Hankins, J., and

McLaughlin, J. S. (1979). Pancoast's tumor: irradiation or surgery? *Ann. Thorac. Surg.* **28**(6)**:**578–586.

Bloedorn, F.G. (1961). Combined therapy: irradiation and surgery in the treatment of bronchogenic carcinoma. *Am. J. Roentgenol.* **85**(5)**:**875–885.

Bromley, L. L., and Szur, L. (1955). Combined radiotherapy and resection for carcinoma of the bronchus. Experiences with 66 patients. *Lancet* **11:**937–941.

Carney, D. N., Mitchel, J. B., and Kinsella, T. J. (1983). *In vitro* radiation and chemotherapy sensitivity of established cell lines of human small cell lung cancer and its large cell morphological variants. *Cancer Res.* **43:**2806–2811.

Cox, J. D., and Yesner, R. A. (1979). Adenocarcinoma of the lung: recent results from the Veterans Administration Lung Groups. *Am. Rev. Respir. Dis.* **120:**1025–1029.

Cox, J. D., Azarnia, N., Byhardt, R. W., Shin, K. H., Emami, B., and Pajak, T. F. (1990). A randomized phase I/II trial of hyperfractionated radiation therapy with total doses of 60.0 Gy to 79.2 Gy: possible survival benefit with $\geqslant$ 69.6 Gy in favorable patients with radiation therapy oncology group stage III non-small cell lung carcinoma: report of Radiation Therapy Oncology Group 83-11. *J. Clin. Oncol.* **8:**1543–1555.

Devine, J. W., Mendenhall, W. M., Million, R. R., and Carmichael, M. J. (1986). Carcinoma of the superior pulmonary sulcus treated with surgery and/or radiation therapy. *Cancer* **57:**941–943.

Dillman, R. O., Seagren, S. L., Propert, K. J., Guerra, J., Eaton, W. L., Perry, M. C., Carrey, R. W., and Frei, E. F. (1990). A randomized trial of induction chemotherapy plus high-dose radiation versus radiation alone in stage III non-small-cell lung cancer. *N. Engl. J. Med.* **323:**940–945.

Fowler, J. F. (1989). The linear–quadratic formula and progress in fractionated radiotherapy. *Br. J. Radiol.* **62:**679–694.

Hilaris, B. S., Martini, N., Wong, G. Y., and Nori, D. (1987). Treatment of superior sulcus tumor (Pancoast tumor). *Surg. Clin. North Am.* **67**(5)**:**965–977.

Hilaris, B. S., and Martini, N. (1988). The current state of intraoperative interstitial brachytherapy in lung cancer. *Int. J. Radiat. Oncol. Biol. Phys.* **15:**1347–1354.

Katz, H. R., and Alberts, R. W. (1983). A comparison of high-dose continuous and split-course irradiation in non-oat-cell carcinoma of the lung. *Am. J. Clin. Oncol.* **6:** 445–457.

Kirsh, M. M., Dickerman, R., Fayos, J., Lampe, I., Pellegrini, R. V., Gago, O., and Sloan, H. (1973). The value of chest wall resection in the treatment of superior sulcus tumors of the lung. *Ann. Thorac. Surg.* **15**(4)**:**339–346.

Komaki, R., Roh, J., Cox, J. D., and da Conceicao, A. L. (1981). Superior sulcus tumors: results of irradiation of 36 patients. *Cancer* **48:**1563–1568.

Lad, T., Rubinstein, L., and Sadeghi, A., of the Lung Cancer Study Group (1988). The benefit of adjuvant treatment for resected locally advanced non-small cell lung cancer. *J. Clin. Oncol.* **6:**9–17.

Libshitz, H. E. (1990). Computed tomography in bronchogenic carcinoma. *Semin. Roentgenol.* **25**(1)**:**64–72.

Little, C. D., Nau, M. M., Carney, D. N., Gazdar, A. F., and Minna, J. D. (1983). Amplification and expression of the v-myc oncogene in human lung cancer cell lines. *Nature* **306:**194–196.

McKenna, W. G., Weiss, M. C., Endlich, B., et al. (1990). Synergistic effect of the c-myc oncogene with H-ras on radioresistance. *Cancer Res.* **50:**97–102.

Miller, J. I., Mansour, K. A., and Hatche, C. R. (1978). Carcinoma of the superior pulmonary sulcus. *Ann. Thorac. Surg.* **28**(1)**:**44–46.

Mira, J. G., Miller, T. P., and Crowley, J. J. (1990). Chest irradiation (RT) vs chest RT and chemotherapy ± prophylactic brain RT in localized non-small cell lung cancer: a Southwest Oncology Group randomized study. *Int. J. Radiat. Oncol. Biol. Phys.* **19** (suppl 1)**:**145.

Mountain, C. F. (1986). A new international staging system for lung cancer. *Chest* **4:**225S–233S.

Noordijk, E. M., v.d. Poest Clement, E., Hermans, J., Wever, A. M. J., and Leer, J. W. H. (1988). Radiotherapy as an alternative to surgery in elderly patients with resectable lung cancer. *Radiother. Oncol.* **13:**83–89.

Paulson, D. C. (1979). Carcinoma in the superior pulmonary sulcus. *Ann. Thorac. Surg.* **28:**3–4.

Paulson, D. C. (1975). Carcinomas in the superior pulmonary sulcus. *J. Thorac. Cardiovasc. Surg.* **70:**1095–1104.

Perez, C. A., Stanley, K., Rubin, P., Kramer, S., Brady, L., Perez-Tamayo, R., Brown, G. S., Concannon, J., Rotman, M., and Seydel, H. G. (1980). A prospective randomized study of various irradiation doses and fractionation schedules in the treatment of inoperable non-oat-cell carcinoma of the lung. *Cancer* **45:**2744–2753.

Regaud, C., and Nogier, T. (1911). Sterilization roentgenienne totale et definitive, sans radiodermite, des testiculées du Belier adulte; conditions de sa réalisation. *C. R. Soc. Biol.* **70:**202–203.

Rissanen, P. M., Tikka, U., and Holsti, L. R. (1968). Autopsy findings in lung cancer treated with megavoltage radiotherapy. *Acta Radiol.* **7:**433–442.

Sandler, H. M., Curran, W., and Turrisi, A. T. (1990). The influence of tumor size and pretreatment staging on outcome following radiation therapy alone for Stage I non-small cell lung cancer. *Int. J. Radiat. Oncol. Biol. Phys.* **19:**9–13.

Saunders, M. I., Dische, S. (1990). Continuous, hyperfractionated, accelerated radiotherapy (CHART) in non-small cell carcinoma of the bronchus. *Int. J. Radiat. Oncol. Biol. Phys.* **19:**1211–1215.

Schaake-Koning, M. B., Van Houtte, P., Van den Bogaert, W., Dalesio, O., Kirkpatrick, A., and Bartelink, H. (1990). Radiotherapy combined with low-dose cis-diammine dichloroplatinum (II) (CDDP) in inoperable nonmetastatic non-small cell lung cancer (NSCLC): a randomized three arm phase II study of the EORTC lung cancer and radiotherapy cooperative groups. *Int. J. Radiat. Oncol. Biol. Phys.* **19:**967–972.

Shields, T. W. (1972). Preoperative radiation therapy in the treatment of bronchial carcinoma. *Cancer* **30:**1388–93.

Skarin, A., Jochelson, M., Sheldon, T., et al. (1989). Neoadjuvant chemotherapy in marginally resectable stage III M_0 non-small cell lung cancer: long term follow-up in 41 patients. *J. Surg. Oncol.* **40:**266–274.

Stanford, W., Barnes, R. P., and Tucker, A. R. (1980). Influence of staging in superior sulcus (pancoast) tumors of the lung. *Ann. Surg.* **29:**406–409.

Umsawasdi, T., Barkley, H. T., Booser, D. J., et al. (1982). Role of prophylactic brain irradiation (PBI) during combined chemoradiotherapy (CCRT) for inoperable adeno and squamous cell lung cancer (ASCLC). *Proc. ASCO*, 148.

Van Houtte, P., Rocmans, P., Smets, P., Goffin, J. C., Lustman-marechal, J., Vanderhoeft, and Henry, J. (1980). Postoperative radiation therapy in lung cancer: a controlled trial after resection of curative design. *Int. J. Radiat. Oncol. Biol. Phys.* **6:**983–986.

Van Houtte, P., MacLennan, I., Poulter, C., and Rubin, P. (1984). External radiation in the management of superior sulcus tumor. *Cancer* **54:**223–227.

Warram, J. (1975). Preoperative irradiation of cancer of the lung: final report of a therapeutic trial. A collaborative study. *Cancer* **36:**914–925.

Weisenburger, T. H., and Gail, M. (1986). The Lung Cancer Study Group: effects of postoperative mediastinal radiation on completely resected stage II and stage III epidermoid cancer of the lung. *N. Engl. J. Med.* **315**(22):1377–1381.

Wright, C. D., Monscure, A. C., Shepard, J. A. O., Wilkins, E. W., Mathiesen, D. J., and Grillo, H. C. (1988). Superior sulcus lung tumors. *J. Thorac. Cardiovasc. Surg.* **94:** 69–74.

25

Investigational Therapies in Disseminated Non-Small-Cell Lung Cancer

PAUL J. HESKETH

Boston University Medical Center
Boston, Massachusetts

Lung cancer is the single most common cause of cancer death in the United States in men and women, with 145,000 projected deaths in 1991 (Boring et al., 1991). Non-small-cell lung cancer (NSCLC), consisting of the histologic subtypes adenocarcinoma, large cell undifferentiated carcinoma, and squamous cell carcinoma, makes up 75–80% of all cases (Minna et al., 1989). Surgical resection is the only treatment modality with a reasonable chance of imparting cure when applied to appropriately selected patients. Only approximately 40% of patients have resectable disease at presentation, and only one-quarter of these (10–12% overall) are alive at 5 years and apparently cured of their disease (Miller, 1990).

Therefore, the great majority of patients with NSCLC have disseminated disease and require systemic treatment. Conventional systemic therapies in NSCLC are quite limited. Unlike small cell lung cancer, which initially is responsive to chemotherapy in most patients, NSCLC has proven to be much more resistant. Efforts are underway to optimize current chemotherapy approaches and to discover new agents. Attempts to translate recent insights into the biology of lung cancer into therapeutic options such as the biological response modifiers, monoclonal antibodies, and growth factor–toxin conjugates hold the promise for significant progress in the future. This chapter will review a number of promising investigational treatment strategies for NSCLC.

I. Conventional Chemotherapy

Only a handful of the more than four dozen drugs tested have demonstrated significant single-agent activity, defined as overall response rates of greater than 15%, in advanced NSCLC (Kris et al., 1985). These include cisplatin, mitomycin, vindesine, and ifosfamide (Table 1). Nearly all responses have been partial, of short duration, and have not clearly imparted any survival benefit.

There have been many attempts to improve upon the modest success achieved with single agents by the use of various combinations of the most active drugs. The response rates achieved with the best combinations are fairly consistently superior to those obtained with single agents. Over the past decade, the majority of the most active combinations have been cisplatin based (Table 2). Despite the higher response rates seen with the combinations, median survival consistently ranges between 5 to 9 months and it remains unclear whether such combinations confer any survival benefit.

A number of trials have been conducted attempting to assess the impact of chemotherapy on overall survival. Only two of these have enrolled reasonably large numbers of patients and employed modern cisplatin-based chemotherapy regimens (Table 3). These include one trial conducted in the United Kingdom and Australia (Woods et al., 1990) and another run by the National Cancer Institute of Canada (Rapp et al., 1988). Two hundred and one patients with stage IIIB or IV disease were entered into the British-Australian study. Patients were randomized to receive chemotherapy with cisplatin and vindesine or best supportive care alone without chemotherapy. Both groups could receive radiotherapy or other palliative therapies as required. Patients on the chemotherapy arm had a longer median survival than those receiving best supportive care, but this difference was not statistically significant. Patients with stage IIIB disease, treated with chemotherapy, fared the best with a survival difference approaching significance. Unfortunately, no attempt was made to measure quality of life in this study.

In the Canadian trial, 251 patients with stage IIIB or IV disease were

Table 1 Active Chemotherapy Agents in NSCLC[a]

Agent	Patients, no.	Significant response, %
Cisplatin	126	24
Ifosfamide	196	20
Mitomycin	115	18
Vindesine	449	18

[a]Significant response rate >15% in phase II trials totaling >100 patients (Kris et al., 1985).

Table 2 Cisplatin-Based Chemotherapy Regimens in Disseminated NSCLC

Regimen	Patients, no.	Significant response, %	Reference
PVd	636	32	Bunn, 1989
CAP	443	28	Bunn, 1988
EP	974	30	Bunn, 1989
MVP	604	51	Bunn, 1989

P, cisplatin; Vd, vindesine; C, cyclophosphamide; A, doxorubicin; E, etoposide; M, mitomycin; V, vinblastine or vindesine

entered. Patients were randomized to receive either cyclophosphamide, doxorubicin, and cisplatin (CAP), or vindesine and cisplatin (VP), or best supportive care alone. Despite very modest objective response rates of 15.3% with CAP, and 25.3% with VP, survival benefits were seen with chemotherapy in both active treatment arms. Treatment with VP resulted in the largest survival difference compared with best supportive care. This translated into a 4 month median survival prolongation. Poor compliance with planned quality of life measures prevented any conclusions from being drawn about this issue. A cost–benefit analysis was carried out, however, and it was of interest that chemotherapy was found to be reasonably cost-effective compared with best supportive care (Jaakkimainen et al., 1990).

A review of the results of these last two randomized trials gives us a reasonable overview of the status of conventional chemotherapy in patients with advanced NSCLC. Despite some clear progress, the overall impact of chemotherapy remains limited. At best it confers a modest survival benefit and was, at

Table 3 Chemotherapy vs. Supportive Care Only in Advanced NSCLC

Trial location[a]	Regimens	Response, %	Median survival, weeks	
UK/Australia	PV	28	27	p = 0.33
	BSC	—	17	
NCI-Canada	CAP	15	25	p = 0.05
	VP	25	33	p = 0.01
	BSC	—	17	

[a]UK/Australia (Woods et al., 1990); NCI-Canada (Rapp et al., 1988).
P, cisplatin; V, vindesine; C, cyclophosphamide; A, doxorubicin; BSC, best supportive care.

least in one large randomized study, cost-effective compared with supportive care alone. The impact of chemotherapy on quality of life in patients with disseminated NSCLC remains completely undefined. Thus there is considerable room for improvement in the treatment of disseminated NSCLC. New approaches are needed.

II. Investigational Approaches to Disseminated NSCLC

In seeking ways to improve therapeutic outcome in disseminated NSCLC, a number of potential directions can be envisioned, including optimizing the use of conventional agents, discovering new active drugs, or exploring fundamentally different approaches (Table 4).

A. Optimizing the Use of Conventional Agents

Two possible means to improve the activity of conventional therapies include chemotherapy dosage intensification and the use of pharmacologic modulators.

1. Dosage Intensification

To date, most efforts to explore chemotherapy dosage intensification in lung cancer have been conducted with small cell lung cancer, an intrinsically more chemosensitive disease, in which the results of such approaches have been mixed (Souhami et al., 1983, 1985; Cohen et al., 1977; O'Donnell et al., 1985; Figueredo et al., 1985; Hande et al., 1982). There is a relative paucity of such data in NSCLC. Systematic studies investigating a potential dose–response effect for the active single agents in NSCLC are, for the most part, nonexistent.

Cisplatin is arguably the single most active agent in NSCLC. A review of prior single-agent cisplatin trials in NSCLC, in which a minimum of 20 evaluable patients have been included, suggests a positive dose–response relationship (Britell et al., 1978; Pannettiere et al., 1983; Bhuchar and Lanzotti, 1982; Vogl et al., 1982; Dejager et al., 1980; Gandara et al., 1989) (Table 5). With the exception of the study by Bhuchar and Lanzotti, a consistent trend towards

Table 4 Investigational Therapies in Disseminated NSCLC

Optimizing use of conventional agents
New agents
Novel approaches

Table 5 Single-Agent Cisplatin in NSCLC

Planned dosage intensity, mg/m^2/week	Patients, no	Response, %	Reference
18.75	22	9	Britell et al., 1978
25	145	13	Panettiere et al., 1983
25–35	24	0	Bhuchar and Lanzotti, 1982
37.5	30	33	Vogl et al., 1982
40	61	26	DeJager et al., 1980
50	76	36	Gandara et al., 1989

improved response is noted as planned dosage intensity increased from 18–25 mg/m^2/week to 37.5–50 mg/m^2/week.

Studies attempting to define the importance of cisplatin dosage when used in combination regimens have had mixed results. Gralla and co-workers (1981) compared vindesine plus low-dosage cisplatin (60 mg/m^2) with vindesine plus high-dosage cisplatin (120 mg/m^2) in a randomized trial of patients with NSCLC. Median duration of response and survival were significantly better on the higher-dosage cisplatin arm. Klastersky and colleagues (1986), however, were unable to find any difference when cisplatin dosage was increased from 60 to 120 mg/m^2 in patients with disseminated NSCLC treated with a cisplatin–etoposide combination.

A major limiting factor with dosage-intensive cisplatin regimens, particularly those at a dosage of 150–200 mg/m^2, is toxicity. The use of hypertonic saline and aggressive hydration has limited renal toxicity, but neurologic and hematologic toxicity remains considerable. Gandara and co-workers (1989) employed a novel administration schedule in an attempt to lessen such toxicity. They administered cisplatin at a dosage of 100 mg/m^2 on day 1 and day 8 of a 28 day treatment cycle to 92 patients with stage IIIB and stage IV NSCLC. The response rate among the 76 evaluable patients was 36%, including 6 complete responses. Minimal myelosuppression was encountered, although peripheral neuropathy was still dosage limiting. The Southwest Oncology Group has conducted a subsequent randomized trial that attempted to determine whether cisplatin administered in this dosage and schedule is superior to the conventional-dosage (50 mg/m^2 day 1 and day 8) cisplatin. Accrual is now completed and the results of this very important trial are eagerly awaited.

Attempts to escalate chemotherapy dose more substantially in NSCLC have been limited by bone marrow toxicity. Two potential means to lessen this problem include the use of autologous bone marrow support and/or recombinant hematopoietic growth factors. Despite preclinical evidence of steep dose–response curves and occasional non-cross-resistance with a number of alkylating agents, the results with high-dosage chemotherapy combined with autologous bone marrow transplantation (ABMT) have been disappointing (Williams et al., 1989; Lazarus et al., 1990). Response rates of approximately 50% can be achieved with this approach in patients with NSCLC refractory to conventional chemotherapy. Response durations have averaged 3 months, and nonhematologic toxicity has been severe.

The recent availability of recombinant hematopoietic growth factors offers a potentially less cumbersome means of chemotherapy dosage intensification. A major problem with this approach, as with ABMT, is that nonhematologic toxicities quickly become dosage limiting. No substantive data are currently available on this approach in NSCLC, although a number of trials combining hematopoietic growth factors with chemotherapy are currently underway.

2. Pharmacologic Modulation

Modulating the activity of chemotherapy agents by the use of additional agents with no intrinsic antineoplastic activity (pharmacologic modulation) is an area of intense interest. The best example of a significant clinical advance evolving from such an approach is the modulation of 5-fluorouracil's (5-FU) activity by leucovorin in the treatment of colon cancer. The combination of 5-FU and leucovorin has been shown to be superior to 5-FU alone with respect to response and survival in a number of trials (Erlichman et al., 1988; Petrelli et al., 1989; Poon et al., 1989).

Most of the current interest in pharmacologic modulation in the treatment of cancer relates to attempts to overcome chemotherapy drug resistance, or, to a lesser extent, protect normal host tissues from chemotherapy-induced toxicity. Specific mechanisms of resistance to individual chemotherapy agents, such as that seen with amplified dihydrofolate reductase gene expression in methotrexate-resistant tumor cells, have been described (Curt et al., 1983; Trent et al., 1984). A more significant problem often seen in lung cancer treatment is multidrug resistance: neoplastic cells become resistant to multiple cytotoxic agents including agents, to which the tumor cells have not yet been exposed. Unlike small cell lung cancer, in which resistance is usually acquired, most NSCLC tumors are intrinsically resistant to a host of agents. One of the best characterized forms of multidrug resistance occurs with the overexpression of a 170,000 dalton membrane protein (P-glycoprotein) encoded by the MDR1 gene (Ling and Thompson, 1974; Fojo et al., 1985; Pastan and Gottesman, 1987). The P-glycoprotein is able to facilitate the removal of many cytotoxic drugs from the tumor cell through its capacity to act as an energy-dependent efflux pump (Ling et al., 1988). The MDR1 gene is expressed in a number of different normal tissues as well as a variety of neoplastic cells (Fojo et al., 1987; Goldstein et al., 1989; Salmon et al., 1989; Kartner and Ling, 1989). Agents that block the function of the P-glycoprotein, such as verapamil, have been used successfully in several clinical situations to enhance neoplastic cell sensitivity to chemotherapy (Dalton et al., 1989; Miller et al., 1991).

It appears unlikely that MDR1 plays any significant role in resistance to chemotherapy in NSCLC. Lai and co-workers (1989) noted that almost all nontumorous lung tissues, lung cancer tumors, and cell lines expressed low levels of MDR1 RNA. Mechanisms of resistance other than MDR1 overexpression appear to be operative in most patients with NSCLC. A primary focus of a number of investigators is defining the mechanisms associated with resistance to alkylating agents (AA), including platinum compounds (Table 6). These are more likely to be relevant to NSCLC and may offer targets for modulation of chemotherapy activity. A number of mechanisms have been described in association with resistance to alkylating agents. These include decreased intracellular accumulation (Teicher et al., 1986; Bungo et al., 1990; Bernal et al., 1990), enhanced inactivation by intracellular detoxification systems (Kelley et al., 1988; Carmichael et al., 1988), the adverse effect of neoplastic cell hypoxia upon AA effect (Mulcahy, 1988), and altered DNA repair (Masuda et al., 1988).

The glutathione (GSH)/glutathione transferase system (GST) is an intracellular detoxification system that has evolved as a means of inactivating free radicals. Elevated levels of GSH have been noted in a number of AA-resistant neoplastic cell lines, including some NSCLC lines (Ozols et al., 1988; Carmichael et al., 1988). A reduction in cellular levels of GSH can be achieved with buthionine sulfoximine (BSO), an irreversible inhibitor of g-glutamylcysteine synthetase, an enzyme required for GSH biosynthesis. Addition of BSO to AA-resistant cell lines has been associated with substantial reversal of drug resistance (Green et al., 1984; Ozols et al., 1987). Early clinical trials are now underway using BSO in combination with alkylating agents in drug-resistant ovarian cancer.

Elevated glutathione transferase levels have been noted in a number of AA-resistant tumor cell lines (Teicher et al., 1987; Bedford et al., 1987). Many structurally unrelated compounds are effective inhibitors of GST activity (Mannervik and Danielson, 1988). Of particular interest are the diuretic ethacrynic acid and the prostaglandin I1 analog piriprost. Enhanced neoplastic killing can be achieved with the addition of nontoxic doses of these two compounds to chlorambucil in certain neoplastic cell lines (Tew et al., 1988).

Table 6 Resistance to Alkylating Agents: Potential Targets for Pharmacologic Modulation

Mechanism of resistance	Potential intervention
Increased intracellular levels of glutathione	Buthionine sulfoximine (BSO)
Increased intracellular levels of glutathione transferase	Ethycrinic acid Prostaglandins
Neoplastic cell hypoxia	Nitroimidazoles
Enhanced DNA repair	Aphidicolin

Another approach to pharmacologic modulation involves attempts to exploit the oxygenation differences between tumors and normal tissues. In the presence of hypoxic neoplastic cells, the nitroimidazole compounds can selectively potentiate the antineoplastic effect of certain bifunctional alkylating agents (Mulcahy, 1988; Coleman et al., 1988a). A number of clinical trials have been carried out testing this approach (Mulcahy and Trump, 1988). With a single exception (Coleman et al., 1988b), all of these trials have failed to show a substantial benefit for the addition of a nitroimidazole sensitizer. Most of these studies were not optimally designed, however, and therefore may not constitute an adequate test of this concept. In the one positive trial reported to date, Coleman and colleagues (1988b) treated 100 patients with NSCLC with melphalan alone or combined with oral misonidazole. A significantly higher response rate was noted with the combination treatment.

Increased DNA repair activity has been noted in some AA-resistant cell lines (Masuda et al., 1988). This constitutes another potential target for therapeutic intervention. Aphidicolin, an inhibitor of the DNA polymerases alpha and beta, decreases DNA repair activity and can partially restore the sensitivity of cisplatin-resistant cell lines to this agent (Masuda et al., 1988). A related compound, aphidicolin succinate, is now in clinical trials in Europe as an antineoplastic agent. Adding this agent to conventional cytotoxics might be a useful approach in patients with refractory malignancies.

It is unlikely, given the multifactorial nature of resistance to cytotoxic agents, that any interventional strategy simply targeting one potential mechanism of resistance will have substantial benefit. Instead, combinations of modulators are more likely to be successful. Given the relative lack of toxicities of these agents, this may be a viable therapeutic approach as the mechanisms of drug resistance are better elucidated.

B. New Chemotherapy Agents in NSCLC

Given the limited number of agents with significant activity in NSCLC, another logical direction for investigative efforts is in new drug discovery. A number of agents have demonstrated promising activity in early phase II clinical trials, and warrant further evaluation (Table 7).

1. Antifolates

A number of new antifolates are currently undergoing clinical evaluation. These include the lipophilic antifolate trimetrexate and the water-soluble analog of methotrexate, edatrexate. Two phase II trials assessing the single-agent activity of trimetrexate in NSCLC have noted mixed results (Kris et al., 1989a; Maroun, 1988). The larger of the two studies was a multi-institutional trial that noted a response rate of 19% in 70 chemotherapy-naive patients with advanced NSCLC

Table 7 New Chemotherapy Agents in NSCLC

Agent	Evaluable patients, no.	Response, %	Reference
Edatrexate	19	32	Shum et al., 1988
Teniposide (VM-26)	34	21	Giaccone, 1988
Vinorelbine	69	33	Depierre et al., 1989
CPT-11	22	41	Fukuoka et al., 1990

(Maroun, 1988). A smaller trial conducted at Memorial–Sloan Kettering Cancer Center (MSKCC) showed no activity in 14 patients (Kris et al., 1989a). The dosage-limiting toxicity with this compound was myelosuppression.

Another antifolate that appears to have a more promising future is edatrexate. In a small phase II trial conducted at MSKCC, edatrexate demonstrated both a very encouraging response rate (32%) and duration of response (13 months) (Shum et al., 1988). Unlike with trimetrexate, myelosuppression was infrequent, with mucositis being the dosage-limiting toxicity. Recently, the Memorial group has reported the preliminary results of a dosage-escalating trial in an attempt to determine the optimal dosage of edatrexate when combined with mitomycin C and vinblastine (Kris et al., 1989b). The overall major response rate was 60% in 30 evaluable patients. The regimen was well tolerated with a moderate degree of myelosuppression.

2. *Teniposide*

Teniposide (VM-26) is a podophyllotoxin derivative that has been evaluated in a number of neoplastic diseases. In small cell lung cancer it appears to be a very active agent, with an overall response rate of 90% in one phase II trial (Bork et al., 1986). Giaccone (1988) treated 48 patients with advanced NSCLC with VM-26 in a phase II dosage-ranging trial. A response rate of 21% was noted in the 34 chemotherapy-naive patients. The European Organization for Research and Treatment of Cancer (EORTC) has initiated a trial comparing single agent VM-26 with a combination of VM-26 and cisplatin.

3. *Vinorelbine*

Vinorelbine is the first of a group of semisynthetic vinca alkaloids chosen for clinical trials. Preclinical evaluation demonstrated activity for vinorelbine against a variety of human NSCLC xenografts in nude mice (Cros et al., 1989). In a large phase II study conducted in France, Depierre and colleagues (1989) administered 30 mg/m^2 of vinorelbine intravenously on a weekly basis to 78 patients with advanced NSCLC. In the 69 evaluable patients, 23 (33.3%) achieved an objective response, with a median response duration of 34 weeks. Leukopenia was dosage-limiting, although significant thrombocytopenia was not encountered. This agent appears to be less neurotoxic than the other vinca alkaloids vincristine and vindesine.

4. CPT-11

Another plant alkaloid derivative, CPT-11, is currently undergoing evaluation. This agent is derived from the plant alkaloid camtothecin. It appears to exert its antineoplastic effect by inhibiting the DNA repair enzyme topoisomerase I. The results of a phase II trial with this agent in patients with previously untreated NSCLC were recently reported by Fukuoka and co-workers (1990). They used CPT-11 at a dosage of 100 mg/m^2 administered as a 90 minute intravenous (iv) infusion on a weekly basis. Nine of the 22 evaluable patients (40.9%) achieved a partial response. The most frequent toxicities were leukopenia, nausea/vomiting, diarrhea, and alopecia.

C. Novel Therapeutic Approaches

All of the therapeutic options discussed to this point have focused in some way on chemotherapy as the primary component. It would appear from the significant number of studies done to date that with the possible exception of efforts to overcome resistance to chemotherapy with modulating agents, significant progress will likely require fundamentally different approaches. Examples of such new approaches include the use of biological response modifiers alone or combined with cytotoxic chemotherapy, monoclonal antibodies, and growth factor–toxin conjugates (Table 8).

1. Biological Response Modifiers

Despite the theoretical promise of the biological response modifiers, they have had minimal impact to date in NSCLC. The adoptive immunotherapy approach utilizing lymphokine-activated killer (LAK) cells and systemic interleukin 2 (IL-2) has been ineffective in NSCLC (Rosenberg et al., 1985, 1987; West et al.,

Table 8 Novel Therapeutic Approaches in NSCLC

Biological response modifiers ± chemotherapy
Monoclonal antibodies
Growth factor–toxin conjugates

1987; Kradin et al., 1987). Despite the limited number of studies conducted to date, it would appear unlikely that any biological employed alone will have significant activity. Instead, the use of combinations of biologicals or biologicals combined with other modalities appears to be a potentially more fruitful approach. In this regard, Yang and colleagues (1990) have conducted a preliminary study combining low-dosage IL-2 with tumor necrosis factor in 16 patients with advanced NSCLC. Neither agent in the dosages employed had demonstrated any clinical activity in lung cancer previously. One partial and 3 minor responses were seen in the 12 evaluable patients. This regimen was reasonably well tolerated, with thrombocytopenia being the dosage-limiting toxicity.

Interferons administered alone have been completely ineffective in inducing tumor regression in NSCLC (Gruneberg et al., 1985; Olesen et al., 1987; Schiller et al., 1989). Recently, however, there has been growing interest in a possible role for the interferons in combination with cytotoxic chemotherapy (Wadler and Schwartz, 1990). Of particular interest has been the combination of interferon-α and fluorouracil. Encouraging results with this combination have been noted in the treatment of patients with colorectal cancer (Wadler et al., 1989). Although there is considerable speculation, the precise mechanisms of action and optimal dosing and sequencing of interferon when combined with chemotherapy are unclear.

One combination that may be relevant for NSCLC is the addition of cisplatin to interferon-α. A number of observations suggest that this combination might be worthy of further investigation. Carmichael and co-workers (1986) noted a considerable augmentation of cisplatin's activity when it was combined with interferon-α in human NSCLC xenografts. Smyth and colleagues (1988) extending upon these observations noted a 23% response rate with the combination of cisplatin and interferon-α in a small phase II trial of patients with advanced NSCLC. Recently, Rosso and co-workers (1990) reported the preliminary results of an Italian trial in which the combination of cisplatin, cyclophosphamide, and doxorubicin was administered alone or in combination with interferon-α in 179 patients with NSCLC. The rate of tumor regression in the combination arm was twice that achieved with chemotherapy alone.

2. *Monoclonal Antibodies*

The use of monoclonal antibodies (Mabs) directed against tumor-associated antigens is another possible means of designing therapeutic strategies for NSCLC. Several groups have used radiolabeled Mabs and demonstrated uptake at sites of neoplastic disease in NSCLC (Chan et al., 1986; Perkins et al., 1986; Kalofonos et al., 1988; Divgi et al., 1991). Divgi and colleagues, utilizing an indium-111-labeled monoclonal antibody raised against the epidermal growth factor (EGF) receptor in patients with squamous cell carcinoma of the lung, demonstrated imaging of presumed metastases 1 cm or greater in diameter with Mab doses of 40 mg or more. Even with Mab doses up to 300 mg, no appreciable toxicity was noted in this study.

Most monoclonal antibodies to tumor-associated determinants have little or no intrinsic activity against tumors by themselves and therefore must be used in combination with other agents such as radioisotopes, toxins, and chemotherapy agents (monoclonal antibody conjugates). Only a handful of very preliminary trials have attempted such an approach in NSCLC to date (Goodman et al., 1990; Elias et al., 1990).

A number of potential obstacles limit the application of Mab therapy, including lack of specificity, very low antibody uptake in tumor (usually in the range of 0.01–0.001% of the injected dose/g tumor), and the host immune response to the nonhuman proteins employed (Goldenberg, 1991). The use of human antibodies should help with the latter problem (James, 1990).

Another fundamentally different approach to the development of targeted cytotoxins has recently been introduced. Recombinant DNA technology has been used as a means of conjugating potent bacterial toxins (diphtheria toxin, *Pseudomonas* exotoxin A) to a variety of cellular growth factors (Murphy, 1988; Chaudhary et al., 1987, 1988; Lorberboum-Galski et al., 1988; Siegall et al., 1988). Using this approach, Murphy (1988) has constructed fusion genes in which the receptor-binding domain of diphtheria toxin has been deleted and replaced with DNAs encoding for growth factors such as α-melanocyte-stimulating hormone (MSH) and IL-2. The fusion protein formed by these fusion genes will bind to specific growth factor receptors on the target cell of interest. The fusion protein is then internalized by receptor-mediated endocytosis, with subsequent inhibition of protein synthesis by ADP-ribosylation, ultimately resulting in cell death (Williams et al., 1990).

Early clinical trials are underway using the fusion protein IL-2–diphtheria toxin in the treatment of hematologic malignancies in which high-affinity IL-2 receptor expression has been identified (Hesketh et al., 1990; Lemaistre et al., 1990). To date, this approach has been generally well tolerated and evidence of antineoplastic efficacy has been noted. It is unclear at present whether a role for growth factor–toxin conjugates will be defined in NSCLC. It is clear, however, that receptors for a number of autocrine growth factors such as transforming growth factor (TGF)-α (Imanishi et al., 1988), insulin-like growth factor (Natale et al., 1988), and epidermal growth factor (EGF) (Haeder et al., 1988; Veale et al., 1989; Dazzi et al., 1989) have been identified in several NSCLC cell lines. EGF receptor expression on NSCLC cell lines has been the particular focus of a number of investigators.

The function(s) of epidermal growth factor is not well characterized. It appears to be involved in both cell growth and differentiation (Cohen, 1986; Gusterson et al., 1984; Ozanne et al., 1986). Receptors for EGF are found on normal and malignant cells of epidermal or mesenchymal origin (Gulick et al.,

1986; Real et al., 1986) and on all NSCLC histologic types (Veale et al., 1987). Higher concentrations of EGF receptors are found on tumors than in normal lung tissue, a difference that may be exploitable therapeutically. Shaw and co-workers have developed a fusion gene whose product is a hybrid protein consisting of diphtheria toxin linked to epidermal growth factor. The hybrid protein displaces high-affinity [^{125}I]EGF binding and induces tryosine phosphorylation of the EGF receptor in a manner similar to native EGF. It is also capable of inhibiting protein synthesis in a variety of EGF-receptor positive human tumor cell lines (Shaw et al., 1990). Preclinical evaluation of this agent with human tumor xenografts is currently underway.

In summary, despite some progress, the treatment of disseminated NSCLC remains unsatisfactory. There is a consistent trend toward a modest prolongation of survival when cisplatin-based combination chemotherapy is compared to best supportive care only. The impact of chemotherapy on the quality of patients' life has not been adequately assessed. Efforts are underway to optimize current chemotherapy approaches and to discover new agents. The therapeutic gains to be realized from these efforts are likely to be modest. Novel approaches utilizing biological response modifiers, monoclonal antibodies, and growth factor–toxin conjugates should be pursued. More significant advances await a better understanding of the biology of lung cancer and the mechanisms of resistance to treatment.

References

Bedford, P., Walker, M. C., Sharma, H. L., Perera, A., McAuliffe, C. A., Masters, J. R. W., and Hill, B. (1987). Factors influencing the sensitivity of two human bladder carcinoma cell lines to cis-diamminedichloroplatinum (II). *Chem. Biol. Interact.* **61:** 1–15.

Bernal, S. D., Speak, J. A., Boeheim, K., Dreyfuss, A. I., Wright, J. E., Teicher, B. A., Rosowsky, A., Tsao, S. W., and Wong, Y. C. (1990). Reduced membrane protein associated with resistance of human squamous carcinoma cells to methotrexate and cis-platinum. *Mol. Cell. Biochem.* **95:**61–70.

Bhuchar, V. K., and Lanzotti, V. J. (1982). High-dose cisplatin for lung cancer. *Cancer Treat. Rep.* **66:**375–376.

Boring, C. C., Squires, T. S., and Tong, T. (1991). Cancer statistics. *Ca* **41:**19–36.

Bork, E., Hansen, M., Dombernowsky, P., Hansen, S. W., Pedersen, A. G., and Hansen, H. H. (1986). Teniposide (VM-26), an overlooked highly active agent in small cell lung cancer. Results of a phase II trial in untreated patients. *J. Clin. Oncol.* **4:**524–527.

Britell, J. C., Eagan, R. T., Ingle, J. N., Creagan, E. T., Ruben, J., and Frytak, S. (1978). Cis-dichlorodiammine platinum (II) alone followed by adriamycin plus cyclophosphamide at progression versus cis-dichlorodiammine platinum (II), adriamycin, and cyclophosphamide in combination for adenocarcinoma of the lung. *Cancer. Treat. Rep.* **62:**1207–1210.

Bungo, M., Fujiwara, Y., Kasahara, K., Nakagawa, K., Ohe, Y., Sasaki, Y., Irino, S., and Saijo, N. (1990). Decreased accumulation as a mechanism of resistance to cis-diamminedichloroplatinum (II) in human non-small cell lung cancer cell lines: relation to DNA damage and repair. *Cancer Res.* **50:**2549–2553.

Bunn, P. A. (1988). Lung cancer: current understanding of biology, diagnosis, staging and treatment (monogr). Wallingford, CT, Bristol-Myers. pp. 1–67.

Bunn, P. A., Jr. (1989). The expanding role of cisplatin in the treatment of non-small cell lung cancer. *Semin. Oncol.* **16**(Suppl)**:**10–21.

Carmichael, J., Fergusson, R. J., Wolf, C. R., Balkwill, F. R., and Symth, J. F. (1986). Augmentation of cytotoxicity of chemotherapy by human α-interferons in human non-small cell lung cancer xenografts. *Cancer Res.* **46:**4916–4920.

Carmichael, J., Mitchell, J. B., Friedman, N., Gazdar, A. F., and Russo, A. (1988). Glutathione and related enzyme activity in human lung cancer lines. *Br. J. Cancer* **58:**437–440.

Chan, S. Y. T., Evan, G. I., Ritson, A., Watson, J., Wraight, P., and Sikora, K. (1986). Localization of lung cancer by a radiolabeled monoclonal antibody against the c-myc oncogene product. *Br. J. Cancer* **54:**761–769.

Chaudhary, V. K., Fitzgerald, D. J., Adhya, S., and Pastan, I. (1987). Activity of a recombinant fusion protein between transforming growth factor type alpha and *Pseudomonas* toxin. *Proc. Natl. Acad. Sci. U.S.A.* **84:**4538–4542.

Chaudhary, V. K., Mizukami, T., Fuerst, T. R., Fitzgerald, D. J., Moss, B., Pastan, I., and Berger, E. A. (1988). Selective killing of HIV infected cells by recombinant human CD4-*Pseudomonas* exotoxin hybrid protein. *Nature* **335:**369–375.

Cohen, M. H., Creaven, P. J., Fossieck, B. E., Jr., Broder, L. E., Selawry, O. S., Johnston, A. V., Williams, C. L., and Minna, J. D. (1977). Intensive chemotherapy of small cell bronchogenic carcinoma. *Cancer. Treat. Rep.* **61:**349–364.

Cohen, S. (1986). Isolation of a mouse submaxillary gland protein accelerating incisor eruption and eyelid opening in newborn mice. *J. Biol. Chem.* **237:**1555–1562.

Coleman, C. N., Bump, E. A., and Kramer, R. A. (1988a). Chemical modifiers of cancer treatment. *J. Clin. Oncol.* **6:**709–733.

Coleman, C. N., Carlson, R. W., Halsey, J., Kohler, M., Gribble, M., Sikic, B. I., and Jacobs, C. (1988b). Enhancement of the clinical activity of melphalan by the hypoxic cell sensitizer misonidazole. *Cancer Res.* **48:**3528–3532.

Cros, S., Wright, M., Morimoto, M., Lataste, H., Couzinier, J. P., and Krikorian, A. (1989). Experimental antitumor activity of Navelbine (5-nor-anhydrovinblastine, vinorelbine). *Semin. Oncol.* **16**(Suppl):15–20.

Curt, G. A., Carney, D. N., Cowan, K. H., Jolivet, J., Bailey, B. D., Drake, J. C., Kao-Shan, C. S., Minna, J. D., and Chabner, B. A. (1983). Unstable methotrexate resistance in human small cell carcinoma associated with double minute chromosomes. *N. Engl. J. Med.* **308:**199–202.

Dalton, W. S., Grogan, T. M., Meltzer, P. S., Scheper, R. J., Durie, B. G., Miller, T. P., and Salmon, S. E. (1989). Drug resistance in multiple myeloma and non-Hodgkin's lymphoma: detection of P-glycoprotein and potential circumvention by addition of verapamil to chemotherapy. *J. Clin. Oncol.* **7:**415–424.

Dazzi, H., Haselton, P. S., Thatcher, N., Barnes, D. M., Wilkes, S., Swindell, R., and

Lawson, R. A. M. (1989). Expression of epidermal growth factor receptor (EGF-R) in non-small cell lung cancer. Use of archival tissue and correlation of EGF-R with histology, tumour size, node status and survival. *Br. J. Cancer* **59:**746–749.

DeJager, R., Longeval, E., and Klatersky, J. (1980). High-dose cisplatin with fluid and mannitol-induced diuresis in advanced lung cancer. A phase II clinical trial of the EORTC Lung Cancer Working Party (Belgium). *Cancer Treat. Rep.* **64:**1341–1346.

Depierre, A., Lemarie, E., Dabouis, G., Garnier, G., Jacoulet, P., and Dalphin, J. C. (1989). Efficacy of Navelbine (NVB) in non-small cell lung cancer (NSCLC). *Semin. Oncol.* **16**(Suppl)**:**26–29.

Divgi, C. R., Welt, S., Kris, M., Real, F. X., Yeh, S. D. J., Gralla, R., Merchant, B., Schweighart, S., Unger, M., Larson, S. M., and Mendelsohn, J. (1991). Phase I and imaging trial of indium III-labeled anti-epidermal growth factor receptor monoclonal antibody 225 in patients with squamous cell lung carcinoma. *J. Natl. Cancer. Inst.* **83:**97–104.

Elias, D. J., Hirshowitz, L., Kline, L. E., Kroener, J. F., Dillman, R. O., Walker, L. E., Robb, J. A., and Timms, R. M. (1990). Phase I clinical comparative study of monoclonal antibody KS 1/4 and KS 1/4-methotrexate immunoconjugate in patients with non-small cell lung carcinoma. *Cancer Res.* **50:**4154–4159.

Erlichman, C., Fine, S., Wong, A., and Elhakim, T. (1988). A randomized trial of fluorouracil and folinic acid in patients with metastatic colorectal carcinoma. *J. Clin. Oncol.* **6:**469–475.

Figueredo, A. T., Hryniuk, W. M., Strautmanis, I., Frank, G., and Rendell, S. (1985). Cotrimoxazole prophylaxis during high-dose chemotherapy of small-cell lung cancer. *J. Clin. Oncol.* **3:**54–64.

Fojo, A. T., Whang-Peng, J., Gottesman, M. M., and Pastan, I. (1985). Amplification of DNA sequences in human multidrug-resistant KB carcinoma cells. *Proc. Natl. Acad. Sci. U.S.A.* **82:**7661–7665.

Fojo, A., Ueda, K., Slamon, D. J., Poplack, D. G., Gottesman, M. M., and Pastan, I. (1987). Expression of a multidrug-resistant gene in human tumors and tissues. *Proc. Natl. Acad. Sci. U.S.A.* **84:**265–269.

Fukuoka, M., Negoro, S., Niitani, H., and Taguchi, T. (1990). A phase II study of a new camptothecin derivative, CPT-11 in previously untreated non-small cell lung cancer. *Proc. Am. Soc. Clin. Oncol.* **9:**226.

Gandara, D. R., Wold, H., Perez, E. A., Deisseroth, A. B., Doroshow, J., Meyers, F., McWhirter, K., Hannigan, J., and DeGregorio, M. W. (1989). Cisplatin dose intensity in non-small cell lung cancer: phase II results of a day 1 and day 8 high-dose regimen. *J. Natl. Cancer. Inst.* **81:**790–794.

Giaccone, G. (1988). The European Organization for Research and Treatment of Cancer (EORTC) trials of new agents for advanced non-small cell lung cancer. *Semin. Oncol.* **15**(Suppl)**:**46–48.

Goldenberg, D. M. (1991). Challenges to the therapy of cancer with monoclonal antibodies. *J. Natl. Cancer Inst.* **83:**78–79.

Goodman, G. E., Hellstrom, I., Brodzinsky, L., Nicaise, C., Kulander, B., Hummel, D., and Hellstrom, K. E. (1990). Phase I trial of murine monoclonal antibody L6 in breast, colon, ovarian, and lung cancer. *J. Clin. Oncol.* **8:**1083–1092.

Goldstein, L. J., Galski, H., Fojo, A., Willingham, M., Lai, S., Gazdar, A., Pirker, R., Green, A., Cossman, J., Gottesman, M. M., and Pastan, I. (1989). Expression of a multidrug resistance gene in human cancers. *J. Natl. Cancer Inst.* **81:**116–124.

Gralla, R. J., Casper, E. S., Kelsen, D. P., Braun, D. W., Jr., Dukeman, M. E., Martini, N., Young, C. W., and Golbey, R. B. (1981). Cisplatin and vindesine combination chemotherapy for advanced carcinoma of the lung. A randomized trial investigating two dosage schedules. *Ann. Intern. Med.* **95:**414–420.

Green, J. A., Vistica, D. T., Young, R. C., Hamilton, T. C., Rogan, A. M., and Ozols, R. F. (1984). Potentiation of melphalan cytotoxicity in human ovarian cancer cell lines by glutathione depletion. *Cancer Res.* **44:**5427–5431.

Gruneberg, S. M., Kempf, R. A., Itri, L. M., Venturi, C. L., Boswell, W. D., Jr., and Mitchell, M. S. (1985). Phase II study of recombinant alpha interferon in the treatment of advanced non-small cell lung carcinoma. *Cancer Treat. Rep.* **69:**1031–1032.

Gulick, W. J., Marsden, J. J., Whittle, N., Ward, B., Bobrow, L., and Waterfield, M. D. (1986). Expression of epidermal growth factor receptors on human cervical, ovarian, and vulval carcinomas. *Cancer Res.* **46:**285–292.

Gusterson, B. A., Cowley, G., Smith, J. A., and Ozanne, B. (1984). Cellular localization of human epidermal factor receptors. *Cell. Biol. Int. Rep.* **8:**649–658.

Haeder, M., Rothsch, M., Bepler, G., Hennig, C., Havemann, K., Heimann, B., and Moelling, K. (1988). Epidermal growth factor receptor expression in human lung cancer cell lines. *Cancer Res.* **48:**1132–1136.

Hande, K. R., Oldham, R. K., Fer, M. F., Richardson, R. L., and Greco, F. A. (1982). Randomized study of high-dose versus low-dose methotrexate in the treatment of extensive small cell lung cancer. *Am. J. Med.* **73:**413–418.

Hesketh, P., Caguioa, P., Bulger, K., Koh, H., Pihan, G., Carey, R., Mihm, M., Parker, K., Woodworth, T., and McCaffrey, R. (1990). Clinical response in cutaneous T-cell lymphoma to an IL-2 diphtheria hybrid toxin ($DAB_{486}IL2$). *Blood* **76**(Suppl)**:**352a.

Imanishi, K., Yamaguchi, K., Honda, S., and Abe, K. (1988). Transforming growth factor-α as a possible autocrine growth factor for human adenocarcinoma of the lung. In: *Progress in Endocrinology*. Edited by H. Imura, K. Shizume, and S. Yoshida. Amsterdam, Elsevier, pp. 1363–1368.

Jaakkimainen, L., Goodwin, P. J., Pater, J., Warde, P., Murray, N., and Rapp, E. (1990). Counting the costs of chemotherapy in a National Cancer Institute of Canada randomized trial in non-small cell lung cancer. *J. Clin. Oncol.* **8:**1301–1309.

James, K. (1990). Human monoclonal antibodies and engineered antibodies in the management of cancer. *Semin. Cancer. Biol.* **1:**243–253.

Kalofonos, H. P., Sivolapenko, G. B., Courtenay-Luck, N. S., Snook, D. E., Hooker, G. R., Winter, R., McKenzie, C. G., Taylor-Papadimitrou, J. J., Lavender, P. J., and Epenetos, A. A. (1988). Antibody guided targeting of non-small cell lung cancer using ^{III} In-labeled HMFG $F(ab)_2'$ fragments. *Cancer Res.* **48:**1977–1984.

Kartner, N., and Ling, V. (1989). Multidrug resistance in cancer. *Sci. Am.* **260:**44–51.

Kelley, S. L., Basu, A., Teicher, B. A., Hacker, M. P., Hamer, D. H., and Lazo, J. S. (1988). Over-expression of metallothionein confers resistance to anticancer drugs. *Science* **241:**1813–1815.

Klastersky, J., Sculier, J. P., Ravez, P., Libert, P., Michel, J., Vandermoten, G., Rocmans, P., Bonduelle, Y., Mairesse, M., Michiels, T., Thiriaux, J., Mommen, P., and Dalesio, O. (1986). A randomized study comparing a high and standard dose of cisplatin in combination with etoposide in the treatment of advanced non-small cell lung carcinoma. *J. Clin. Oncol.* **4:**1780–1786.

Kradin, R. L., Boyle, L. A., Preffer, F. I., Callahan, R. J., Barlai-Kovach, M., Strauss, H. W., Dubinett, S., and Kurnick, J. T. (1987). Tumor-derived interleukin-2 dependent lymphocytes in adoptive immunotherapy of lung cancer. *Cancer Immunol. Immunother.* **24:**76–85.

Kris, M., Cohen, E., and Gralla, R. (1985). An analysis of 134 Phase II trials in non-small cell lung cancer (NSCLC). IV World Conference on Lung Cancer, Toronto, p. 133 (abstr.).

Kris, M. G., D'Acquisto, R. W., Gralla, R. J., Burke, M. T., Marks, L. D., Fanucchi, M. P., and Hellan, R. T. (1989a). Phase II trial of trimetrexate in patients with stage III and IV non-small-cell lung cancer. *Am. J. Clin. Oncol.* **12:**24–26.

Kris, M. G., Gralla, R. J., Potanovitch, L. M., Marks, L. A., and Hellan, R. T. (1989b). Incorporating 10-ethyl-10-deazaaminopterin (EDAM) into combination therapy with mitomycin (M) and vinblastine (V) for patients with advanced non-small cell lung cancer. *Proc. Am. Soc. Clin. Oncol.* **8:**227.

Lai, S. L., Goldstein, L. J., Gottesman, M. M., Pastan, I., Tsai, C. M., Johnson, B. E., Mulshine, J. L., Ihde, D. C., Kayser, K., and Gazdar, A. F. (1989). MDR1 gene expression in lung cancer. *J. Natl. Cancer Inst.* **81:**1144–1150.

Lazarus, H. M., Spitzer, T. R., and Creger, R. J. (1990). Phase I trial of high-dose etoposide, high-dose cisplatin, and reinfusion of autologous bone marrow for lung cancer. *Am. J. Clin. Oncol.* **13:**107–112.

LeMaistre, F., Rosenblum, M., Reuben, J., Parkinson, D., Meneghetti, C., Parker, K., Shaw, J., Deisseroth, A., and Woodworth, T. (1990). Phase I study of genetically engineered DAB_{486}IL-2 in IL-2 receptor expressing malignancies. *Blood* **76**(Suppl)**:**360a.

Ling, V., and Thompson, L. H. (1974). Reduced permeability in CHO cells as a mechanism of resistance to colchicine. *J. Cell. Physiol.* **83:**103–116.

Ling, V., Juranka, P. F., and Endicott, J. A. (1988). Multidrug resistance and P-glycoprotein expression. In: *Mechanisms of Drug Resistance in Neoplastic Cells.* Edited by P. V. Wooley and K. D. Tew. San Diego, Academic Press, pp. 197–209.

Lorberboum-Galski, H., Fitzgerald, D., Chaudhary, V., Adhya, S., and Pastan, I. (1988). Cytotoxic activity of an interleukin 2–*Pseudomonas* exotoxin chimeric protein produced in *Escherichia coli. Proc. Natl. Acad. Sci. U.S.A.* **85:**1922–1926.

Mannervik, B., and Danielson, U. H. (1988). Glutathione transferases—structure and catalytic activity. *Crit. Rev. Biochem.* **23:**283–287.

Maroun, J. (1988). Clinical response to trimetrexate as sole therapy for nonsmall cell lung cancer. *Semin. Oncol.* **15**(Suppl)**:**17–21.

Masuda, H., Hamilton, T. C., and Ozols, R. F. (1988). Increased DNA repair as a mechanism of acquired resistance to L-phenylanine mustard and cisdiammine-dichloroplatinum (II) in human ovarian cancer cell lines. *Cancer Res.* **48:**5713–5716.

Miller, T. P. (1990). Rationale for the use of chemotherapy in non-small cell lung cancer. *Semin. Oncol.* **17**(Suppl)**:**11–13.

Miller, T. P., Grogan, T. M., Dalton, W. S., Spier, C. M., Scheper, R. J., and Salmon, S. E. (1991). P-glycoprotein expression in malignant lymphoma and reversal of clinical drug resistance with chemotherapy plus high-dose verapamil. *J. Clin. Oncol.* **9:**17–24.

Minna, J. D., Pass, H., Glatstein, E., and Ihde, D. C. (1989). Cancer of the lung. In: *Cancer: Principles and Practice of Oncology*. Edited by V. T. DeVita, Jr., S. Hellman, and S. A. Rosenberg. Philadelphia, J. B. Lippincott, pp. 591–705.

Mulcahy, R. T. (1988). Update: the potential for chemosensitization of alkylating agents by nitroimidazoles. *Oncology* **2:**17–27.

Mulcahy, R. T., Trump, D. L. (1988). Clinical chemosensitization by misonidazole and related compounds: a critical evaluation. *J. Clin. Oncol.* **6:**569–573.

Murphy, J. R. (1988). Diphtheria-related peptide hormone gene fusions: a molecular genetic approach to chimeric toxin development. In: *Immunotoxins*. Edited by A. E. Frankel. Norwell, Kluwer Academic Publishers, pp. 123–159.

Natale, R. B., Cuttita, F., Nakanishi, Y., Minna, J., Gazdar, A., and Mulshine, J. (1988). IGF-I can stimulate proliferation of non-small cell lung cancer cell lines in vitro. *Proc. Am. Soc. Clin. Oncol.* **7:**197.

O'Donnell, M. R., Ruckdeschel, J. C., Baxter, D., McKneally, M. F., Caradonna, R., and Horton, J. (1985). Intensive induction chemotherapy for small cell anaplastic carcinoma of the lung. *Cancer Treat. Res.* **69:**571–575.

Olesen, B. K., Ernst, P., Nissen, M. H., and Hansen, H. H. (1987). Recombinant interferon A (IFL-rA) therapy of small cell and squamous cell carcinoma of the lung. A phase II study. *Eur. J. Cancer Clin. Oncol.* **23:**987–989.

Ozanne, B., Richards, C. S., Hendler, F., Burns, D., and Gusterson, B. (1986). Overexpression of the EGF receptor is a hallmark of squamous cell carcinoma. *J. Pathol.* **149:**9–14.

Ozols, R. F., Louie, K. G., Plowman, J., Behrens, B. C., Fine, R. L., Dykes, D., and Hamilton, T. C. (1987). Enhanced melphalan cytotoxicity in human ovarian cancer in vitro and in tumor-bearing mice by buthionine sulfoximine depletion of glutathione. *Biochem. Pharmacol.* **36:**147–153.

Ozols, R. F., Hamilton, T. C., Masuda, H., and Young, R. C. (1988). Manipulation of cellular thiols to influence drug resistance. In: *Mechanisms of Drug Resistance in Neoplastic Cells*. Edited by P. V. Woolley and K. W. Tew. San Diego, Academic Press, pp. 289–306.

Panettierre, F. J., Vance, R. B., and Stuckey, W. J. (1983). Evaluation of single-agent cisplatin in the management of non-small cell carcinoma of the lung: a Southwest Oncology Group Study. *Cancer Treat. Rep.* **67:**399–400.

Pastan, I., and Gottesman, M. (1987). Multiple-drug resistance in human cancer. *N. Engl. J. Med.* **316:**1388–1393.

Perkins, A. C., Pimm, M. V., Morgan, D. A., Wastie, M. L., Reynolds, J. R., and Baldwin, R. W. (1986). ^{131}I and ^{111}In-labeled monoclonal antibody imaging of primary lung carcinoma. *Nucl. Med. Commun.* **7:**729–739.

Petrelli, N., Douglas, H. O., Jr., Herrera, L., Russell, D., Stablein, D. M., Bruckner, H. W., Mayer, R. J., Schinella, R., Green, M. D., Muggia, F. M., Megibow, A., Greenwald, E. S., Bukowski, R. M., Harris, J., Levin, B., Gaynor, E., Loutfi, A., Kalser, M. H.,

Barkin, J. S., Benedetto, P., Woolley, P. V., Nauta, R., Weaver, D. W., and Leichman, L. P. (1989). The modulation of fluorouracil with leucovorin in metastatic colorectal carcinoma: a prospective randomized phase III trial. *J. Clin. Oncol.* **7:**1419–1426.

Poon, M. A., O'Connell, M. J., Moertel, C. G., Wieand, H. S., Cullinan, S. A., Everson, L. K., Krook, J. E., Mailliard, J. A., Laurie, J. A., Tschetter, L. K., and Wiesenfeld, M. (1989). Biochemical modulation of fluorouracil: evidence of significant improvement of survival and quality of life in patients with advanced colorectal cancer. *J. Clin. Oncol.* **7:**1407–1417.

Rapp, E., Pater, J. L., Willan, A., Cormier, Y., Murray, N., Evans, W. K., Hodson, D. I., Clark, D. A., Feld, R., Arnold, A. M., Ayoub, J. I., Wilson, K. S., Latreille, J., Wierzbicki, R. F., and Hill, D. P. (1988). Chemotherapy can prolong survival in patients with advanced non-small-cell lung cancer—report of a Canadian multicenter randomized trial. *J. Clin. Oncol.* **6:**633–641.

Real, F. X., Rettig, W. J., Chesa, P. G., Melamed, M. R., Old, L. J., and Mendelsohn, J. (1986). Expression of epidermal growth factor receptor in human cultured cells and tissues: relationship to cell lineage and stage of differentiation. *Cancer Res.* **46:** 4726–4731.

Rosenberg, S. A., Lotze, M. T., Muul, L. M., Leitman, S., Chang, A. E., Ettinghauser, S. E., Matory, Y. L., Skibber, J. M., Shiloni, E., Vetto, J., Seipp, C. A., Simpson, C., and Reichert, C. M. (1985). Observations on the systemic administration of autologous lymphokine-activated killer cells and recombinant interleukin-2 to patients with metastatic cancer. *N. Engl. J. Med.* **313:**1485–1492.

Rosenberg, S. A., Lotze, M. T., Muul, L. M., Chang, A., Aves, F. P., Leitman, S., Linehan, W. M., Robertson, C. N., Lee, R. E., Ruben, J. T., Seipper, C. A., Simpson, C. G., and White, D. E. (1987). A progress report on the treatment of 157 patients with advanced cancer using lymphokine-activated killer cells and interleukin-2 or high dose interleukin-2 alone. *N. Engl. J. Med.* **316:**889–897.

Rosso, R., Ardizzoni, A., Salvati, F., Rinaldi, M., Rubagotti, A., Pennucci, C., Tonachella, R., DeMarinis, F., Cruciani, A. R., Mantellini, E., Soresi, E., Ferrara, G., Romano, F., Bandera, M., Martini, M., and Fortini, C. (1990). Combination chemotherapy and recombinant (R) alfa interferon (IFN) for metastatic non-small cell lung cancer (NSCLC): a randomized FONICAP trial. *Proc. Am. Soc. Clin. Oncol.* **9:**227.

Salmon, S. E., Grogan, T. M., Miller, T., Scheper, R., and Dalton, W. S. (1989). Prediction of doxorubicin resistance in vitro in myeloma, lymphoma, and breast cancer by P-glycoprotein staining. *J. Natl. Cancer Inst.* **81:**696–701.

Schiller, J. H., Storer, B., Dreicer, R., Rosenquist, D., Frontiera, M., and Carbone, P. P. (1989). Randomized phase II-III trial of combination beta and gamma interferons and etoposide and cisplatin in inoperable non-small cell cancer of the lung. *J. Natl. Cancer. Inst.* **81:**1739–1743.

Shaw, J. P., Arrigo, D., Rhoad, A., Thomas, J., Akiyoshi, D., Nichols, J., and Bacha, P. (1990). Specificity and mechanism of action of a genetically engineered hybrid protein composed of epidermal growth factor and a fragment of diphtheria toxin. Second International Symposium on Immunotoxins. Lake Buena Vista, FL.

Shum, K. Y., Kris, M. G., Gralla, R. J., Burke, M. T., Marks, L. M., and Heelan, R. T.

(1988). Phase II study of 10-ethyl-10-deaza-aminopterin in patients with stage III and IV non-small-cell lung cancer. *J. Clin. Oncol.* **6**:446–450.

Siegall, C. B., Chaudhary, V. J., Fitzgerald, D. J. P., and Pastan, I. (1988). Cytotoxic activity of an interleukin 6–*Pseudomonas* exotoxin fusion protein on human myeloma cells. *Proc. Natl. Acad. Sci. U.S.A.* **85**:9738–9742.

Smyth, J., Fergusson, R., Stewart, M., Cornbleet, M., Gregor, A., and Leonard, R. (1988). Alpha interferon potentiates cisplatin in patients with non-small cell lung cancer (NSCLC). *Proc. Am. Soc. Clin. Oncol.* **7**:201.

Souhami, R. L., Harper, P. G., Linch, D., Trask, C., Goldstone, A. H., Tobias, J. S., Spiro, S. G., Geddes, D. M., and Richards, J. D. (1983). High-dose cyclophosphamide with autologous marrow transplantation for small cell carcinoma of the bronchus. *Cancer. Chemother. Pharmacol.* **10**:205–207.

Souhami, R. L., Finn, G., Gregory, W. M., Birkhead, B. G., Buckman, R., Edwards, D., Goldstone, A. H., Harper, P. G., Spiro, S. G., Tobias, J. S., and Geddes, D. (1985). High-dose cyclophosphamide in small-cell carcinoma of the lung. *J. Clin. Oncol.* **3**: 958–963.

Teicher, B. A., Cucchi, C. A., Lee, J. B., Flatow, J. L., Rosowsky, A., and Frei, E. (1986). Alkylating agents: in vitro studies of cross-resistance patterns in human cell lines. *Cancer Res.* **46**:4379–4383.

Teicher, B. A., Holden, S. A., Kelley, M. J., Shea, T. C., Cucchi, C. A., Rosowsky, A., Henner, W. D., and Frei, E. III. (1987). Characterization of a human squamous carcinoma cell line resistant to cis-diamminedichloroplatinum (II). *Cancer Res.* **47**: 388–393.

Tew, K. D., Bomber, A. M., and Hoffman, S. J. (1988). Ethacrynic acid and piriprost as enhancers of cytotoxicity in drug resistant and sensitive cell lines. *Cancer Res.* **48**: 3622–3625.

Trent, J. M., Buick, R. N., Olson, S., Horns, R. C., Jr., and Schimke, R. T. (1984). Cytologic evidence for gene amplification in methotrexate-resistant cells obtained from a patient with ovarian adenocarcinoma. *J. Clin. Oncol.* **2**:8–15.

Veale, D., Ashcroft, T., Marsh, C., Gibson, G. J., and Harris, A. L. (1987). Epidermal growth factor receptors in non-small cell lung cancer. *Br. J. Cancer* **55**:513–516.

Veale, D., Kerr, N., Gibson, G. J., and Harris, A. L. (1989). Characterization of epidermal growth factor receptor in primary human non-small cell lung cancer. *Cancer Res.* **49**: 1313–1317.

Vogl, S. E., Berenzweig, M., Camacho, F., Berenzweig, M., Greenwald, E., and Kaplan, B. H. (1982). Efficacy study of intensive cisplatin therapy in advanced non-small cell bronchogenic carcinoma. *Cancer* **50**:24–26.

Wadler, S., and Schwartz, E. L. (1990). Antineoplastic activity of the combination of interferon and cytotoxic agents against experimental and human malignancies: a review. *Cancer Res.* **50**:3473–3486.

Wadler, S., Schwartz, E. L., Goldman, M., Lyver, A., Rader, M., Zimmerman, M., Wiernik, P. H., Itri, L., and Weinberg, V. (1989). 5-Fluorouracil and recombinant α-2a-interferon: an active regimen against colorectal carcinoma. *J. Clin. Oncol.* **7**: 1769–1775.

West, W. H., Tauer, K. W., Yannelli, J. R., Marshall, G. D., Orr, D. W., Thurman, G. B., and Oldham, R. K. (1987). Constant infusion recombinant interleukin-2 in adoptive immunotherapy of advanced cancer. *N. Engl. J. Med.* **316:**898–905.

Williams, S. F., Bitran, J. D., Hoffman, P. C., Robin, E., Fullem, L., Beschorner, J., Golick, J., and Golomb, H. M. (1989). High-dose, multiple-alkylator chemotherapy with autologous bone marrow reinfusion in patients with advanced non-small cell lung cancer. *Cancer* **63:**238–242.

Williams, D. P., Wen, Z., Watson, R. S., Boyd, J., Strom, T. B., and Murphy, J. R. (1990). Cellular processing of the interleukin-2 fusion toxin DAB $_{486}$-IL-2 and efficient delivery of diphtheria fragment A to the cytosol of target cells requires Arg^{194}. *J. Biol. Chem.* **265:**20673–20677.

Woods, R. L., Williams, C. J., Levi, J., Page, J., Bell, D., Byrne, M., and Kerestes, Z. L. (1990). A randomized trial of cisplatin and vindesine versus supportive care only in advanced non-small cell lung cancer. *Br. J. Cancer* **61:**608–611.

Yang, S. C., Owen-Schaub, L., Menidiguren-Rodriguez, A., Grimm, E. A., Hong, W. K., and Roth, J. A. (1990). Combination immunotherapy for non-small cell lung cancer. Results with interleukin-2 and tumor necrosis factor-α. *J. Thorac. Cardiovasc. Surg.* **99:**8–13.

PART VII

SMALL CELL LUNG CANCER: CRITICAL ASSESSMENT OF TREATMENT STRATEGIES

26

Chemotherapy of Small Cell Lung Cancer

HEINE H. HANSEN and PAUL E. G. KRISTJANSEN

Finsen Institute, Rigshospitalet
Copenhagen, Denmark

I. Introduction

The management of patients with small cell lung cancer (SCLC) has undergone major changes during the past 20 years. Before 1970, surgery and radiotherapy were the most common forms of treatment, but these local methods provided only rarely effective long-term control, when used as single treatments. Appreciation of the frequency and extent of metastases coupled with the sensitivity of SCLC to a variety of chemotherapeutic agents has led to the present emphasis upon the central role of systemic chemotherapy. These changes have resulted in a fivefold increase in median survival and a long-term disease-free survival of >3 years in 5–10% of the group as a whole, and in 15–20% of patients presenting with limited disease extent and other favorable prognostic factors (Hansen, 1987). Even though considerable progress has been achieved, there is still no standardized treatment for SCLC. Work is being carried out in many centers and in national and international groups to obtain further knowledge of the special biological features of this disease entity, including the search for alternative treatments, with the hope that it will become a more readily curable disease.

II. Prognostic Factors

With the available therapy it is important, before initiating therapy, to have its purpose in mind. In elderly patients palliation might be most important, while in other patients long-term survival or cure is the ultimate goal in spite of a more pronounced toxicity of the treatment. It is therefore important to evaluate patients carefully with respect to the main prognostic factors before instituting treatment (Østerlind, 1986). Some of the most important prognostic factors are listed in Table 1. The two key factors are pretreatment performance status and extent of disease. With respect to age and gender, patients below 60 years of age do better than those above 60 and women appear to have a better prognosis than men. A pretreatment weight loss of more than 3 kg indicates a significantly worse prognosis.

The prognostic value of the histopathologic subclassification of SCLC according to the World Health Organization (WHO) classification of 1982 is somewhat confusing, and there is disagreement regarding the prognostic impact of the various subtypes. This may reflect a lack of consistency of the different pathologic findings rather than a genuine difference in the biology of the various subtypes. It is noteworthy that Carney et al. in 1981 observed an especially poor prognosis for patients with small cell carcinoma, characterized before treatment as tumors with small cell and large cell components.

These tumors have always been difficult to classify, which was one of the reasons for the recent proposal by the International Association for the Study of Lung Cancer for a new classification (Hirsch et al., 1988). In this revised system, the tumors are categorized into three groups: pure small cell carcinoma, small cell/large cell, and combined tumors with SCLC components. With the use of this recommendation, which is more simple than the previous, the former inconsistencies are avoided and the present prognostic knowledge is taken into account. With

Table 1 Prognostic Factors in SCLC

Stage: limited or extensive
Performance status
Gender[a]
Age
Subclassification[b]
Bone metastases
Liver metastases
Blood biochemical values, especially lactate dehydrogenase

[a]The prognostic impact of gender seems to have lessened along with the increase in incidence of SCLC in women (Østerlind, unpublished observation).

[b]Especially poor prognosis if large cell elements are observed.

respect to the impact on survival of the anatomical stage, bone marrow metastases and CNS involvement per se result in a poor prognosis.

III. Staging

The recognition of SCLC as a systemic disease has rendered the anatomical staging of patients as the basis of treatment outside an experimental setting less important. To assess prognosis and compare results from different trials, staging procedures are still important, although it is now evident that patients can be stratified into distinct prognostic groups on the basis of biochemical evaluation, including levels of lactate dehydrogenase (LDH), albumin, and alkaline phosphatases, in combination with other descriptive data (Østerlind, 1986). The anatomical stage is important for deciding whether to apply additional local treatment such as surgery and/or radiotherapy as part of the overall treatment plan. The tumor–node–metastases (TNM) system recommended by the Union International Contre Cancer (UICC) has not traditionally been considered well suited for SCLC because more than 95% of the patients will be classified in the worst stage. The recent modification of the TNM system (Mountain, 1987) has changed the situation. Two systems are now available for the staging of patients with SCLC: the classic V.A. Lung Cancer Study Group (VALG) system of "limited" or "extensive" disease, and the recently revised TNM system. In the VALG system, the classification of patients with contralateral mediastinal or supraclavicular nodes and of patients with ipsilateral pleural effusions has not been uniformly handled by different investigators. A recent international workshop on SCLC (Stahel et al., 1989) reached consensus on the following recommendation. The *limited* disease classification includes patients with disease restricted to one hemithorax with regional lymph node metastases including hilar, ipsilateral and contralateral mediastinal, and/or supraclavicular nodes. In addition, patients with ipsilateral pleural effusion are included, whether the cytologic findings are positive or negative. Contralateral nodes in the mediastinum and the supraclavicular region are included because the prognostic influence of these metastatic sites is less than that of distant metastases and also because the revised TNM system groups these patients into stage III and not in stage IV. The *extensive* disease classification includes all patients with disease sites not eligible for the limited stage, and this category is equivalent to stage IV. Stages I–III of the revised TNM then offer a subdivision of the limited disease category, which may be useful when local treatment modalities are evaluated.

IV. Chemotherapy of SCLC

The main treatment modality is chemotherapy, while the exact role of radiotherapy and surgery in combination with chemotherapy in the treatment of SCLC remains unclear.

The ideal therapeutic goal in SCLC is to reach the highest percentages of long-term disease-free survival (cures) with the lowest possible morbidity. We are still far from this despite the fact that many antineoplastic agents have been shown to have antitumor activity in SCLC and to produce initial responses in up to 90% of patients when given single or in combination.

For some time it has been considered evident that drug combinations with three or four drugs are superior to single agents, based on theoretical considerations as well as clinical investigations. Nevertheless recent results have suggested that epipodophyllotoxins, either as single agents or in a two-drug combination with platinum, might be effective as multidrug combinations in producing initial responses (Bunn et al., 1989).

The cytostatic treatment of SCLC is constantly subject to change and refinement. During the 1970s, the median survival was prolonged by four to five times and possible cure was obtained in 5–10% of all patients. Major additional improvement has not been observed in the last decade, but a vast amount of studies has consolidated the early results. Many agents have exhibited antitumor activity, a list is shown in Table 2. The majority of studies include compounds such as etoposide, vincristine, cis-platinum, cyclophosphamide, doxorubicin, CCNU, and methotrexate. Among the most commonly used combinations are: cisplatinum and etoposide; vincristine, etoposide, and cyclophosphamide; cyclophosphamide, CCNU, vincristine, and etoposide; and cyclophosphamide, doxorubicin, and vincristine. Examples of these regimens, including scheduling and the actual dosages, are given in Table 3. Etoposide has, during the last few years, increasingly been used in the initial treatment, since randomized studies have shown that combinations including this drug are superior to those without (Hirsch et al., 1987; Jackson et al., 1983).

When given aggressively, the regimens will result in a response rate in excess of 80% for both stages of SCLC. Complete response is produced in 30–40% of patients with limited disease and in 15–20% of patients with extensive disease. A variety of options to improve treatment are under investigation. These include alternating "non-cross-resistant" chemotherapy, scheduling drug admin-

Table 2 Active Agents in SCLC

Epipodophyllotoxins	Vinca alkaloids	Others
Etoposide	Vincristine	Doxorubicin
Teniposide	Vindesine	Epirubicin
Alkylating agents	Vinblastine	CCNU
Cyclophosphamide	Platinum derivatives	ACNU
Ifosfamide	Cisplatinum	BCNU
Nitrogen mustard	Carboplatinum	Methotrexate
Hexamethylmelamine		

Table 3 Commonly Used Regimens in SCLC

Cisplatinum	80 mg/m^2 i.v. q 3 weeks, day 1
Etoposide	80 mg/m^2 i.v. daily on days 1–3 q 3 weeks
Cyclophosphamide	1000 mg/m^2 i.v. q 4 weeks, day 1
CCNU	70 mg/m^2 p.o. q 4 weeks day 1
Vincristine	1.3 mg/m^2 (max 2.0 mg) q 4 weeks day 1, except first 4 weeks when administered weekly
Etoposide	70 mg/m^2 p.o. daily on days 2–5 q 4 weeks
Etoposide	50 mg/m^2 i.v. daily on days 1–5 q 3 weeks
Doxorubicin	45 mg/m^2 i.v. q 3 weeks
Cyclophosphamide	1000 mg/m^2 i.v. q 3 weeks
Cyclophosphamide	1500 mg/m^2 i.v. q 3 weeks
Doxorubicin	40 mg/m^2 i.v. q 3 weeks
Vincristine	2 mg i.v. q 3 weeks.

istration based on cell cycle analysis, use of anticoagulants in combination with chemotherapy, incorporation of new agents with high activity in the combination chemotherapy regimens, intensive high-dosage chemotherapy with or without bone marrow support or transplantation, use of biological response modifiers.

A. Alternating vs. Sequential Chemotherapy

1. Background

Despite the initial chemosensitivity of SCLC, resistant clones present at diagnosis or emerging during therapy cause treatment failures in most patients. Evidence for a correlation between primary and emerging heterogeneity and clinical resistance has been derived from clinical investigations as well as from cell lines and human xenografts (Vindeløv et al., 1980; Roed et al., 1988). A simple mathematical model based on a probabilistic nature of spontaneously arising resistant clones has been proposed by Goldie and co-workers (1982). With an assumption of exponential growth and a log kill at each dose of chemotherapy, the course of therapy with two truly non-cross-resistant regimens, compared with sequential chemotherapy with the same regimens, was investigated by a computer simulation. If there was symmetry in the two regimens (i.e., same log kill and similar mutation rates producing resistance against each regimen), the alternating principle resulted in a greater cure rate in the model. Fulfillment of the symmetry criteria cannot be proved in the clinical setting, and non-cross-resistance has proved very difficult to ascertain.

2. Clinical Experience

A review by Elliot et al. (1984) concluded that treatment schedules using cyclic alternating non-cross-resistant drug combination in SCLC yield tumor responses comparable to those obtained with continuous regimens with a similar level of toxicity; controlled trials have failed to demonstrate major advantages in terms of improved survival. Details of trial design and especially the timing may be of critical importance; further controlled studies are warranted. Careful attention to the trial design with elimination of confounding variables such as radiotherapy, re-evaluation of disease-free status, and prolonged follow-up of larger numbers of patients will be necessary; and, finally, increased recognition of tumor cell heterogeneity as a major reason for treatment failure together with in vitro determination of drug sensitivity in cross-resistance may lead to a more rational application of alternating chemotherapy in the future.

A more recent updated review by Østerlind (1989) did not change the conclusions of Elliot et al. (1984). In the 1984 review none of the trials published at that time were able to demonstrate a convincing advantage of alternating chemotherapy. Results from six large controlled trials have been published since then (Daniels et al., 1984; Feld et al., 1987; Havemann et al., 1987; Østerlind et al., 1986; Pedersen et al., 1987; Roth et al., 1989; Ettinger et al., 1990) (Table 4). Schedules and regimens vary too much to make a meta-analysis feasible. The trials found small advantages of alternating chemotherapy for either limited-stage disease (Østerlind et al., 1986; Pedersen et al., 1987), extensive-stage disease (Daniels et al., 1984), or both stages (Havemann et al., 1987), but no impressive differences. In addition to results shown in Table 4, the latest and one of the largest studies (Ettinger et al., 1990) found a 2 year survival of 10% in the alternating arm (CAV-HEM) compared with 4% in the sequential arm (CAV). It has been suggested (Fukuoka et al., 1988; Batist et al., 1986) that the etoposide–platinum (EP) combination, when given initially, seems to be associated with a greater response rate than the CAV (cyclophosphamide, doxorubicin, vincristine) combination. This is likely to be a reflection of the fact that there is increasing evidence for an asymmetrical cross-resistance between EP and CAV, since patients in whom treatment fails or who do not respond to EP generally do worse after crossover to CAV than do patients who receive EP as secondary treatment (Evans et al., 1985; Zacharaski et al., 1981). Another explanation for the lack of realization of the Goldie-Coldman predictions is a type II error problem of overlooking existing differences. The number of patients required in a two-armed trial, in which the new treatment is supposed to result in a median survival of 18 months compared to 12 months in the control arm, is 448 patients (224 per arm) if the level of significance is the conventional 5% and the statistical power 0.75 (Østerlind, 1989). Although the current clinical experience does not contradict or even weaken the Goldie-Coldman model, it is evident that alternating chemotherapy has not been a great step forward. The primary reason is probably the failure to fulfill the criteria of the theoretical model.

B. Scheduling of Drugs Based on Cell Kinetic Observations

This has been the subject of a single clinical trial (Hirsch et al., 1987). The superiority of etoposide scheduling based on data from flow cytometric DNA analyses was demonstrated.

C. Anticoagulants

The role of anticoagulants was the subject of a small prospective randomized study by the VA Lung Cancer Study Group in the early 1980s (Zacharaski et al., 1981). Fifty patients were randomized to receive chemotherapy and radiotherapy with or without warfarin. Median survival was 24 weeks for control-treated patients and 50 weeks for the warfarin-treated group. The difference related to warfarin was particularly evident in the subgroup of patients with disseminated disease at the time of randomization and could not be explained by an imbalance of such prognostic factors as performance status, stage of disease, age, and sex. The warfarin-treated group also demonstrated a significant increase in time before progression, which suggested an influence of warfarin treatment on the metastatic potential of the tumor. The use of warfarin in combination chemotherapy regimens has since been under large-scale evaluation by several cooperative groups in the United States. A larger Cancer and Acute Leukemia Group B (CALGB) study on this topic (Chahinian et al., 1990) was published recently, comprising 328 patients, 294 evaluable, with extensive SCLC. Advantage was found in objective response rates for the warfarin-treated group, while overall survival also was better in the warfarin-treated group, but without reaching the conventional levels of significance. The use of warfarin should still remain experimental.

D. New Drugs

The most active of the new drugs include carboplatin (JM-8) (Smith et al., 1985) and the podophyllotoxin derivatives, VP-16 (etoposide) and VM-26 (teniposide). The latter compound was recently shown to be highly active, with a response rate of 90%, in untreated patients with SCLC (Bork et al., 1986). The marked difference in response rates observed for the same compound (e.g., VM-26, in untreated (90%) and previously treated (18%) patients is important. This reveals that there are major methodologic problems in the design and execution of clinical phase II trials with new agents in a highly chemosensitive tumor.

In the identification of active drugs selected for phase II trials, the importance of useful experimental models has been emphasized, although the correlation of drug activity between human cancer and animal and in vitro results is still

Table 4 Regimens and Results in Six Controlled Trials of Sequential (S) versus Alternating (A) Chemotherapy in SCLC

	Regimens, no. of patients			Results: Survival (mo)			Results: Complete response rates, %		
	Limited	All	Extensive	Limited	All	Extensive	Limited	All	Extensive
Stanford study, 1984 (Daniels et al., 1984)									
S: CVLPz × 2 Irr CVLPz . . . 18 mo	28 pts		56 pts	10		7	54		20
				NS		$p = 0.001$	NS		$p = 0.03$
A: EAM × 3 Irr CVLPz + EAM + CVLPz	28		50	16		10	42		44
Canadian studies, 1987 (Feld et al., 1987)									
S: CAV ×3+EP ×3 (+Irr)	146 pts		144 pts	15.5		8.0	45		27
				NS		$p = 0.03$	NS		$p < 0.05$
A: CAV + EP × 3 (+ Irr)	154		145	15.0		9.6	52		39
German study, 1987 (Havemann et al., 1987)									
S: CAV × 8 + Irr	53 pts		99 pts	11.1		8.9	33		15
						$p < 0.05$			
A: EVI + PAV × 3 + CML × 2 + Irr	51		99	13.4		9.9	52		28

Danish study, 1986–7 (Østerlind et al., 1986; Pedersen et al., 1987)							
S: CLVE . . . + P/A/Vd/M/H for 19 mo	154	71	9.5	7.5		44	21
A1: CLVM + EAAV . . . for 18 mo	151	66	11.5	7.5	$p < 0.05$		37
A2: CLVM + EAV + PVdH . . . for 18 mo	152	66	12.0	8.0		41	21
American Joint study, 1989 (Roth et al., 1989)							
S1: EP×4		344		9.5			17
S2: CAV × 6				9.5			12
A: EP + CAV × 3				9.5			17
ECOG study, 1990 (Ettings et al., 1990)							
S: CAV × 6–8		294		10.6			16
				$p < 0.002$ (after adjustment for prognostic factors)			$p = 0.03$
A: CAV + HEM × 3–4		283		11.5			23

S, sequential; A, alternating; Irr, irradiation; NS, not significant.
Agents: A, doxorubicin; C, cyclophosphamide; E, etoposide; H, hexamethylmelamine; I, ifosfamide; L, lomustine; M, methotrexate; P, cisplatin; Pz, procarbazine; V, vincristine; Vd, vindesine.

poor (Roed et al., 1986). It is important to note that newer active agents for years now have all been analogs of agents previously shown to be active in the treatment of SCLC. A major breakthrough probably will require the introduction of agents with new mechanisms of action.

E. Special Clinical Situations

With respect to certain clinical situations that have an effect on the management of SCLC, including CNS metastases, superior vena cava syndrome, and treatment at relapse, the recent literature has shed further light on the usefulness of chemotherapy. The palliation of symptoms related to paraneoplastic syndromes, such as inappropriate ADH syndrome, still almost exclusively depends on the general responsiveness to the systemic therapy.

1. *CNS Metastases*

The management of primary CNS involvement at the start of systemic treatment is generally concomitant radiotherapy, since most cytostatic agents are presumed not to penetrate sufficiently into brain metastases. Recent observations have questioned this concept (Kristjansen and Hansen, 1988; Kantharjian et al., 1984; Lee et al., 1989; Twelves et al., 1990), since patients with brain metastases verified by computed tomographic (CT) scan from the start of treatment apparently do (at least initially) as well without as with irradiation, provided that chemotherapy is given initially. Complete responses on CT scans of the brain and subsequent neurologic alleviation after induction chemotherapy suggest that initial brain metastases respond as frequently as metastatic SCLC tumors in other sites. The precise impact of these observations on the overall management awaits prospective analysis of large groups of patients. Also brain relapses have responded to chemotherapy with regimens containing etoposide or teniposide (Postmus et al., 1989a; Giaccone et al., 1988). Treatment of leptomeningeal carcinoma is generally disappointing. This may be due partially to the frequent occurrence of concurrent multiple metastases. The poor prognosis of these patients along with the lack of reliable objective parameters to monitor treatment outcome makes the evaluation of various approaches difficult. Intrathecal methotrexate remains the most widely used treatment. The information on the use of other cytostatic agents is sparse. Intravenous high-dosage etoposide therapy has been used with some effect, but again with considerable systemic toxicity (Postmus et al., 1989b).

2. *Superior Vena Caval Obstruction*

When superior vena cava syndrome is part of the initial presentation, radiotherapy was previously considered essential. Studies (Dombernowsky and Hansen, 1978; Kane et al., 1976) have shown that systemic chemotherapy alone in almost all cases produces sufficient relief from this condition, with the effect usually observed within a few days.

3. *Treatment at Relapse*

Results of second-line treatment with combination chemotherapy are generally disappointing, which is a major problem because most patients will relapse within 10–12 months. The first recognizable clinical relapse may be either locally or in metastatic sites and subsequent treatment depends on this localization. A multifocal relapse will usually lead to change of chemotherapy to include other active agents not used in the primary treatment. The response rates with such assumed non-cross-resistant regimens are 20–25%, with a median duration of 3–4 months. Provided there was a chemotherapy-free interval before relapse, reinduction therapy with a combination that has produced response earlier in the course of treatment seems to be considerably more efficient, with response rates exceeding 50% when analyzed retrospectively (Giaccone, 1989; Andersen et al., 1990). If the patient with relapse has not received etoposide + cisplatinum earlier, this combination may also produce response rates of 50%.

F. Duration and Intensity of Treatment

There is a tendency to shorten the duration of therapy, provided that it is very intensive. A common policy is to re-evaluate patients at the end of the planned number of treatment cycles with careful restaging. This re-evaluation should include, at least, bronchoscopy and repetition of the initial staging procedures. If this examination indicates that the patient is in complete remission, treatment can be discontinued and the patient observed closely. About one-third of patients with a complete remission after 1 year will eventually relapse.

Several studies have therefore focused on the role of maintenance chemotherapy in prolonging time to relapse or even avoiding relapse. Different trial designs are applied in these studies (Bunn et al., 1989). In some studies patients completing their induction chemotherapy received no further treatment, even at the time of disease progression in responding patients. These trials sometimes demonstrated a small survival advantage for the maintenance arm. Most trials have employed reinduction chemotherapy at time of disease progression, either with the original regimen or with other combinations. In this group of trials there has been no survival benefit for maintenance chemotherapy. At present there is a consensus that six cycles of the most active regimens constitute an acceptable standard (Bunn et al., 1989).

The drug delivery can be intensified by increasing the dosages or by reducing the intervals between treatments. The so-called intensive therapy covers several different approaches as listed in Table 5. Table 6 lists five randomized studies testing the effects of increased doses of drugs in the same combination

Table 5 Intensification Strategies

Multiple drug therapy
Consolidation
Alternating regimens
High-dosage chemotherapy
Initial
Late
Continuous chemotherapy

(Cohen et al., 1977; Figueredo et al., 1985; O'Donnell et al., 1985; Wolff et al., 1986; Ihde et al., 1987). Dosage escalation studies, supported by autologous bone marrow transfusion, have yielded considerable toxicity but so far no therapeutic advantage, neither when given as part of the initial treatment nor as late intensification therapy. A recent update (Klastersky and Sculier, 1989) reviewed all available studies dealing with this issue. Most studies included only a very small number of patients and there were no prospective randomized trials. Intensification studies that included more than 25 patients are listed in Table 7 (Souhami et al., 1983; Thatcher et al., 1985a,b). Preliminary reports on weekly chemotherapy suggest slight advantages but the follow-up is short and there are still no randomized comparisons.

V. Toxicity of Chemotherapy

Since it is necessary to administer maximal chemotherapy with or without irradiation, a considerable level of treatment-induced complications should be anticipated. These include drug-specific effects (e.g., renal toxicity from platinum and neural toxicity from vinca alkaloids) in addition to myelosuppression with serious infectious episodes during leukopenic episodes. The concept of improving the well-being of patients by means of parenteral hyperalimentation has failed to be confirmed in large randomized trials from several centers (Weiner et al., 1985). On the contrary, the hyperalimentated patients did significantly worse in experiencing unpleasant complications such as sepsis, fluid overload, hyponatremia, and hyperglycemia requiring insulin. Infection prophylaxis by use of cotrimoxazole allowed for the use of higher dosages in outpatients in a recent investigation (Figueredo et al., 1985). Overall results were not improved and side effects were increased. It seems that myelosuppression leads to serious problems in fewer than 25% and that lethal effects occur in fewer than 5% of patients in aggressive combination chemotherapy studies. Tardive side effects have recently emerged in the increasing group of long-term survivors. An increased tendency to secondary

Table 6 Randomized Trials Testing Drug Dosages in the Same Combination

Reference		Regimen and dosage (mg/m²)			Response No.	Response Rate (%)	CR	PR	MST, mos.	Statistical analysis of survival
Cohen et al., 1977		CCNU	MTX	CTX						
	I + II	100	15	1000	23	96	7	15		N.R.
	III	50	10	500	9	45	—	4		
Figueredo et al., 1985		ADR	VCR	CTX						
	I	60	1	1500–2000	52	50	11	15		N.S.
	II	50	1	1000	51	39	11	9		N.S.
O'Donnell et al., 1985		CTX	VCR	meCCNU						
	I	2000	2	100	14	43	3	3	10.75	N.S.
	II	750	2	75	14	71	8	2	9	
Wolff et al., 1986		VP–16								
	I	100	day 1–3		26	4	—	1	3.1	
	II	200	day 1–3		27	7	—	2	5	
	III	300	day 1–3		26	4	—	1	5.6	N.S.
Ihde et al., 1987		VP–16	CDDP							
	I	80 × 5d	27 × 5d		21	86	6	12	13	
	II	80 × 3d	80 × 1d		25	88	8	14	11	N.S.

CR, complete response; PR, partial response; MST, median survival time; N.R., not reported; N.S., not significant; MTX, methotrexate; CTX, cyclophosphamide; ADR, doxorubicin; VCR, vincristine; VP–16, etoposide; CDDP, cisplatin.

Table 7 Dose Intensification Studies (n > 25) Testing Megadosages as Induction Chemotherapy

Reference	Regimens and dosage: CTX	Regimens and dosage: VP-16	Stage	Patients, no.	CR (%)	PR (T)	MST, mos.	2-Yr survival (%)
Souhami et al., 1983	200 mg/kg 2 courses	4–600 mg/m^2	LD	26	50	31	9.65	15 (DFS)
Thatcher et al., 1985a	1.5–3.5 g/m^2	480 mg/m^2	LD	111	56	25	11	13
Thatcher et al., 1985b	2.5 g/m^2	480 mg/m^2	LD	78	54	25	11	

CTX, cyclophosphamide; VP–16, etoposide; CR, complete response; PR, partial response; MST, median survival time; DFS, disease–free survival leukemia, especially acute myeloblastic leukemia (AML), in patients with SCLC treated with regimens including alkylating agents (Pedersen-Bjergaard et al., 1985) has been recognized. Second primary tumors, including non-small-cell lung cancers, should be looked for and confirmed histologically since they are potentially curable by surgery.

VI. Hematopoietic Growth Factors

Hematopoietic growth factors are glycoprotein hormones that regulate the proliferation and differentiation of hematopoietic progenitors and the function of mature blood cells. Several substances have been applied in clinical studies: erythropoietin, granulocyte–macrophage colony-stimulating factors (GM-CSF), granulocyte colony-stimulating factor (G-CSF), macrophage colony-stimulating factor (M-CSF), and interleukin-3.

A. Clinical Effects with Special Regard to SCLC

G- and GM-CSF are at present being tested in several clinical trials including patients with SCLC. With regard to SCLC, only one full study has been published (Bronchud et al., 1987). Twelve patients with advanced SCLC were subjected to continuous infusion of G-CSF at the following dosage levels: 1, 5, 10, 20, and 40 μg/kg/day for 5 days starting 7 days before chemotherapy in a phase I study. In all 12 patients the number of peripheral neutrophils increased rapidly to a maximum of 100×10^9/L at 10 μg/kg/day. The neutrophils were shown to be functionally normal in tests of their mobility and bactericidal activity. The chemotherapy was a combination of doxorubicine, ifosfamide/mesna, and etoposide. Nine of 12 patients entered the phase II part of the study, and G-CSF was given to each patient for 14 days on alternate cycles of chemotherapy. The median duration of absolute neutropenia was reduced by 80%, with a return to normal, or above normal, neutrophil counts within 2 weeks after day 1 of chemotherapy. Six severe infectious episodes were observed during the cycles of chemotherapy that did not include G-CSF, while no infectious episodes occurred when patients were treated with G-CSF. No toxicities resulted from the treatment. Recently, Crawford et al. (1990) reported an interim analysis of a double-blind randomized trial of 126 of a planned total of 240 patients with SCLC, who received recombinant human G-CSF (r-metHuG-CSF) as a self-administered subcutaneous bolus during chemotherapy with cyclophophamide, doxorubicin, and etoposide. The dosage was 230 μg/m^2/day on days 4–17 of a 21-day cycle, unless the neutrophil count exceeded 10×10^9/L after day 12, in which case the r-metHuG-CSF was discontinued. Patients who developed febrile neutropenia during the first course of therapy were unblinded and continued on open-label CSF.

This open unilateral crossover design makes a comparison of the treatment and placebo group beyond the first cycle very difficult, especially with regard to the endpoints: response and survival. However, significant differences in duration of neutropenia and the incidence of neutropenic fever were demonstrable in favor of G-CSF. A new parameter, the "area over the curve" (AOC), was applied as an integrated measure of the severity of the neutropenia. AOC was defined in a semilogarithmic plot of absolute neutrophil count (ANC) against time as the AOC between the descending and the ascending intercept with a baseline ANC value of $0.5 \times 10^9/L$. Mild bone pain in 15% was the only observed toxicity related to r-metHuG-CSF.

A preliminary report (Schiller et al., 1990) on a randomized comparison of cyclophosphamide, doxorubicin, and etoposide plus or minus GM-CSF subcutaneously, 10–20 μg/kg on days 3–14 in 22 patients with SCLC described similar reductions in the myelosuppression but also cases of grade 3–4 toxicity.

VII. Conclusion

Small cell lung cancer is a systemic disease and systemic chemotherapy forms the backbone of the overall therapeutic management. Many agents are active and several two- to four-drug combinations produce comparable results. Overall results have been unchanged for some years, with complete or partial remissions being obtained in 80–90% of all patients with a median duration of 9–11 months. Median survival is dependent on the initial stage and other prognostic factors and is at present 11–16 months. In good-prognosis subgroups, long-term survival, and potential cure, is obtained in about 20%, while the overall long-term survival does not exceed 10%. Elimination of resistant cells after initial response is the main obstacle to further improvement of treatment outcome. None of the newer approaches aimed at this seem to have improved the overall results significantly. New drugs with alternative mechanisms of action are needed, but critical reappraisals of known strategies may also be beneficial since we still have much to learn about the available tools in systemic therapy.

From the clinical data on CSF application published so far, it is reasonable to believe that CSF may serve to reduce treatment-related myelotoxicity. Whether this would reduce or only modify the overall morbidity is uncertain at present. If we consider that myelosuppression seems to lead to serious problems in fewer than 25% and that lethal effects occur in fewer than 5% of patients in aggressive combination chemotherapy studies, reduced neutropenia is likely to decrease the incidence and severity of infections. A survival benefit obtained by avoiding reductions and delays of doses or by preparing the way for dosage escalation or intensification of chemotherapy by, for example, shortening the interval between courses, is possible and is presently being investigated in randomized trials.

To evaluate the potential usefulness of CSFs, future studies should focus on clinically relevant endpoints such as survival and/or quality of life, depending on which basic assumptions are made. A survival benefit, achieved by an intensified therapy, made possible by CSF, would appear only if there really is a continuous dose–response relationship in SCLC, and only if no other toxicities are potentially dosage limiting. The palliative viewpoint assumes that myelosuppression is a major cause of morbidity that justifies prolonged prophylactic medication with CSF. Studies that follow this train of thought should compare CSF treatment with other means of prophylaxis, such as oral antibiotics.

References

Andersen, M., Kristjansen, P. E. G., and Hansen, H. H. (1990). Second line chemotherapy in small cell lung cancer. *Cancer Treat. Rev.* **17:**427–436.

Batist, G., Carney, D. N., Cowan, K. H., et al. (1986). Etoposide and cisplatin in previously treated small-cell lung cancer: clinical trial and in vitro correlates. *J. Clin. Oncol.* **4:** 982–986.

Bork, E., Hansen, M., Dombernowsky, P., et al. (1986). Teniposide (VM-26). An overlooked highly active agent in small cell lung cancer. Results of a phase II trial in untreated patients. *J. Clin. Oncol.* **4:**524–528.

Bronchud, M. H., Scarffe, J. H., Thatcher, N., et al. (1987). Phase I/II study of recombinant human granulocyte colony-stimulating factor in patients receiving intensive chemotherapy for small cell lung cancer. *Br. J. Cancer* **56:**809–813.

Bunn, P. A., Cullen, M., Fukuoka, M., et al. (1989). Chemotherapy in small cell lung cancer: a consensus report. *Lung Cancer* **5:**127–134.

Carney, D. N., Matthews, M. J., Ihde, D. C., et al. (1981). Influence of histological subtype of small cell carcinoma of the lung on clinical presentation, response to therapy and survival. *J. Natl. Cancer Inst.* **65:**1225–1229.

Chahinian, A. P., Propert, K. J., Ware, J. H., Zimmer, B., Perry, M.C., et al. (1990). A randomized trial of anticoagulation with warfarin and of alternating chemotherapy in extensive small cell lung cancer by the Cancer and Leukemia Group B. *J. Clin. Oncol.* **7:**993.

Cohen, M. H., Creaven, P. J., Fossieck, B. E., et al. (1977). Intensive chemotherapy of small cell bronchogenic carcinoma. *Cancer Treat. Rep.* **61:**349–354.

Crawford, J., Ozer, H., Johnson, D., and the G-CSF study group. (1990). Granulocyte colony stimulating factor: prevention of chemotherapy induced febrile neutropenia in patients with small cell lung cancer. A randomized double blind placebo controlled trial. *Proc. ASCO*, 884.

Daniels, J. R., Chak, L. Y., Sikic, B. I., et al. (1984). Chemotherapy of small cell carcinoma of the lung: a randomized comparison of alternating and sequential combination chemotherapy programs. *J. Clin. Oncol.* **2:**1192–1199.

Dombernowsky, P., and Hansen, H. H. (1978). Combination chemotherapy in the management of superior vena caval obstruction in small cell anaplastic carcinoma of the lung. *Acta Med. Scand.* **204:**513–516.

Elliot, J. A., Østerlind, K., and Hansen, H. H. (1984). Cyclic alternating "non cross resistant" chemotherapy in the management of small cell anaplastic carcinoma of the lung. *Cancer Treat. Rev.* **11:**103–114.

Ettinger, D. S., Finkelstein, D. M., Abeloff, M. D., Ruckdeschel, J. C., Aisner, S. C., and Eggleston, J. C. (1990). A randomized comparison of standard chemotherapy versus alternating chemotherapy and maintenance versus no maintenance therapy for extensive-stage small cell lung cancer: a phase III study of the Eastern Cooperative Oncology Group. *J. Clin. Oncol.* **8:**230–240.

Evans, W. K., Osoba, D., Feld, R., et al. (1985). Etoposide and cisplatin: an effective treatment for relapse in small cell lung cancer. *J. Clin. Oncol.* **3:**65–71.

Feld, R., Evans, W. K., Coy, P., et al. (1987). Canadian multicenter randomised trial comparing sequential and alternating administration of two non-cross resistant chemotherapy combinations in patients with limited small cell carcinoma of the lung. *J. Clin. Oncol.* **5:**1401–1409.

Figueredo, A. T., Hryniuk, W. M., Strautmanis, I., Frank, G., and Rendell, S. (1985). Cotrixamole prophylaxis during high-dose chemotherapy of small cell lung cancer. *J. Clin. Oncol.* **3:**54–64.

Fukuoka, M., Furuse, K., Saijo, N., et al. (1988). A randomized study in the treatment of small cell lung cancer: cyclophosphamide, adriamycin and vincristine vs. cisplatin and etoposide vs. cyclophosphamide, adriamycin and vincristin alternating with cisplatin and etoposide. *Lung Cancer* **4** (suppl.)**:**A101.

Giaccone, G. (1989). Second line chemotherapy in SCLC. *Lung Cancer* **5**(4–6)**:**207–213.

Giaccone, G., Donadio, M., Bonardi, G. M., Testore, F., and Calciati, A. (1988). Teniposide (VM-26): an effective treatment for brain metastases of small cell carcinoma of the lung. *Eur. J. Cancer Clin. Oncol.* **24:**1905–1906.

Goldie, J. H., Coldman, A. J., Gudauskas, G. A. (1982). Rationale for the use of alternating non-cross resistant chemotherapy. *Cancer Treat. Rep.* **66:**439–449.

Hansen, H. H. (1987). Chemotherapy of small cell carcinoma: a review. *Q. J. Med.* **63** (240)**:**275–282.

Havemann, K., Wolf, M., Holl, R., et al. (1987). Alternating versus sequential chemotherapy in small cell lung cancer. A randomized German multicenter trial. *Cancer* **59:**1072–1082.

Hirsch, F. R., Hansen, H. H., Hansen, M., et al. (1987). The superiority of combination chemotherapy including etoposide based on in vivo cell cycle analysis in the treatment of extensive small cell lung cancer. *J. Clin. Oncol.* **5:**585–591.

Hirsch, F. R., Matthews, M. J., Aisner, S., et al. (1988). Histopathologic classification of small cell lung cancer. *Cancer* **62:**973–977.

Ihde, D. C., Johnson, B. E., Mulshine, J. L., et al. (1987). Randomized trial of high dose versus standard dose etoposide and cisplatin in extensive disease stage small cell lung cancer. Proceedings, 23rd ASCO meeting, abstr. no. 71a.

Jackson, D. V., Zekan, P. J., Caldwell, R. D., et al. (1983). VP-16-213 in combination chemotherapy with chest irradiation for small cell lung cancer: a randomised trial of the Piedmont Oncology Association. *J. Clin. Oncol.* **2:**1343–1351.

Kane, R. C., Cohen, M. H., Broder, L. E., and Bull, M. J. (1976). Superior vena cava obstruction due to small cell anaplastic carcinoma. *JAMA* **235:**1717.

Kantharjian, H., Farha, P. A. M., Spitzer, G., et al. (1984). Systemic combination chemotherapy as primary treatment of brain metastases from lung cancer. *South Med. J.* **77:**426–429.

Klastersky, J. A., and Sculier, J.-P. (1989). Intensive chemotherapy of small cell lung cancer. *Lung Cancer* **5:**196–206.

Kristjansen, P. E. G., and Hansen, H. H. (1988). Brain metastases from small cell lung cancer treated with combination chemotherapy. *Eur. J. Cancer Clin. Oncol.* **24:** 545–549.

Lee, J. S., Murphy, W. K., Glisson, B. S., Dhingra, H. M., Holoye, P. Y., et al. (1989). Primary chemotherapy of brain metastases in small cell lung cancer. *J. Clin. Oncol.* **7:**916–920.

Mountain, C. F. (1987). Staging of lung cancer: the new international system. *Lung Cancer* **3:**4–11.

O'Donnell, M. R., Ruckdeschel, J. C., Baxter, D., McKneally, M. F., Caradonna, R., and Horton, J. (1985). Intensive induction chemotherapy for small cell anaplastic carcinoma of the lung. *Cancer Treat. Rep.* **69:**571–575.

Østerlind, K. (1986). Prognostic factors in small cell carcinoma. An analysis of 874 consecutive patients. In: *Lung Cancer: Basic and Clinical Aspects*. Edited by H. H. Hansen. Boston, Martinus-Nijhoff, pp. 129–152.

Østerlind, K. (1989). Alternating versus sequential chemotherapy in small cell lung cancer. *Lung Cancer* **5:**173–177.

Østerlind, K., Pedersen, A. G., Vindeløv, L. L., et al. (1986). Alternating or continuous chemotherapy of extensive stage small cell lung cancer. Results of a controlled trial on 204 patients. *Lung Cancer* **2:**127–128.

Pedersen-Bjergaard, J., Østerlind, K., Hansen, M., et al. (1985). Acute non-lymphocytic leukemia, preleukemia, and solid tumors following intensive chemotherapy of small cell carcinoma of the lung. *Blood* **66:**1393–1897.

Pedersen, A. G., Østerlind, K., Vindeløv, L. L., et al. (1987). Alternating or continuous chemotherapy of small cell lung cancer. A three armed randomized trial. *Proc. Am. Soc. Clin. Oncol.* **6:**195.

Postmus, P. E., Holthuis, J. J. M., Haaxma-Reiche, H., et al. (1989a). High dose etoposide for brain metastases of small cell lung cancer. A phase II study. *Br. J. Cancer* **59:** 254–256.

Postmus, P., Haaxma-Reiche, H., Berendsen, H. H., and Sleifer, D. T. (1989b). High-dose etoposide for meningeal carcinomatosis in patients with small cell lung cancer. *Eur. J. Cancer Clin. Oncol.* **25:**377–378.

Roed, H., Vindeløv, L. L., Spang-Thomsen, M., and Engelholm, S. Å. (1986). Limitations and potentials of in vitro sensitivity testing of human small cell carcinoma of the lung. In: *Lung Cancer III*. Edited by H. H. Hansen. Boston, Martinus Nijhoff, pp. 77–89.

Roed, H., Vindeløv, L. L., Christensen, I. J., Spang-Thomsen, M., and Hansen, H. H. (1988). The cytotoxic activity of cisplatin, carboplatin and teniposide alone and combined determined on four human small cell lung cancer cell lines by the clonogenic assay. *Eur. J. Clin. Oncol.* **24:**247–253.

Roth, B. J., Johnsen, D. H., Greco, F. A., et al. (1989). A phase III trial of etoposide and cisplatin versus cyclophosphamide, doxorubicin, and vincristine versus alternation of the two therapies for patients with extensive small cell lung cancer: preliminary results. *Proc. Am. Soc. Clin. Oncol.* **8**:225.

Schiller, J. H., Storer, B., Oken, M. M., et al. (1990). Randomized trial of granulocyte macrophage colony stimulating factor in patients with small cell carcinoma of the lung. *Proc. ASCO*, 943.

Smith, I. E., Harlund, S. J., Robinson, B. A., et al. (1985). A very active new cisplatinum analogue in the treatment of small cell lung cancer. *Cancer Treat. Rep.* **69**:43–46.

Souhami, R. L., Harper, P. G., Linch, D., et al. (1983). High-dose cyclophosphamide in small cell carcinoma of the lung. *J. Clin. Oncol.* **3**:958–963.

Stahel, R. A., Ginsberg, R., Havemann, K., et al. (1989). Staging and prognostic factors in small cell carcinoma of the lung. Consensus report. *Lung Cancer* **5**:119–126.

Thatcher, N., James, R. D., Steward, W. P., et al. (1985a). Three months treatment with cyclophosphamide, VP-16 followed by methotrexate and thoracic radiotherapy for small cell lung cancer. *Cancer* **56**:1332–1336.

Thatcher, N., Stout, D. R., Smith, D. B., et al. (1985b). Three months treatment with chemotherapy and radiotherapy for small cell lung cancer. *Br. J. Cancer* **52**: 327–332.

Twelves, C. J., Souhami, R. L., Harper, P. G., Spiro, S. G., Earl, H. M., Tobias, J. S., Quinn, H., and Geddes, D. M. (1990). The response of cerebral metastases in small cell lung cancer to systemic chemotherapy. *Br. J. Cancer* **61**:147–150.

Vindeløv, L. L., Hansen, H. H., Christensen, I. J., et al. (1980). Clonal heterogeneity of small cell anaplastic carcinoma of the lung demonstrated by flow cytometric DNA analysis. *Cancer Res.* **40**:4295–4300.

Weiner, R. S., Kramer, B. S., Clamon, G. H., et al. (1985). Effects of hyperalimentation during treatment in patients with small cell lung cancer. *J. Clin. Oncol.* **3**:949–957.

Wolff, S. N., Birch, R., Sama, P., and Greco, F. A. (1986). Randomized dose–response evaluation of etoposide in small cell carcinoma of the lung: a Southeastern Cancer Study Group Trial. *Cancer Treat. Rep.* **70**:583–587.

Zacharaski, L. R., Henderson, W. G., Rickles, F. R., et al. (1981). Effect of warfarin in small cell carcinoma of the lung. *JAMA* **245**:831–835.

27

Controversies in the Treatment of Small Cell Lung Cancer

ROBERT L. SOUHAMI

University College and Middlesex School of Medicine
London, England

I. Introduction

When results of treatment of small cell lung cancer are presented, it is usual to find that patients have been entered into studies in which the maximum follow-up is 3–4 years. It is quite common to find that survival based on 2 or 3 years of follow-up is quoted as if this represented the cure rate of small cell lung cancer. For patients with limited disease, such "survival" figures are typically 10–15% of those treated. Very few studies have addressed the question of the true cure rate of small cell lung cancer with long, continued follow-up of large groups of patients. In the study by Davis et al. (1985), 1580 patients were followed for up to 10 years after diagnosis and treatment in community practice. The results showed that only 2.4% of patients were alive at 5 years. Patients were more likely to be alive if they had limited disease and had undergone surgical resection (the latter implying extremely limited disease). Østerlind et al. (1986) restaged patients at 18 months after treatment and then evaluated patients for up to 5 years beyond this point. Of 874 patients with small cell lung cancer, only 7.6% were alive at 18 months and deaths continued throughout the subsequent 5 year period of follow up. At the end of this period, only 2.5% were alive.

We have recently undertaken, on behalf of the Lung Cancer Working Party of the United Kingdom Coordinating Committee on Cancer Research, a long-term follow-up of 3681 patients who were entered into studies at centers in the United Kingdom during the period 1978–1986 (Souhami and Law, 1990). The studies were both randomized and nonrandomized and the only requirement was that electronic databases existed for these patients. Follow-up was either through the trial office itself or through the National Health Service registry. Causes of death were taken from hospital notes or from death certificates. This study has recently been published (Souhami and Law, 1990). Of the total number of patients, only 5.9% were alive at 2 years, 8.5% of those with limited disease and 2.2% of those with extensive disease. The survival following 2 years is shown in Figure 1 for all patients and the cause of death is classified in Figure 2 according to whether it was due to small cell lung cancer or some other cause, including other cancers or any other cause of death. From these figures it can be seen that death continues beyond 2 years but reaches a plateau at 7 years, at which point only 40% of the 2 year survivors are alive. This represents a total of 3% of the entire population. In Figure 2 it can be seen that deaths from small cell lung cancer are uncommon after 6 years of follow-up, but that other causes of death continue and at 8 years equal those from small cell lung cancer. These other causes of death are other cancers (such as non-small-cell lung cancer, bladder cancer) and vascular disease and respiratory failure associated with cigarette smoking.

These depressing figures indicate how far we have to go in treatment. However, they conceal the fact that chemotherapy, for many patients, prolongs

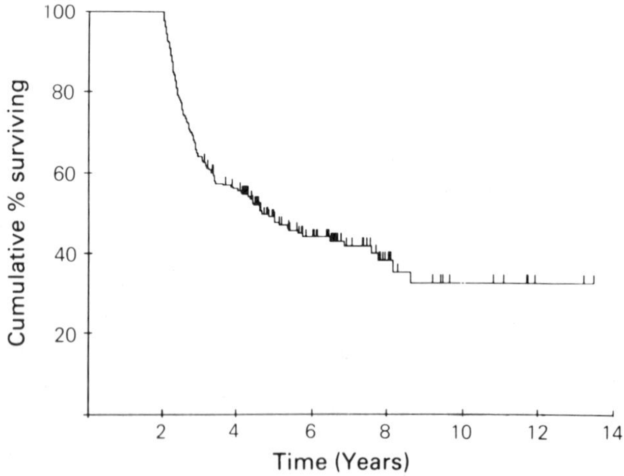

Figure 1 Post-2-year survival in SCLC, all causes of death considered (from Souhami and Law, 1990, with permission).

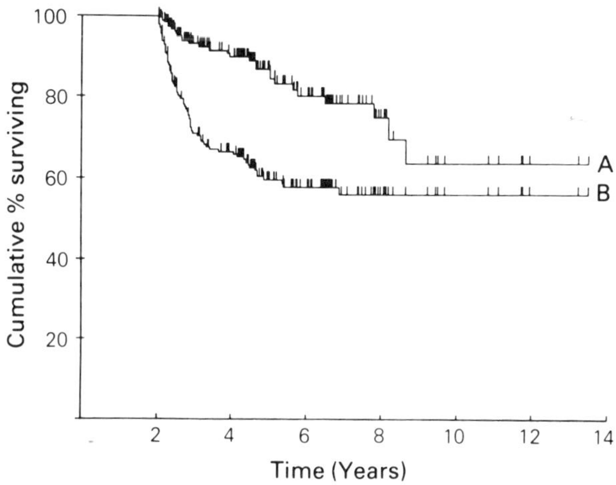

Figure 2 Post-2-year survival in SCLC. (A) Deaths not due to SCLC. (B) Deaths from SCLC (from Souhami and Law, 1990, with permission).

survival even if it does not result in cure. Furthermore, they indicate that some patients are cured by treatment. This can be interpreted as meaning that an unknown quantity of patients are nearly cured by current methods and might be if new agents or more intensive treatments were introduced.

These data imply that there is no "gold standard" of treatment for patients with small cell lung cancer either with limited disease or extensive disease. For the vast majority of patients, treatment is palliative. This allows us to think of new methods of treatment and of trial designs that would not only be of value for patients with small cell lung cancer but might also indicate general principles that are of importance for cancer treatment generally.

II. What is the Contribution of Thoracic Radiation to Survival?

Several randomized trials have been carried out in which patients treated with chemotherapy have been randomly allocated to receive, or not receive, radiation to the primary tumor (Bunn et al., 1987; Fox et al., 1980; Perez et al., 1984; Perry et al., 1987; Souhami et al., 1984). The design of these studies has varied greatly since radiotherapy has been given before chemotherapy, after chemotherapy has been completed, or in the middle of the chemotherapy program. In the latter case the chemotherapy program may have been interrupted by the radiation or the radiation might have been given concurrently with chemotherapy. These issues and that of radiation dosage have been discussed by Turrisi (1988). Some of these studies have shown no improvement in survival at 2 years or beyond (Fox et al., 1980; Souhami et al., 1984) while others have shown a modest survival benefit (Perry et al., 1987).

When a clinician considers the value of a particular treatment program, it is important not just to show that a statistically significant difference exists in favor of one treatment or another. For the result of the trial to be clinically interpretable, the *size* of the difference must be known with confidence. This obvious point is sometimes forgotten. A 1% improvement in 5 year survival in favor of thoracic radiation would not be considered compelling evidence for its use while a 10% improvement in survival (i.e., a doubling of present survival rates) would be considered by most to be a significant advance. It is sad that none of the studies has achieved anything like the size to allow such differences, if any, to be stated with confidence. In perhaps the best known of these trials, that of the Cancer and Leukemia Group B (CALGB) (Perry et al., 1987), patients were randomized to receive either chemotherapy alone or radiotherapy either early or late during the chemotherapy program.

The overall survival data are shown in Figure 3 and the local recurrence data

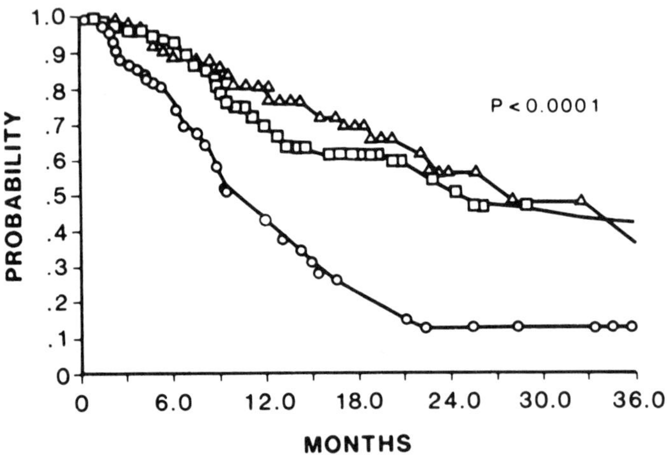

INDUCTION RX	CENSORED	FAILED	TOTAL	MEDIAN
Regimen I	99	26	125	26.8
Regimen II	106	39	145	25.5
Regimen III	58	71	129	10.1

Figure 3 Effect of two regimens of thoracic irradiation on survival in limited stage SCLC in the CALGB trial (from Perry et al., 1987, with permission).

in Figure 4. It can be seen that the late radiotherapy program produced a slight but significant survival advantage at 3 years, while the earlier radiotherapy did not. On the other hand, the local control rates were the same. This study, the largest of its kind, still only has 120 patients in each arm. This is insufficient to give a precise estimate of the size of the benefit. Indeed, in the late radiotherapy arm the survival advantage might be due to statistical chance, since the local control rates are the same in both radiotherapy arms. On the other hand, the result might indicate that there is an interaction of radiation and chemotherapy that results in improved survival with one kind of radiation program but not the other. The reader will notice that the follow-up is short and that results at 6–8 years are likely to show no difference in long-term survival, given that the curves appear to be coming together at 4 years. Long-term survival results would be interesting.

None of this should be taken as a criticism of the CALGB study, which is the best of its kind and certainly superior in size to that my own group carried out (Souhami et al., 1984). The main problem in all studies is lack of statistical power. This may be overcome by a proposed overview analysis to be carried out at the Institut Gustave Roussy (Arriagada and Pignon, personal communication), but it contains a lesson for the future in the design of this kind of study in which an

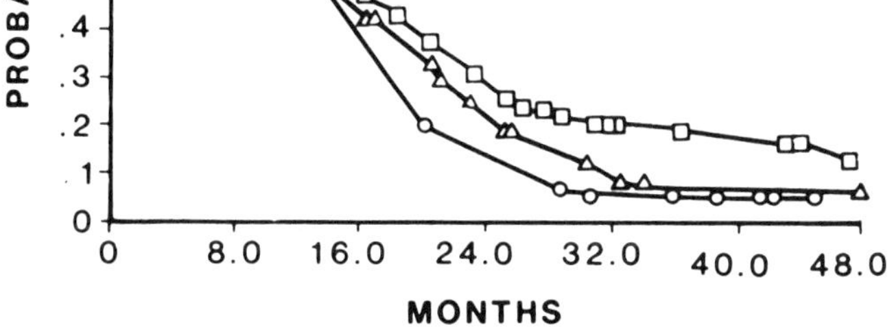

INDUCTION RX	CENSORED	FAILED	TOTAL	MEDIAN
△–△ Regimen I	21	104	125	13.1
□–□ Regimen II	32	113	145	14.6
○–○ Regimen III	11	118	129	13.6

Figure 4 Local recurrence with and without thoracic irradiation in SCLC in the CALGB trial (from Perry et al., 1987, with permission).

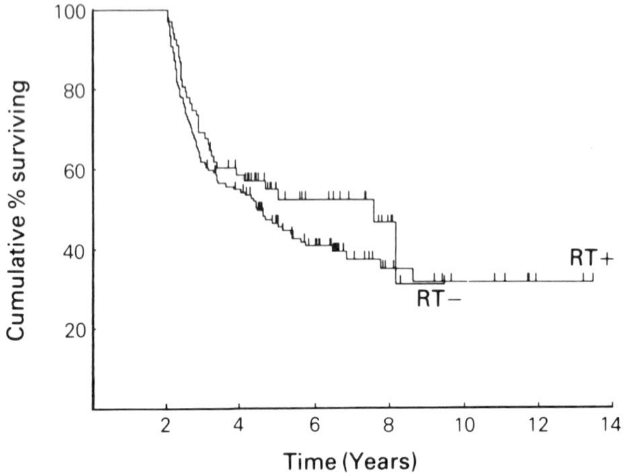

Figure 5 Post-2-year survival in SCLC according to whether the treatment protocol did (RT+) or did not (RT−) include thoracic radiation. All causes of death considered (from Souhami and Law, 1990, with permission).

important issue of treatment is being addressed. In the follow-up study carried out in the United Kingdom alluded to earlier, there was no difference in long-term survival whether or not the protocol contained thoracic irradiation (Fig. 5). This of course is not a randomized comparison between radiation and no irradiation, but it perhaps indicates that the effects of thoracic irradiation on survival are likely to be relatively small when patients are evaluated beyond 5 years.

Even if survival is affected only marginally, thoracic radiotherapy has a useful role in the treatment of limited-stage SCLC. Almost all the studies show that local control rates in the thorax are superior if radiation is given. This is a further justification for the use of thoracic irradiation in treatment of limited-stage disease when patients are showing a partial or complete response to chemotherapy.

III. What is the Contribution of Prophylactic Cranial Irradiation?

Several studies have indicated that 20–30% of patients with SCLC will develop cerebral metastases (Komaki et al., 1983; Nugent et al., 1979). For the most part, these metastases are solid, vascularized tumor masses and not leptomeningeal spread. Patients who develop cerebral metastasis are particularly disadvantaged. The consequences are socially very difficult. Fits, raised intracranial pressure, hemiplegia, dementia, and personality disturbances are difficult for both patients and relatives. We have shown (Felletti et al., 1985) that patients developing brain metastasis as the first site of relapse spent a greater proportion of the rest of their lives in hospital than those whose disease relapsed in the liver as the first site.

Prophylactic cranial irradiation (PCI) reduces the likelihood of intracerebral relapse. This has been shown both in unrandomized and randomized studies (Bleehen et al., 1983). The rate of intracerebral relapse falls from 22% to about 6% with the use of PCI. On the other hand, PCI is itself unpleasant for some patients (Feld et al., 1985) and there have been some anxieties about long-term neurologic sequelae (Johnson et al., 1985) although these have been felt to be less frequent by others. So far no study has shown a significant survival advantage in favor of PCI, although the randomized studies conducted so far have been much too small to demonstrate any realistic survival advantage. Two large-scale randomized trials are currently addressing this issue.

However, the issue is not survival alone. The social morbidity of brain metastasis may be worth preventing even if survival is not prolonged (Felletti et al., 1985). Perhaps we should not be too surprised that there is little impact on survival since there is increasing evidence that brain metastasis represents a failure of control of systemic disease by chemotherapy and is thus an indication that relapse is likely to occur at other sites, even if prevented in the brain by PCI. It is now clear that the brain is not a "sanctuary site" for chemotherapy. While drugs will not penetrate the cerebrospinal fluid (CSF) and are unlikely to be effective against leptomeningeal spread of tumors, there is ample evidence that vascularized tumors in the brain respond to chemotherapy in the same way as metastases at any other site (Twelves and Souhami, 1991). In the long-term follow-up study in the United Kingdom no survival difference was seen for those patients who had received PCI compared with those who had not (Fig. 6). Once again, this is not a randomized comparison but it does indicate that the survival advantage of PCI is likely to be small when follow-up is prolonged.

IV. Will Dosage Intensification Increase Cure Rate?

Some patients, albeit a few, are cured by current chemotherapy programs. Patients are more likely to be cured if they have small, localized tumors and are of good performance status at the time of diagnosis (Souhami et al., 1985). It is therefore reasonable to ask whether an increase in the intensity of chemotherapy is feasible in this population of middle-aged or elderly cigarette smokers, and, if it is, whether it results in an increase in cure rate. While several studies have looked at the effect of alternating different combinations of chemotherapy, these have not really addressed the question of the intensity of the chemotherapy program. In the study by Johnson et al. (1987), a very intensive program failed to achieve an increase in survival rate in a small number of patients with extensive disease. This

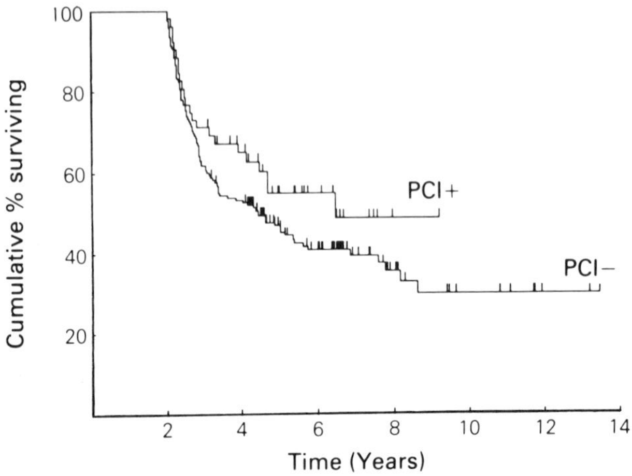

Figure 6 Post-2-year survival in SCLC according to whether the treatment protocol did (PCI+) or did not (PCI−) include PCI. All causes of death considered ($p = 0.163$) (from Souhami and Law, 1990, with permission).

study used conventional chemotherapy cycles in which the dosages were given to the point of significant myelosuppression. A recent South West Oncology Group study (Taylor et al., 1990) has used weekly chemotherapy in an attempt to increase the amount of drug given over time. This study, which was not randomized, shows an overall response rate of 82% (complete response [CR] 47%, partial response [PR] 38%). Myelosuppression was the major problem. A similar study using different agents has been reported by Miles et al. (1991). In this weekly myelosuppressive program the overall response rate was 92% (51% CR, 41% PR). This study included patients with limited disease and those with extensive disease with relatively good prognostic features (good performance status, normal liver enzyme levels). This group is currently carrying out a randomized study of weekly chemotherapy of this kind compared with conventional combination chemotherapy using PE/CAV in alternating cycles. Other groups are studying the role of hematopoietic growth factors in limiting the effect of neutropenia between chemotherapy doses. These might allow either larger dosages of drug to be given, or a shortened time interval between each cycle, thus increasing the overall intensity of the program. To date no study has yet been reported in which a randomized comparison of these approaches has been made with conventional chemotherapy.

Very high dosage chemotherapy has also been used in the treatment of SCLC, both as induction treatment (Souhami et al., 1989) and as late intensification (Spitzer et al., 1986). Although a high response rate is obtained when high-dosage induction chemotherapy is used, thus far no survival advantage has been seen. The only randomized trial of the late intensification procedure was carried out by Humblet et al. (1987). In this study 101 patients were treated with combination chemotherapy. Of these, 45 who were responding either completely or partially to the chemotherapy program were randomized to receive either high-dosage chemotherapy as a single cycle or else the same drugs in a single low-dosage cycle. The study showed that for patients with limited disease, there was a slight prolongation of survival, especially if the high-dosage procedure was carried out in complete responders. The numbers were, however, very small and it is difficult to be confident of the results. One problem with this study is that the drugs used as induction chemotherapy (cyclophosphamide, etoposide, doxorubicin, methotrexate, vincristine, cisplatin) included some of those used in the intensification procedure (cyclophosphamide, etoposide, BCNU). The exception was that BCNU was also added in the intensification procedure. The difficulty here is that it seems improbable that a tumor resistant to several cycles of these drugs when given in conventional dosages would nonetheless be cured when these were given in a single high-dosage cycle as late intensification. Nevertheless, this approach might have some value if drug combinations could be found that were either non-cross-resistant or only partially cross-resistant and with which it was reasonably likely that following remission induction with one group of drugs, the second might be able to consolidate the remission. The definition of what we mean by non-cross-resistance can perhaps be defined better in studies in patients with extensive disease.

It has not yet been shown that increasing the intensity of chemotherapy results in a greater proportion of long-term survivors. This is largely due to the paucity of clinical trials in this area. This is one aspect of clinical research in small cell lung cancer that will be explored by many groups in the future.

V. What Treatment Should be Offered to Patients with Extensive Disease?

Some patients with extensive disease are so unwell and have such a short prognosis that it is unrealistic to ask questions of treatment intensity in this group. These patients are characterized by poor performance status, a very high serum alkaline phosphatase or lactate dehydrogenase (LDH) level, a low plasma albumin level, and a low plasma sodium level (Souhami et al., 1985). In these patients it appears reasonable to assess new drugs for their response in previously untreated patients. Although anxieties have been expressed about the possible effect on response to subsequent conventional therapy, significant detriment to the patient does not seem likely provided responses are assessed early and the patient then given conventional chemotherapy. In other patients with extensive disease, chemotherapy may be reasonably well tolerated. In these patients it seems opportune to ask questions about drug scheduling and dosage, in particular whether the same total dose of drugs can be given in a form that allows for entirely outpatient treatment, in which toxicity is reduced. We must also assess whether, under these circumstances, response rates and survival can be maintained. These questions of schedule and intensity will be of importance not just in small cell lung cancer but in a variety of other tumors. As mentioned earlier, in this group of patients a definition of cross-resistance between chemotherapy regimens can be made.

References

Bleehen, N. M., Bunn, P. A., Cox, J. D., et al. (1983). Role of radiation therapy in small cell anaplastic carcinoma of the lung *Cancer Treat. Rep.* **67:**11–19.

Bunn, P. A., Lichter, A. S., Makuch, et al. (1987). Chemotherapy alone or chemotherapy with chest irradiation therapy in limited stage small cell lung cancer: a prospective randomized trial. *Ann. Intern. Med.* **106:**655–662.

Davis, S., Wright, P. W., Schulman, S. F., et al. (1985). Long-term survival in small cell carcinoma of the lung: a population experience. *J. Clin. Oncol.* **3:**80–87.

Feld, R., Channon, G. H., Blunn, R., et al. (1985). Short course prophylactic cranial irradiation for small cell lung cancer. *Am. J. Clin. Oncol.* **8:**371–376.

Felletti, R., Souhami, R. L., Spiro, S. G., et al. (1985). Social consequences of brain or liver relapse in small cell carcinoma of the bronchus. *Radiother. Oncol.* **4:**335–339.

Fox, R. M., Woods, R. L., Brodie, G. M., et al. (1980). A randomized study: small cell anaplastic lung cancer treated by combination chemotherapy and adjuvant radiotherapy. *Int. J. Radiat. Oncol. Biol. Phys.* **6:**1083–1085.

Humblet, Y., Symann, M., Bosky, A., et al. (1987). Late intensification chemotherapy with autologous bone marrow transplantation in selected small cell carcinoma of the lung: a randomized study. *J. Clin. Oncol.* **5:**1864–1871.

Johnson, B. E., Becker, B., Goff, W. B., et al. (1985). Neurologic, neuropsychologic and computed cranial tomography scan abnormalities in 2- to 10-year survivors of small cell lung cancer. *J. Clin. Oncol.* **3:**1659–1667.

Johnson, D. H., De Leo, M. J., Hande, K. R., et al. (1987). High dose induction chemotherapy with cyclophosphamide, etoposide and cisplatin for extensive-stage small cell lung cancer. *J. Clin. Oncol.* **5:**703–709.

Komaki, R., Cox, J. D., Holoye, P. Y., and Hyhardt, R. W. (1983). Changes in the relative risk and sites of central nervous system metastasis with effective combined chemotherapy and radiation therapy for small cell carcinoma of the lung. *Am. J. Clin. Oncol.* **6:**515–521.

Miles, D. W., Earl, H. M., Souhami, R. L., et al. (1991). Intensive weekly chemotherapy for good prognosis patients with small cell lung cancer (SCLC). *J. Clin. Oncol.* **9:** 280–285.

Nugent, J. L., Bunn, P. A., Matthews, M., et al. (1979). CNS metastases in small cell bronchogenic carcinoma. Increasing frequency and changing pattern with lengthening survival. *Cancer* **44:**1885–1893.

Østerlind, K., Hansen, H. H., Hansen, M., and Dombernowsky, P. (1986). Mortality and morbidity in long-term surviving patients treated with chemotherapy with or without irradiation for small cell lung cancer. *J. Clin. Oncol.* **4**:1044–1051.

Perez, C. A., Einhorn, L., Oldham, R. K., et al. (1984). Randomised trial of radiotherapy to the thorax in limited small cell carcinoma of the lung treated with multiagent chemotherapy and elective brain irradiation. A preliminary report. *J. Clin. Oncol.* **2:** 1200–1208.

Perry, M. C., Eaton, W. L., Propert, K. J., et al. (1987). Chemotherapy with or without radiation therapy in limited small cell carcinoma of the lung. *N. Engl. J. Med.* **316:** 912–918.

Souhami, R. L., and Law, K. (1990). Longevity in small cell lung cancer. *Br. J. Cancer* **61:**584–589.

Souhami, R. L., Geddes, D. M., Spiro, S. G., et al. (1984). Radiotherapy in small cell cancer of the lung treated with combination chemotherapy: a controlled trial. *Br. Med. J.* **288:**1643–1646.

Souhami, R. L., Bradbury, I., Geddes, D. M., et al. (1985). Prognostic significance of laboratory parameters measured at diagnosis in small cell carcinoma of the lung. *Cancer Res.* **45:**2878–2882.

Souhami, R. L., Hadjichristou, H. J., Miles, D. W., et al. (1989). Intensive chemotherapy with autologous bone marrow transplantation for small cell lung cancer. *Cancer Chemother. Pharmacol.* **24:**321–325.

Spitzer, G., Farha, P., Valdivieso, M., et al. (1986). High dose intensification therapy with autologous bone marrow support for limited small cell bronchogenic carcinoma. *J. Clin. Oncol.* **4:**4–13.

Taylor, C. W., Crowley, J., Williamson, S. K., et al. (1990). Treatment of small cell lung cancer with an alternating chemotherapy regimen given at weekly intervals: a South West Oncology Group pilot study. *J. Clin. Oncol.* **8:**1811–1817.

Turrisi, A. T. (1988). Combined-modality treatment of limited small cell lung cancer. *Adv. Oncol.* **4:**17–25.

Twelves, C. J., and Souhami, R. L. (1991). Should cerebral metastases be treated by chemotherapy alone? *Ann. Oncol.* **2:**15–17.

AUTHOR INDEX

Italic numbers give the page on which the complete reference is listed.

A

B

E

F

I

J

K

L

Mc

M

N

O

P

S

T

U

V

X

Y

Z

SUBJECT INDEX

A

B

D

E

F

G

H

I

K

L

M

N